An Illustrated Chinese Materia Medica in Hong Kong

香港中藥材圖鑑

谢志伟 题

Zhao Zhongzhen

An Illustrated Chinese Materia Medica in Hong Kong

General Editor: Zhao Zhongzhen

Published/Edited by: School of Chinese Medicine, Hong Kong Baptist University

Printed by: Chung Hwa Book Co., (H.K.)Ltd.
Unit 1, 2/F., Fu Hang Building,
1 Hok Yuen Street East, Hunghom,
Kowloon, H.K.

ISBN: 988-97448-2-1
Printed in Hong Kong

The publishers wish to thank Eu Yan Sang (Hong Kong) Limited for sponsoring the publication and production of this book.

First Edition, May 2004

General Editor

Dr. Zhao Zhongzhan is currently the course director of the Bachelor of Pharmacy (Hons) in Chinese Medicine, School of Chinese Medicine, Hong Kong Baptist University. He is also a member of the Chinese Medicines Board of the Chinese Medicine Council of Hong Kong and a member of the HKSAR Department of Health Scientific Committee on Hong Kong Chinese Materia Medica Standards. Dr. Zhao has long been engaged in the study of Chinese medicines resources, species and quality.

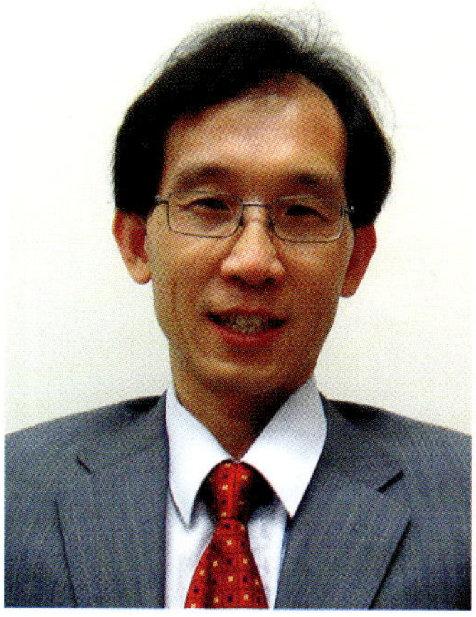

- 1982:graduated from the Beijing University of Traditional Chinese Medicine and Pharmacology with a bachelor's degree in Chinese medicine
- 1985:obtained a Master's degree in Chinese medicines from the China Academy of Traditional Chinese Medicine
- 1992:obtained his PhD degree in Pharmacy from the Tokyo University of Pharmacy and Life Science in Japan
- 1989:commissioned by the World Health Organization as Main Editor of *Medicinal Plants in China*
- 1999:commissioned by The State Pharmacopoeia Commission of the People's Republic of China as Chief Editor of A Colored Atlas of Microscopic Identification of *Chinese Materia Medica in Powdered Form as Specified in Pharmacopoeia of the People's Republic of China.*

Editorial Staff

This book is published with the strong editorial support and expert guidance of Hong Kong Baptist University scholars and Hong Kong Hospital Authority professionals as well as the participation and support of the local Chinese medicines industry.

An Illustrated Chinese Materia Medica in Hong Kong (Chinese Version)

Editorial Committee

General Editor: Zhao Zhongzhen

Senior Editors: Wu Jialin, Yan Zhongkai

Editorial Committee Members:
Zhao Zhongzhen
Tam Hungpun
Alice Wong
Kim Wu
Rosalind Chan
Wu Jialin
Yan Zhongkai

Assistants to Editor-in-Chief:
Hu Yani
Song Yue

Authors & Editors:
Zhao Zhongzhen
Wu Jialin
Yan Zhongkai
Tam Hungpun
Jiang Zhihong
Hu Yani
Song Yue
Yu Tao
Bian Zhaoxiang
Li Min
Peng Yong
Kim Wu
Tong Tak Wing
Wu Wenying

Copy Editor: Lawrence W.C. Lo

Photographers:
Tong Tak Wing
Lam Yuen Chi
Wu Wenying
Shum Chung Yin
Wong Kai Man
Cho Ting Fai
Man Sui Cheung
Lui Miu Man

Editorial Assistants:
Zhang Hong
Selina L M Ming
Nicole W F Shum
Ian K Mok
Echo P W Lau
Cheung Tony

Cover Inscription: Daniel C. W. Tse

The Chinese materia medica presented in this book are mainly provided by Eu Yang Sang (Hong Kong) Limited.

An Illustrated Chinese Materia Medica in Hong Kong

General Editor: Zhao Zhongzhen

Editorial Team

Editor-in-Chief of English Translation: Martha P.Y. Cheung

Senior Editors:
William W.L. Che
Agnes W.L. Chen
Jane C.C. Lai

Editors:
Ester S.M. Leung
Tam Hung Pun *(for 'Indications')*
Tan Zaixi
Jiang Zhihong *(for 'Chemical Composition')*

Academic Editor: Hu Yani

Copy Editor: Lawrence W.C. Lo

Project Coordinators:
William W.L. Che
Hu Yani

Research Supporters
Wu Wenying
Peng Yong
Chen Jun
Song Yue

Translation Team Members:
Agnes W.L. Chen
Jane C.C. Lai
Ken Y.F. Wu
Alvin T.S. Leung
Mamie S.M. Chan
William W.L. Che
Edwin H.K. Ng
Flora S. T. Tong
Sarah L.H. So
Jacque S. T. Wong
Esther H.S. Kwok
Chau Yeuk Kei
Cheung Kim Man
Cheung Wing Man
Ching Siu Ching
Choi Suk Man
Choi Sze Nga
Chui Wai Ying
Fan Hin Yi
Tony H.K. Cheung
Claudia L.M. Ho
Nana M.N. Ko
Kwok Wing Shan
Emily K.W. Lam
Lam Sze Wun
Law Kin Lung
Rachelle S.L. Lee
Li Chui Yi
Phebe H.P. Loo
Ng Man Ting
Pang So Fan
Natalie K.Y. Shin
Brenda C.K. Shum
Siu Yuen Ling
So Ching Man
Tang Ho Ying
Wong Ching Man
Wong Yee Man
Cherry Y.Y. Wong
Yip Ming Tak
Yiu Ting Ting
Ng Ka Wing
Martha P.Y. Cheung

Translator for 'Indications': Echo P.W. Lau

Translators for 'Chemical Composition': Tam Yui Hin, Leung Chiu Yin, Chu Yuen Shan

Sketch Drawing: Cheng Xuan Xuan

Contents

Animal Medicines

Mineral Medicines

Foreword 1

The use of Chinese medicine has been well accepted by the community of Hong Kong. Our society is increasingly aware of the benefits of healthy lifestyle and recognizes the importance of health promotion. Chinese medicine, with its focus on preserving and promoting health and unique concept in disease prevention and treatment, is often regarded as a discipline with potential for high growth in economic development. The Chinese medicine sector generally considers that the strategy in developing Chinese medicine should focus on the regulation, modernization, industrialization and globalization. Over the past few years, a solid foundation has been laid for the statutory control, education and applied research for Chinese medicine.

For thousands of years, Chinese herbs have been used under Chinese medicine theory and represent a unique and distinct body of knowledge and treatment methods. The earliest literature on "*Chinese herbs*" 「神農本草經」could be dated back over 1800 years ago towards the end of the East Han Dynasty. It contained 365 types of herbs, many of which are still being used. As the collection in medical literatures grows over the centuries, it is now important to summarize, analyze and refine the contents and adopt a scientific approach in developing reference materials for the Chinese medicine sector.

The book "*An Illustrated Chinese Materia Medica in Hong Kong*" published by the Baptist University of Hong Kong is the first book on the commonly used herbs in Hong Kong. It is the results of dedicated work of a team of Chinese medicines researchers. It is produced after meticulous review and presented in a concise manner with illustration on a rich collection of photograph on the specimens. It will certainly serve as a very useful reference for practitioners and traders in Chinese medicine locally and overseas. This book, first published in Chinese, is now translated into English. This will help people from different cultures to understand Chinese medicine and facilitate its promotion globally.

It is with great pleasure that I write this foreword for this book which contains description of over 500 commonly used Chinese herbs. This is a publication which will be treasured by many who practise or use Chinese medicine for promotion of health.

Dr. T.H. Leung, *JP*
March 2004.

Foreword 2

I have travelled to Hong Kong on business trips many times in recent years and have witnessed the rapid development of Chinese medicine there. What impresses me most is the significance Hong Kong attaches to the infrastructure of the industry: Chinese medicine in Hong Kong has already stepped onto the path of regulation and legalisation; the teaching of Chinese medicine and the nurturing of talents have been greatly enhanced; the standards for Chinese medicines in Hong Kong have been established and the scientific research of Chinese medicine enthusiastically encouraged. All these developments have laid a solid foundation for attaining the visionary goal of bringing into reality an international Chinese medicine centre.

Hence, when I finished reading 《香港中藥材圖鑑》*(An Illustrated Chinese Materia Medica in Hong Kong)*, I felt all the more the commitment and industrious work of those in the Hong Kong Chinese medicines industry in ensuring a healthy development of the local Chinese medicines sector.

The findings and retrospects of this publication turned an illustrious page in the history of the Hong Kong Chinese medicines industry: it showed with evidence that Hong Kong's acquisition of its status as an international Chinese medicines distributing and logistic centre was through the provision of quality crude drugs and its strong attachment to credibility and reliability. These contents not only fill up the vacuum in the history of Chinese medicines development, but they also clearly illustrate that Hong Kong has the capability and the potential to shoulder the heavy responsibility of being an international trading centre for Chinese medicines in the future.

Of course, to accomplish the lofty mission of becoming an international Chinese medicine centre, Hong Kong faces an arduous task and a long road ahead. The standardisation of Chinese medicines, however, is still a crucial part. At present, the research team led by Dr. Zhao Zhongzhen is doing solid work for the development of pharmacognosy in Hong Kong and is working closely with the local Chinese medicines industry. In addition, a Chinese medicines centre has been established in Hong Kong Baptist University. All this contributes enormously to building a technical platform for the development of Chinese medicine in Hong Kong. The publication of 《香港中藥材圖鑑》 (*An Illustrated Chinese Materia Medica in Hong Kong*) has even become a congratulatory event for the Chinese medicines industry in Hong Kong.

A thorough review of the book finds the provision of detailed and accurate materials with strong scientific evidence. Through colourful photographs, the book vividly and concisely reveals before the eyes of the readers the crude drugs and decoction pieces used by local Chinese and sold in Hong Kong. These, coupled with the simple and succinct descriptions, help the readers to know accurately the authentication characteristics of each crude drug and therefore pave the way for reaching the ultimate goal of genuine authentication. Accordingly, this is an excellent and practical reference book for those involved in the teaching, research, sale, trading and clinical work of Chinese medicine.

The unique position of Hong Kong on the global map will allow the complementary and harmonious development of Chinese medicine with industries such as tourism, information, trading and high technology. This will gradually lead to making Hong Kong a window for the display of Chinese medicine and a bridge between Chinese medicine and the international world. I have full confidence in the future development of Chinese medicine in Hong Kong.

I am pleased to learn the heartening news that the English translation of this book is now published. It is a great pleasure for me to write this foreword in addition to extending my congratulations.

Prof. Xiao Peigen

Academician

Chinese Academy of Engineering

Oct 2003

A Guide to the Use of This Book

1. This publication documents 506 items of commonly used Chinese materia medica in Hong Kong. The selection list is based on 'Schedule 1' and 'Schedule 2' of the Chinese Medicine Ordinance announced by the Chinese Medicine Council of Hong Kong, on the 2000 edition of the *Pharmacopoeia of the People's Republic of China (C.P.)*, and on a field survey of the circulation of Chinese medicines in the Hong Kong market today.

2. The entries are divided into three parts and arranged in the following order: plants (443 items), animals (41 items) and minerals (22 items). The items in each part are arranged alphabetically according to their Latin name.

3. For each documented Chinese materia medica, the information given includes:

(i) Name: including Latin name, English name, *pinyin* of Chinese common name and Chinese common name.

(ii) Source: including the family name, the species name and, for animal and plant-originated species, the part used for medicinal purposes.

(iii) Distribution: including the main distribution regions of the documented Chinese materia medica. When Hong Kong is one of the regions, it will be specified.

(iv) Harvest and Processing: the processing method(s) used in the main distribution regions.

(v) Description: a detailed description of the characteristics of the crude drug. The Chinese materia medica that are typically used in Hong Kong are stated in the 'Note' section.

(vi) Indications: documenting the main indications of the Chinese materia medica.

(vii) Chemical Composition: listing the main chemical components of the Chinese materia medica.

4. When documenting those Chinese materia medica with multiple sources, the representative species commonly used in Hong Kong are usually described in the main text. Those species that have other sources and are listed in *C.P.* are only briefly mentioned in the 'Note' section. Those species not yet clarified are not included in this publication.

5. For Chinese materia medica with multiple sources, those species mentioned in the 'Note' section belong to the same genus as the one indicated in the 'Source' section if the first part of the species name is written with the same initial. An example is Radix Paeoniae Rubra, the root of *Paeonia lactiflora* Pall. In the 'Note' section, it is stated that according to C.P., also used for medicinal purposes is the root of *P. veitchii* Lynch. The initial *P.* here indicates that the two *species Paeonia lactiflora* Pall. and *P. veitchii* Lynch belong to the same genus.

6. For clarity of meaning and provision of up-to-date information, items of Chinese materia medica listed in 'Schedule 1' and 'Schedule 2' of the Chinese Medicine Ordinance announced by the Chinese Medicine Council of Hong Kong are indicated in the 'Note' section as Category I (Toxic/Potent) and Category II Chinese Materia Medica respectively.

7. With regard to the processed items, those with similar source(s) are not individually listed but are specified in the 'Note' section instead. An example is Radix Aconiti Lateralis Preparata and the processed Radix Aconiti Lateralis Preparata.

8. All the photographs printed in this publication are of authenticated Chinese materia medica. The magnification of the published photograph is specified with a measuring scale. All the photographed items are kept in the Bank of China (Hong Kong) Chinese Medicines Centre, School of Chinese Medicine, Hong Kong Baptist University.

9. This publication includes a Latin name index of the source animals or plants of the Chinese materia medica, and an English name index, a *pinyin* index and a Chinese name index of the Chinese materia medica.

10. The measurement units adopted in this publication are official and universally adopted. For example, metres (m), centimetres (cm) and millimetres (mm) are used to describe the length of the Chinese materia medica.

11. The editor specifies in the 'Note' section the current practice in Hong Kong.

12. In this publication, the *Pharmacopoeia of the People's Republic of China will be referred to as C.P.*

13. A number of pen-and-ink drawings have been provided to acquaint the common readers with the different parts of plants described in this publication.

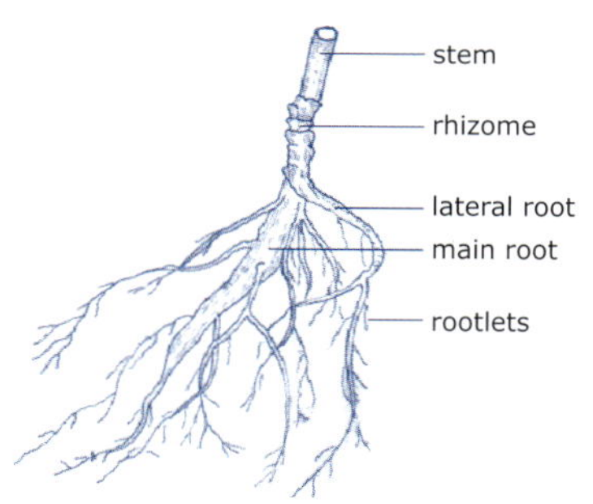

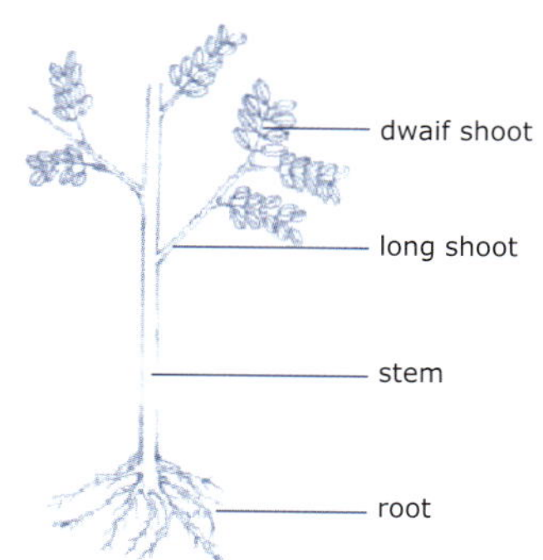

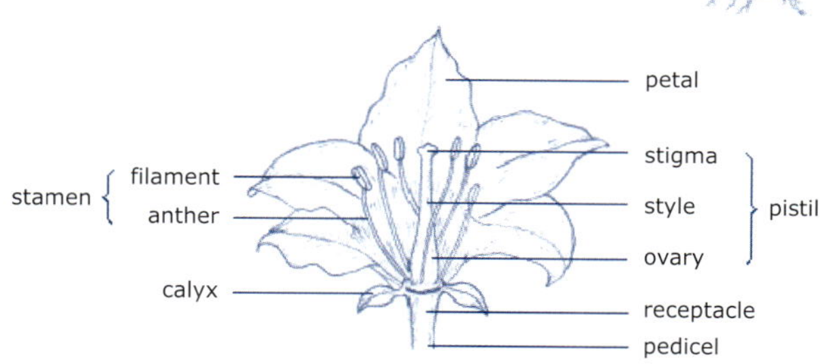

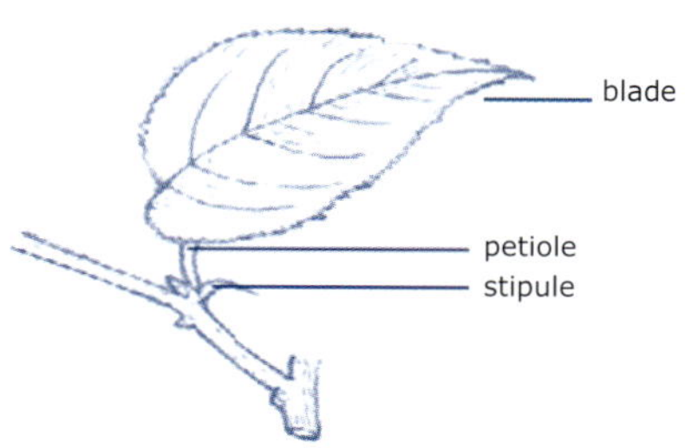

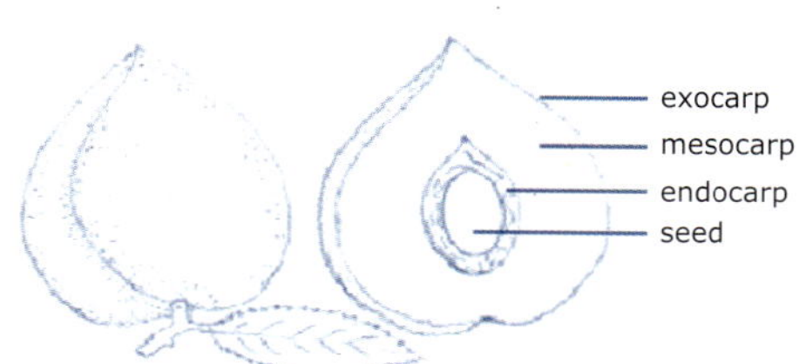

Preface by Dr. Zhao Zhongzhen

It was barely half a year ago when An Illustrated Chinese Materia Medica in Hong Kong saw daylight. We have since received enthusiastic responses from practitioners in the field of Chinese medicine, both from within our country and from other parts of the world; and with our readership covering profession personnel to individuals who are curious towards the discipline. At a time when Hong Kong is taking its first strides in placing Chinese medicine under statutory control, the publishing of this book bears practical significance towards building up an industrial standard amongst our peers.

On its own, the Chinese version of An Illustrated Chinese Materia Medica in Hong Kong is not enough to enable Chinese medicine to take on a significant role on the global stage. As a place where the cultures of East and West meet and intermingle, the city of Hong Kong is arguably best suited for assisting Chinese medicine towards achieving this goal.

The translating of Chinese materia medica opens up a whole new sphere of interest worthy of closer scrutiny. Yet it is also an enormously challenging task. Such an undertaking would require unreserved exchanges and sincere collaborations between professionals across the boundaries of the academia - one specializing in Chinese medicine, the other in language. The Hong Kong Baptist University enjoys a unique edge in this respect. The English edition of An Illustrated Chinese Materia Medica in Hong Kong cannot have been completed without the full support of Professor Martha Cheung and the many professional translators from the Centre for Translation, and the participation of the many specialists from the School of Chinese Medicine in the university.

The path to the standardization of Chinese medicines is guided by two elements - the nomenclature of the drugs as the signpost, and the precision usage of the crude drugs as the milestone. The weight of An Illustrated Chinese Materia Medica in Hong Kong bears in its identification of the Chinese crude drugs - a small yet significant step - through the coadunation of illustrations and texts to an end of a rigorous standard in employing identification methods and technical jargons. As regards the 'nature and action' (性味功效) of the crude drugs, there has yet to be a universal standard even within the scope of the Chinese medicine practices. These shall await more in-depth investigation and further research.

To assist readers in their approach to the text, in the course of producing the English Edition of An Illustrated Chinese Materia Medica in Hong Kong certain adjustments have been made with regards to the Chinese Edition. These include the addition of pen-and-ink drawings and indexes.

The production of the English Edition has again received the generous sponsorship from Eu Yan Sang Ltd. A word of gratitude again for their contribution.

Zhao Zhongzhen
School of Chinese Medicine, Hong Kong Baptist University
28 March 2004

Introduction

By Zhao Zhongzhen
Translated by Martha P.Y. Cheung

Chinese medicine[1] in Hong Kong is a key component of Chinese medicine in China. Likewise, the Chinese medicines[2] trading industry in Hong Kong forms a branch of the development of the Chinese medicines trading industry in China. Hong Kong, moreover, is a window through which the world can understand Chinese medicines and an important channel for the introduction of Chinese medicines to the world.

1. Reclaimed land turned into a Chinese medicines trading centre

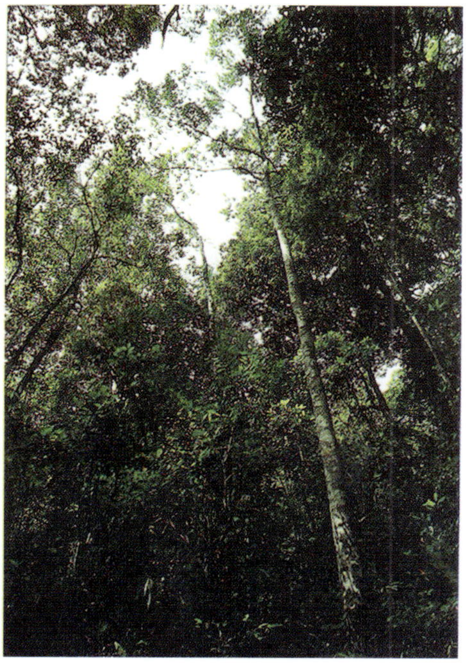

Aquilaria sinensis **(Lour.) Gilg. (Fam. Thymelaeaceae)**

Chinese medicines occupy an integral part of the history of Hong Kong. From the very beginning, Hong Kong has played a crucial role in the trading of Chinese medicines. There is in fact an interesting story about how Hong Kong (variously interpreted as 'incense port' or 'fragrant harbour') acquired her name. In the old days, Dongguan County of Guangdong Province in China grew a type of tree - *Aquilaria sinensis* (Lour.) Gilg. (Incense Tree) - that was often used as a substitute for Aquilaria agallocha Roxb. (Eaglewood). Its resin - used as raw material for incense and also known for its medicinal value - was called 'Guanxiang' (莞香) (meaning 'the fragrance [xiang] of Dongguan'). Because of her geographical advantage, Hong Kong soon became a trading centre for the import and re-export of 'Guanxiang' to different parts of China. As time went by, this port for transporting incense and Chinese medicines was simply referred to as 'fragrant port', and its transliteration, which was based on the dialect spoken by the boat people who first identified the island for the British, became the name by which the city is known all over the world - 'Hong Kong'.

---

1 'Chinese medicine' (zhongyi, 中醫) is a broad term referring to the art and science of healing based on the philosophy and theory developed by the Chinese people since antiquity, and to the use of Chinese medicinal materials which are of herbal, animal, or mineral origin for the treatment, prevention or alleviation of disease or symptoms of disease in human beings, or for the regulation of the functional states of the human body. [Translator's note]

2 'Chinese medicines' (zhongyao, 中藥), as explained in the main text, refers to the medicines prescribed in accordance with the principles and theories of orthodox Chinese medicine. It has three main components: crude drugs (yuanyaocai, 原藥材), decoction pieces (yinpian, 飲片), and proprietary Chinese medicines (zhongchengyao, 中成藥). Crude drugs and decoction pieces are often collectively referred to as 'Chinese materia medica' (中藥材) although 'Chinese materia medica' also carries a broader meaning denoting the study of the sources, nature, properties and preparation of the crude drugs used in medicine. [Translator's note]

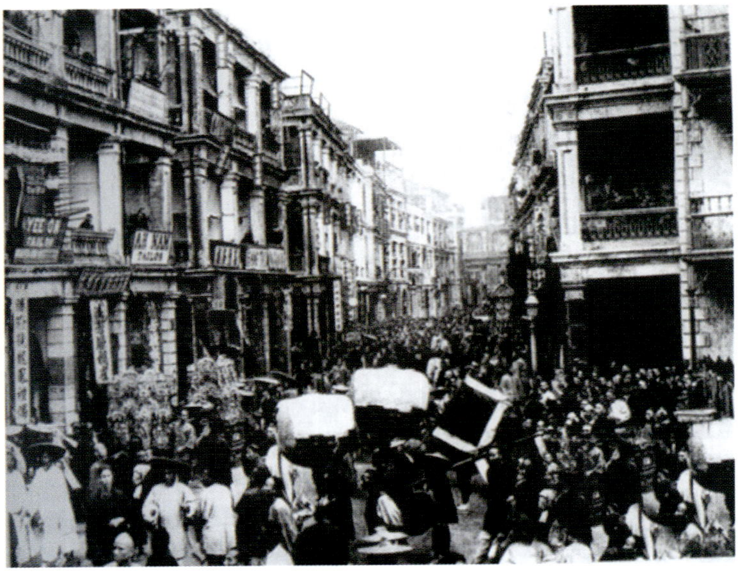

A street in the neighbourhood of Nam Pei Hong in the early 20th century

Hong Kong is comprised of Hong Kong island, the Kowloon peninsula, and the New Territories. The total land area is about 1,096 square kilometres, with about 60 square kilometres of reclaimed land.

Land reclamation began in the year 1852, about a decade after Hong Kong was officially opened as a trading port. The first strip of reclaimed land was located north of Queen's Road Central (皇后大道中). In those years, most of the economic activities were concentrated in the waterfront area (i.e. along Bonham Strand [文咸東街], Bonham Strand West [文咸西街], Wing Lok Street [永樂街], and Ko Shing Street [高陞街]), where the shops for the trading of sundry goods via the southern and northern routes were. The southern route dealt mainly with the trading of local produce from South East Asia, while the northern route was mainly engaged in the trading of China-made exports from different parts of the Mainland. The proximity to the sea facilitated the loading and unloading of goods, especially of Chinese medicines from the piers, customs clearance, inventory taking, and delivery. On this tiny stretch of reclaimed land, a unique distribution centre for Chinese medicines was born, unique even amongst other such distribution centres in China.

On the Chinese mainland, the distribution centres for Chinese medicines used to be located along the old historical routes; nowadays, they are mostly in areas along the major rivers or the coast. Going from north to south, the major distribution centres by the sea include Dalian, Yingkou, Tianjin, Yantai, Shanghai, Hangzhou, Ningbo, Wenzhou, Quanzhou and Guangzhou. All through history, Hong Kong's prosperity depended heavily on her close relation with Guangzhou. In the early years, Hong Kong was no more than an extension of the Chinese medicines trading industry of Guangzhou. After Britain took over Hong Kong in 1841, she opened Hong Kong as a trading port. With the arrival of trading vessels and capitals, Hong Kong developed rapidly as an entrepot and trading centre. The rapid growth of the Chinese medicines trading industry in Hong Kong took place in the 1950s. The trade embargo imposed on China as a result of the outbreak of the Korean War brought a halt to the export of precious crude drugs such as the resin of *Aquilaria agallocha* Roxb. (Eaglewood) from the South East Asian countries into China. Likewise, the export of Chinese crude drugs from China directly to those countries was also stopped. Hong Kong took

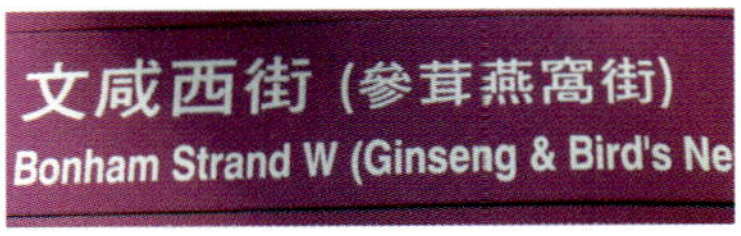

Bonham Strand West, known for selling Ginseng, Pilose Antler, and Bird's Nest

the opportunity and served as the link, and Ko Shing Street (高陞街) rose to become a world famous distribution centre of Chinese medicines.

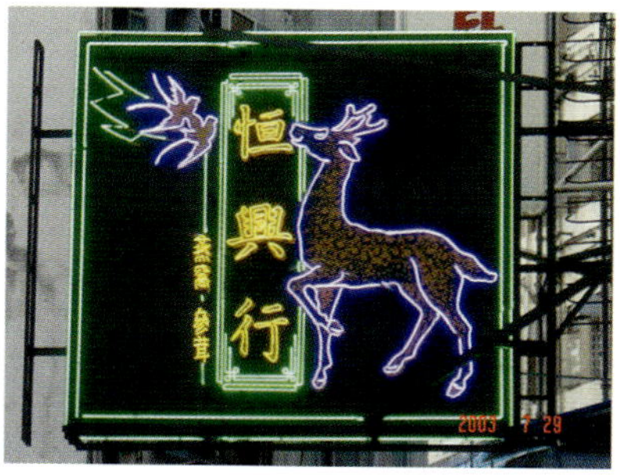

Neon lights in Ko Shing Street advertising Bird's Nest and Pilose Antler

Like attracts like. One shop opens, another follows. This is how business grows and such a characteristic is even more evident in Hong Kong. People go to Fa Hui Park in Mongkok to buy flowers, Hollywood Road to buy antiques, and Bonham Strand West (文咸西街) and Ko Shing Street for Chinese medicines. According to the recollection of those who have run a business there, from after the Second World War to the early 1980s, the companies in that area - known collectively as Nam Pei Hong (南北行, literally 'south and north companies') because they were all in the trading business, either with South East Asia or with China - had its own security guards. The cost of hiring these guards, who were armed with shotguns when they patrolled the streets, was evenly shared amongst the shops and the overall arrangement was the responsibility of the administrative office of Nam Pei Hong. Such a system of self-regulation was effective and a particularly important feature of the Chinese medicines trading industry in Hong Kong. This was because the British government in Hong Kong had always adopted a laissez faire attitude towards the existence, development and regulation of Chinese medicine and Chinese medicines alike. In fact, for a long time, members of the Chinese Medicines Merchants Association all had a cabinet of their own, and the names of those dealing business with them on credit would be taped on the cabinet until the debts had been honoured. The Man Mo Temple (文武廟), which in the old days served as a meeting place for the local gentries and dignitaries to deliberate on important matters, was also a place where major issues regarding the Chinese medicines trading industry would be discussed and the decisions made by this 'council' commanded high respect from the public. In the absence of government regulations, these two measures ensured the smooth operation of the self-regulatory system.

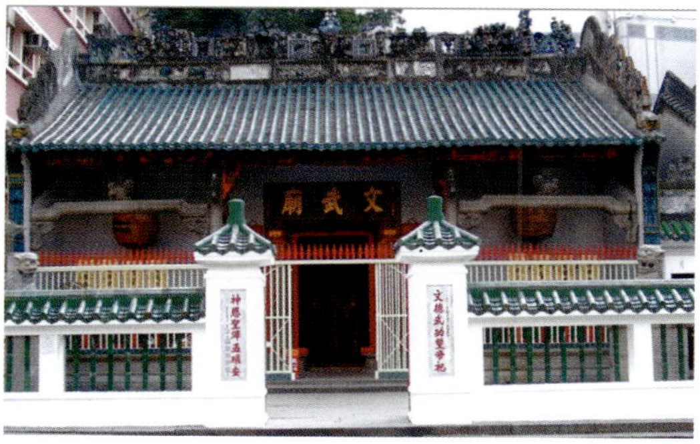

The 'council' of the Chinese medicines trading industry in the past

Before the Second World War, the Chinese medicines shops were mostly gathered in Bonham Strand West and its vicinity. As rents went up, these shops moved to Ko Shing Street while Bonham Strand West became the home of shops that sold more expensive items such as Nidus Collocaliae Esculentae (Bird's Nest, Yanwuo, 燕窩), Radix Ginseng (Ginseng, Rensen, 人參) and Cornu Cervi Pantotrichum (Pilose Antler, Lurong, 鹿茸). The Pau Sau Tong Ginseng & Antler Association Hong Kong Limited, established in 1912, largely consisted of members that sold Moschus (Musk, Shexiang, 麝香), Calculus Bovis (Cow-Bezoar, Niuhuang, 牛黃), Fel ursi (Bear Bile, Xiongdan, 熊膽), Radix Panacis Quinquefolii (American Ginseng, Xiyangshen, 西洋參), Nidus Collocaliae Esculentae (Bird's Nest), and other such precious crude drugs. The plaque bearing the Association's name is still visible on a wall in Bonham Strand West today.

Even though retail Chinese medicines shops can be seen in many parts of Hong Kong today, Ko Shing Street is still the hub for wholesale trade and for import and export business. The street, less than 300 metres long, is lined with shops, and the air is filled with the fragrance of Chinese materia medica. Inside the shops, crude drugs of all types stand in elegant display;

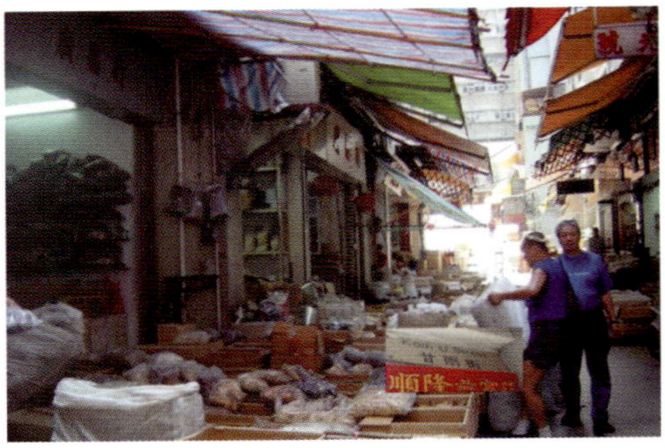

Kom U Street (甘雨街), a little alley, a treasure trove of Chinese medicines

outside, neon signs, posters, and advertisements half cover the sky. There is even an inconspicuous side alley called 'Kom U Street' (甘雨街). Less than a hundred metres long, it is a real treasure trove of Chinese materia medica.

The Hong Kong Chinese Medicines Merchants Association was established in 1928. Its members are mostly based in Bonham Strand West and Ko Shing Street. These streets truly deserve the reputation of being a Chinese medicines trading centre. Standing there, you could feel how deeply Hong Kong people rely upon and appreciate Chinese medicines; you would discover a living Who's Who of Chinese medicines in Hong Kong. The entire place is like a museum of Chinese medicines, a dynamic museum that captures the pulsing rhythm of the Chinese medicines trading industry in Hong Kong.

In 2004, a Chinese medicines theme garden will be set up at the intersection of Bonham Strand West and Ko Shing Street. Bringing together folk customs and Chinese medicines, the theme garden will add new excitement to a Chinese medicines street rich in history and tradition.

2. Geographical advantage put to good use

Hong Kong is situated at the southeastern tip of the Chinese mainland - a kingdom of natural medicines - and is also close to Taiwan and South East Asia. A continuous supply of Chinese crude drugs from the north can arrive by land while the precious crude drugs from South East Asia can arrive by sea. Hong Kong's natural harbour is big and deep enough for a few hundred cargo ships to load and unload at the same time. With such a geographical advantage, Hong Kong has for long done well in the Chinese medicines trade. In particular, she has excelled as an entrepot for the trading of Chinese medicines between the Chinese mainland, Taiwan, and the Western world.

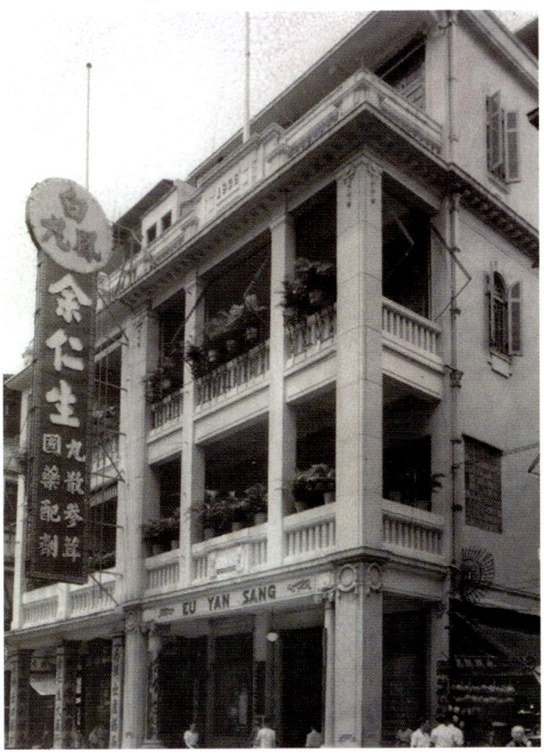

Century-old Eu Yan Sang - exterior of the shop in the early years

Hong Kong's development into an international centre for commerce, finance, communications and shipping is to be traced not just to her geographical location and her natural harbour. Hong Kong's independent judicial system, sound accounting system and healthy banking system all work to instill confidence in investors from abroad. In addition, with her highly developed information technology, Hong Kong provides quick and immediate access to prices, thus allowing buyers of commercial products in Chinese medicines to respond quickly to the demands of the market and place their orders accordingly. In July 2003, the Cato Institute of the United States, in conjunction with the Fraser Institute of Canada, ranked Hong Kong for the ninth consecutive time as the freest economy amongst 123 regions in the world -

yet another international affirmation of the superiority of the systems in Hong Kong.

Anyone can do business in Hong Kong, as long as he/she abides by the law. And since most imported goods are tax free, goods from all over the world find their ways here to compete for sale. The prices of some imported medicines are cheaper than those on the Chinese mainland, and this further strengthens the development of entrepot trade in Hong Kong.

The Chinese medicines trading industry in Hong Kong has had its good times and bad times, just like the economy of Hong Kong. In the 1970s and 1980s, when the economy was at its peak and there was a boom in the property market, the financial industry and tourism, Hong Kong developed into a major international financial centre. Likewise, the Chinese medicines trading industry entered its golden period.

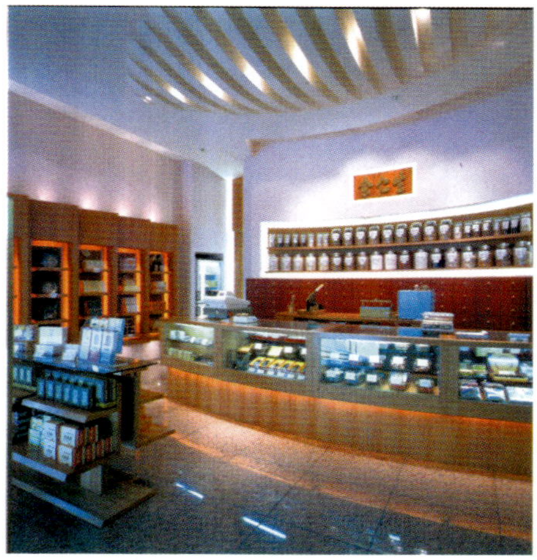

Modern Eu Yan Sang - one of the 82 chain stores spread throughout Hong Kong and Southeast Asia

The Chinese medicines trading industry in Hong Kong has three components: import and export, wholesale, and retail. It has a workforce of over 10,000 people. Retail shops alone exceed three hundred in number.

Hong Kong has always played the role of a major entrepot for Chinese crude drugs and decoction pieces. Over 95% of the Chinese medicines in Hong Kong are imported. As many as 900 kinds of crude drugs are sold in local Chinese medicines shops. Of the 10,000 kinds of proprietary Chinese medicines on sale in Hong Kong, about 2,000 kinds are manufactured locally.

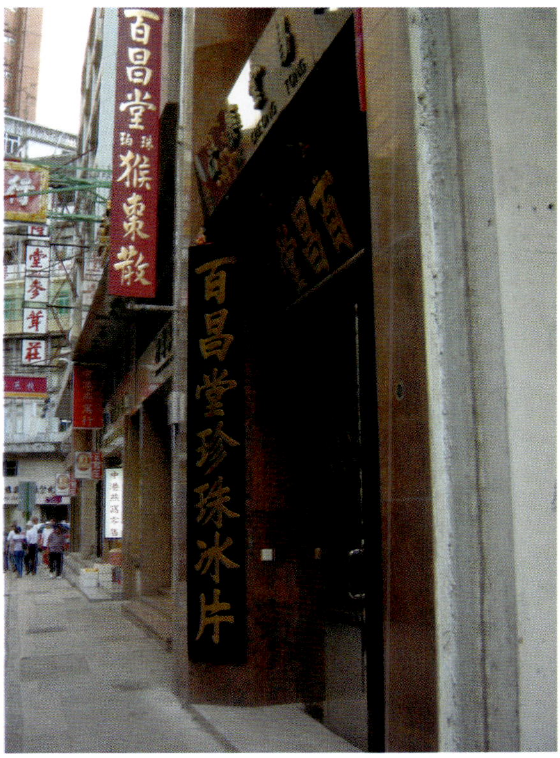

Bak Tseung Tong, a century-old Chinese medicines shop in Nam Pei Hong

Hong Kong is the largest market for Chinese medicines exported from the Mainland. Apart from re-exporting them to other countries and regions, Hong Kong also thrives on entrepot trade of Chinese crude drugs and decoction pieces from other places to China. In the past few years, import of Chinese crude drugs and decoction pieces into Hong Kong reached an annual average of over 2 billion Hong Kong dollars while export reached an annual average of 1.6 to 1.9 billion Hong Kong dollars. Of the Chinese crude drugs and decoction pieces imported into Hong Kong every year, only a small portion was absorbed by the local market, the rest were re-exported to the Mainland and other places such as Taiwan, Japan, South East Asia, Europe and the United States.

There are a few special features pertaining to the Chinese medicines trade in Hong Kong. Chinese crude drugs and decoction pieces imported from the Mainland are large in quantity and low in value, while those re-exported to the Mainland are the reverse. This is largely because the Mainland is not the main distributor of expensive items such as Radix Ginseng (Ginseng - cultivated or naturally grown), Calculus Bovis (Cow-Bezoar), Cornu Cervi Pantotrichum (Pilose Antler), and the resin of Aquilaria agallocha Roxb. (Eaglewood) and these items account for 70% of the total worth of Chinese medicines imported into Hong Kong. On the other hand, items such as Radix Angelicae Sinensis (Chinese Angelica, Danggui, 當歸), Radix Codonopsis (Pilose Asiabell Root, Dangshen, 黨參), Radix Astragali (Milkvetch Root, Huangqi, 黃芪), Rhizoma Dioscoreae (Common Yam Rhizome, Shanyao, 山藥), Radix Rehmanniae (Rehmannia Root, Dihuang, 地黃), Flos Chrysanthemi (Chrysanthemum Flower, Juhua, 菊花), and Fructus Lycii (Barbary Wolfberry Fruit, Gouqizi, 枸杞子) are inexpensive, even though they are almost exclusively imported from the Mainland.

Due to high rents and high wages, the prices of Chinese crude drugs in Hong Kong are considerably higher than those on the Mainland. Hong Kong, therefore, hones her competitive edge by focusing on quality and reliability. Hong Kong merchants trading in Chinese crude drugs are known for being particular about quality, not prices. Their strategy works and Hong Kong enjoys high international reputation with her customers.

3. Precious crude drugs and Chinese herbal tea - something for everyone

One characteristic of the use of Chinese medicines in Hong Kong is how widely Chinese medicines feature in the daily life of the people of Hong Kong: Chinese crude drugs are frequently used for preparing soups, and Hong Kong people are in the habit of drinking Chinese herbal tea.

Many supermarkets are stocked with packets of Chinese herbal medicinal preparations and health-enhancing crude drugs. People can buy them to make soups or tea. 'Support what is right and dispel evil' is the fundamental philosophy of Chinese medicine. The eight treatment methods in Chinese medicine - 'sweating', 'vomiting', 'downward ejection', 'harmonizing', 'warming', 'clearing', 'dispersing', and 'enhancing' - can be grouped into two broad categories based on the principles of reinforcing and draining.[3] As a principle, 'reinforcing' encompasses methods to supply insufficiencies of yin (陰), yang (陽), qi (氣) and xue (血), while 'draining' encompasses methods to dispel dampness, and to clear heat and eliminate fire. Chinese medicinal soups have a warming effect on the body and serve a health-reinforcing function; Chinese herbal tea operates in a reverse manner and produces its effect through clearing and draining. It would not be too much of an exaggeration to say that together, Chinese medicinal soups and Chinese herbal tea encapsulate in them the treatment methods of Chinese medicine.

Chinese medicines shops in Hong Kong all pride themselves on the sale of Radix Ginseng (Ginseng) and Cornu Cervi Pantotrichum (Pilose Antler) - well-known for their health-reinforcing effects. The sale of Radix Ginseng (Ginseng), Cornu Cervi Pantotrichum (Pilose Antler), and Radix Astragali (Milkvetch Root) is high, while proprietary Chinese medicines with fanciful names

---

3 A useful reference in English is A Practical Dictionary of Chinese Medicine, Second Edition, ed. Nigel Wiseman & Feng Ye. It provides explanations of the eight treatment methods and of the concepts in Chinese medicine referred to in this 'Introduction', e.g. yin (陰), yang (陽), qi (氣), xue (血), 'dampness', 'heat', 'fire', etc.. It should be noted, however, that in this book, two of the treatment methods are translated differently from Wiseman and Ye's dictionary. 'Downward ejection' is used in place of Wiseman and Ye's 'precipitation' because the former translation could convey the meaning much more readily and more clearly than the latter. And while Wiseman and Ye use 'supplementing' to translate the eighth treatment method, it is rendered here as 'enhancing' in order to avoid the associative meanings which the word 'supplement' has in Western medicine, e.g. vitamin supplement, dietary supplement. [Translator's note]

such as Eight Immortals Pill (Baxian Wan, 八仙丸), Perfection Major Supplementation Pill (Shiquan Dabu Wan, 十全大補丸), Black-bone Chicken and White Phoenix Pill (Wujibaifengwan, 烏雞白鳳丸), and Deer's Tail Pill (Luweiba Wan, 鹿尾巴丸) are also popular in Hong Kong. Having soup made with health-enhancing Chinese crude drugs is as much a custom of the local Chinese as taking milk is for the Westerners. Most Chinese restaurants in Hong Kong, big or small, serve soup of the day. In canteens, one often finds dishes with health-promoting ingredients such as Radix Glehniae (Coastal Glehnia Root, Beishashen, 北沙參), Rhizoma Polygonati Odorati (Fragrant Solomonseal Rhizome, Yuzhu, 玉竹), Semen Coicis (Coix Seed, Yiyiren, 薏苡仁), Semen Ginkgo (Ginkgo Seed, Baiguo, 白果), Bulbus Lilii (Lily Bulb, Baihe, 百合), and Fructus Lycii (Barbary Wolfberry Fruit, Gouqizi, 枸杞子). In classy restaurants and hotels, nutritious and often expensive items such as black-bone chicken, soft-shelled turtle, Cordyceps (Chinese Caterpiller Fungus, Dongchongxiacao, 冬蟲夏草), Bird's Nest, and shark's fin feature prominently in the menu. In fact, in autumn and winter, one can do good business by selling soups. Some restaurants even provide delivery service. Just ring them up and they will deliver the soups to your office. In recent years, health food has become very popular and courses in Chinese medicine run by universities on food therapy and medicinal diet are also well attended. This is probably because consumers in Hong Kong are health-conscious, even as they delight in yielding to the pleasure of the palate.

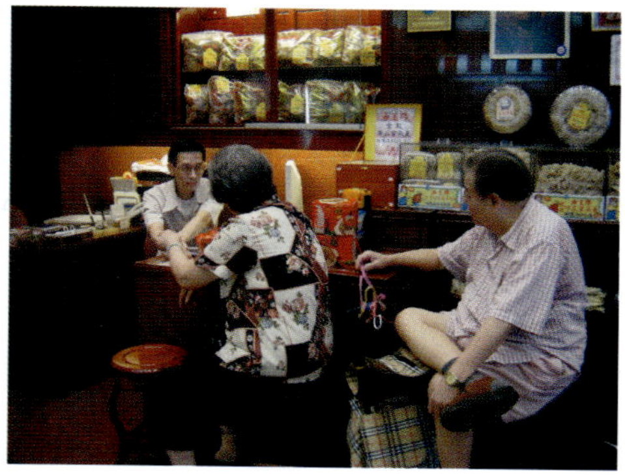

Chinese medicines shops also provide consultation service

In Hong Kong, health-reinforcing crude drugs are mostly imported from the Chinese mainland, while the crude drugs for making Chinese herbal tea are mostly obtained locally. The ingredients of Chinese herbal tea can be collected when fresh or when they are dried. Moreover, they vary depending on the season. They also vary in number - from as few as a single herb to as many as twenty four. These ingredients are mostly herbs for dispelling dampness and for clearing heat, for example, Herba Houttuyniae (Heartleaf Houttuynia Herb, Yuxingcao, 魚腥草), Herba Abri (Canton Love-Pea Vine, Jigucao, 雞骨草), Herba Lobeliae Chinensis (Chinese Lobelia Herb, Banbianlian, 半邊蓮), Herba Plantaginis (Plantain Herb, Cheqiancao, 車前草), Fructus Bruceae (Java Brucea Fruit, Yadanzi, 鴉膽子), Radix Ilicis Pubescentis (Pubescent Holly, Maodongqin, 毛冬青), Fructus Rosae Laevigatae (Cherokee Rose Fruit, Jinyingzi, 金櫻子), Herba Lysimachiae (Christina Loosestrife, Jinqiancao, 金錢草), Fructus Mornordicae Charantiae (Balsam Pear, Kugua, 苦瓜), Cortex Schefflerae Octophyllae (Ivy Tree Bark, Yajiaomu, 鴨腳木), Radix Helicteris (Narrowleaf Screwtree Root, Shanzhima, 山芝麻), Herba Polygoni Chinensis (Chinese Knotweed Herb, Huotanmu, 火炭母), Folium Mori (Mulberry Leaf, Sangye, 桑葉), Cortex Ilicis Rotundae (Ovateleaf Holly Bark, Jiubiying, 救必應), Semen Oroxyli (Indian

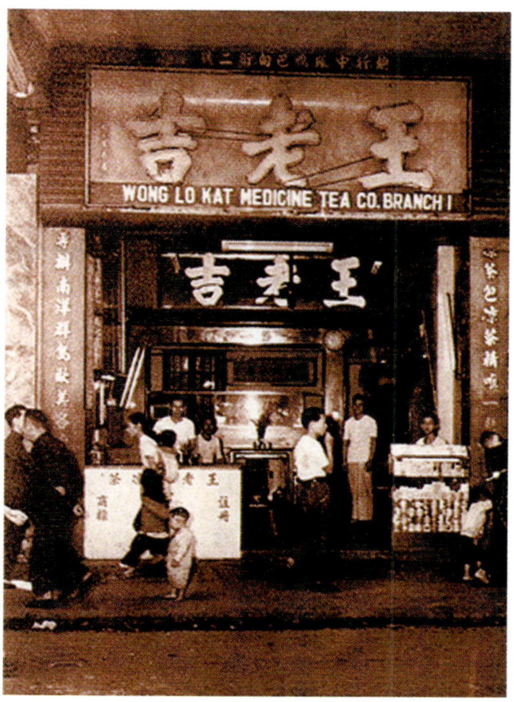

Age-old Chinese herbal tea shop - Wong Lo Kut

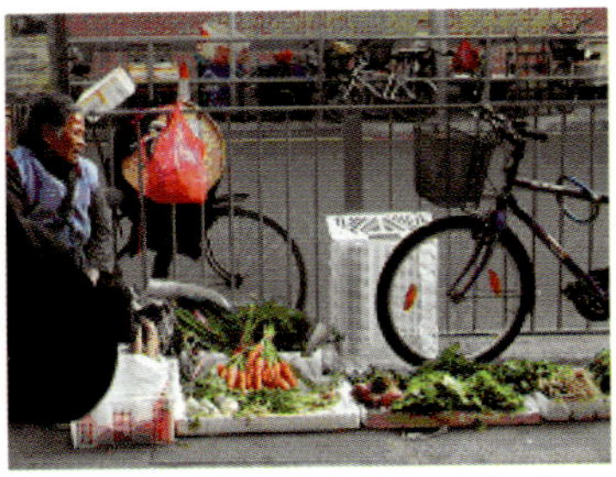

A street stall selling medicinal herbs

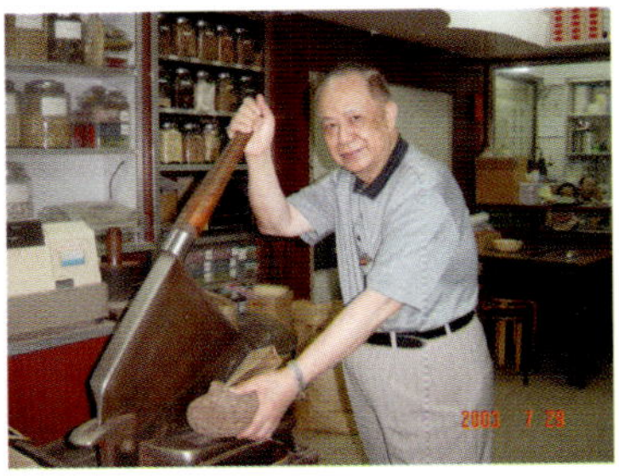

The authority of a Chinese medicines shop processing Poria (Fuling, 茯苓)

Trumpetflower Seed, Muhudie, 木蝴蝶), Herba Elephantopi Scaberis (Scabrous Elephant-foot Herb, Didantou, 地膽頭), Rhizoma Imperatae (Lalang Grass Rhizome, Baimaogen, 白茅根), Herba Lophatheri (Lophatherum Herb, Danzhuye, 淡竹葉), and Spora Lygodii (Japanese Climbing Fern Spore, Haijinsha, 海金沙).

'Take some Chinese herbal tea to clear the damp-heat in your body' - they say. Indeed, Chinese herbal tea is very much a part of the daily life of Hong Kong Chinese. In the market in early morning, it is easy to find stalls selling fresh medicinal herbs. There are few Hong Kong Chinese who have not taken a bowl or two of Chinese herbal tea, and few who could not name the names of a few crude drugs. In the last century, there was even an 'Association for Hong Kong and Kowloon traders in Chinese herbal tea'. At its peak, it boasted a membership of over 400. Chris Patten, the last British governor of Hong Kong, also paid a visit to a Chinese herbal tea shop as part of an image-building exercise - an indicative sign of how popular Chinese herbal tea is with the locals.

Chinese herbal tea shops can be seen everywhere in Hong Kong. The selling of ready-made Chinese herbal tea seems to be a practice unique to Hong Kong and Guangdong Province. Even though modern technology has led to the introduction of soluble granules to make the preparation of Chinese herbal tea much easier, the tea shops are still frequented by many faithful customers.

The frequency with which Hong Kong people take Chinese medicinal soups and Chinese herbal tea explains why the consumption of Chinese medicines per capita in Hong Kong is higher than that in other regions. The average life expectancy of Hong Kong people is among the highest in the world. Perhaps that has something to do with the soup-and-tea combination, which embraces the two fundamental treatment principles of Chinese medicine - reinforcing and draining.

4. 'Decoction Pieces' (yinpian, 飲片) - unique processing methods and attractive packaging

'Decoction pieces' are crude drugs cut to size in preparation for decoction. Depending on their shapes, and in order to comply with the requirements of doctor's prescription, of efficient dispensing and proper decoction, the crude drugs are often processed into the form of slices, sections, slivers, and pieces.

The Internal Canon of Medicine of the Yellow Emperor (《黃帝內經》) , a canonical Chinese medicine text produced in the pre-Qin period (21st century B.C.E.-221C.E.), contains records of medicines for 'biting and masticating' - the earliest form of decoction pieces. As for the term '飲片' (yinpian, decoction pieces), it can be traced to a Southern Song Dynasty (1127 - 1279 C.E.) text, to the description, 'processed crude drugs take the form of powder, crude drugs that of decoction pieces (yinpian, 飲片)'. Decoction pieces were called into being by clinical needs, and became more sophisticated with improvements in cutting and slicing techniques.

In Hong Kong, the traditional methods of processing were largely based on those of Guangzhou. As time went by, Hong Kong evolved a distinct processing style of her own. Apart from selecting quality crude drugs, attention is paid to packaging for commercial purposes. A kaleidoscope of innovative measures are used, including for example, specially designed

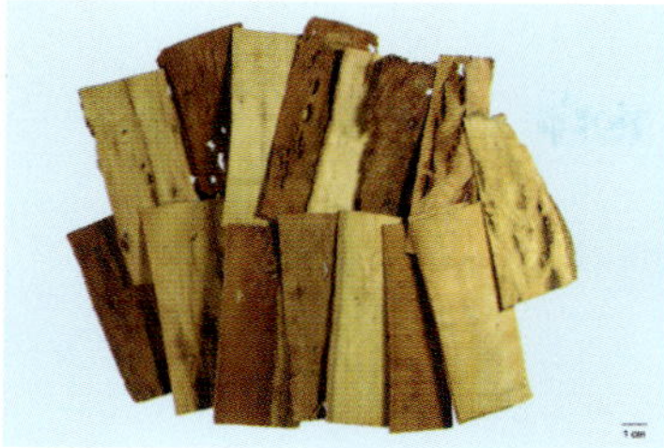

In Hong Kong, Cortex Phellodendri (Huangbo, 黃柏) is customarily used in the form of slices.

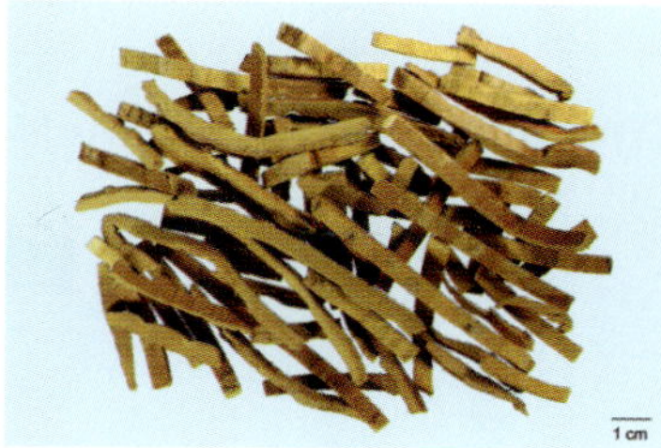

On the Mainland, Cortex Phellodendri (Huangbo, 黃柏) is mostly used in the form of fine sticks.

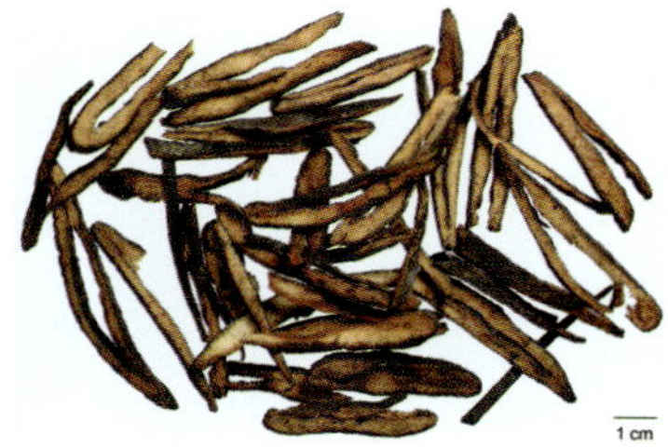

Fructus Aurantii (Zhiqiao, 枳殼) - transformed in appearance after processing.

containers. In addition, the crude drug Radix Notoginseng (Sanchi, Sanqi, 三七) is coloured black and the bark is then given a polished look; Fructus Aurantii (Orange Fruit, Zhiqiao, 枳殼) is pounded flat and then cut into strips; Radix Angelicae Sinensis (Chinese Angelica), Rhizoma Gastrodiae (Tall Gastrodia Tuber, Tianma, 天麻), and Radix Salviae Miltiorrhizae (Danshen Root, Danshen, 丹參) are all compressed and then cut length-wise into slices. Processed decoction pieces often assume a new look, not only in shape but also in colour, and bear little resemblance to their counterparts sold on the Mainland. For this reason, the identification and authentication of crude drugs can no longer be based simply on knowledge built on long years of experience in the trade.

In 1988, the Mainland implemented national standardization measures for processed Chinese medicines. A total of 554 items of processed crude drugs are included. Of the 522 items of commonly used Chinese materia medica collected in the 2000 edition of the Pharmacopoeia of the People's Republic of China, there are, listed under the heading 'Processing', 120 kinds of crude drugs to be cut into slices, over 100 kinds to be cut into sections, over 20 kinds to be shaved into slivers, over 10 kinds to be cut into lumps, and over 30 kinds to be pounded. Since the beginning of this century, the mainland authorities have been implementing standardization practices in factories for the production of decoction pieces. Guidelines are established for Good Manufacture Practice (GMP) and factories have to upgrade their technology to obtain a license.

In Hong Kong, regulations on the quality standards for processed decoction pieces have yet to be introduced. The relative merits of the decoction pieces produced in Hong Kong and those produced on the Mainland will have to be ascertained later on through comparative studies based on clinical observations, pharmacological study and chemical tests.

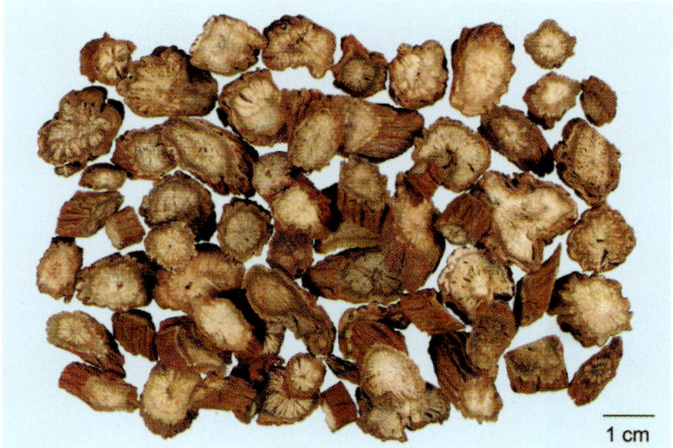

On the Mainland, Radix Salviae Miltiorrhizae (Danshen, 丹參) is mostly used in the form of cross-cut slices.

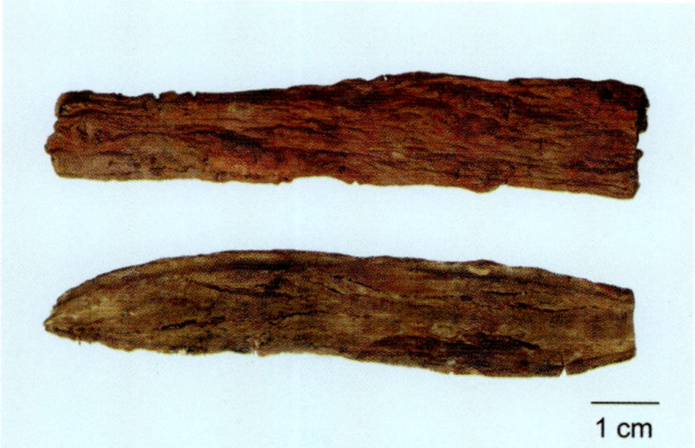

In Hong Kong, Radix Salviae Miltiorrhizae (Danshen, 丹參) is customarily used in the form of length-wise cut slices.

Table 1 Comparison of decoction pieces processed in Hong Kong and the Mainland[4]

Decoction Pieces	Mainland	Hong Kong
Radix Angelicae Sinensis (Donggui, 當歸)	Upper part: cut into pieces Axial root: cut length-wise into slices Branch roots: tie into a bundle and cut into slices	Upper part: cut length-wise into thin slices
Radix Salviae Miltiorrhizae (Danshen, 丹參)	Cross-cut into slices, or cut into sections	Compress and cut length-wise
Radix Notoginseng (Sanqi, 三七)	Cut, or grind into fine powder	Colour crude drug black and give the bark a polished look
Radix Paeoniae Alba (Baishao, 白芍)	Cross-cut into thin slices	Cut length-wise
Rhizoma Polygonati Odorati (Yuzhu, 玉竹)	Cross-cut	Shave
Radix Vladimiriae (Chuanmuxiang, 川木香)	Cross-cut into thin slices	Cut length-wise into thin slices
Rhizoma Smilacis Glabrae (Tufuling, 土茯苓)	Cut into thin, suborbicular slices	Cut length-wise into thin slices
Radix Asparagi (Tiandong, 天冬)	Slant cut into thin slices	Cut open longitudinally, remove woody core and compress
Radix Polygoni Multiflori (Heshouwu, 何首烏)	Cut into irregular, thick slices or sections	Mostly processed and then cut length-wise into slices
Radix Scutellariae (Huangqi, 黃芩)	Cut into thin, suborbicular or irregular slices	Cut length-wise into thin slices
Cortex Phellodendri (Huangbo, 黃柏)	Cut into fine sticks	Cut trunk bark into rectangular slats and then cut slats length-wise into thin slices
Fructus Aurantii (Zhiqiao, 枳殼)	Cross-cut into halves	Pound flat with a hammer and cut

4 English names of the Chinese materia medica referred to in the table will not be provided since the problem of confused nomenclature, described in Section 5, is not unique to the Chinese linguistic community but also to the English linguistic community. For the same reason, Section 5 will not carry the English names of any Chinese materia medica in the discussion.

5. Custom-drugs and confused nomenclature

In Hong Kong, the Chinese crude drugs sold in the market often pose a challenge to the discerning buyer. Different crude drugs are referred to by the same common name in Chinese, or the same crude drug is referred to by different common names. There are also counterfeit products. Although the Chinese Medicine Council of Hong Kong has, in Schedules 1 and 2 of the Chinese Medicine Ordinance passed in 1999, specified two lists of Chinese crude drugs[5], with one list containing 31 Chinese crude drugs known to be Toxic/Potent, and the other list 574 Chinese crude drugs commonly used in Hong Kong, there are a number of crude drugs the basic origin of which has not yet been determined. The problem of quality is still to be solved.

'Regional custom-drugs' refer to the substitutes, used in some regions, of certain authentic Chinese crude drugs. Having been used as a substitute in a particular region and having thus built up some reputation for being effective, custom-drugs belong to a strange category: they cannot be endorsed, and yet they cannot be dismissed without adequate research data. Be that as it may, doctor's prescription should be required before custom-drugs are used.

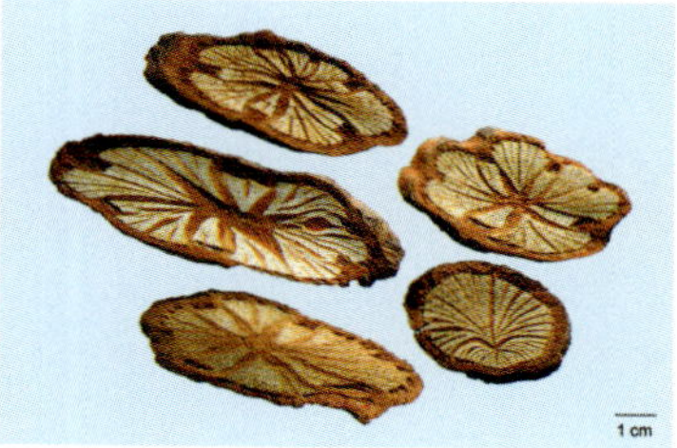

Decoction pieces of Caulis Sargentodoxae (Daxueteng, 大血藤).

As for 'confused nomenclature', the term describes a situation whereby some crude drugs are referred to by the same common names in Chinese as those designated for their counterpart proper or for regional custom-drugs. Whether confused nomenclature is caused by mistaken identity or by the existence of counterfeit products, their very presence constitutes a threat to the health of the populace and a violation of the safety standard for the use of Chinese medicines. Standardization measures are urgently needed.

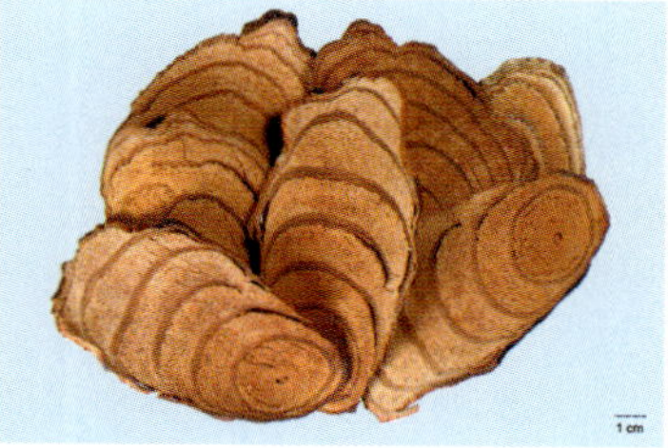

Decoction pieces of Caulis Spatholobi (Jixueteng, 雞血藤)

In the Preface of the Chinese text of *A Compendium of Materia Medica* (《本草綱目》, Ming Dynasty, 16th century), Li Shizhen, the author, had specially included a section on confused nomenclature and listed a large number of examples as illustration. It is obvious that the problem of different crude drugs being referred to by the same Chinese name has existed for centuries, though it is much more acute today. The problem exists on the Chinese mainland, in Hong Kong, and overseas. It arises because of a number of reasons:

(5.A.)Historical and geographical reasons

China is a large country with huge climatic differences between the north and the south; plants therefore differ greatly in variety, depending on their habitats. In the days when transportation was slow and delivery uncertain, local crude drugs had to be used as substitutes when the proper ones could not arrive. Guangdong Province is a case in point. Separated by Dayu Mountain, it falls outside the Yangtze River valley and Yellow River valley. Consequently, a lot of

5 In the Chinese Medicine Ordinance in Hong Kong, the translation for '中藥材' (zhongyaocai) is 'Chinese herbal medicines'. This term, however, is too narrow to embrace the full range of ingredients used in Chinese medicines, which do not only consist of herbs and plants but also of minerals and animals. The term could perhaps be more appropriately used as a literal translation of another Chinese term, '中草藥' (zhongcaoyao). [Translator's note]

local herbal medicines are used for treatment purposes and eventually, this gives rise to the 'Lingnan' school of practice in Chinese medicine. Below are a few examples of local crude drugs used as regional custom-drugs:

(5.A.i.)In northern China, Radix Isatidis (Banlangen, 板藍根) is mostly the dried root of *Isatis indigotica* Fort. (Fam. Cruciferae); in Hong Kong, Rhizoma et Radix Baphicacanthis Cusiae (Nanbanlangen, 南板藍根) is used instead and it is the dried root of *Baphicacanthus cusia* (Nees.) Bremek. (Fam. Acanthaceae). In the Pharmacopoeia of the People's Republic of China, the two are listed separately, i.e. as two separate crude drugs.

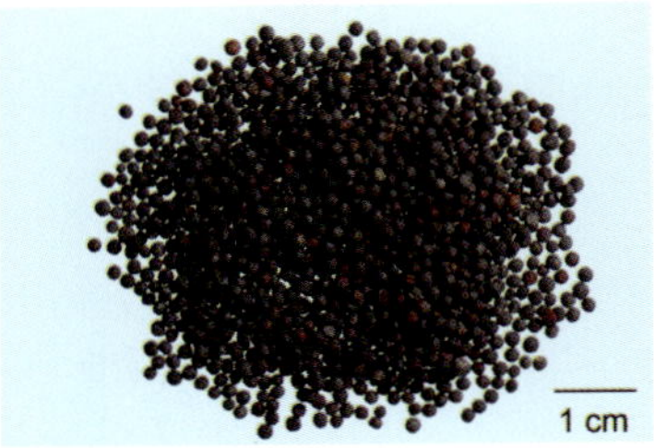

Semen Vaccariae (Wangbuliuxing, 王不留行)

(5.A.ii.)Semen Vaccariae (Wangbuliuxing,王不留行), according to the *Pharmacopoeia of the People's Republic of China*, is the seed of *Vaccaria segetalis* (Neck.) Garcke (Fam. Caryophyllaceae). But the crude drug customarily used in Hong Kong, called Guangdong Wangbuliuxingke (廣東王不留行殼), is Fructus Fici Pumilae, which is the pericarp of *Ficus pumila* L. (Fam. Moraceae). The two crude drugs bear certain resemblance in their Chinese names but are remote in taxonomic relationship. Whether one could be used as a substitute for the other is a highly debatable question.

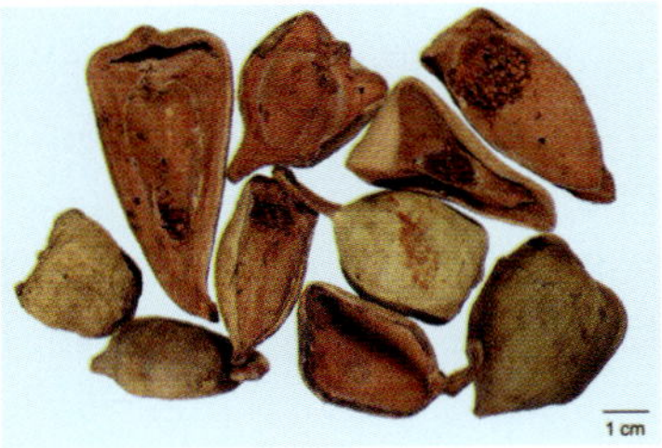

Fructus Fici Pumilae (Guangdong Wangbuliuxingke, 廣東王不留行殼)

(5.A.iii.)Again, according to the *Pharmacopoeia of the People's Republic of China*, Rhizoma Cimicifugae (Shengma, 升麻), should be the rhizome of *Cimicifuga heracleifolia* Kom. (Fam. Ranunculaceae). A crude drug sold in Hong Kong - Radix Serratulae Chinensis - is customarily called Guangdong Shengma (廣東升麻), but it is in fact the root of *Serratula chinensis* S. Moore (Fam. Compositae). The two crude drugs are sometimes interchangeably used in prescriptions.

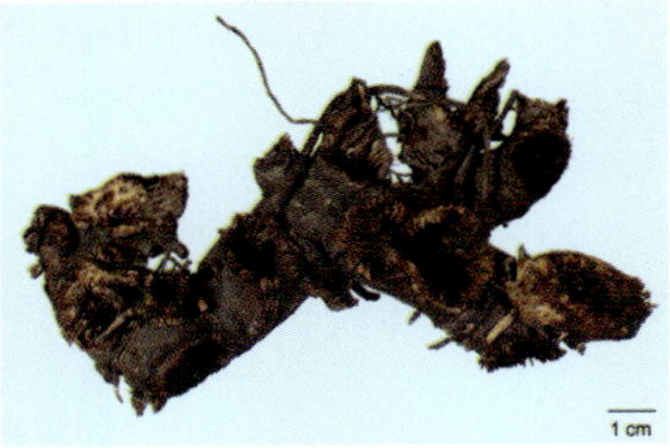

Rhizoma Cimicifugae (Shengma, 升麻)

(5.B.)Factors relating to the Chinese language and the Chinese writing system

The Chinese common name, 'Mutong' (木通) is often used to describe three kinds of plant crude drug used in Chinese medicines. These include Caulis Akebiae Quinatae (Mutong, 木通; source plant: *Akebia quinata* [Thunb.] Decne, [Fam. Lardizabalaceae]), Caulis Clematidis Armandii (Chuan Mutong, 川木通; source plant: *Clematis armandii* Franch. [Fam. Ranunculaceae], or Clematis Montana Buch.-Ham. [Fam. Ranunculaceae]), and Caulis Aristolochia Manshuriensis (Guan Mutong, 關木通; source plant: Aristolochia manshuriensis Kom. [Fam. Aristolochiaceae]). In the Chinese medicine tradition, Caulis Akebiae Quinatae has always been used as Mutong (木通). But in the 2000 edition of the *Pharmacopoeia of the People's Republic of China*, it is Caulis Aristolochia Manshuriensis (Guan Mutong, 關木通) and Caulis Clematidis Armandii (Chuan Mutong, 川木通) that get listed. Japan, however, follows the tradition from ancient times, and the *Japanese Pharmacopoeia* lists Caulis Akebiae Quinatae (source plant: *Akebia quinata* [Thunb.] Decne, [Fam. Lardizabalaceae]) and not the two found in the *Pharmacopoeia of the People's Republic of China*. Rectification of the situation is needed and the *Pharmacopoeia of the People's Republic of*

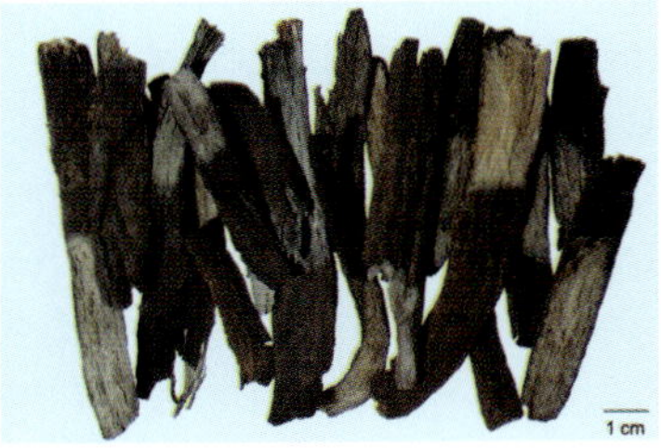

Radix Serratulae Chinensis (Guangdong Shengma, 廣東升麻)

China should seriously re-examine that entry in its next edition. It was reported in the international press that over use of aristolochic acid would lead to renal failure. The drug that in fact causes renal failure is Caulis Aristolochia Manshuriensis (Guan Mutong, 關木通; source plant: *Aristolochia manshuriensis* Kom. [Fam. Aristolochiaceae]). However, since it has the Chinese characters '木通' (Mutong) in its Chinese name, the other two crude drugs with these two Chinese characters in their names (mentioned above) are mistaken as the culprit drug.

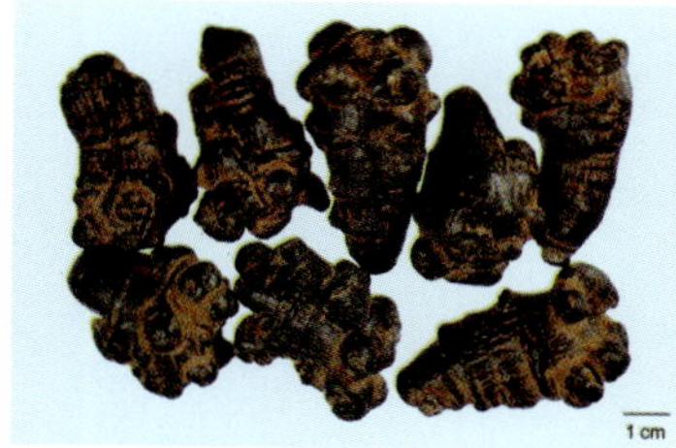

Radix Notoginseng (Sanqi, 三七)

Radix Notoginseng (Sanqi, 三七) and Rhizoma Tupistrae Chinensis (Chuan Sanqi, 川三七) come from totally different sources. The source of the former is *Panax notoginseng* (Burk.) F .H. Chen (Fam. Araliaceae); while that of the latter, *Tupistra chinensis Bak* (Fam. Liliaceae). In Hong Kong, these two crude drugs get mixed up with each other and, when used interchangeably, will produce toxic side effects. The confusion arises because both crude drugs have the Chinese characters '三七' (Sanqi) in their names.

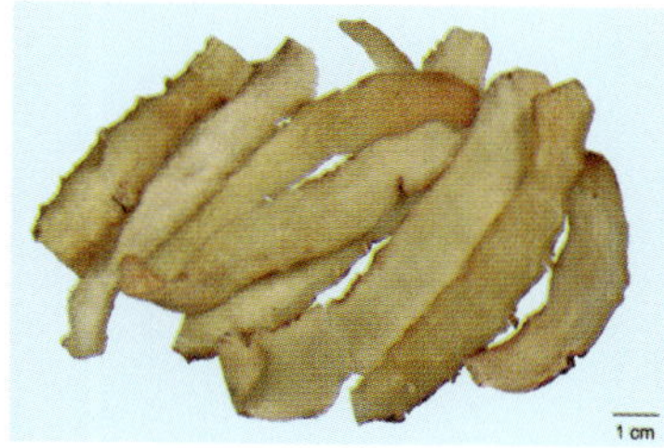

Rhizoma Tupistrae Chinensis (Chuan Sanqi, 川三七)

Confused nomenclature does not appear overnight, and it will not disappear overnight. It takes time and vigorous identification measures to separate those with genuine medicinal functions from those that are useless or harmful to humans. And in order to root out confusion, those crude drugs that have been found to possess genuine medical functions should be listed separately. For example, Radix Serratulae Chinensis (Guangdong Shengma, 廣東升麻) and Rhizoma Cimicifugae (Shengma, 升麻) - discussed in (5.A.iii.) above - must be clearly distinguished from each other and must not be used interchangeably simply because both have the Chinese characters '升麻' (Shengma) in their names.

(5.C.)Similar in shape and appearance, totally different in property

The principal species of Radix Clematidis (Weilingxian, 威靈仙) should be the roots of *Clematis chinensis Osbeck* (Fam. Ranunculaceae). However, at one time in the Hong Kong market, Radix et Rhizoma Sinopodophylli Emodi (Guijiu, 鬼臼), which are the roots of *Sinopodophyllum emodi* (Wall.) Ying (Fam. Berberidaceae) were used as Radix Clematidis because the two roots look alike in shape. The mistake had led to drug poisoning.

Another example. Radix Cynanchi Atrati (Baiwei, 白薇) and Rhizoma Cynanchi Stauntonii (Baiqian, 白前) are of the same family (Fam. Asclepiadaceae). Ancient herbal medicine texts give little descriptions of the macroscopic characteristics of these two crude drugs. Often they are compared to Herba Asari (Xixin, 細辛) and Radix Achyranthis Bidentatae (Niuxi, 牛膝). Alternatively, they are distinguished by the colour on the outer surface of the root and by its texture - one is yellow, the other is white; one is pliable, the other is fragile. The descriptions are too brief to be of use in differentiating the two crude drugs. Those in the profession use terms such as 'hollow' to describe Rhizoma Cynanchi Stauntonii (Baiqian, 白前) and 'solid' to describe Radix Cynanchi Atrati (Baiwei, 白薇). But, in some regions, the jargon could be used in just the reversed manner for these two crude drugs. In Hong Kong, the two are often mixed up. Another crude drug, Herba Gerberae Piloselloidis (Baimeicao, 白眉草), is often confused with Radix Cynanchi Atrati (Baiwei, 白薇) because the first two Chi-

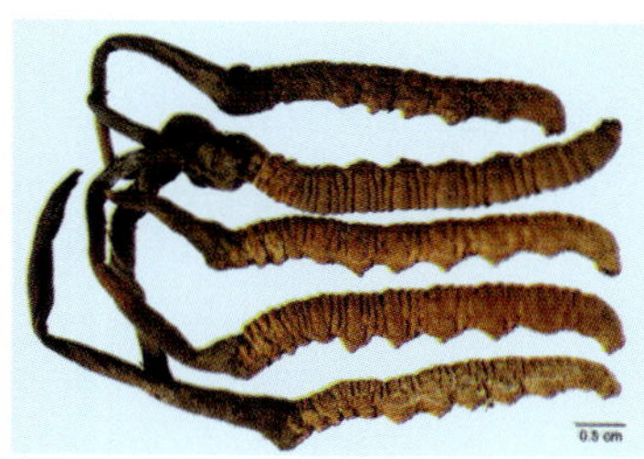

Cordyceps (Dongchongxiacao, 冬蟲夏草)

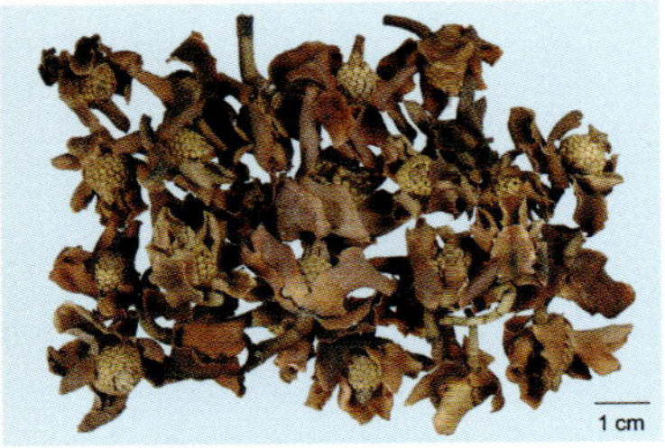

Flos Magnoliae Cocinis (Yehehua, 夜合花)

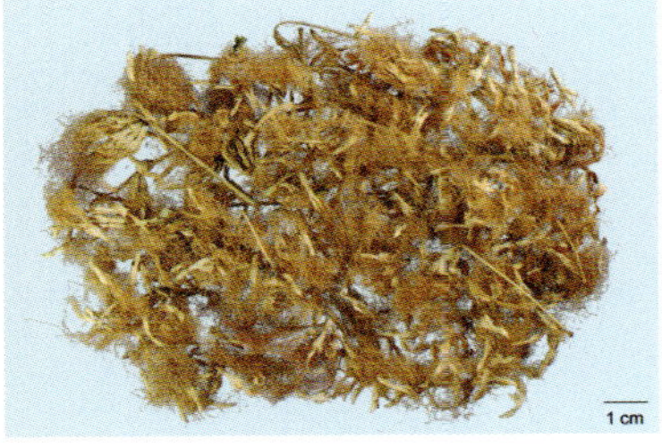

Flos Albiziae (Hehuanhua, 合歡花)

nese characters of Herba Gerberae Piloselloidis (白眉) are identical in Cantonese pronunciation to the Chinese name of Radix Cynanchi Atrati (白薇).

(5.D.) Counterfeit products - wilful deception

Because precious crude drugs are expensive, many yield to the temptation of making a quick profit by manufacturing counterfeit products. For precious crude drugs such as Moschus (Musk), Calculus Bovis (Cow-Bezoar), Fel ursi (Bear Bile), and Cornu Saigae Tataricae (Pronghorn, Lingyangjiao, 羚羊角), counterfeit products made from plastic material, natural analogous material, and other such substances are particularly numerous. The more precious and rare the crude drug is, the more likely it will be that counterfeit products would find their way into the market. Cordyceps (Chinese Caterpiller Fungus, Dongchongxiacao, 冬蟲夏草) is a classic example. It is a crude drug of the Hepialidae family. It grows on the Qinghai-Tibet Plateau and has its natural habitat in the snow line area 3000 metres above sea level. Nowadays, unscrupulous merchants use Rhizoma Stachydis Geobombycis, rhizome of *Stachys geobombycis* C.Y. Wu (Dican, 地蠶) (Fam. Labiatae), and pass it off as Cordyceps (Dongchongxiacao, 冬蟲夏草). Other counterfeit products of Cordyceps (Dongchongxiacao, 冬蟲夏草) that have been found in the market are produced by putting gypsum, wheat flour, soybean flour and corn flour into moulds for compression.

As can be seen from the above analysis, the phenomenon of different crude drugs with the same common name in Chinese is largely caused by historical and geographical factors, and by the age-old practice of using custom-drugs. The confusion thus arisen is of course compounded by the existence of counterfeit products. But, dishonesty aside, much of the problem is to be traced to the nomenclature of Chinese crude drugs. The standardization of names, therefore, must be enforced if the problem is to be solved. To give one more example. Flos Albiziae (Hehuanhua, 合歡花) refers to the flower buds of *Albizia julibrissin* Durazz. (Fam. Leguminosae). In Hong Kong, however, '合歡花' (Hehuanhua, Flos Albiziae) is called '夜合花' (Yehehua, Flos Magnoliae Cocinis) - probably because the Chinese characters '合' (he) and '花' (hua) appear in both Chinese names - while '夜合花' (Yehehua, Flos Magnoliae Cocinis), which refers to the flowers of *Magnolia coco* (Lour.) DC (Fam. Magnoliaceae), is called '合歡花' (Hehuanhua, Flos Albiziae). In other words, A is mistaken as B and B is mistaken as A. To traders of Chinese medicines and to the general public, therefore, the establishment of standardized Chinese names for Chinese crude drugs is likely to be more important than the establishment of standardized Latin names for those drugs. And, needless to say, the establishment of a systematic nomenclature system for Chinese medicines provides the foundation for the standardization of Chinese medicines as a whole.

The examples of custom-drugs and confused nomenclature cited above are not exhaustive. Further cases of lack of discrimination in the use of crude drugs or of crude drugs being administered by mistake will be studied in detail in the future, and modern scientific methods would be used for identification, analysis and assessment. Crude drugs that fail to produce the specified treatment effects set down by the established standards should be eliminated. Those that can produce the specified treatment effects should be given a proper place in the domain of Chinese medicines.

6. Retrospect and prospects

'Chinese medicines' (zhongyao, 中藥) is an umbrella term referring to the medicines prescribed in accordance with the principles and theories of orthodox Chinese medicine. It has three main components: crude drugs, decoction pieces, and proprietary Chinese medicine.

History shows that one strand of human civilization consists of the continuous discoveries, advances in understanding, summation of knowledge and new breakthroughs made in Chinese medicines by the Chinese people. The first and earliest surviving text on Chinese materia medica is *Shen Nong's Herbal Classic* (《神農本草經》), written aboat 2,000 years ago. The text, written in the name of Shen Nong (a mythic figure of antiquity said to have discovered the curative virtues of plants), describes 365 kinds of crude drugs and establishes the basic theory and treatment principles of Chinese medicines. Since then, a number of related texts appeared - *Annotated Shen Nong's Herbal Classic* (《本草經集註》) (5th century), *The Newly-revised Materia Medica* (《新修本草》) (7th century), *Proved and Classified Materia Medica* (《證類本草》) (11th -12th century), *Compendium of Materia Medica* (《本草綱目》) (16th century), etc. They take Shen Nong's Herbal Classic as the primary text and revolve round it, critique it, elaborate upon it, forming a treasury of canonical texts on Chinese medicine. Each a magnificent achievement, these works epitomize the various historical climactic points in the development of Chinese medicine in China. They also represent important milestones in the development of traditional folk medicines of the world.

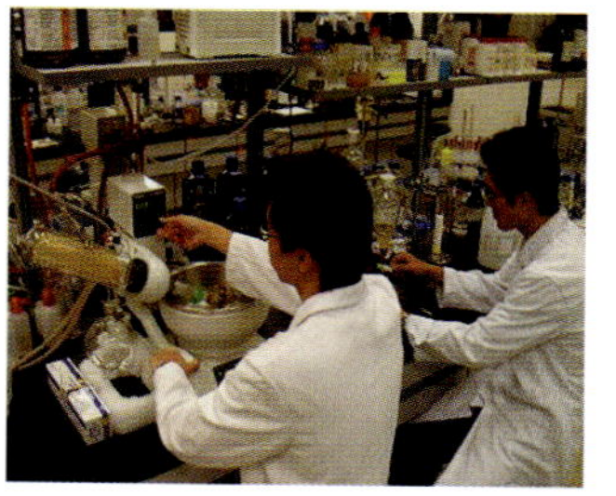

Chinese medicine education develops rapidly.

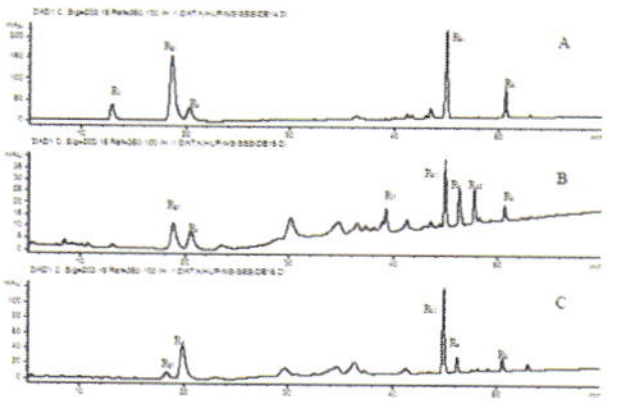

HPLC fingerprint chromatograms of Radix Panacis Quinquefolii (Xiyangshen, 西洋參), Radix Ginseng (Rensen, 人參) and Radix Notoginseng (Sanqi, 三七)

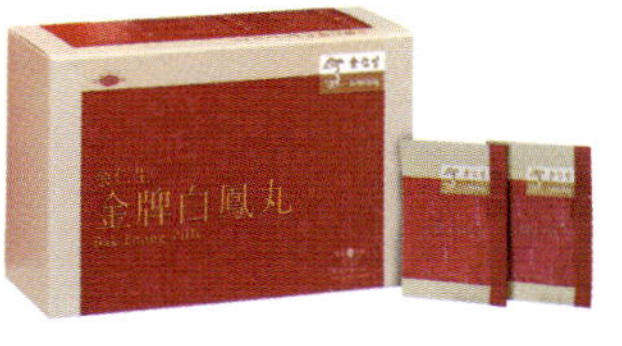

A new-generation Chinese medicines products developed with the assistance of the Innovation & Technology Commission

The establishment of the People's Republic of China ushered in a new era for the growth and development of Chinese medicine as a whole. Important reference works are compiled and published, including *Chinese Materia Medica Dictionary* (《中藥大辭典》) (1977), *A Compilation of Chinese Medical Herbs* (《全國中草藥匯編》) (1975/1996), *Modern Chinese Materia Medica* (《中藥誌》) (1982-1988), *Chinese Materia Medica* (《中華本草》) (1999). So far, over 10,000 kinds of Chinese medicines have been recorded.

Another monumental project is the compilation of the Pharmacopoeia of the People's Republic of China. It was first published in 1963 as a single volume. In 1977, legislation was introduced making it obligatory to update the Pharmacopoeia every five years. Now, the Pharmacopoeia of the People's Republic of China is the only pharmacopoeia in the world that observes such a vigorous process of continuous updating. From Shen Nong's Herbal Classic to the Pharmacopoeia of the People's Republic of China - the achievements of the Chinese people in Chinese medicines are enshrined in these two canonical texts. Together, they show how far Chinese medicines have traveled, both in theory and in practice.

All through the years when Hong Kong was a British colony, Chinese medicine and Chinese medicines were basically left on their own - to thrive or to die. Hong Kong's return to Chinese sovereignty on 1st July 1997, however, marked the dawning of a new era for Chinese medicine in Hong Kong - an era of steady progress based on the gradual introduction of regulatory

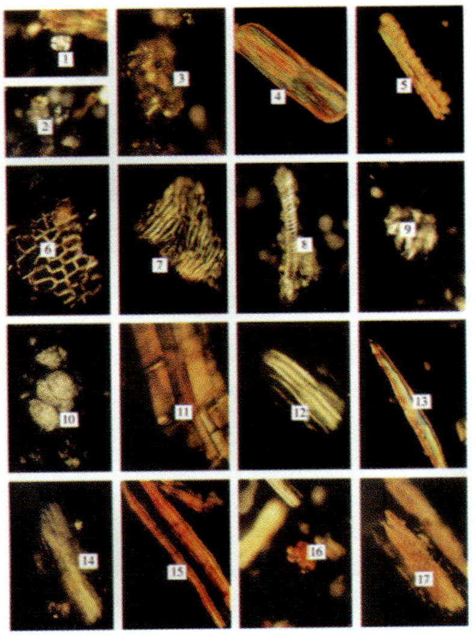

1. Microscopic Iaentification of Proprietary Chinese Medicines.
2. The age of identification chaos in Chinese medicines has passed.

measures. Within a few years, legislations on the trading of Chinese medicines and on the practice of Chinese medicine in Hong Kong were passed, certificate and degree courses in Chinese medicine and Chinese medicines were offered by local universities, regulations relating to the licensing of Chinese medicines traders and to the registration of proprietary Chinese medicines were introduced, and out-patient units for Chinese medicine were set up in some public hospitals. All these are concrete and effective measures to ensure that both Chinese medicine and Chinese medicines develop healthily in Hong Kong.

The first and most crucial step in the establishment of standards for Chinese medicines is the identification and authentication of the source of different species of Chinese crude drugs and the establishment of a systematic nomenclature. If Chinese medicines are to be introduced to the world at large, it is a matter of compelling urgency that proper standards are set up to rectify the somewhat chaotic situation caused by the use of custom-drugs and by confused nomenclature.

Under the initiative of the Department of Health in Hong Kong, local and overseas scholars are now working in collaboration with specialists in the field on a standardization project - 'Hong Kong Standard of Chinese Materia Medica'. The deployment of the latest state-of-the-art technology in this project will contribute significantly to the internationalization of Chinese medicines.

As Hong Kong moves forward into the twenty-first century, and as socio-economic factors change and consumers' tastes and habits also change, Chinese medicines shops are likely to become more diversified in their modes of operation. But Hong Kong's position as an entrepot and a distribution centre of Chinese medicines will remain as strong as ever. In fact, it can be envisaged that Hong Kong will assume a pivotal role in promoting and enhancing the process of modernization and internationalization of Chinese medicines in the years ahead.

Arillus Longan

Longan Aril
Longyanrou

龍眼肉

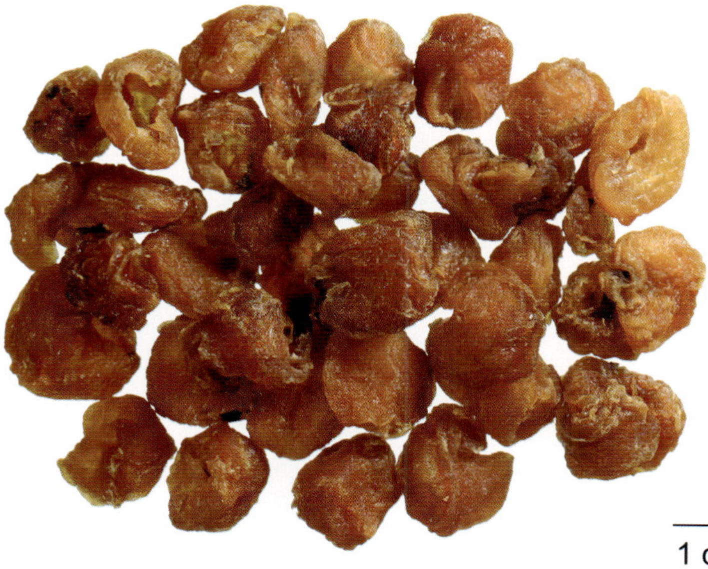

1 cm

Crude Drug

Source The aril of *Dimocarpus longan* Lour. (Fam. Sapindaceae).

Distribution Mainly in Chinese provinces such as Fujian, Guangxi, Guangdong and Yunnan; also in Hong Kong.

Harvest & Processing Harvest fruits after maturation in summer; dry under the sun until nearly dry; peel off arils, dry under the sun or by heat. Alternatively, boil fruits in water for 10 minutes; dry under the sun; roast with fire; peel off arils and dry under the sun.

Description Irregular pieces, often stuck together in clusters; 1-1.5 cm long, 1-3.5 cm wide, about 1mm thick; yellowish-brown; translucent. Outer surface (the side near to pericarp) shrivelled and uneven; inner surface (the side attached to the seed) lustrous, marked with fine longitudinal wrinkles. Soft and smooth; sticky. Odour: slightly fragrant; taste: quite sweet.

Indications 1. Palpitation, insomnia, forgetfulness, dizziness 2. Debility during convalescence and after delivery

Chemical Composition Adenine and choline exist in the dried fruit; the seeds contain 2-amino-4-methylhex-5-ynoic acid and 2-amino-4-hydroxymethylhex-5-ynoic acid.

Benzoinum

Benzoin
Anxixiang

安息香

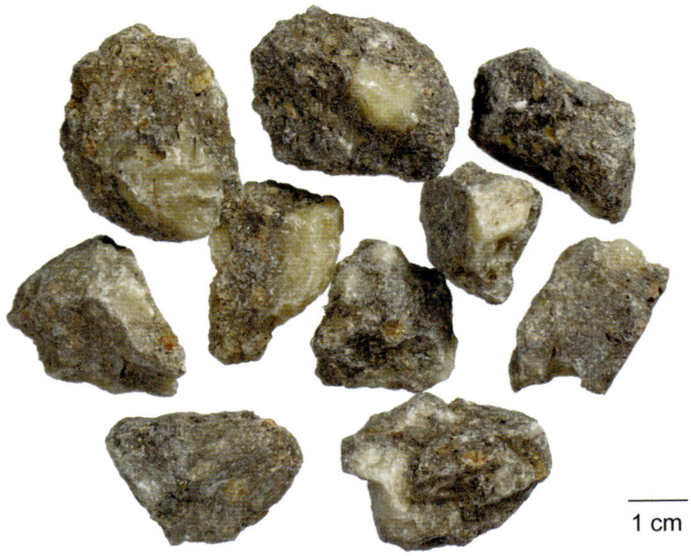

Crude Drug

Benzoinum

Source The botany bar gum of *Styrax tonkinensis* (Pierre) Craib ex Hart. (Fam. Styracaceae).

Distribution Mainly in Chinese provinces such as Guangxi, Yunnan and Guangdong. Imported benzoin is mainly produced in Indonesia and Thailand.

Harvest & Processing From April to September, choose trees 5-10 years old and use knife to make several triangular cuts about 40 cm from the ground around each tree trunk; let drip and collect the white resin secreted from the wounds; dry in shaded areas. At every other following month or one and a half months, make similar cuts 4 cm above the last ones. Repeat the process around the cuts to collect solidified milk-white resin.

Description Resin from natural secretion: small irregular pieces, slightly flat, often cohered into lumps; outer surface orange-yellow, with waxy lustre. Resin from induced injury: irregular cylindrical pieces or flat pieces; outer surface greyish-white to pale yellowish-white. Brittle, break easily. When broken, surface smooth and milk-white; after exposure to air, surface gradually turns pale yellowish-brown, yellowish-brown and then reddish-brown. When heated, resin softens and melts. Odour: aromatic; taste: slightly acrid, gritty when chewed.

Indications 1. Impairment of consciousness 2. Chest and abdominal pain 3. Skin ulcer (external use).

Chemical Composition Contains 70-80% resin with coniferyl benzoate.

Borneolum Syntheticum

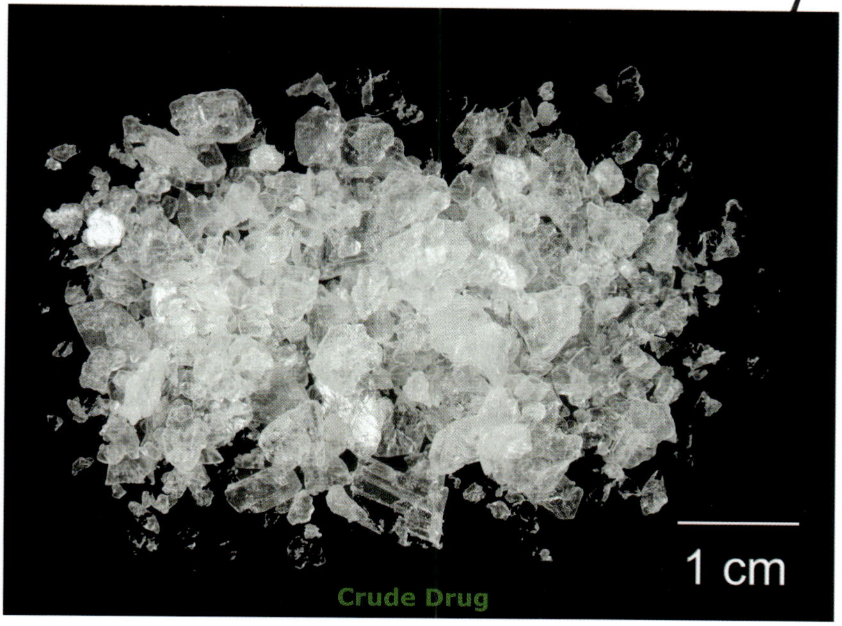

Borneol
Bingpian
冰片

Source The crystallised compound formed naturally from the resin of *Dryobalanops aromatica* Gaertn. f. (Fam. Dipterocarpaceae).

Distribution Mainly in places such as Sumatra of Indonesia. Mostly imported into China through Hong Kong.

Harvest & Processing Collect dried resin from clefts in the trunks of *Dryobalanops aromatica* and then process. Alternatively, chop down trunks and branches; cut into fragments; distil and sublimate with steam; let cool to crystallise into "*Meihua bingpian*"(Plum Flower-like Borneol).

Description Colourless and transparent, or white and translucent crystals, polygonal and lamellar (like a thin plate), or granular. Brittle. Odour: fresh and fragrant; taste: acrid, fresh. Melt slowly when chewed. Volatile; when lit, produce bright flames and heavy fumes.

Indications 1. Impairment of consciousness 2. Sore throat, toothache, aphthous ulcer, otopyorrhoea, cervical erosion, skin infection (external use) 3. External oculopathy (external use).

Chemical Composition Borneol.

Note Also commercially sold as *Bingpian* are "*Aipian*"(Borneol from *Blumea balsamifera* DC. [Fam. Compositae]) and "*Jipian*" (Machine-Made Borneol), the latter being a synthetic.

Borneolum Syntheticum

Bulbus Allii Macrostemonis

Longstamen Onion Bulb
Xiebai

薤白

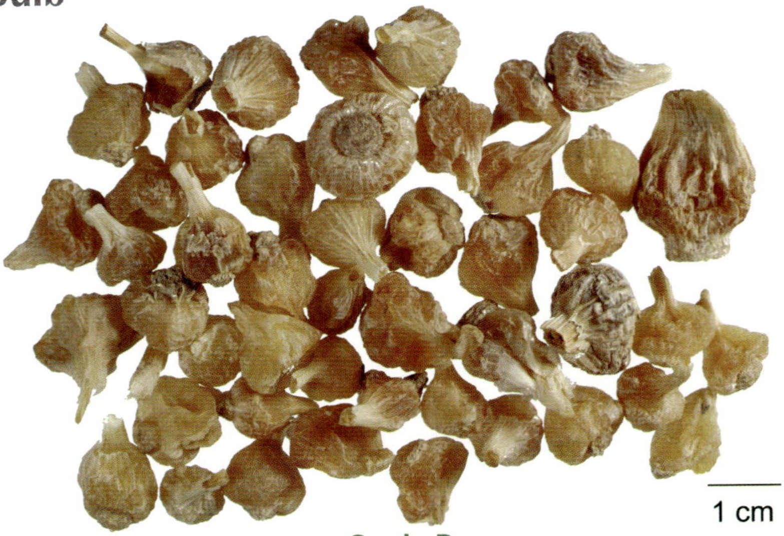

Crude Drug

Source The bulb of *Allium macrostemon* Bge. (Fam. Liliaceae).

Distribution Mainly in Chinese provinces such as Hebei, Jiangsu and Hubei, and in northeastern China.

Harvest & Processing Harvest bulbs in summer and autumn; wash clean; remove fibrous roots; steam thoroughly, or boil thoroughly in boiling water; dry under the sun.

Description Irregular and ovoid (egg-shaped); 0.5-1.5 cm thick, 0.5-1.8 cm in diameter. Outer surface yellowish-white or pale yellowish-brown, shrivelled, translucent, covered with off-white membranous scales; base marked with a protuberant plateau. Hard; cuticular. Odour: with a bad smell of garlic; taste: slightly sour.

Indications
1. Chest pain, cough and dyspnoea, abdominal distension
2. Dysentery with tenesmus.

Chemical Composition Mainly contains macrostemonosides A, D, E, F.

Note According to *C.P.*, also used for medicinal purposes is the bulb of *A. chinensis* G. Don.

Bulbus Fritillariae Cirrhosae

Tendrilleaf Fritillary Bulb
Chuanbeimu

川貝母

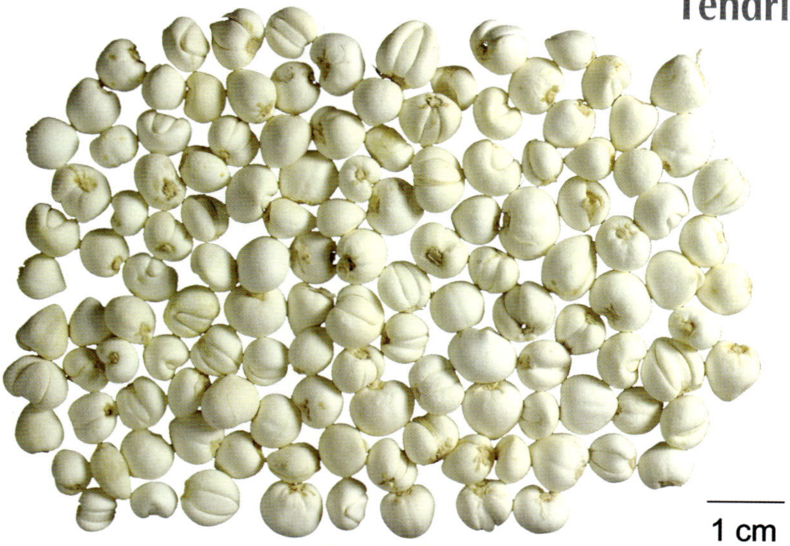

Crude Drug

Source The bulb of *Fritillaria cirrhosa* D.Don (Fam. Liliaceae).

Distribution Mainly in Chinese provinces such as Sichuan, and in Tibet, and Yunnan.

Harvest & Processing Dig up bulbs in summer and autumn, or when snow melts; remove foreign matter; dry under the sun or dry at low temperatures.

Description Subconical or subspherical; 3-8 mm tall, 3-9 mm in diameter. Outer surface off-white. Paired outer scale leaves, with one bigger than the other; the larger blade partially embracing the smaller one, with the unwrapped part crescent in shape. Top part tightly closed, encasing a subcylindrical central bud with relatively pointed apex and 1-2 scale leaflets. Apex obtuse or slightly pointed; base flat, slightly dented; core with 1 dull greyish-brown plateau; occasionally with remnants of fibrous roots. Hard and brittle; when broken, surface white and highly starchy. Odour: faint; taste: slightly bitter.

Indications 1. Cough with thick and yellowish sputum 2. Carbuncles

Chemical Composition Mainly contains a variety of steroidal alkaloids.

Note According to *C.P.*, also used as *Bulbus Fritillariae Cirrhosae* for medicinal purposes is the bulb of *F. unibracteata* Hsiao *et* K. C. Hsia, of *F. przewalskii* Maxim. and of *F. delavayi* Franch.

Bulbus Fritillariae Thunbergii

Thunberg Fritillary Bulb

Zhebeimu

浙貝母

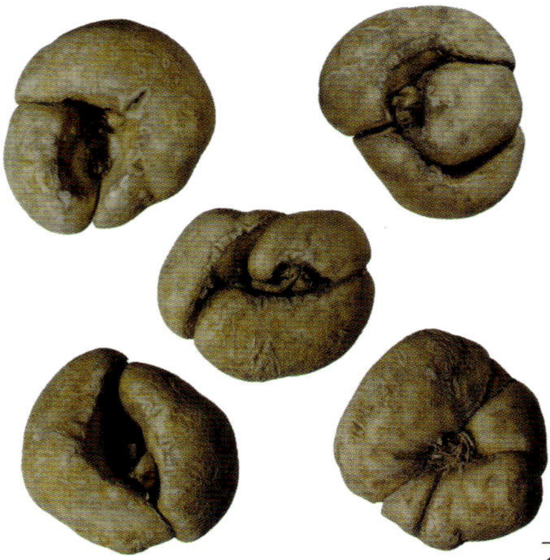
1 cm

Crude drug

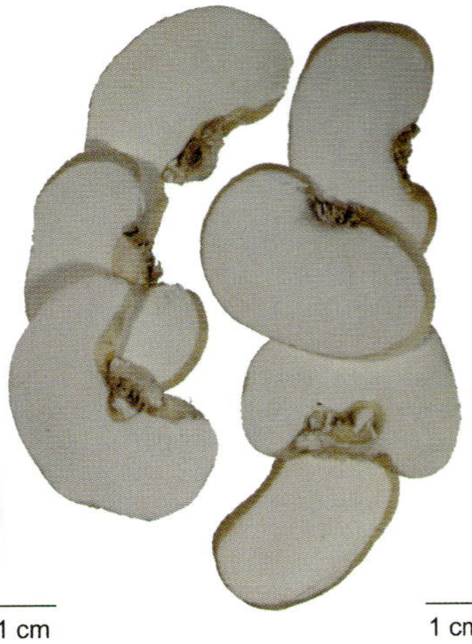
1 cm

Decoction Pieces

Bulbus Fritillariae Thunbergii

Source
The bulb of *Fritillaria thunbergii* Miq. (Fam. Liliaceae).

Distribution
Mainly in Chinese provinces such as Zhejiang; also in Jiangsu, Anhui and Hunan.

Harvest & Processing
Dig out bulbs in early summer when plants have withered. Classify according to size; those with central buds removed are processed to produce '*Zhubei*'(Pearl Thunberg Fritillary). Put bulbs collected in specially-made wooden barrels to shake off the bark; mix bulbs with calcined shell powder to absorb the pulp; dry under the sun or dry by heat. Alternatively, cut bulbs regardless of size; wash clean; remove central buds; cut into thick slices while fresh; wash clean again and dry to produce '*Zhebeipian*'(Thunberg Fritillary Slice).

Description
Zhubei is the whole bulb of Thunberg Fritillary. Flattened and spherical; 1-1.5 cm thick, 1-2.5 cm in diameter. Outer surface off-white; 2 scale leaves in outer layer, plump, slightly reniform (kidney-shaped), holding to each other and containing 2-3 small scale leaves and dried, shrivelled stem remnants. Hard and brittle, breaks easily; when broken, surface white to yellowish-white, highly starchy. Odour: faint; taste: bitter.

Indications
1. Cough with thick and yellowish sputum, lung abscess 2. Skin infection, subcutaneous nodule, scrofula, goiter.

Chemical Composition
Mainly contains steroidal alkaloids such as verticine and verticinone.

Bulbus Fritillariae Ussuriensis

Ussuri Fritillary Bulb
Pingbeimu

平貝母

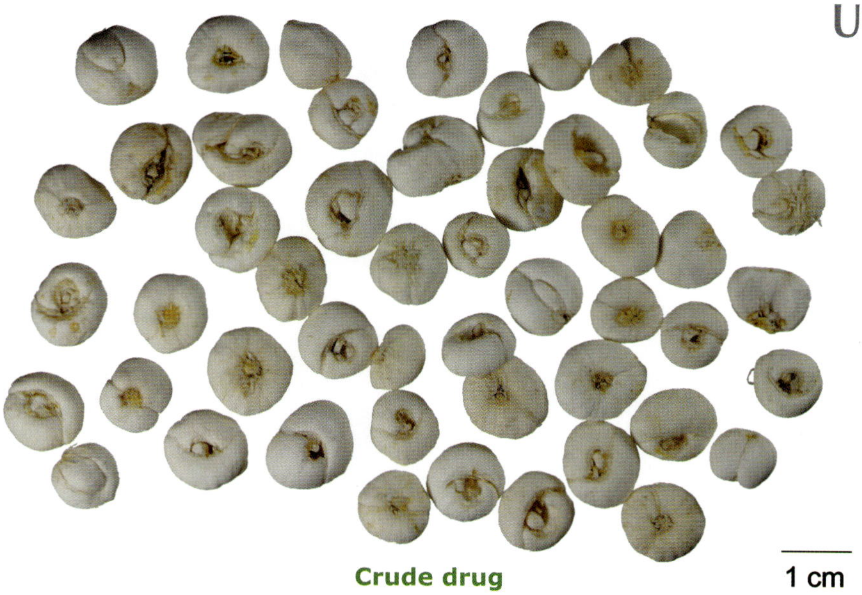

Crude drug

Source The bulb of *Fritillaria ussuriensis* Maxim. (Fam. Liliaceae).

Distribution Mainly in Chinese provinces such as Heilongjiang and Jilin.

Harvest & Processing Dig up bulbs of 3-4 year old in the early half of June when the above-ground parts wither; remove bark, fibrous roots, soil and sand; dry.

Description Disc-like; 0.5-1 cm thick, 0.8-2 cm in diameter. Outer surface milky-white or pale yellow. 2 scale leaves in the outer layer, plump, of about the same size or with one larger than the other, holding to each other; top end slightly flat or a little dented, often slightly acrocidal (split on top).The scale leaves in the centre small. Solid and brittle; broken surface starchy. Odour: faint; taste: bitter.

Indications Cough with yellowish sputum

Chemical Composition Mainly contains alkaloids such as pingbeimine A, B, C, and pingbeimine glucoside.

Bulbus Lilii

Lily Bulb
Baihe

百合

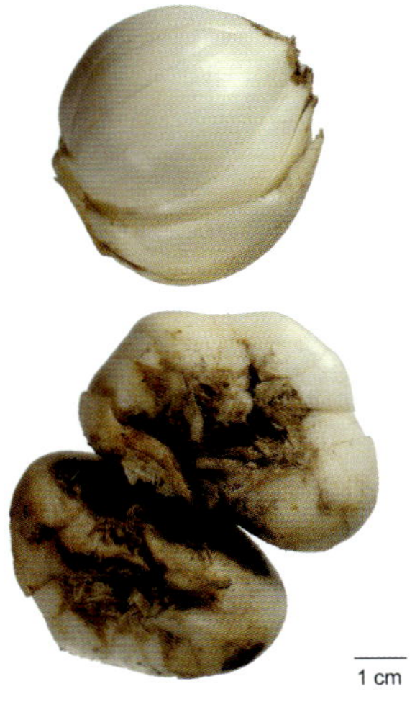

Crude Drug

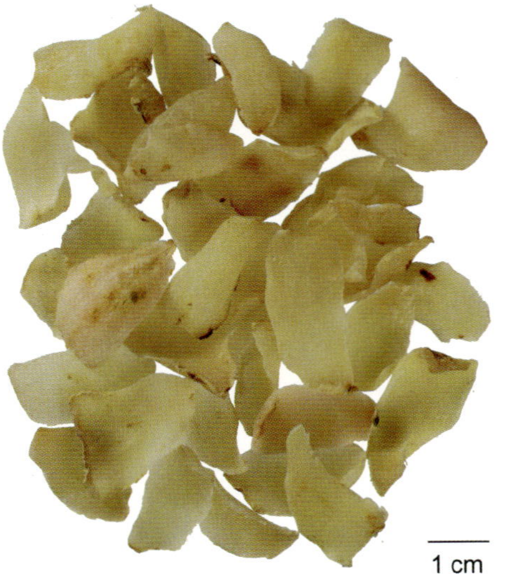

Decoction Pieces

Source The bulb of *Lilium brownii* F. E. Brown var. *viridulum* Baker (Fam. Liliaceae).

Distribution Mainly in Chinese provinces such as Hebei, Henan, Anhui, Jiangxi, Zhejiang, Hubei, Hunan and Shaanxi.

Harvest & Processing In the second year after transplantation, dig up bulbs in September and October after leaves wither; remove haulms and fibrous roots; reserve bulbules for seeding purpose; wash clean large bulbs; make a cross-section cut at the base; separate the scale leaves; boil in water for 5-10 minutes; when scale leaves soften at the edges and slightly crack in the back, scoop up immediately and put in fresh water to wash away the mucilage; spread thinly and dry under the sun or by heat.

Description Scale leaf oblong and elliptical. Apex pointed, base relatively wide; slightly undulate (wavy), involute (with the margins rolled inwards towards the upper side); 1.5-3 cm long, 0.5-1 cm wide, about 4 mm thick; with 3-5 venous (vein-like) striae, some indistinct. Outer surface white or pale yellow; smooth and translucent; hard and brittle, breaks easily; broken surface smooth, cuticular. Odourless; taste: slightly bitter.

Indications 1. Cough, haemoptysis 2. Irritability, insomnia, excessive dreams, palpitation, forgetfulness 3. Convalescence of febrile diseases

Chemical Composition Mainly contains glycosides such as regaloside A.

Note According to *C.P.*, also used for medicinal purposes is the bulb of *L. lancifolium* Thunb. and *L. pumilum* DC.

Bulbus Lycoridis Radiatae

Shorttube Lycoris Bulb

Shisuan

石蒜

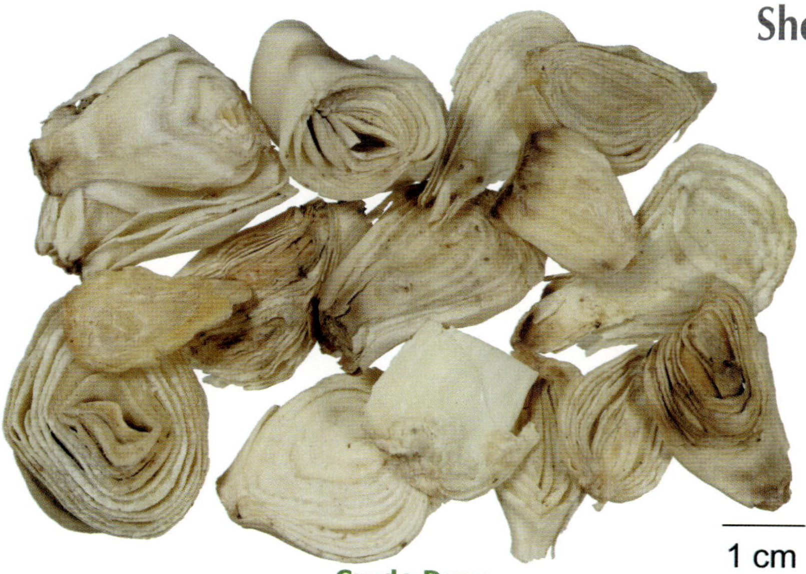

Crude Drug

Source The bulb of *Lycoris radiate* (L'Herit.) Herb. (Fam. Amaryllidaceae).

Distribution Mainly in regions south of the Yangtze River in China.

Harvest & Processing Dig out bulbs in autumn; wash clean larger ones and dry under the sun for medicinal purposes. For plants naturally grown, collect bulbs at season; use while fresh, or wash clean and dry under the sun.

Description Oval or subspherical; 4-5 cm long, 2.5-4 cm in diameter. Top end marked with remnants of leaf base about 3 cm long; base with numerous white fibrous roots. Bulb wrapped by 2-3 outer layers of dried, dull brown membranous scales and 10-20 inner layers of glutinous, white fleshy scales; yellowish-white buds sprouting from short, shrunken plateau. Commonly sold in the market in the form of length-wise cut or cross-cut slices. Odour: distinctive and slightly pungent; taste: extremely bitter.

Indications 1. Sore throat, tonsillitis, copious expectoration 2. Ascitis, hydrothorax, 3. Haemorrhoid 4. Scrofula, carbuncle, sores, tinea, burn and scald 5. Trauma, arthralgia, snakebite

Chemical Composition Mainly contains alkaloids.

Cacumen Platycladi

Chinese Arborvitae Twig and Leaf
Cebaiye

侧柏葉

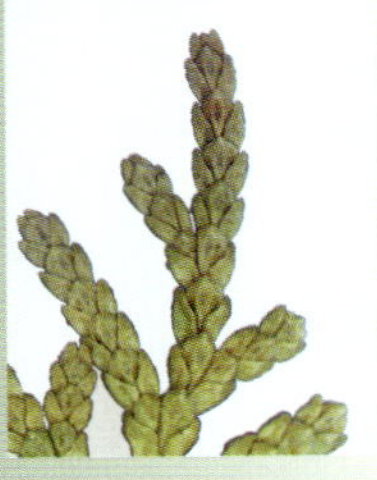

Chinese Arborvitae Twig and Leaf Magnified

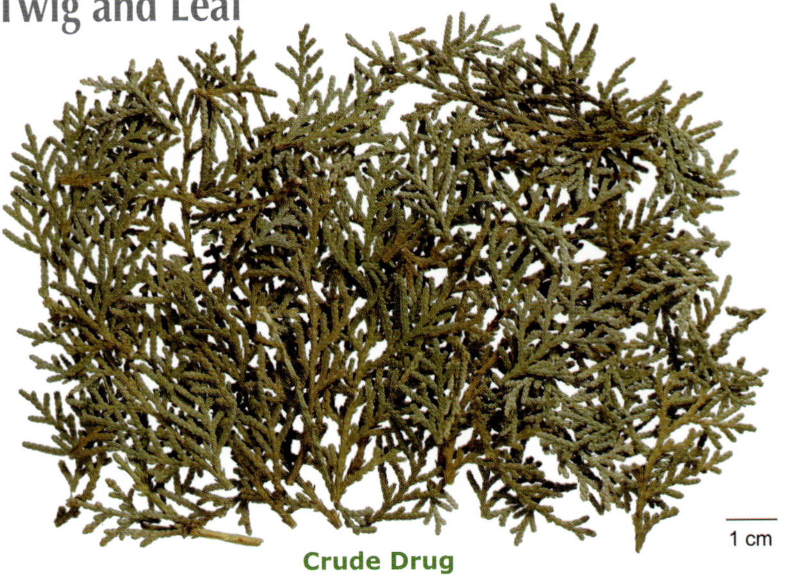

Crude Drug

Source The twig and leaf of *Platycladus orientalis* (L.) Franco (Fam. Cupressaceae).

Distribution In most regions of China, including Hong Kong.

Harvest & Processing Collect young branches and leaves anytime during the year, mostly in summer and autumn; dry in shaded areas.

Description Twig ramose (with many branches), flat; varying in length; pale reddish-brown. Leaves small, squamiform (scale-like). Apex obtuse. Leaves opposite (borne in pairs at each node), densely and closely attached to twigs; lateral leaves cariniform (keel-shaped), covering the middle leaves. All leaves dark green or yellowish-green. Twig brittle; breaks easily; when broken, surface yellowish-white. Odour: fresh and fragrant; taste: bitter-astringent, slightly acrid.

Indications 1. Haematemesis, epistaxis, gastrointestinal bleeding, haematuria, dysfunctional uterine bleeding 2. Chronic bronchitis 3. Alopecia, baldness.

Chemical Composition Mainly contains essential oils such as α-thujone,and flavonoids such as quercitrin.

Note Can be prepared for medicinal purposes by carbonizing.

Cacumen Tamaricis

Chinese Tamarisk Twig
Xiheliu

西河柳

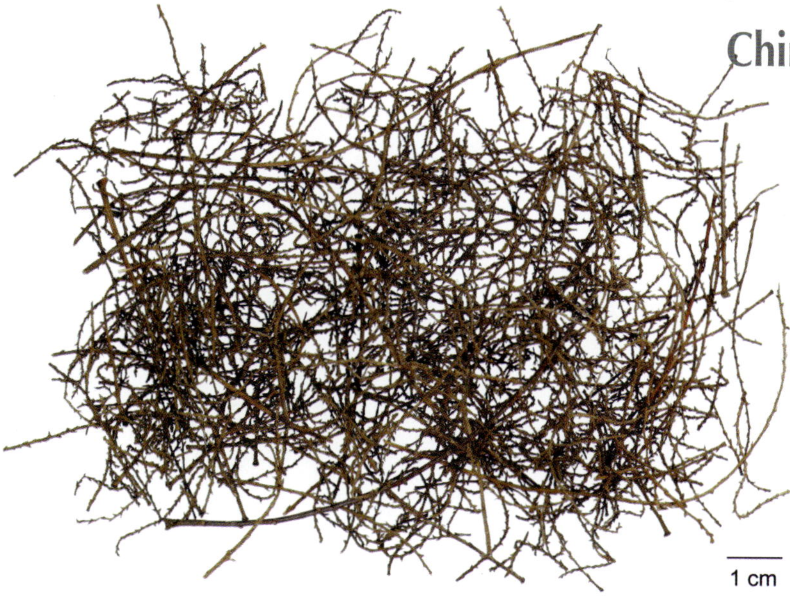

Crude Drug

Source The young twig and leaf of *Tamarix chinensis* Lour. (Fam. Tamaricaceae).

Distribution In most regions of China, including Hong Kong.

Harvest & Processing Collect young twigs before efflorescence; dry in shaded areas.

Description Twig cylindrical in shape. Young twigs slender; 0.5-1 mm in diameter, length uneven; outer surface greyish-green or yellowish-green; brittle, break easily. Leaves alternate (borne singly at each node); blades small and squamiform (scale-like), ovate (egg-shaped in outline and attached at the broad end) and triangular. Apex pointed, base accrete (grown or joined together). Outer surface of thick twigs yellowish-brown or reddish-brown; leaves often fall off, leaving remnants of protuberant leaf base; thick twigs break easily; when broken, surface even, yellowish-white, with pith in the centre. Odour: faint; taste: mild.

Indications 1. Measles and other eruptive exanthem 2. Arthralgia

Chemical Composition Mainly contains tamarixinol, tamarixone and tamarixol.

Cacumen Tamaricis

Carpophorum Calvatial Lilacinae

Lilactic Puffball

Mabo

馬勃

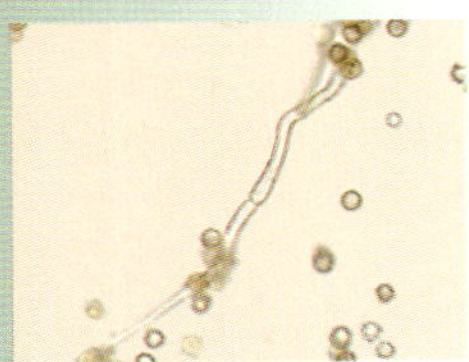

Lilactic Puffball Magnified

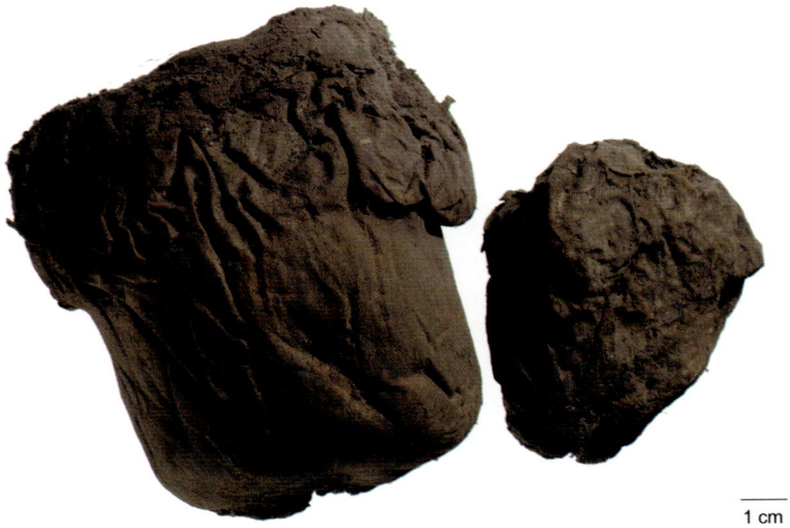

Crude Drug

Source: The sporophore of *Calvatia lilacina* (Mont. et Berk.) Lloyd (Fam. Lycoperdaceae).

Distribution: Mainly in Chinese provinces such as Jilin, Liaoning, Hebei, Shandong and Qinghai, and in Xinjiang.

Harvest & Processing: Harvest fruiting bodies promptly at maturation in summer and autumn; remove sand and soil; dry under the sun.

Description: Sporophore flattened and spherical when intact, cupulate (cup-shaped) when broken; 5-12 cm in diameter; sterile base well-developed, stipitate (with a stalk). Exoperidium thin, dull purplish-brown, with heavy wrinkles and orbicular (round) indentations; purple spore clusters exposed when upper part of exoperidium falls off. Light in weight; elastic; when twiddled with fingers, spores burst into the air in abundance. Spores visible under a microscope. Odour: faint; taste: mild.

Indications: 1. Sore throat, cough, aphronia. External use for traumatic bleeding, skin ulcer and frostbite.

Chemical Composition: Mainly contains calvatic acid.

Note: According to *C.P.*, also used for medicinal purposes is the sporophore of *Calvatia gigantea* (Batsch ex Pers.) Lloyd and *Lasiosphaera fenzlii* Reich., both of which belong to the same family as *Calvatia lilacina* (Mont. et Berk.) Lloyd.

Caulis Akebiae Quinatae

Akebia Stem
Mutong
木通

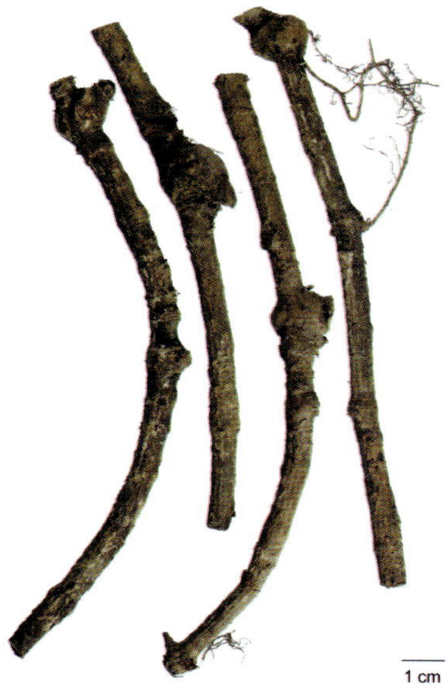

Crode drug

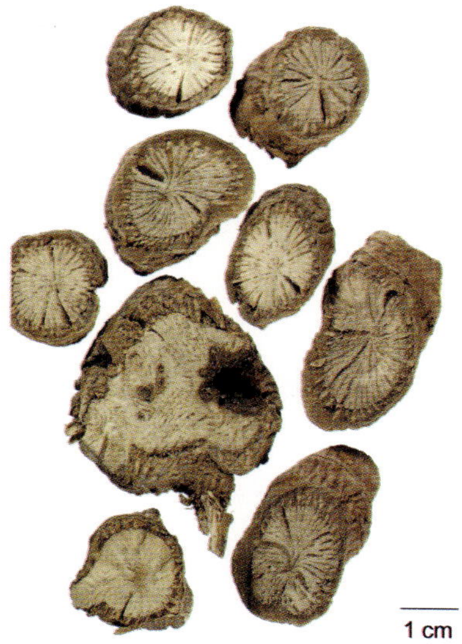

Decoction Pieces

Source Mainly the vine of *Akebia trifoliate* (Thunb.) Koidz. *var. australis* (Diels) Rehd. (Fam. Lardizabalaceae).

Distribution Mainly in southwestern and eastern China.

Harvest & Processing Cut off old vines in autumn and winter 5-6 years after transplantation and when plants start to bear fruits; dry the vines under the sun or by heat.

Description Cylindrical, slightly twisted; 2-5 mm in diameter. Outer surface greyish-brown, marked with shallow longitudinal grooves; lenticels protuberant, orbicular (round), or transverse, oblong and orbicular, around 1 mm in diameter; marked also with branch scars. Hard and brittle, breaks quite easily; when broken transversely, surface relatively smooth; cortex thin, reddish-brown; xylem greyish-white; vessel pores arranged densely and irregularly; rays narrow and indistinct; central pith orbicular and conspicuous. Odour: faint; taste: mild and slightly acrid.

Indications 1. Oedema and dysuria 2. Aphthous ulcer, irritability, insomnia and oliguria with reddish urine 3. Amenorrhoea, galactostasis 4. Arthralgia, joint stiffness

Chemical Composition Mainly contains triterpene saponins such as akeboside Sta, St Stc.

Caulis Bambusae in Taeniam

Bamboo Shavings
Zhuru

竹茹

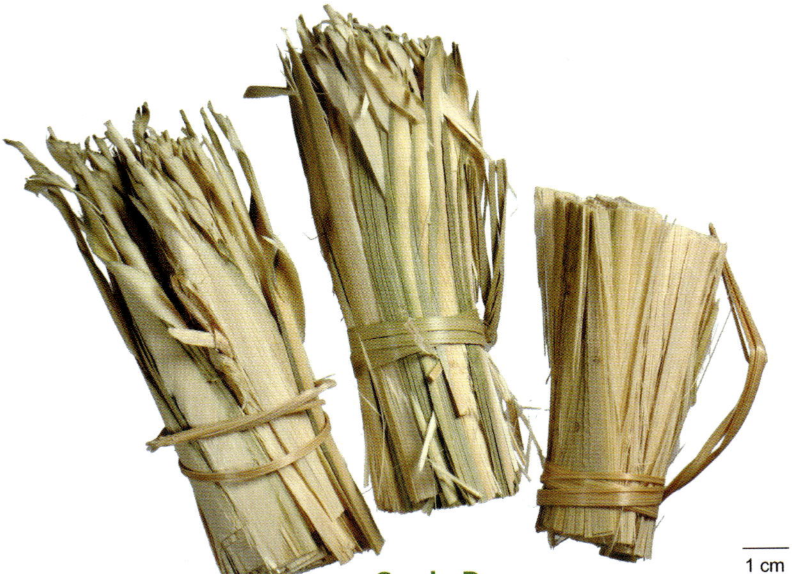

Crude Drug

Source — The shavings of the stems of *Bambusa tuldoides* Munro (Fam. Gramineae).

Distribution — Mainly in Chinese provinces such as Shandong, Jiangsu, Anhui, Zhejiang, Jiangxi, Henan, Hunan and Hubei.

Harvest & Processing — In winter, cut the new bamboo stems grown during the year; remove branches and leaves; saw stems into sections; scrape off green bark; scrape middle layer into shavings.

Description — Irregular, filiform (thread-like) or taenioid (ribbon-like), often rolled up and interwoven into balls, or in the form of wood shavings; varying in length, 5-7 mm wide, 3-5 mm thick. Colour of shavings: pale yellowish-white, light green, greenish-yellow, dull yellowish-green, yellowish-green or golden-yellow; outer surface rough, marked with fine longitudinal striae. Broken surface highly fibrous. Light in weight; pliable and elastic. Odour: slightly fresh and fragrant; taste: slightly sweet.

Indications — 1. Cough with thick and yellow sputum 2.Vexation, feeling of oppression in the chest, insomnia, palpitation 3.Vomiting, bitter taste in the mouth 4. Bleeding

Chemical Composition — Contains 2, 5-dimethoxy-p-benzoquinone, p-hydroxybenzaldehyde and syringaldehyde.

Note — According to *C.P.*, also used for medicinal purposes are the shavings of the stems of *Phyllostachys nigra* (Lodd. ex Lindl.) Munro var. *henonis* (Mitf.) Stapf et Rendle and *Sinocalamus beecheyanus* (Munro) McClure var. *pubescens* P. F. Li, both of which belong to the same family as *Bambusa tuldoides* Munro.

Caulis Clematidis Armandii

Armand Clematis Stem
Chuanmutong
川木通

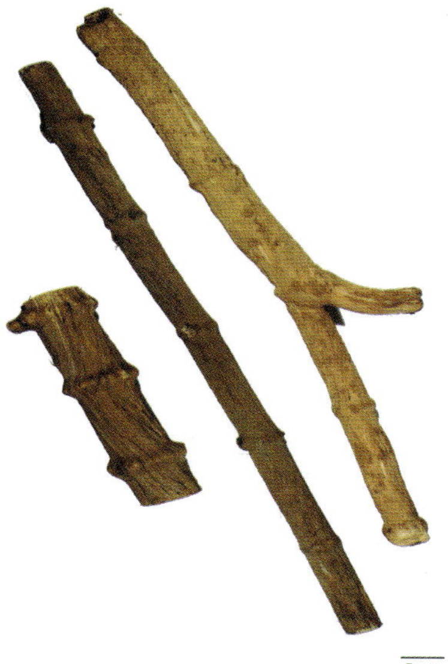

Crude Drug

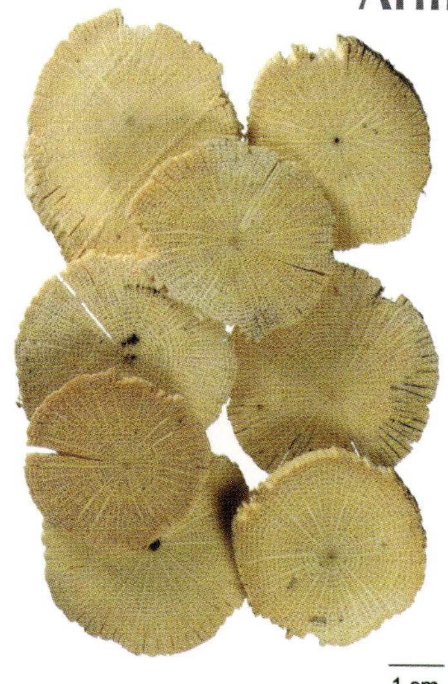

Decoction Pieces

Source The vine of *Clematis armandii* Franch. (Fam. Ranunculaceae).

Distribution Mainly in Chinese provinces such as Sichuan, Hunan, Shaanxi, Guizhou and Hubei.

Harvest & Processing Collect vines in spring and autumn; remove cork; dry under the sun, or slice into thin pieces while fresh and then dry under the sun.

Description Long and cylindrical, slightly twisted; 3.5-6.5 cm in diameter. Outer surface yellowish-brown or dull yellowish-brown, marked with longitudinal grooves and ridges; nodes bulgy; cortex remnants easily torn off. Hard, does not break easily. When sliced, margin irregular; cortex remnants yellowish-brown; xylem light brown and broad, densely poriferous (with numerous pores), marked with radial yellowish-white striae and cracks; occasionally hollow in the centre. Odourless; taste: mild.

Indications 1. Oedema and dysuria 2. Aphthous ulcer, irritability, insomnia and oliguria with reddish urine 3. Amenorrhoea, galactostasis 4. Arthralgia, joint stiffness

Chemical Composition Mainly contains triterpene saponins.

Note According to *C.P.*, also used for medicinal purposes is the vine of *C. montana* Buch. -Ham.*ex* DC.

Caulis Entadae

Entadae Stem
Guojianglong
過江龍

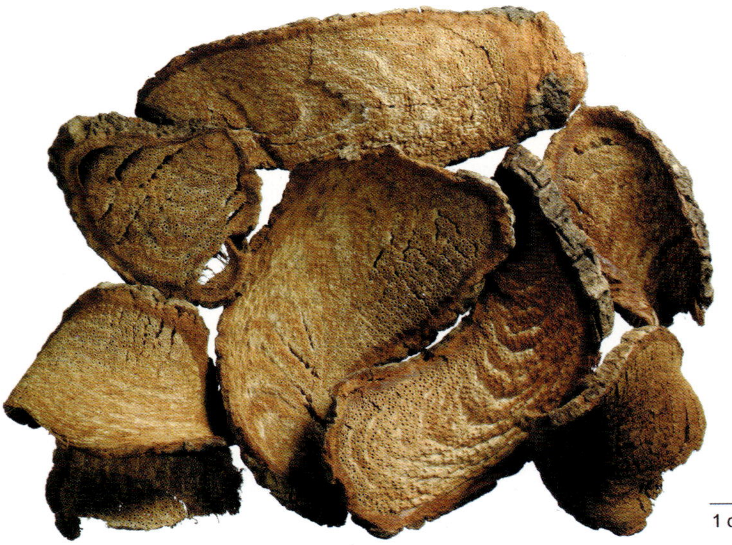

Decoction Pieces

Source The vine of *Entada phaseoloides* (L.) Merr. (Fam. Leguminosae).

Distribution Mainly in Chinese provinces such as Fujian, Guangdong, Hainan, Guangxi and Yunnan; also in Hong Kong.

Harvest & Processing Harvest vines anytime during the year; cut into slices; dry under the sun or use while fresh.

Description Slices of vine irregular in shape and size; 1-2 cm thick. Bark reddish-brown or greyish-brown; rough; marked with lichen markings, conspicuous longitudinal striae or grooves, scars of lateral branches, punctiform (dot-like) lenticels, and often with 1 protuberant ridge. Cut surface shows dark brown cortex with reddish-brown or brownish-black resinoid (resin-like) substance; xylem brown or light brown, poriferous (with numerous pores); pith encircled by reddish-brown resinoid substance arranged in eccentric annulations, and usually with small hollows concentrated on the side with the ridge. Hard, do not break easily. Odour: faint; taste: slightly astringent.

Indications 1. Rheumatism, trauma 2. Lumbar strain, numbness of the extremities

Chemical Composition Bark mainly contains entada saponins II, III, IV.

Caulis Erycibes

Obtuseleaf Erycibe Stem

Dinggongteng

丁公藤

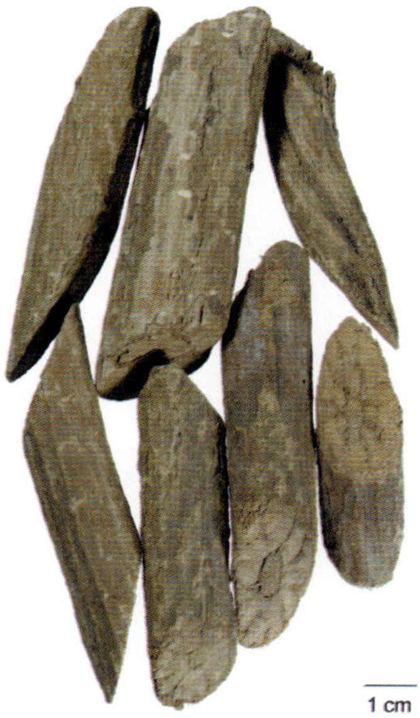

Crude Drug

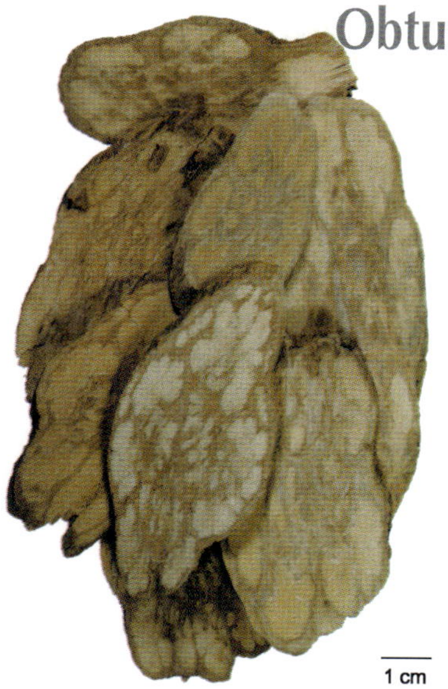

Decoction Pieces

Source The vine of *Erycibe obtusfolia* Benth. (Fam. Convolvulaceae).

Distribution Mainly in central Guangdong and on the offshore islands of China; also in Hong Kong.

Harvest & Processing Harvest vines anytime during the year; cut into sections or slices; dry under the sun.

Description Cylindrical. Outer surface of thick stems greyish-yellow, dull brown or reddish-brown, rough, marked with irregular, dense longitudinal cracks; lenticels numerous, distributed unevenly, yellowish-white, punctiform (dot-like) or verruciform (wart-like), protuberant. Commonly sold in the form of slant-cut sections or slices. Cut surface of thick stems greyish-yellow or pale yellow, with thin cortex and broad xylem; marked with anomalous vascular bundles arranged in several annulations or irregular patterns; xylem of each vascular bundle yellowish-white, slightly protruding, densely packed with vascular pores; pith small, in some cases eccentric. Hard, does not break easily. Odour: faint; taste: mild.

Indications 1. Arthralgia, lumbago and pain of lower extremities, trauma, 2. Abdominal pain 3. Primary glaucoma (external use as eyedrops).

Chemical Composition Mainly contains baogonteng A, scopoletin and scopolin.

Note According to *C.P.*, also used for medicinal purposes and listed as slightly toxic is the vine of *E. schmidtii* Craib.

Caulis et Folium Piperis Hancei

Hance Pepper Stem and Leaf

Shanju

山蒟

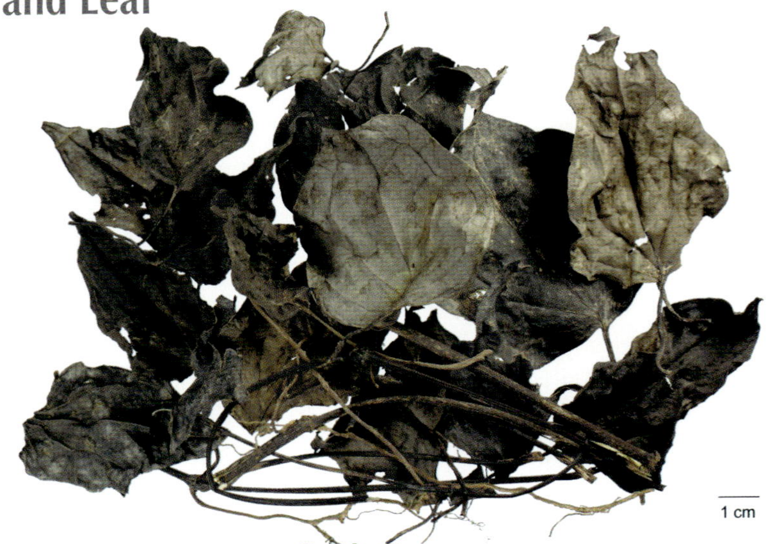

Crude Drug

Source The stem and leaf of *Piper hancei* Maxim. (Fam. Piperaceae).

Distribution Mainly in Chinese provinces such as Fujian, Zhejiang, Jiangxi, Hunan, Guangdong and Hainan; also in Hong Kong.

Harvest & Processing Collect stems and leaves in autumn; cut into segments; use while fresh or dry under the sun.

Description Stem cylindrical and slender; 1-3 mm in diameter; outer surface dull greyish-brown, marked with fine longitudinal striae; nodes bulgy, with adventitious roots; internodes 2-10 cm long; brittle, breaks easily; when broken, surface shows dull greyish-brown cortex and poriferous (with numerous holes) greyish-white xylem. Leaves mostly shrivelled, with some in fragments; when whole and smoothed out, blades narrow and elliptical, or ovate (egg-shaped in outline and attached at the broad end) and lanceolate (lance-head shaped); 4-12 cm long, 2-5 cm wide. Apex acuminate (tapering to a slender point), base somewhat cuneate (wedge-shaped) , often oblique (with unequal sides); upper surface dark green, underside greyish-green. Brittle. Odour: fresh and fragrant; taste: pungent.

Indications 1. Rheumatism 2. Stomachache, dysmenorrhoea, hernia pain 3. Trauma 4. Cough and dyspnoea

Chemical Composition Mainly contains kadsurenone, denudatin B and hancinone.

Caulis Lonicerae

Honeysuckle Stem
Rendongteng

忍冬藤

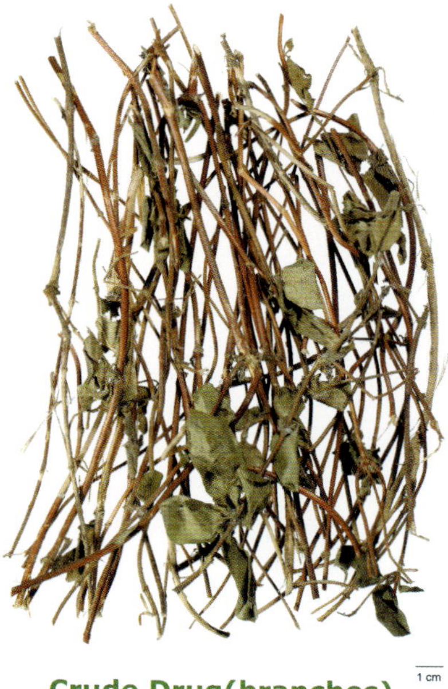

Crude Drug(branches)

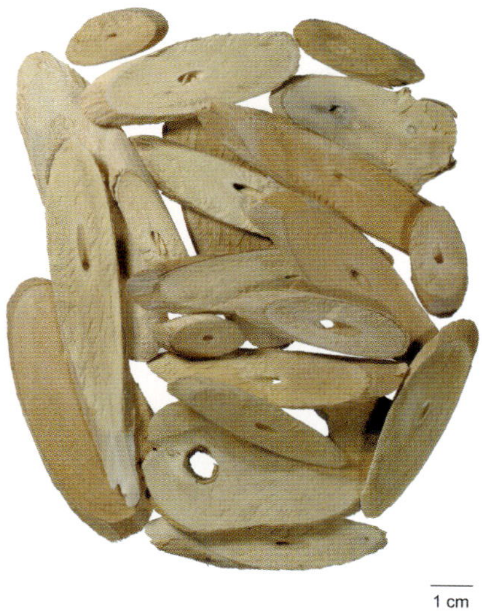

Decoction Pieces(stems)

Source The twig of *Lonicera japonica* Thunb. (Fam. Caprifoliaceae).

Distribution Mainly in Chinese provinces such as Zhejiang, Sichuan, Jiangsu, Henan, Shandong and Guangxi; also in Hong Kong.

Harvest & Processing Cut off stems and branches in autumn and winter; remove foreign matter; tie stems and branches into bundles or roll into heaps; dry under the sun.

Description Often tied into bundles or rolled into heaps; stems long and cylindrical; ramose (with many branches); with remnants and leaf scars. Outer surface brownish-red or dull red, marked with fine longitudinal striae; old branches glabrous (without hairs), young branches covered with pale yellow pubescence; bark easily peels off, exposing greyish-white cortex. Hard and brittle, breaks easily; when broken, surface yellowish-white, with a cavity in the centre. Odour: faint; taste: old branches slightly bitter, young branches mild.

Indications 1. Epidermic febrile diseases, acute dysentery 2. Carbuncles and sores 3. Arthritis

Chemical Composition Contains chlorogenic acid, iridoids and triterpene saponins.

Caulis Perillae

Perilla Stem
Zisugeng

紫蘇梗

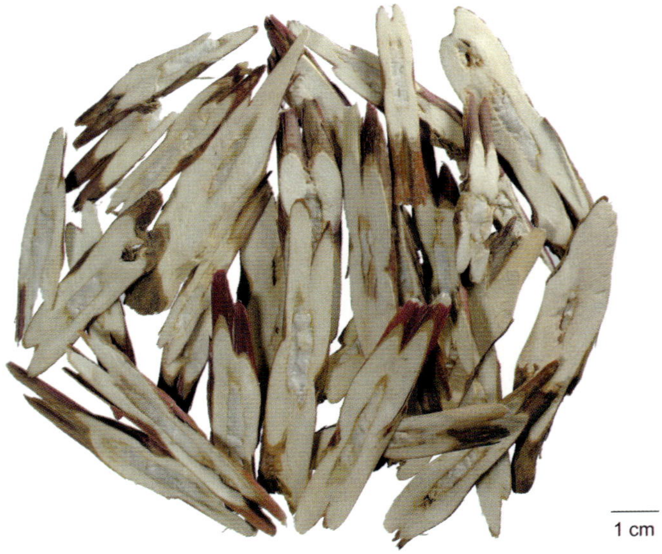

Decoction Pieces

Source The stem of *Perilla frutescens* (L.) Britt. (Fam. Labiatae).

Distribution Mainly in Chinese provinces such as Jiangsu, Hubei, Henan, Zhejiang, Shandong and Sichuan; also in Hong Kong.

Harvest & Processing Cut off above-ground parts in late autumn; remove branchlets, leaf blades and fruits; dry stems under the sun.

Description Quadrangular (four-angled), edges obtuse; varying in length, 0.5-1.5 cm in diameter. Outer surface purplish-brown or dull purple; with longitudinal grooves and fine longitudinal striae on all sides; nodes slightly bulgy, with opposite scars of branchlets and leaves. Light in weight; hard and brittle; broken surface lobate (divided into lobes). Slices 2-5 mm thick, often in the form of slanted oblong cubes; xylem yellowish-white, with fine and dense radial rays; pith white, porous or detached from xylem to form a hollow. Odour: fragrant; taste: mild.

Indications

1. Feeling of oppression in the chest, abdominal distension
2. Morning sickness, threatened abortion

Chemical Composition Perillaketone and egomaketone exist in the upper part.

Caulis Piperis Kadsurae

Kadsura Pepper Stem
Haifengteng

海風藤

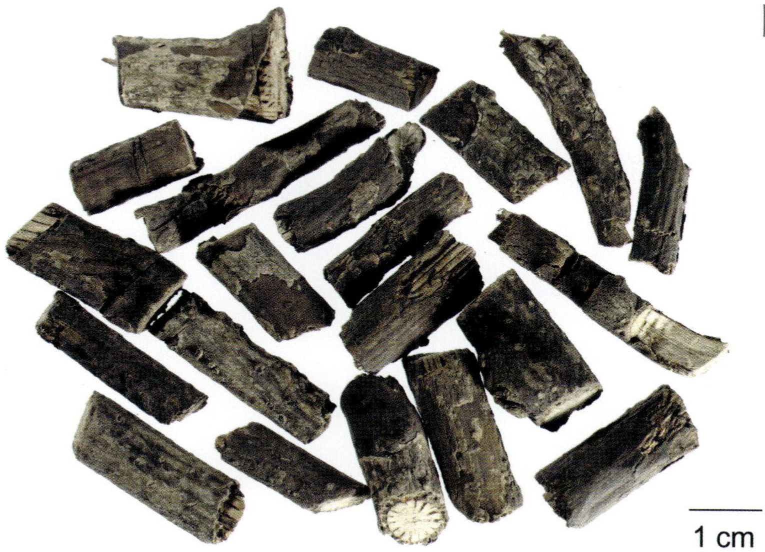

Crude Drug

Source The vine of *Piper kadsura* (Choisy) Ohwi (Fam. Piperaceae).

Distribution Mainly in Chinese provinces such as Fujian, Zhejiang, Guangdong and Taiwan.

Harvest & Processing Cut off vines in summer and autumn; remove roots and leaves; dry under the sun.

Description Flattened and cylindrical, slightly curved; 0.3-2 cm in diameter. Outer surface dull greyish-brown, marked with longitudinal ridges and nodes; internodes 3-12 cm long, nodes bulgy. Light in weight; brittle, breaks easily. When broken, surface uneven; cortex narrow; xylem broad; greyish-yellow xylem and greyish-white rays arranged in a radial form; clefts often found between cortex and xylem; pith in the centre, dull greyish-brown. Odour: fragrant; taste: slightly bitter, acrid.

Indications 1. Rheumatism, arthralgia, stiffness of joints, muscular spasm 2. Cough, dyspnoea, chronic cough

Chemical Composition Mainly contains lignans such as kadsurenin A, B, C.

Caulis Polygoni Multiflori

Tuber Fleeceflower Stem

Shouwuteng

首烏藤

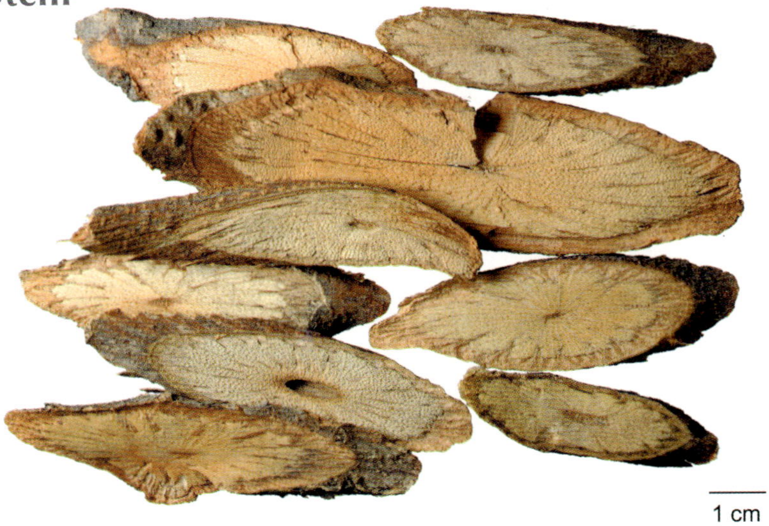

Decoction Pieces

Source The vine of Polygonum multiflorum Thunb. (Fam. Polygonaceae).

Distribution Mainly in Chinese provinces such as Zhejiang, Hubei, Jiangsu and Henan; also in Hong Kong.

Harvest & Processing Cut off vines in autumn and winter; remove leaf remnants; tie up in bundles; dry under the sun or by heat.

Description Long and cylindrical, slightly twisted; varying in length, 3-7 mm in diameter. Outer surface brownish-red or reddish-brown; rough; marked with conspicuous twisting longitudinal wrinkles and small orbicular (round) lenticels. Nodes slightly bulgy, marked with branch scars. Bark thin; peeled off Brittle, breaks easily; when broken, cortex brownish-red; xylem pale yellow; vessel pores conspicuous; pith in the centre white and porous. Odourless; taste: slightly bitter-astringent.

Indications 1. Vexation, insomnia, excessive dreams, insanity and mania 2. Rheumatism 3. Urticaria (external use).

Chemical Composition Mainly contains emodin and physcion.

Caulis Sargentodoxae

Sargentgloryvine Stem

Daxueteng

大血藤

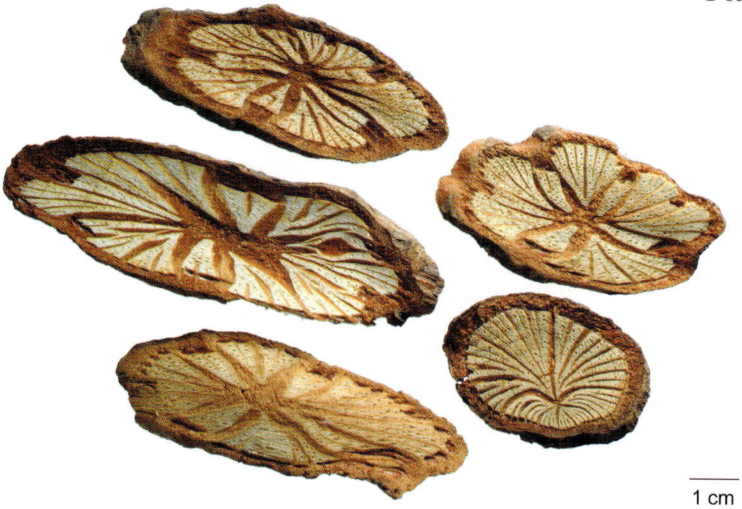

Decoction Pieces

Source The vine of *Sargentodoxa cuneata* (Oliv.) Rehd. et Wils. (Fam. Lardizabalaceae).

Distribution Mainly in Chinese provinces such as Hubei, Sichuan, Jiangxi and Henan.

Harvest & Processing Collect vines in autumn and winter; remove branchlets and leaves; cut into sections or thick slices; dry under the sun.

Description Cylindrical and slightly curved; 1-3 cm in diameter. Outer surface greyish-brown, rough, marked with shallow longitudinal grooves, conspicuous transverse cracks and verruciform (wart-shaped) protuberances; cork would sometimes scale off, exposing dull reddish-brown cortex. Hard; light in weight; breaks easily. When broken, surface shows annular (ring-like) reddish-brown cortex, parts of which extend into the xylem; xylem yellowish-white, poriferous (with numerous pores), with radial reddish-brown striae. Odour: faint; taste: slightly astringent. Commonly used in Hong Kong in the form of angled-cut slices.

Indications 1. Amenorrhoea, dysmenorrhea 2. Appendicitis 3. Rheumatic arthralgia 4. Post traumatic swelling and pain

Chemical Composition Mainly contains emodin, physcion, salidroside and protocatechuic acid.

Note Customarily called '*Jixueteng*' (Suberect Spatholobus Stem) in Hong Kong.

Caulis Sinomenii

Orientvine Stem
Qingfengteng

青風藤

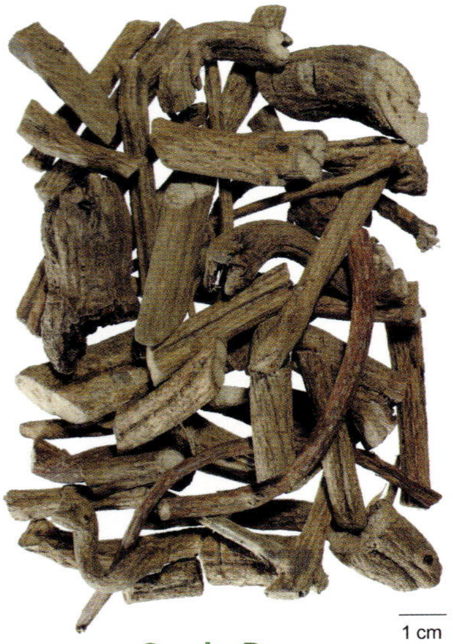

1 cm

Crude Drug

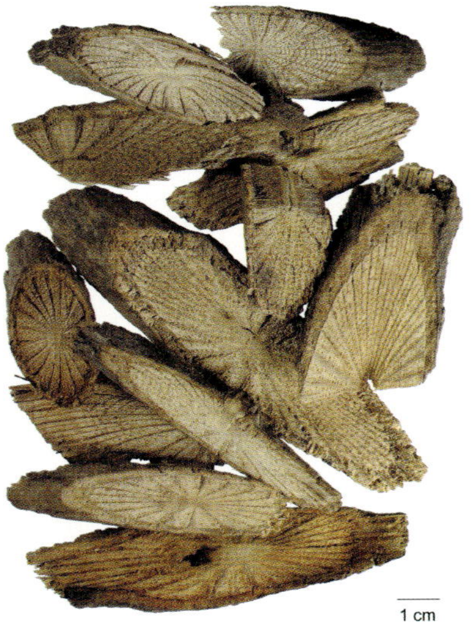

1 cm

Decoction Pieces

Source The vine of *Sinomenium acutum* (Thunb.) Rehd. et Wils. (Fam. Menispermaceae).

Distribution Mainly in southwestern, southern and eastern China.

Harvest & Processing Harvest vines in June and July; remove branchlets and leaves; dry vines under the sun, or soak thoroughly in water; cut into sections and then dry under the sun.

Description Long and cylindrical, slightly curved; 20-70 cm long, 0.5-2 cm in diameter. Thin stems intertwined in bundles; outer surface brownish-green to greyish-brown, marked with longitudinal wrinkles, fine transverse cracks and lenticels; nodes slightly bulgy, with protuberant branch scars or leaf scars. Brittle and fairly hard, breaks rather easily; when broken, surface reveals lobate (lobe-like), greyish-brown xylem. Thick stem hard; broken surface brown; xylem marked with numerous pores and radial striae customarily called 'wheel-spoke lines', small yellowish-white pith at the centre. Odour: faint; taste: slightly bitter.

Indications 1. Rheumatism, rheumatoid arthritis 2. Oedema 3. Hypertension

Chemical Composition Mainly contains a variety of alkaloids, such as sinoacutine and magnoflorine.

Note According to *C.P.*, also used for medicinal purposes is the vine of *S. acutum* (Thunb.) Rehd. et Wils. var. *cinereum* Rehd. et Wils.

Caulis Spatholobi

Suberect Spatholobus Stem

Jixueteng

雞血藤

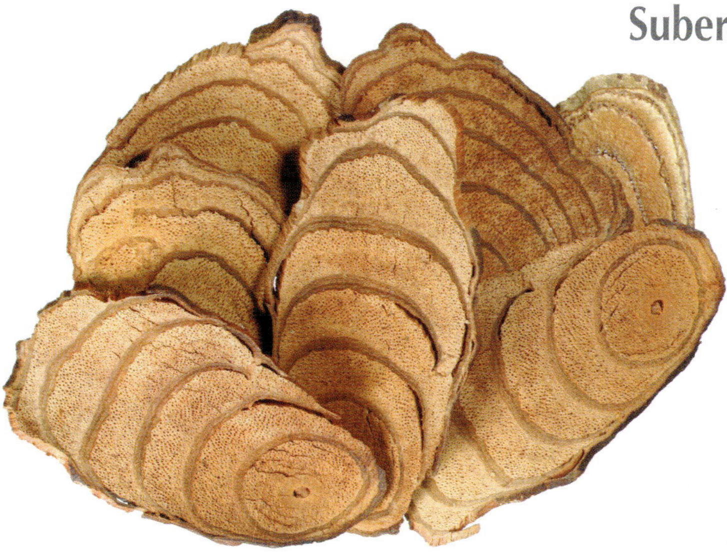

Decoction Pieces

Source The vine of *Spatholobus suberectus* Dunn (Fam. Leguminosae).

Distribution Mainly in Chinese provinces such as Guangdong, Guangxi and Yunnan.

Harvest & Processing Collect vines in autumn and winter; remove branches and leaves; cut into slices or sections; dry under the sun.

Description Flattened and cylindrical. Outer surface greyish-brown, or reddish-brown where cork has fallen off; marked with longitudinal grooves. Cross-section shows pale red xylem with small, irregularly arranged pores; inner side of cortex with dull reddish-brown or blackish-brown resinoid (resin-like) secretion; cortex alternating with xylem, forming eccentric (not positioned directly on the central axis), semi-circular rings; pith small, slanting towards one side. Hard and solid, difficult to break; when broken, surface irregular and lobate (lobe-like). Odour: faint; taste: astringent.

Indications 1. Amenorrhoea, dysmenorrhoea, menstrual disorders
2. Soreness, numbness and stiffness of extremities. 3. Leukopenia

Chemical Composition Mainly contains flavonoids such as formononetin and prunetin.

Caulis Trachelospermi

Chinese Starjasmine Stem
Luoshiteng

絡石藤

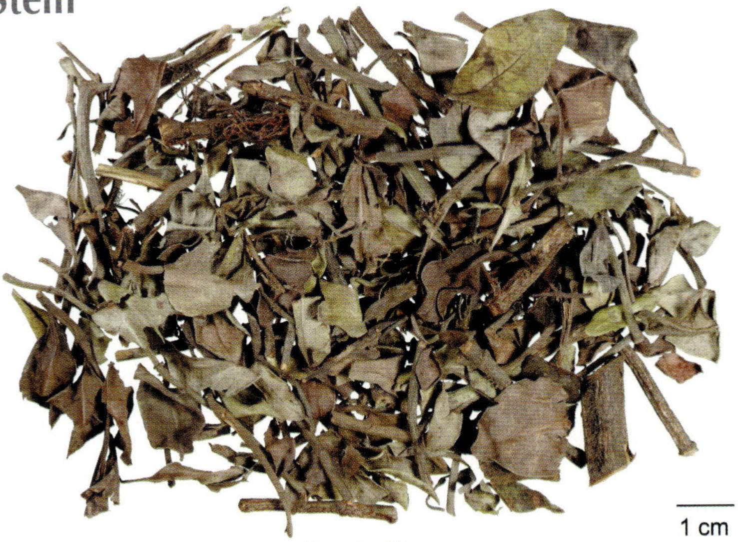

1 cm

Crude Drug

Source The leaf-bearing vine of *Trachelospermum jasminoides* (Lindl.) Lem. (Fam. Apocynaceae).

Distribution Mainly in eastern, northern and southern China; also in Hong Kong.

Harvest & Processing Cut off leaf-bearing vines from winter to the following spring; remove foreign matter; dry under the sun.

Description Cylindrical and slightly curved, ramose (with many branches); varying in length; 1-5 mm in diameter. Outer surface dull reddish-brown or greyish-brown, with small, protuberant, punctiform (dot-like) lenticels and adventitious roots. Hard; when broken, surface pale yellowish-white, often hollow in the centre. Leaves opposite (borne in pairs at each node), with short petioles; when smoothed out, blades elliptical, or ovate (egg-shaped in outline and attached at the broad end) and lanceolate (lance-head shaped); 1-8 cm long, 0.7-3.5 cm wide; entire (with continuous, even margin); slightly recurved (curved backwards); upper surface dull green or brownish-green, underside paler in colour; coriaceous (leathery). Odour: faint; taste: slightly bitter.

Indications 1. Rheumatism, muscular spasm and trauma 2. Skin infection and pharyngitis

Chemical Composition Mainly contains arctiin and tracheloside.

Concretio Silicea Bambusae

Tabasheer
Tianzhuhuang
天竺黄

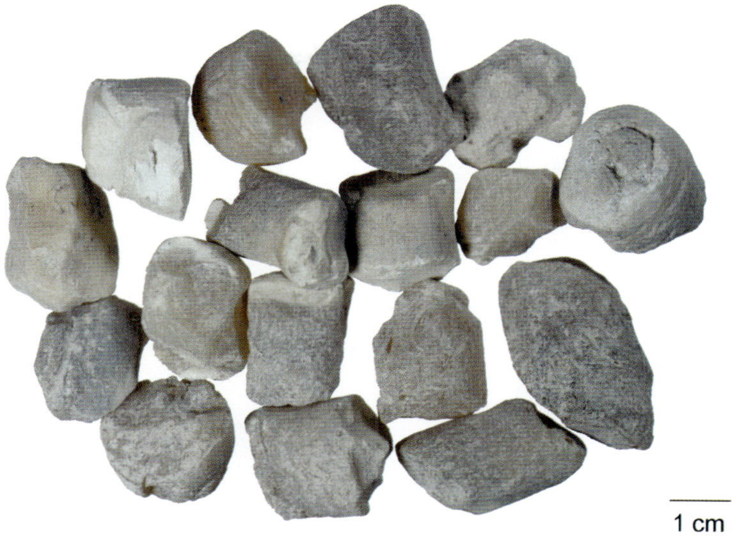

Crude Drug

Source The secretion in the stems of *Bambusa textilis* McClure (Fam. Gramineae).

Distribution Mainly in Chinese provinces such as Yunnan, Guangdong and Guangxi.

Harvest & Processing Chop off bamboo stems in autumn and winter; cut open to get lumps of secretion; dry lumps by airing.

Description Irregular flakes or granules; varying in size. Outer surface greyish-blue, greyish-yellow or greyish-white, in some cases pure white and translucent, in some other cases ivory-coloured and slightly lustrous; surface often covered with powder. Light in weight; hard and brittle, breaks easily; when broken, surface greyish-white, highly hygroscopic (water-absorbent). Odourless; taste: mild, sticky when licked. Produce bubbles when immersed in water, with those pieces ivory in colour gradually turning pale green or sky blue.

Indications 1. Impairment of consciousness in febrile disease 2. Stroke 3. Infantile convulsion and frequent night crying of infants.

Chemical Composition Mainly contains polysaccharides, mannitol and several types of amino acids.

Note According to *C.P.*, also used for medicinal purposes are the lumps of secretion from the stems of *Schizostachyum chinense* Rendle, which belongs to the same family as *Bambusa textilis* McClure.

Cordyceps

Chinese Caterpillar Fungus

Dongchongxiacao

冬蟲夏草

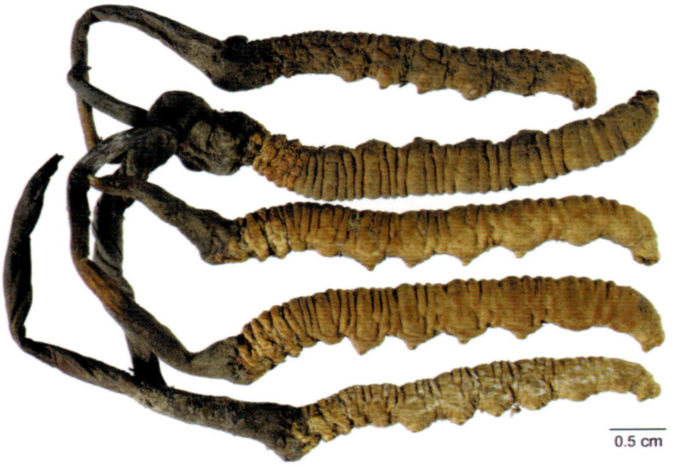

Crude Drug

Source The composite consisting of the stroma of *Cordyceps sinensis* (Berk.) Sacc. (Fam. Clavicipitaceae) parasitizing the larva of insects belonging to the Hepialidae family, and of the larva corpse.

Distribution Mainly in Chinese provinces such as Sichuan, Qinghai and Yunnan, and in Tibet.

Harvest & Processing Dig out stroma-larva composites in early summer when the stromata come out above the ground and before the spores disperse; dry under the sun until nearly dry; remove attached fibrous substances and other foreign matter; dry under the sun or at low temperatures.

Description Larva body joined with a stroma. Larva body resembling a silkworm; outer surface dark yellow to yellowish-brown, with about 20-30 prominent annulations. Legs: 8 pairs; 3 pairs near the head, 4 pairs in the middle and 1 pair near the tail, with the 4 pairs in the middle conspicuous. Head yellowish-red; tail like that of a silkworm. Brittle, breaks easily; broken surface fairly even, pale yellowish-white. Stroma dark brown to reddish-brown, slender and cylindrical, usually longer than the larva body; outer surface marked with fine longitudinal wrinkles. Pliable; broken surface fibrous, off-white. Odour: slightly fishy; taste: slightly bitter.

Indications 1. Chronic cough and asthma, haemoptysis in wasting diseases and pulmonary tuberculosis 2. Impotence and seminal emissions with loin and knee ache

Chemical Composition Contains protein, amino acids, ergosterol, adenine nucleoside, adenine, and D-mannitol.

Cortex Ailanthi

Tree-of-heaven Bark

Chunpi

椿皮

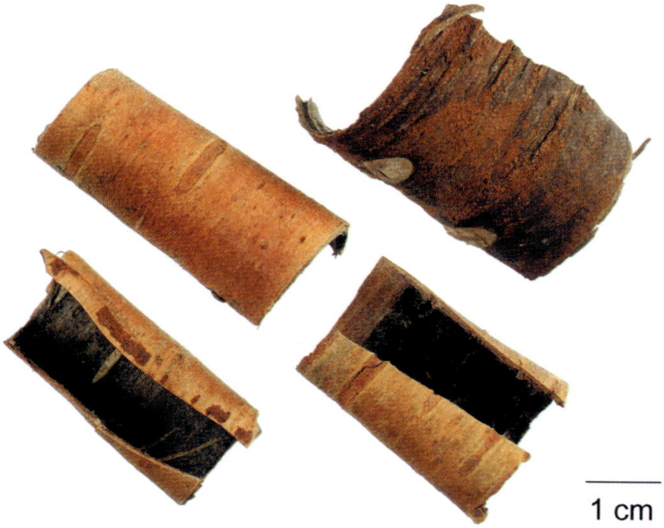

Crude Drug

Source The root bark or stem bark of *Ailanthus altissima* (Mill.) Swingle (Fam. Simarubaceae).

Distribution Mainly in Chinese provinces such as Jiangsu, Zhejiang, Hubei, Hebei, Tianjin and Beijing.

Harvest & Processing Strip off root bark and stem bark in spring and summer; scrape off cork or leave it intact; cut root bark and stem bark into slices or shavings; dry under the sun.

Description Root bark in the form of flat slats or irregular curled sheets. Outer surface greyish-yellow or yellowish-brown, rough; lenticels conspicuous, extending longitudinally, slightly protuberant; inner surface pale yellow, relatively smooth, densely marked with fine angular dots or pits. Hard and brittle. Broken surface strongly fibrous; cortex and bark separate easily. Odour: slightly rancid; when broken, odour intensifies; taste: bitter. Stem bark mostly the shape of flat slats; 3-5 mm or above in thickness. Outer surface dull grey to greyish-black, marked with irregular longitudinal and transverse cracks; lenticels large; pale brownish-red on removal of cork; broken surface granular.

Indications 1. Chronic dysentery, enteritis 2. Melaena 3. Seminal emissions 4. Morbid Leukorrhoea 5. Dysfunctional Uterine bleeding.

Chemical Composition Contains lactone such as ailanthone and amarolide.

Cortex Albiziae

Silktree Albizia Bark

Hehuanpi

合歡皮

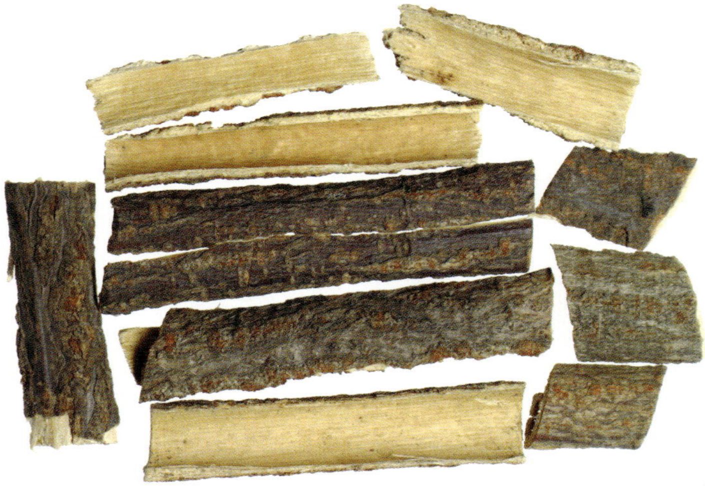

Crude Drug

1 cm

Source The trunk bark of *Albizia julibrissin* Durazz. (Fam. Leguminosae).

Distribution Mainly in Chinese provinces such as Hubei, Jiangsu, Anhui and Zhejiang.

Harvest & Processing Peel off trunk bark in summer and autumn; dry under the sun.

Description Tubular or semi-tubular; 40-80 cm long, 1-3 mm thick. Outer surface greyish-brown to dull greyish-brown; marked with light longitudinal wrinkles and sometimes with shallow cracks; densely covered with conspicuous elliptical transverse lenticels brown or brownish-red in colour; marked occasionally with protuberant transverse ridges or relatively large orbicular (round) branch scars, and often with lichen maculae. Inner surface pale yellowish-brown or yellowish-white; smooth; densely marked with fine longitudinal striae. Hard and brittle, breaks easily; when broken, surface fibrous and lamellate (composed of thin plates), pale yellowish-brown or yellowish-white. Odour: slightly fragrant; taste: mild, slightly astringent and slightly tongue-pricking, then throat-irritating.

Indications 1. Anxiety and insomnia 2. Pulmonary abscess, expectoration 3. Trauma 4. Carbuncle and boils

Chemical Composition Mainly contains triterpene saponins, tannins and flavonoids.

Cortex Cinnamomi

Cassia Bark
Rougui
肉桂

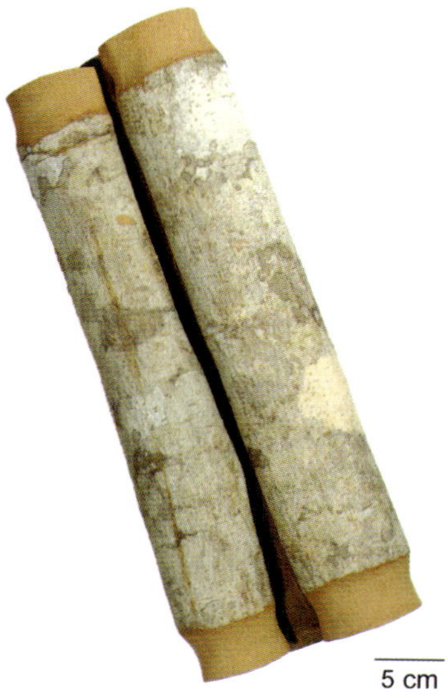

Crude Drug

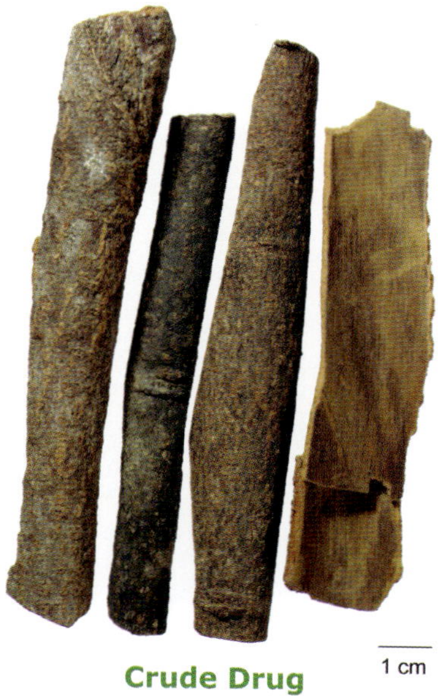

Crude Drug

Source The trunk bark of *Cinnamomum cassia* Presl (Fam. Lauraceae).

Distribution Mainly in Chinese provinces such as Guangxi, Guangdong, Hainan and Fujian; also in Yunnan province.

Harvest & Processing Peel off trunk bark, mostly in autumn; dry in shaded areas.

Description Shallow and sulciform (groove-like), or tubular; 30-50 cm long, 3-10 cm in width or diameter, 2-8 mm thick. Outer surface greyish-brown, slightly rough, marked with irregular fine wrinkles and protuberant transverse lenticels, sometimes with greyish-white maculae; inner surface reddish-brown, fairly even, marked with fine longitudinal striae, and with oil marks when scratched. Hard and brittle, breaks easily. Broken surface uneven; outer layer brown and relatively rough; inner layer reddish-brown, oily and soft, with 1 yellowish-brown stria in between the layers. Odour: heavily aromatic; taste: sweet and hot.

Indications 1. Stomachache, diarrhoea 2. Cough and wheezing 3. Shock, cold and clammy extremities, frostbite. 4. Pain and cold feeling in the lower part of the body 5. Menstrual disorders

Chemical Composition Mainly contains 1.0%-3.5% essential oils with cinnamic aldehyde as the main component; also contains diterpenes such as cinnzeylanine and cinzeylanol.

Cortex Dictamni

Densefruit Pittany Root Bark

Baixianpi

白鲜皮

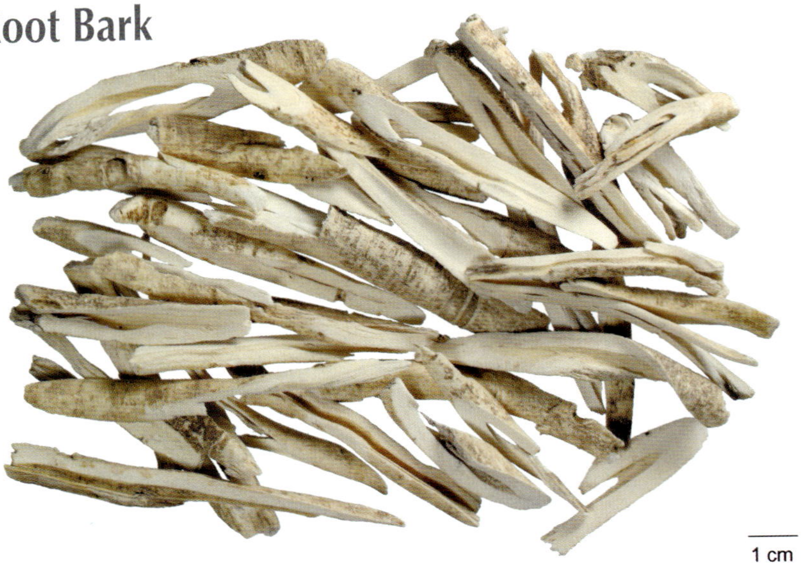

Crude Drug

Source The root bark of *Dictamnus dasycarpus* Turcz. (Fam. Rutaceae).

Distribution Mainly in Chinese provinces such as Liaoning, Hebei and Shandong.

Harvest & Processing Dig out roots in spring and autumn; remove soil, sand and cork; peel off bark and dry it under the sun.

Description Tubular; 5-15 cm long, 1-2 cm in diameter, 2-5 mm thick. Outer surface greyish-white or pale greyish-yellow; marked with fine wrinkles and rootlet scars, and often with granular punctiform (dot-like) protuberances. Inner surface off-white; marked with fine longitudinal striae. Brittle; a burst of white powder when snapped; broken surface uneven, slightly laminiform (consisting of layers); upon removal of cork, small shiny dots visible against the light. Odour: mutton-like; taste: slightly bitter.

Indications 1. Carbuncle, prurigo 2. Scabies and tinea.

Chemical Composition Contains dasycarpamin and trigonelline.

Cortex Eucommiae

Eucommia Bark
Duzhong
杜仲

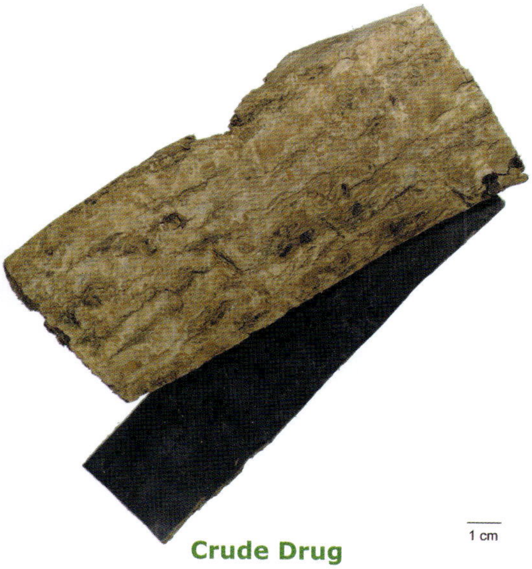

Crude Drug

1 cm

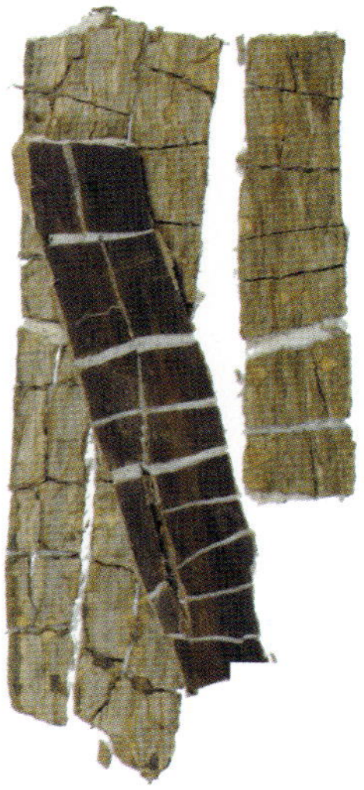

Crude Drug

1 cm

Source The trunk bark of *Eucommia ulmoides* Oliv. (Fam. Eucommiaceae).

Distribution Mainly in Chinese provinces such as Hubei, Sichuan, Guizhou and Yunnan. Mostly cultivated.

Harvest & Processing Peel off trunk bark in spring and summer; scrape away cork from bark while fresh; heap up in layers with inner surfaces of adjacent pieces facing each other; bury deep in hay to let moisture evaporate until cortex turns dull purplish-brown; take out and dry under the sun.

Description Flattened and placoid (plate-like), or slat-like and slightly involute (with the margin rolled inwards); 2-7 mm thick. Bark with cork remnants: outer surface pale greyish-brown or dull greyish-brown; marked with longitudinal grooves or cracks and trapeziform (trapezium-shaped) lenticels, sometimes with lichen maculae. Bark with cork scraped away: pale brown, smooth. Inner surface reddish-purple or dull purplish-brown; smooth. Brittle, breaks easily. Broken surface with interconnected, fine and dense gelatinous silver-white threads; threads elastic, can generally stretch for more than 1 cm before breaking. Odour: faint; taste: slightly bitter; gelatinous when chewed.

Indications
1. Weakness of the lower body and legs, seminal emissions
2. Dizziness due to hypertension.

Chemical Composition Mainly contains lignans such as pinoresinol diglucoside; also contains iridoid glycosides such as ulmoside.

Cortex Fraxini

Ash Bark
Qinpi
秦皮

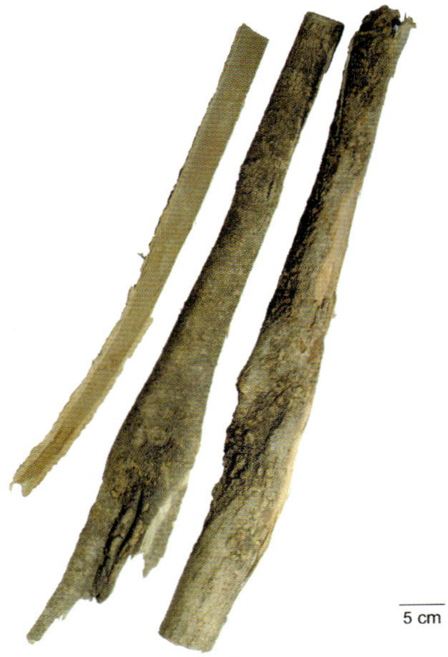

Crude Drug

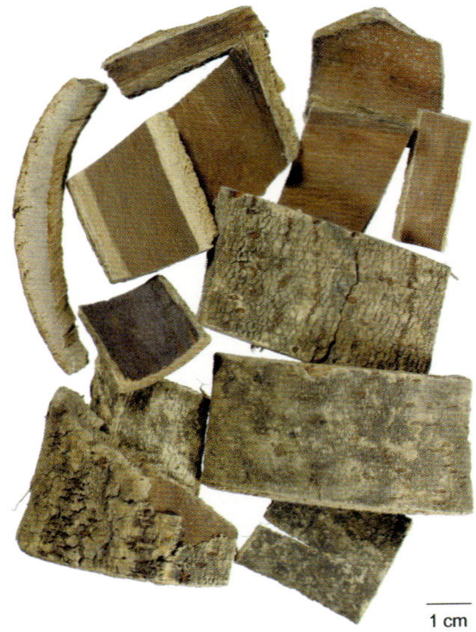

Decoction Pieces

Source The branch bark or stem bark of *Fraxinus rhynchophylla* Hance (Fam. Oleacae).

Distribution Mainly in Chinese provinces such as Heilongjiang, Jilin and Liaoning.

Harvest & Processing Peel off branch bark or stem bark during pruning in spring or autumn; dry under the sun.

Description Branch bark: Tubular or sulciform (groove-like); 1.5-3 mm thick. Outer surface greyish-white, greyish-brown to blackish-brown, or with maculae of these colours; smooth or slightly rough; marked with dense orbicular (round), punctiform (dot-like) greyish-white lenticels and hippocrepiform (horseshoe-shaped) or lunate (crescent-shaped) leaf scars. Inner surface smoother; yellowish-white or yellowish-brown. Hard and brittle; broken surface fibrous. Odour: faint; taste: bitter.
Stem bark: Slat-like pieces; 3-6 mm thick. Outer surface greyish-brown; with rimose (with fissures or cracks) grooves and orbicular or lalongate (transversely elongated) reddish-brown lenticels. Hard; broken surface more fibrous; separates easily in layers and becomes lobate (lobe-like).

Indications 1. Diarrhoea and dysentery especially those with bloody stools 2. Conjunctivitis, nebula 3. Cough and dyspnoea.

Chemical Composition Mainly contains aesculin and aesculetin.

Note According to *C.P.*, also used for medicinal purposes is the branch bark or stem bark of *F. chinensis* Roxb., of *F. szaboana* Lingelsh. and of *F. stylosa* Lingelsh.

Cortex Ilicis Rotundae

Ovateleaf Holly Bark
Jiubiying

救必應

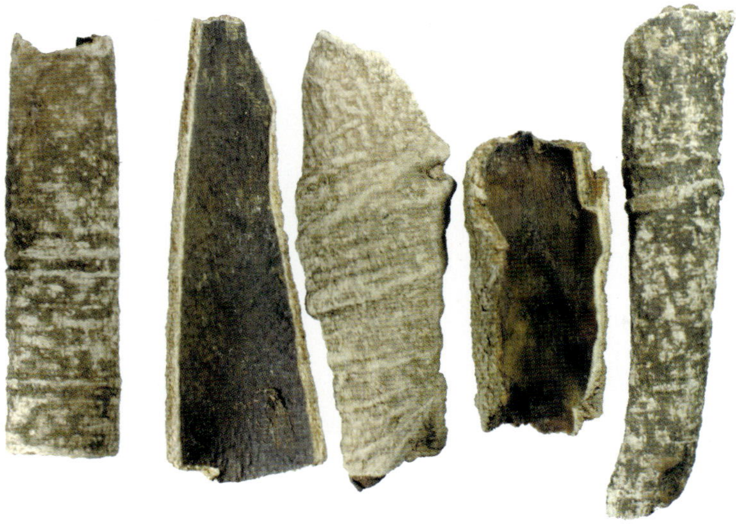

1 cm

Crude Drug

Source The root bark and trunk bark of *Ilex rotunda* Thunb. (Fam. Aquifoliaceae).

Distribution Mainly in regions in China south of Yangtze River valley; also in Hong Kong.

Harvest & Processing Harvest root bark and trunk bark anytime during the year; use while fresh or dry under the sun.

Description Root bark tubular, or slate-like but slightly curled; varying in length, 0.3-1.0 cm thick. Outer surface greyish-yellow or dull greyish-brown, rough, often marked with transverse wrinkles or slightly transverse protuberances; inner surface pale brown or reddish-brown, marked with light longitudinal striae. Hard and brittle; broken surface slightly smooth and a little granular, yellowish-white or pale yellowish-brown. Odour: faint; taste: bitter and slightly astringent. Trunk bark thinner than root bark; slightly involute (with the margins rolled inwards); outer surface marked with quite a large number of protuberant elliptical lenticels.

Indications 1. Common cold high fever, sore throat, conjunctivitis, skin infection, cholecystitis 2. Diarrhoea 3 Bleeding 4. Abdominal pain, stomachache, arthralgia 5. Burn (external use)

Chemical Composition Mainly contains flavonoids glycosides, tannins and triterpene saponins.

Cortex Illicii

Difengpi Bark
Difengpi

地楓皮

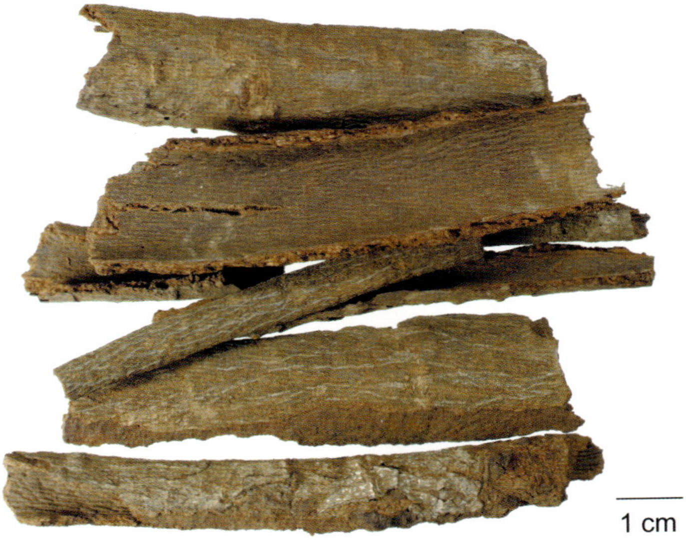

Crude Drug

Source The trunk bark of *Illicium difengpi* K. I. B. et K. I. M. (Fam. Magnoliaceae).

Distribution Mainly in Chinese provinces such as Guangxi.

Harvest & Processing Peel off trunk bark from trees in spring and autumn; dry.

Description Tubular or sulciform (groove-like); 5-15 cm long, 2-3 mm thick. Outer surface greyish-brown to dark brown, marked with conspicuous, criss-crossing longitudinal grooves and sometimes with greyish-white maculae; cork falls off easily, exposing brownish-red cortex; lenticels inconspicuous. Inner surface brown or brownish-red; marked with conspicuous fine longitudinal wrinkles. Texture loose and brittle, breaks easily; when broken, surface granular; no mucilage is produced upon contact with water. Odour: aromatic; taste: slightly astringent.

Indications 1. Rheumatic arthralgia 2. Lumbar muscle strain.

Chemical Composition Mainly contains lignans and phenylpropanoids.

Note Listed as slightly toxic in *C.P.*

Cortex Lycii

Chinese Wolfberry Root-Bark

Digupi

地骨皮

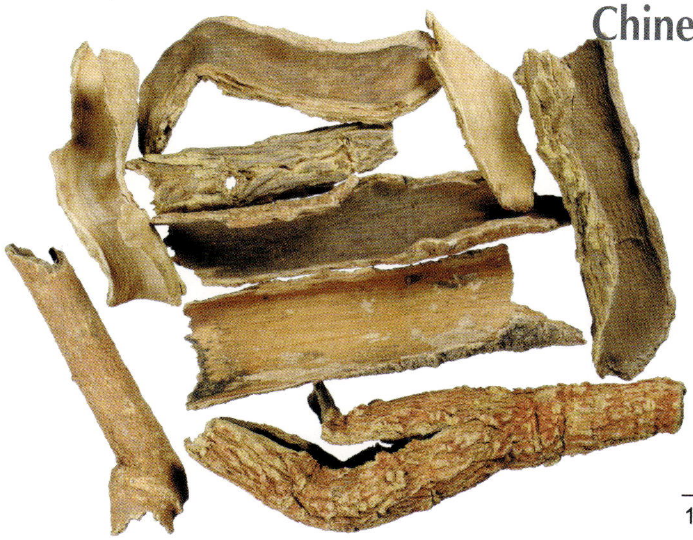

1 cm

Crude Drug

Source The root bark of *Lycium chinensis* Mill. (Fam. Solanaceae).

Distribution Mainly in Chinese provinces such as Hebei, Henan, Shanxi, Zhejiang, Jiangsu and Shaanxi, and Ningxia; also in Hong Kong.

Harvest & Processing Dig out roots anytime during the year; peel off bark and dry it under the sun.

Description Tubular or sulciform (groove-like), or curled sheets irregular in shape; 3-10 cm long, 0.5-1.5 cm in diameter, 1-3 mm thick. Outer surface greyish-yellow to brownish-yellow; rough; marked with longitudinal wrinkles or cracks; scales off easily. Inner surface yellowish-white or greyish-yellow; marked with fine longitudinal striae. Light in weight; brittle, breaks easily. Broken surface uneven; outer layer yellowish-brown, inner layer greyish-white. Odour: faint; taste: slightly sweet, then bitter.

Indications 1. Low-grade fever due to pulmonary tuberculosis, night fever and night sweating, thirst 2. Cough, haemoptysis 3. Epistaxis

Chemical Composition Contains kukoamine A, betaine and lyciumin A, B.

Note According to *C.P.*, also used for medicinal purposes is the root bark of *L. barbarum* L.

Cortex Magnoliae Officinalis

Officinal Magnolia Bark

Houpo

厚樸

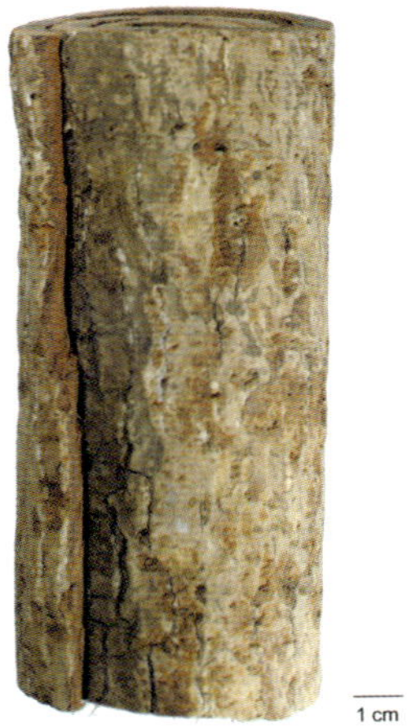

Crude Drug

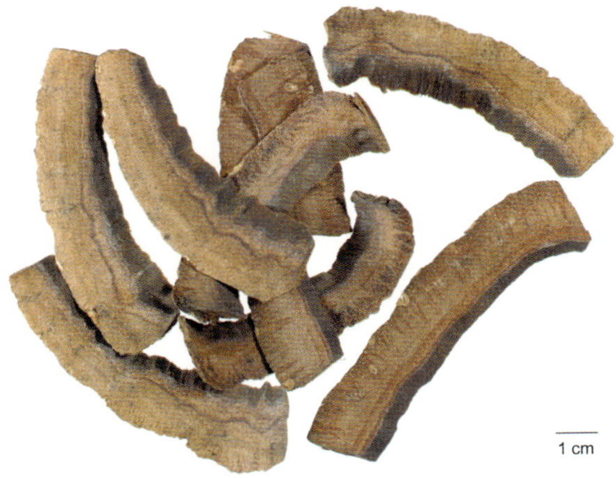

Decoction Pieces

Source The stem bark of *Magnolia officinalis* Rehd. et Wils. (Fam. Magnoliaceae).

Distribution Mainly in Chinese provinces such as Sichuan and Hubei; also in provinces such as Zhejiang, Hunan, Jiangxi and Guizhou. Mostly cultivated.

Harvest & Processing From April to June, collect stem bark from trees 15-20 years old; blanch in boiling water, then heap in an earth pit to let moisture evaporate; when internal moisture has seeped out and inner surface has turned dull purplish-brown or reddish-brown, steam to soften; take out and roll into tubes; dry under the sun.

Description Outer surface greyish-brown or dull greyish-brown; rough; sometimes squamiform (scale-like), peels off easily; marked with conspicuous elliptical lenticels and longitudinal wrinkles; bark with cork scraped off yellowish-brown in colour. Inner surface purplish-brown or dark purplish-brown; densely marked with fine longitudinal striae; oil marks appear when scratched. Hard, does not break easily. When broken, outer surface greyish-brown, granular; inner surface dull purplish-brown or brown, fibrous, highly oleaginous (oily), occasionally with numerous small shiny crystals of magnolol and honokil. Odour: fragrant; taste: pungent and slightly bitter.

Indications 1. Feeling of fullness in the chest and abdomen, dyspepsia
2. Diarrhoea 3. Cough and expectoration.

Chemical Composition Mainly contains lignans such as magnolol and honokil.

Note According to *C.P.*, also used for medicinal purposes are the stem bark, branch bark and root bark of *M. officinalis* Rehd. et Wils. *var. biloba* Rehd. et Wils.

Cortex Meliae

Szechwan Chinaberry Bark

Kulianpi

苦楝皮

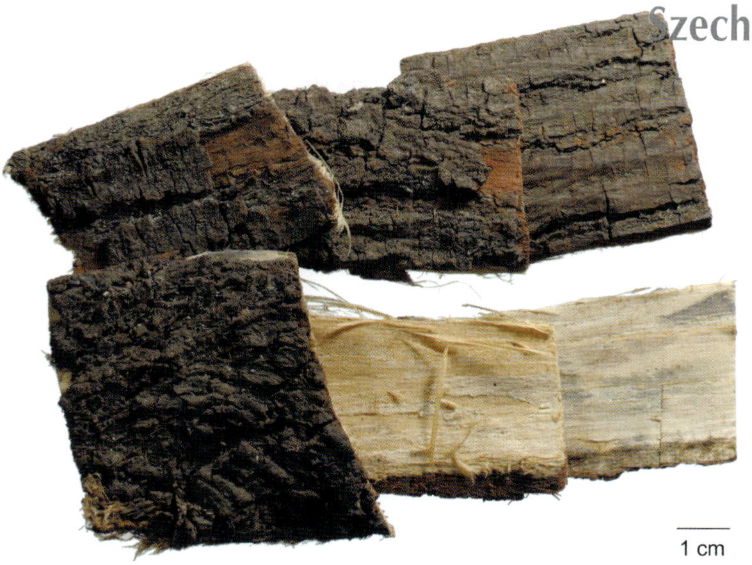

Crude Drug

Source The trunk bark of *Melia toosendan* Sieb. et Zucc. (Fam. Meliaceae).

Distribution Mainly in Chinese provinces such as Sichuan, Yunnan, Guizhou and Gansu.

Harvest & Processing Collect trunk bark in any season. The usual practice is to scrape off cork first and then peel off bark, then dry under the sun or by heat at low temperatures.

Description Irregular slats or curled sulciform (groove-like) sheets; 3-7 mm thick. Old bark with cork still attached: outer surface rough, greyish-brown to reddish-brown; marked with broad longitudinal cracks and fine transverse cracks; with elliptical, transverse, oblong greyish-brown lenticels; cork often scales off. Old bark with cork detached: outer surface pale yellow. Young bark: outer surface purplish-brown, smooth, with a waxy layer; inner surface yellowish-white. Pliable, difficult to break; broken surface fibrous. Breaks into alternating yellow and white layers of slices when folded and rubbed with hands; extremely fine reticulate (net-like) striae on peeled-off slices. Odourless; taste: bitter.

Indications Ascariasis, ancylostomiasis, ringworm infection.

Chemical Composition Mainly contains toosendanin and isotoosendanin.

Note According to *C.P.*, also used for medicinal purposes and listed as toxic are the stem bark and root bark of *M. azedarach* L.

Cortex Mori

White Mulberry RootBark
Sangbaipi

桑白皮

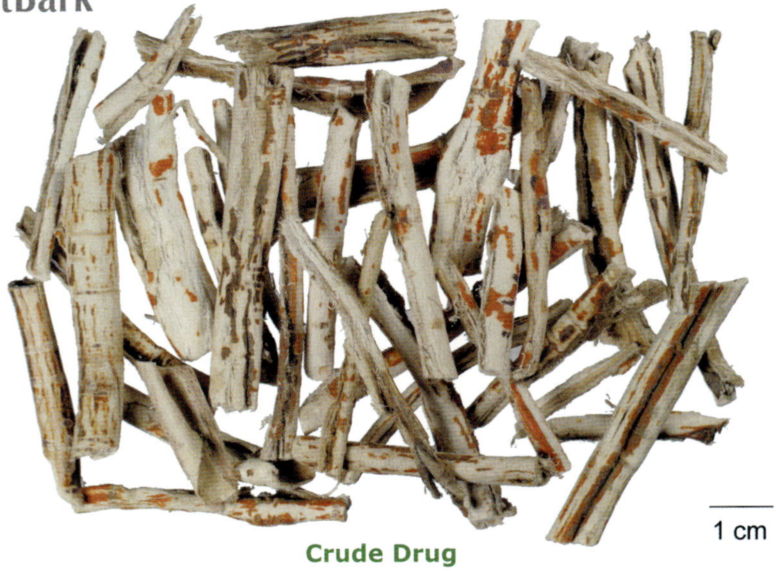

Crude Drug

Source The root bark of *Morus alba* L. (Fam. Moraceae).

Distribution Naturally grown or cultivated in most regions of China; also in Hong Kong.

Harvest & Processing Dig up roots between defoliation in late autumn and germination in the following spring; remove soil and rootlets while roots are fresh; scrape off yellowish-brown cork; cut open cortex longitudinally; peel off bark and dry it under the sun.

Description Twisted and tubular, sulciform (groove-like), or slat-like; 1-4 mm thick, varying in width and length. Outer surface white or pale yellowish-white, smooth, occasionally with remnants of orange-yellow or brownish-yellow squamiform (scale-like) cork; inner surface yellowish-white or pale yellow, marked with fine longitudinal striae. Light in weight; pliable; heavily fibrous; difficult to break but easy to tear off longitudinally, producing a burst of white powder. Odour: faint; taste: slightly sweet.

Indications 1. Cough, dyspnoea 2. Facial dropsy, oedema, oliguria 3. Trauma.

Chemical Composition Mainly contains flavonoids such as mulberrin and morusin.

Cortex Moutan

Tree Peony Root Bark

Mudanpi

牡丹皮

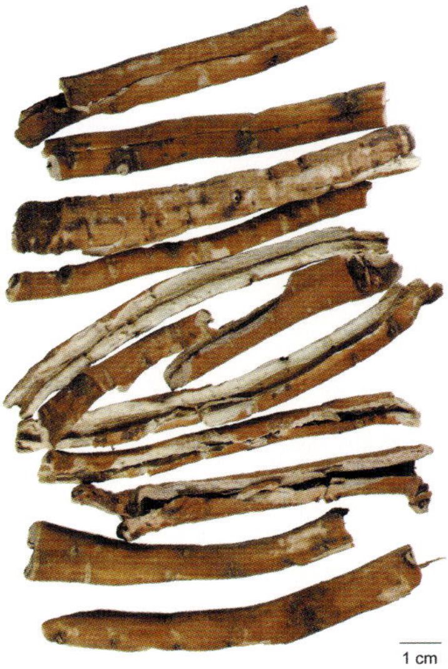

Crude Drug

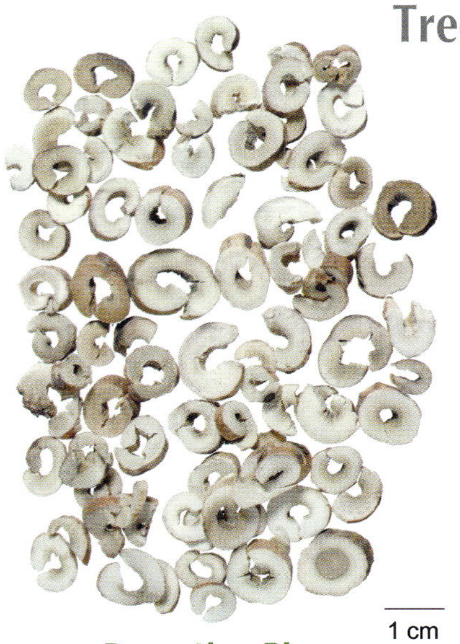

Decoction Pieces

Source The root bark of *Paeonia suffruticosa* Andr. (Fam. Ranunculaceae).

Distribution Mainly in Chinese provinces such as Anhui, Sichuan, Henan and Shandong.

Harvest & Processing Harvest root bark, usually after 3-5 years of cultivation. Dig out roots, mostly in October and November; remove rootlets and caudexes; peel off bark and dry it under the sun.

Description Crude root bark tubular or semi-tubular, with a longitudinal crack caused by a length-wise cut, and curling inwards or slightly outwards; varying in length, usually 5-25 cm long, 0.5-1.2 cm in diameter, 2-4 mm thick. Outer surface dull greyish-brown; marked with numerous slightly dented lalongate (transversely elongated) lenticels and rootlet scars. Inner surface pale greyish-yellow or light brown; marked with noticeable fine longitudinal striae; often covered with shiny crystals of paeonol. Hard and brittle; when broken, surface relatively even, starchy, greyish-white to pink. Odour: with a distinctive fragrance; taste: slightly bitter, astringent.

Indications 1. Febrile diseases, eruptive exanthem, anhidrosis 2. Bleeding 3. Menstrual disorders 4. Peri-appendicular abscess, abdominal mass 5. Skin infection 6. Allergic rhinitis

Chemical Composition Mainly contains paeonol, paeonoside and paeoniflorin.

Cortex Periplocae

Chinese Silkvine Root Bark

Xiangjiapi

香加皮

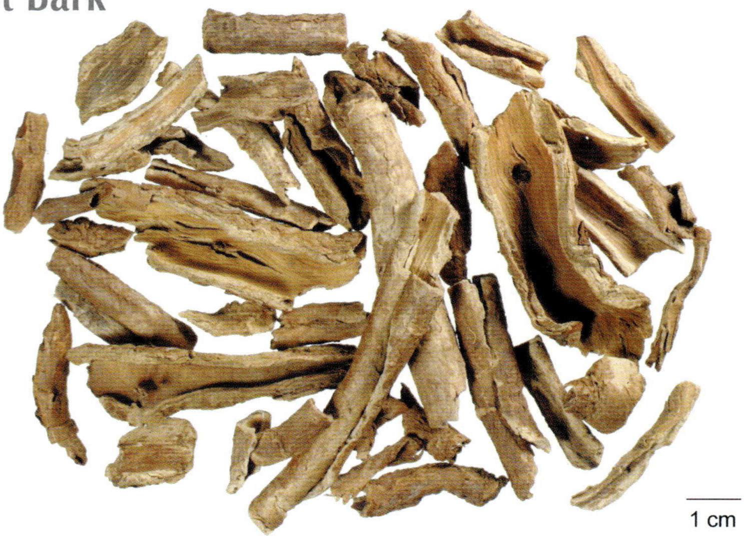

Crude Drug

Source The root bark of *Periploca sepium* bunge (Fam. Asclepiadaceae).

Distribution Mainly in Chinese provinces such as Shanxi, Henan, Hebei, Shandong, Gansu and Hunan.

Harvest & Processing Peel off root bark while fresh in spring and autumn; dry in shaded areas or under the sun.

Description Tubular or sulciform (groove-like), occasionally the shape of irregular chips; 3-10 cm long, 1-2 cm in diameter, 2-4 mm thick. Outer surface greyish-brown or yellowish-brown; cork scales off easily. Inner surface yellowish-white or pale reddish-brown, marked with fine longitudinal striae. Texture loose, brittle; breaks easily. Broken section yellowish-white, uneven. Odour: heavily aromatic; taste: bitter, slightly tongue-numbing.

Indications 1. Rheumatic arthritis with pain and weakness of the loins and knees 2. Palpitaiton, dyspnoea, oedema of the lower extremities.

Chemical Composition Mainly contains periplocin and periploside A, B, C .

Note Listed as toxic in *C.P.*

Cortex Phellodendri

Amur Cork-Tree
Huangbo
黄柏

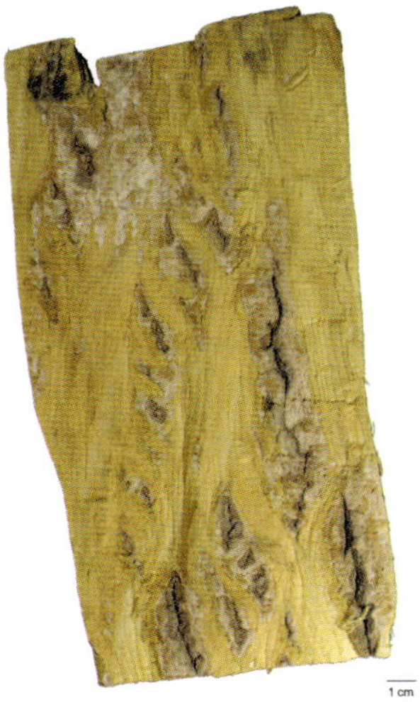

Crude Drug

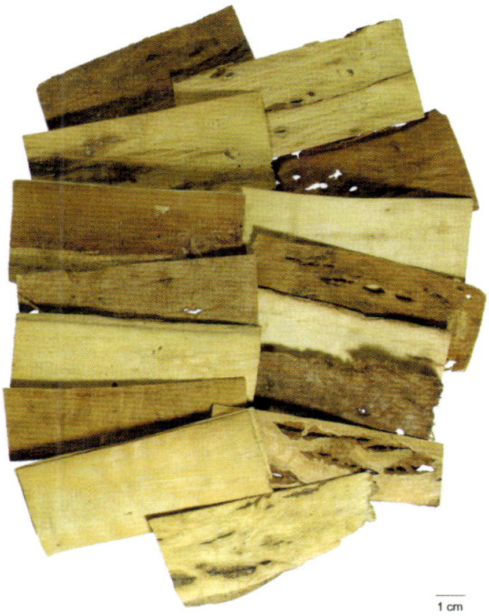

Decoction Pieces

Source The trunk bark of *Phellodendron chinense* Schneid. (Fam. Rutaceae). Customarily called '*Chuan huangbo*'(Sichuan Amur Cork-Tree Bark).

Distribution Mainly in Chinese provinces such as Sichuan and Guizhou; also in provinces such as Shaanxi, Hubei, Yunnan and Hunan.

Harvest & Processing Peel off trunk bark from trees about 10 years old between March and June ; half-dry under the sun; press flat; scrape off cork until it is tinged with yellow but avoid cutting into the cortex; brush clean and dry under the sun; put in dry and well-ventilated places to avoid going mouldy and changing colour. Commonly used in Hong Kong in the form of thin length-wise cut slices.

Description Slat-shaped or shallow and sulciform (groove-like); varying in length and width, 3-7 mm thick. Outer surface yellowish-brown or dull yellowish-brown; relatively smooth; marked with transverse lenticels and irregular longitudinal shallow cracks; occasionally with remnants of dull greyish-brown cork. Inner surface dull yellow or brownish-yellow; densely marked with fine longitudinal ridges. Light in weight; relatively hard. Broken surface dark yellow; lobate (divided into lobes) and layered; fibrous. Odour: faint; taste: bitter; sticky when chewed and turns saliva yellow.

Indications 1. Genitourinary infection, leukorrhoea 2. Diarrhoea 3. Arthralgia 4. Aphthous ulcer 5. Haemorrhoid, dermatitis, eczema, pustules, burns and scalds (external use).

Chemical Composition Mainly contains alkaloids such as berberine and magnoflorine.

Note According to *C.P.*, also used for medicinal purposes and customarily known as '*Guan huangbo*', is the bark of *P. amurense* Rupr.

Cortex Pseudolaricis

Golden Larch Bark
Tujingpi

土荊皮

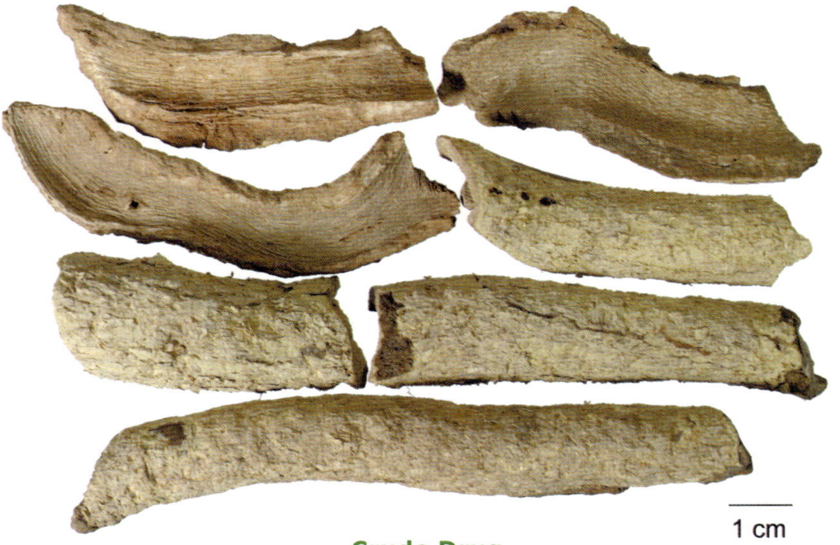

Crude Drug

Source The root bark of *Pseudolarix amabilis* (Nelson) Rehd. (Fam. Pinaceae).

Distribution Mainly in Chinese provinces such as Jiangsu, Zhejiang, Anhui, Jiangxi, Fujian and Hunan.

Harvest & Processing Dig out roots in spring and autumn; peel off root bark; remove cork; wash clean; dry under the sun.

Description Irregular strips, or slightly curled into a groove; varying in length and width, 2-5 mm thick. Outer surface rough, dark greyish-brown, marked with criss-crossing wrinkles and transverse grey-ish-white lenticels; cork often scales off. Inner surface smooth; yellowish-brown to reddish-brown; marked with fine longitudinal striae. Strong and pliable; when broken, surface lobate (lobe-like). Odour: faint; taste: bitter, astringent.

Indications Scabies and tinea.

Chemical Composition Peudolaric acid A, B, C, D and E exist in the roots.

Note Listed as toxic in *C.P.*

Cortex Schefflerae Octophyllae

Ivy Tree Bark

Yajiaomu

鴨腳木

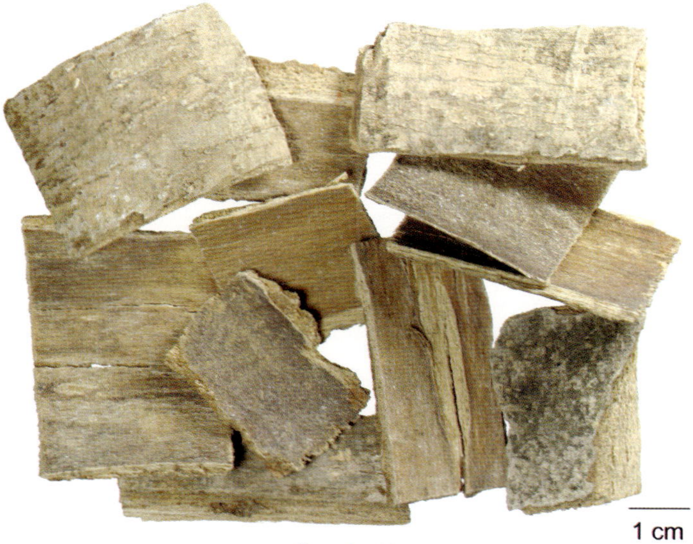

Crude Drug

Source The trunk bark of *Schefflera octophylla* (Lour.) Harms (Fam. Araliaceae).

Distribution Mainly in Chinese provinces such as Guangdong and Guangxi; also in Hong Kong.

Harvest & Processing Collect trunk bark anytime during the year; wash clean; steam thoroughly; cut into slices; dry under the sun.

Description Tubular, or irregular and slate-like; 30-50 cm long, 2-8 mm thick. Outer surface greyish-white or dull grey; rough; often with lichen, and also with suborbicular (almost round), or transverse, oblong and orbicular (round) lenticels. Inner surface greyish-yellow or greyish-brown; marked with fine longitudinal striae. Brittle, breaks easily; broken surface uneven, fibrous. Odour: slightly fragrant; taste: bitter, astringent.

Indications 1. Common cold with fever, pharyngitis 2. Burn and scald, pyogenic skin infection 3. Rheumatism, trauma, fracture

Chemical Composition Mainly contains triterpene saponins such as scheffuroside A, B, C, D.

Exocarpium Benincasae

Chinese Waxgourd Peel
Dongguapi

冬瓜皮

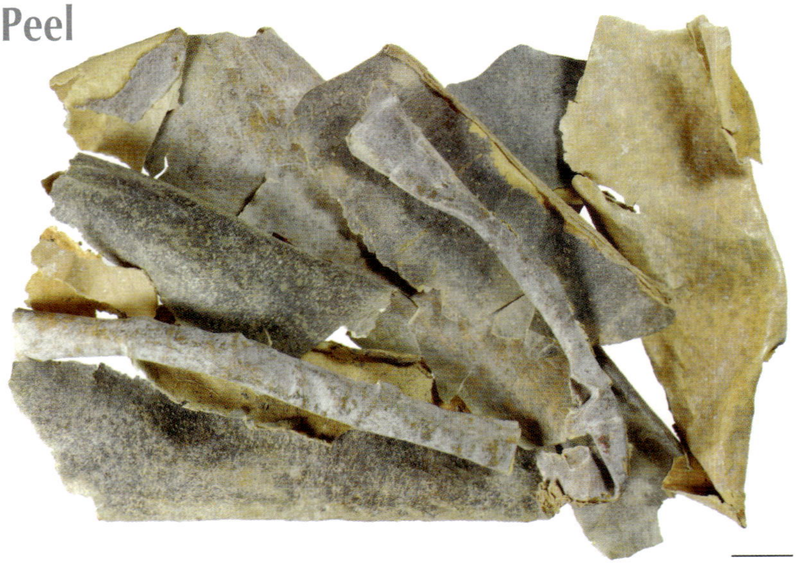

Crude Drug

1 cm

Source The exocarp of *Benincasa hispida* (Thunb.) Cogn. (Fam. Cucurbitaceae).

Distribution Mainly in Chinese provinces such as Hebei, Henan, Anhui, Jiangsu, Zhejiang and Sichuan.

Harvest & Processing Collect exocarp shaved from Chinese waxgourds during food preparation; dry under the sun.

Description Irregular strips, usually involute (with the margins rolled inwards towards the upper side), tubular or double-tubular in shape; varying in size. Outer surface yellowish-white to dull green, smooth or covered with white powder. Inner surface rougher, with venous (vein-like) vascular bundles. Light in weight; brittle, break easily. Odour: faint; taste: mild.

Indications 1. Oedema and dysuria 2. Heat stroke

Chemical Composition Contains volatile compounds such as n-hexanal; also contains triterpene such as glutinol and cucurbita-5, 24-dienol.

Exocarpium Citri Grandis

Pummelo Peel
Huajuhong
化橘紅

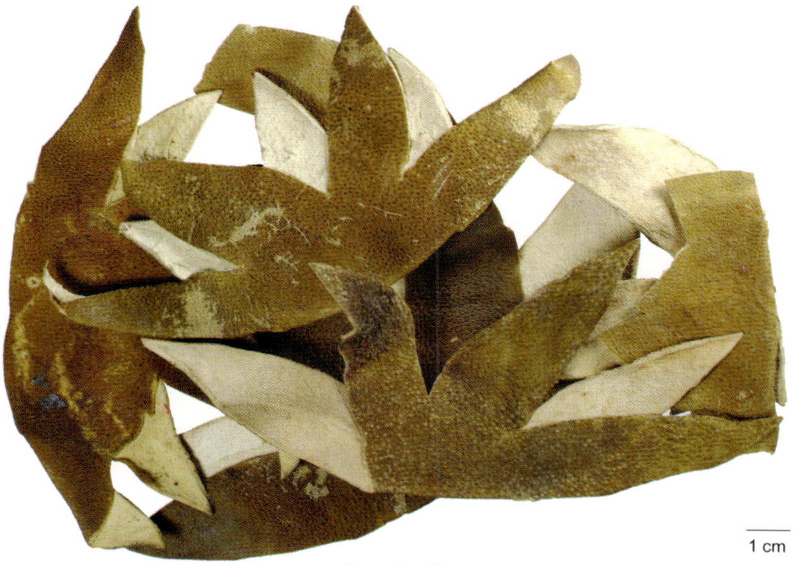

Crude Drug

Source The immature or near-mature exocarp of *Citrus grandis* (L.) Osbeck *var. tomentosa* Hort (Fam. Rutaceae).

Distribution Mainly in Chinese provinces such as Guangdong.

Harvest & Processing Harvest immature fruits before early July; blanch in boiling water; cut pericarp into stars with 7, 5 or 6 points; remove pulp and part of mesocarp; press exocarp into shape; dry under the sun or by heat.

Description The shape of folded seven-pointed stars or smoothed out five-pointed stars; single pieces the shape of willow leaves; when whole and smoothed out, 15-28 cm in diameter, 2-5 mm thick. Outer surface yellowish-green, densely pubescent (covered with short, soft hairs), marked with wrinkles and small oil cavities. Inner surface yellowish-white or pale yellowish-brown, veined. Brittle, break easily. When broken, surface irregular; outer side with a row of irregular, dented oil cavities, inner side fairly pliable and elastic. Odour: aromatic; taste: bitter and slightly acrid.

Indications
1. Cough, itchingness of the throat and copious expectoration
2. Vomiting, epigastric distension, dyspepsia.

Chemical Composition Mainly contains essential oils with citral and linalool as the main components; also contains flavonoids such as naringin.

Note According to *C.P.*, also used for medicinal purposes, and usually known as '*Guang Juhong*' (Glabrous Pummelo Peel), is the exocarp of the immature or near-mature fruit of *C. grandis* (L.) Osbeck.

Flos Albiziae

Silktree Albizia Flower
Hehuanhua

合歡花

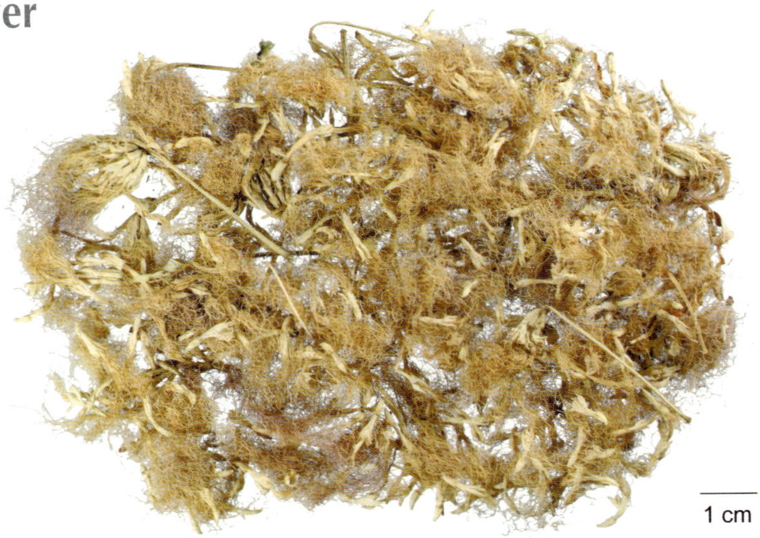

Crude Drug

Source The inflorescence of *Albizia julibrissin* Durazz. (Fam. Leguminosae).

Distribution Mainly in Chinese provinces such as Hebei, Henan, Shaanxi, Zhejiang, Jiangsu, Shangdong, Anhui and Hubei.

Harvest & Processing Collect inflorescences in summer when flowers start to bloom; remove branches and leaves; dry under the sun.

Description Curled into a fluffy mass. Flower slender and curved; 0.7-1 cm long; pale yellowish-brown or pale dull yellowish-brown; with short pedicels. Calyx tubular; sparsely pubescent (covered with short, soft hairs); apex 5-toothed. Corolla tube about twice the length of calyx tube; sparsely pubescent; apex 5-lobed, lobes lanceolate (lance-head shaped). Filaments slender; yellowish-brown or dull yellowish-brown; lower part accrete (grown or joined together), upper part free (not attached to other organs) and sticking out of corolla tube. Light in weight; breaks easily. Odour: slightly fragrant; taste: mild.

Indications 1. Neurasthenia, insomnia, forgetfulness 2. Feeling of oppression in the chest.

Chemical Composition Mainly contains essential oils with linalool oxide and linalool as the main components.

Note Customarily called '*Yehehua*' (Chinese Magnolia Flower) in Hong Kong.

Flos Bombacis Malabarici

Common Bombax Flower
Mumianhua

木棉花

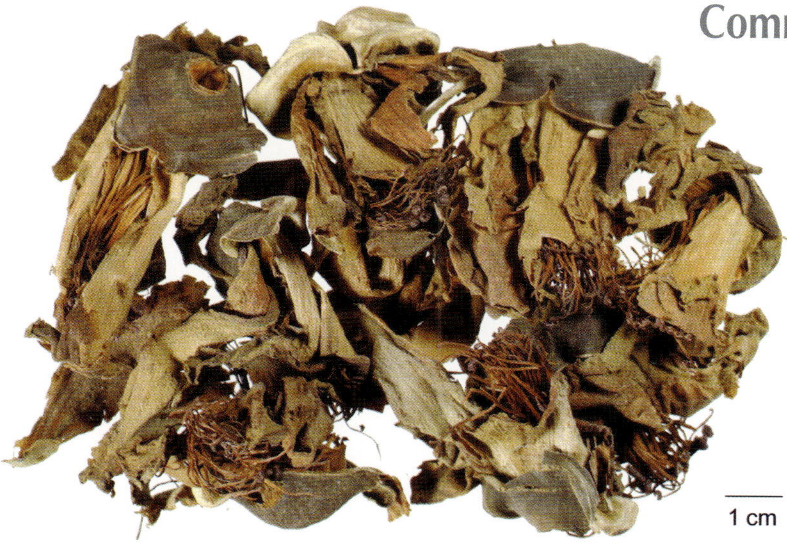

Crude Drug

Source The flower of *Bombax malabaricum* DC. (Fam. Bombacaceae).

Distribution Mainly in Chinese provinces such as Yunnan and Guangdong; also in Hong Kong.

Harvest & Processing Collect flowers in late spring; dry in shaded areas.

Description Dry, shrunken and irregular pieces; ovary and pedicel mostly fallen off. Calyx cupulate (cup-shaped); 2-4.5 cm long; 3- or 5-lobed; lobes obtuse, recurved (curved backwards), thick, coriaceous (leathery), brittle; outer surface reddish-brown or brownish-black, marked with irregular fine wrinkles; inner surface greyish-yellow, densely covered with lustrous silky hairs. Petals 5, shrivelled or in fragments; when whole, obovate (egg-shaped in outline and attached at the narrower end) and elliptical, or lanceolate (lance-head shaped) and elliptical; outer surface brownish-yellow or dark brown, covered with dense stellate (star-shaped) hairs; inner surface purplish-brown or reddish-brown, covered with sparse stellate hairs. Stamens numerous, curled; style remnants fairly thick, slightly longer than stamens. Odour: faint; taste: mild, slightly sweet-astringent.

Indications 1. Rheumatism 2. Diarrhoea, dysentery 3. Chronic gastritis, peptic ulcer 4. Dysfunctional uterine bleeding 5. Boils and sores

Chemical Composition Mainly contains essential oils with 24.7% hexadecanoic acid and 19.68% β-cedrol.

Flos Buddlejae

Pale Butterflybush Flower
Mimenghua

密蒙花

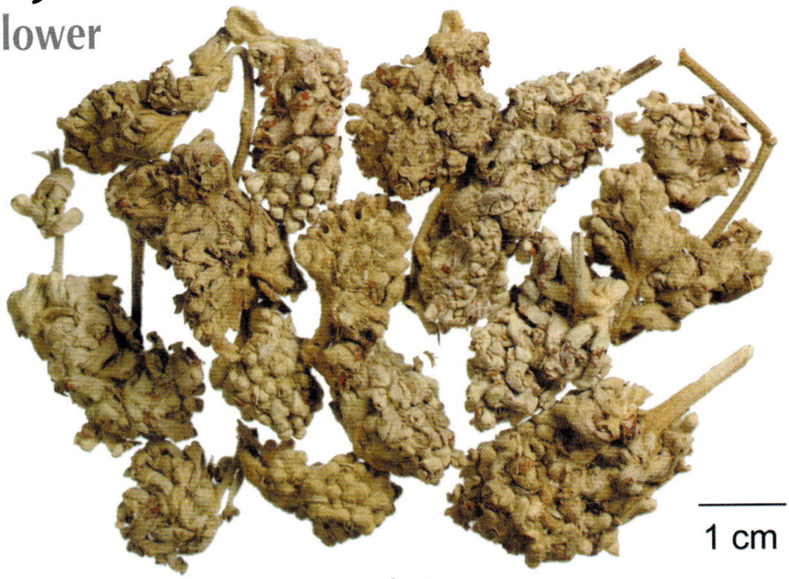

Crude Drug

Source The flower bud and the inflorescence of *Buddleja officinalis* Maxim. (Fam. Loganiaceae).

Distribution Mainly in Chinese provinces such as Hubei, Sichuan, Henan and Shaanxi.

Harvest & Processing Collect flower buds and inflorescences before flowers start to bloom; remove foreign matter; dry under the sun.

Description Mostly inflorescence with dense, clustered flower buds; irregular and obconical (inversely conical); 1.5-3 cm long. Outer surface greyish-yellow or brownish-yellow; densely covered with fine pubescence rusty in colour. Flower buds short and clavate (club-shaped, gradually widening towards the apex); 0.3-1 cm long, 1-2 mm in diameter. Calyx campanulate (bell-shaped); apex 4-toothed. Corolla tubular, same length as calyx or slightly longer; apex 4-lobed, each lobe ovate (egg-shaped in outline and attached at the broad end); stamens 4, grown in the middle part of corolla. Soft. Odour: slightly fragrant; taste: slightly bitter, acrid.

Indications 1. Conjunctivitis, photophobia with lacrimation, Red eyes 2. Blurring of vision 3. Nebula

Chemical Composition Mainly contains glycosides such as linarin, mimengoside and catalposide.

Flos Campsis Grandifloral

Chinese Trumpetcreeper Flower

Lingxiaohua

凌霄花

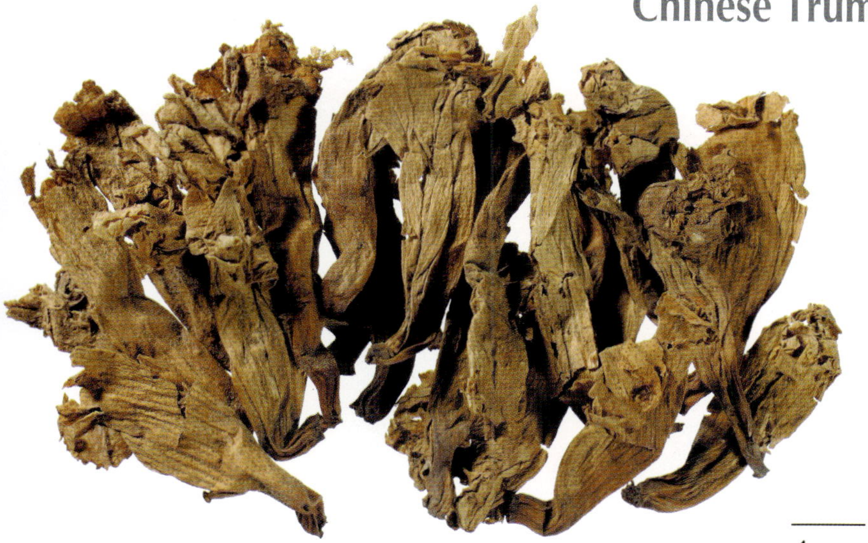

Crude Drug

Source The flower of *Campsis grandiflora* (Thunb.) Loisel ex K. Schum (Fam. Bignoniaceae).

Distribution Mainly in Chinese provinces such as Jiangsu and Zhejiang; also in Hong Kong.

Harvest & Processing Pick freshly-bloomed flowers on sunny days between July and September; dry under the sun.

Description Mostly shrivelled and curled; when intact, 3-5.5 cm long. Calyx campanulate (bell-shaped); about 2 cm long; reddish-brown or brown; thin; apex parted into 5 uneven divisions; lobes triangular and lanceolate (lance-head shaped); outer surface of calyx tube marked with 10 longitudinal veins, 5 of them prominent. Corolla yellowish-brown or brown; when whole and smoothed out, apex 5-lobed; lobes semi-circular, joined at base in a funnelform manner; fine veins visible on outer surface, more prominent on inner surface. Stamens 4, didynamous (two long and two short), blackish-brown. Style 1; stigma orbicular (round) and triangular. Odour: slightly fragrant; taste: slightly bitter, sour.

Indications 1. Menstrual disorders, amenorrhoea with abdominal mass 2. Postpartum abnormal breast swelling 3. Rubella, pruritus, acne.

Chemical Composition Mainly contains oleanolic acid, apigenin and acteoside.

Note According to *C.P.*, also used for medicinal purposes is the flower of *Campsis radicans* (L.) seem.

Flos Carthami

Safflower
Honghua
紅花

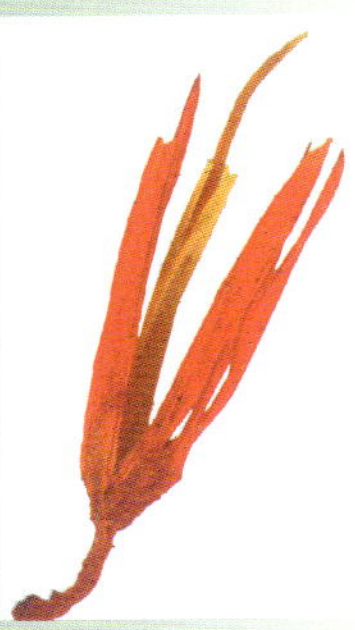

Safflower Magnified

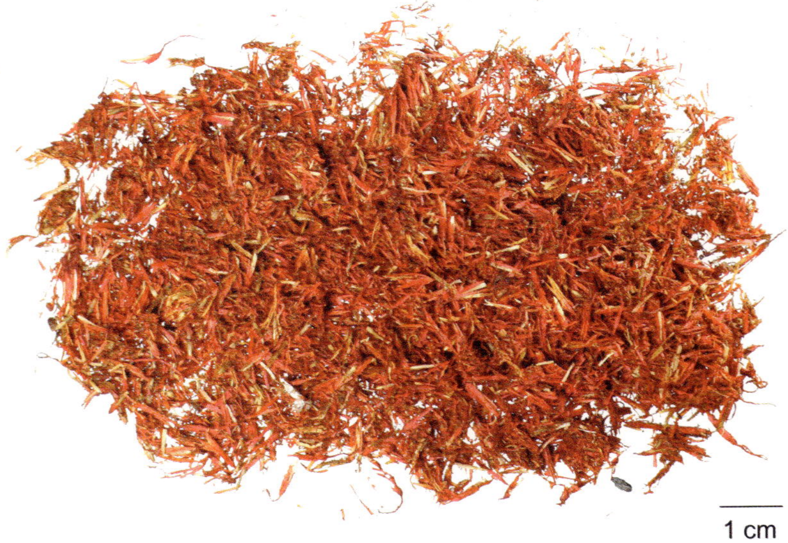

Crude Drug

Source The flower of *Carthamus tinctorius* L. (Fam. Compositae).

Distribution Mainly in Chinese provinces such as Henan, Hebei, Zhejiang and Sichuan. Cultivated.

Harvest & Processing Collect flowers on sunny mornings in summer when corollas turn from yellow to red; dry in shaded areas or under the sun.

Description Tubular flower without an ovary; about 1-2 cm long. Outer surface reddish-yellow or red. Corolla tube slender; apex parted into 5 divisions, each division linear (long and narrow) and 5-8 mm long. Stamens 5; anthers yellowish-white, joined together, forming a tube. Stigma long and cylindrical, extending just beyond anther tube, apex slightly forked. Soft in texture. Odour: slightly fragrant; taste: slightly bitter. When soaked in water, water turns golden-yellow.

Indications 1. Dysmenorrhoea, amenorrhoea 2. Coronary heart disease, angina pectoris 3. Trauma and pain

Chemical Composition Contains pigments such as carthamin (0.3-0.6%) and carthamidin.

Flos Caryophylli

Clove

Dingxiang

丁香

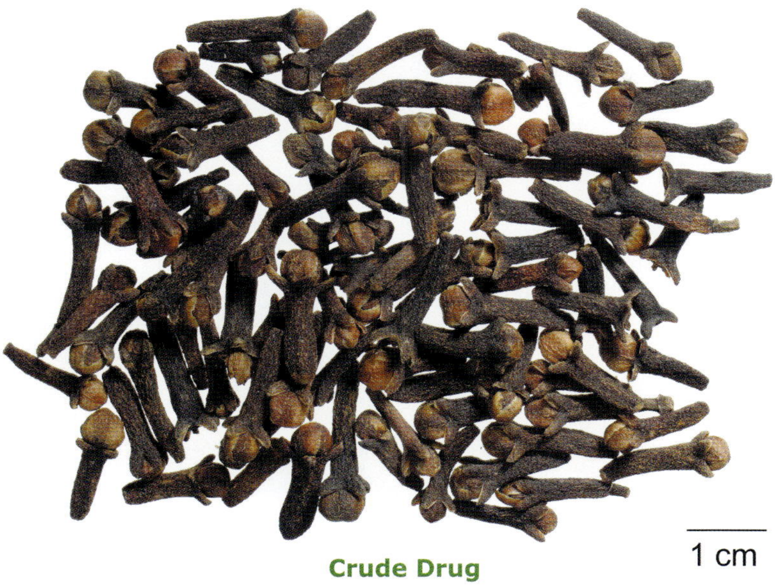

Crude Drug

Source The flower bud of *Eugenia caryophyllata* Thunb. (Fam. Myrtaceae).

Distribution Mainly in Zanzibar Island of Tanzania, and countries such as Malaysia and Indonesia. Introduced into China, the plant is now cultivated in provinces such as Hainan and Guangdong.

Harvest & Processing Collect flower buds when they turn from green to red; dry under the sun.

Description Somewhat pestle-shaped; 1-2cm long. Corolla spherical, 3-5 mm in diameter; petals 4, imbricate (overlapping like tiles on a roof), reddish-brown or dull brownish-yellow; stamens and style inside petals; numerous yellow granular anthers visible after flower buds are rubbed and fall apart. Calyx tube cylindrical, slightly flattened, sometimes slightly curved; 0.7-1.4 cm long; 3-6 mm in diameter; reddish-brown; upper part with 4 triangular sepals stretching out like a cross. Hard, solid and highly oleaginous (oily). Odour: heavily aromatic; taste: pungent and tongue-numbing.

Indications 1. Vomiting, hiccup, anorexia, loose stool 2. Impotence.

Chemical Composition Contains 15-20% essential oils (80-95% eugenol); also contains hydrolysable tannins such as geniin.

Flos Celosiae Cristatae

Cockscomb Flower
Jiguanhua

雞冠花

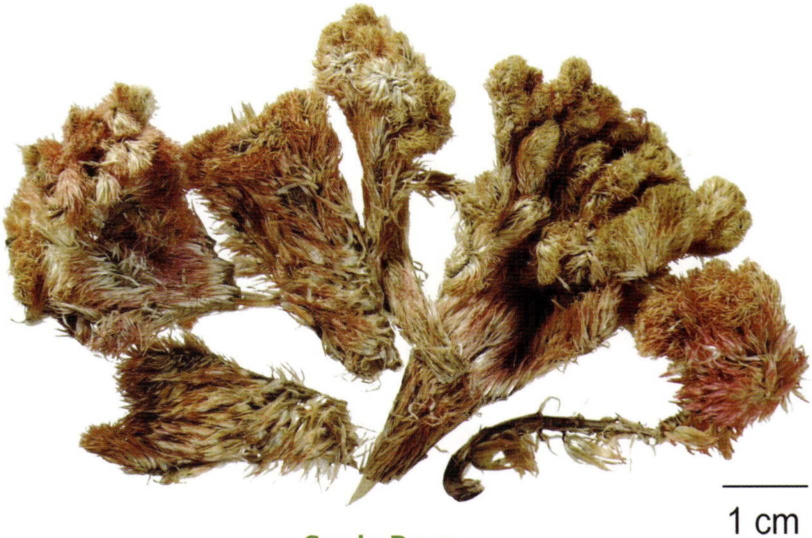

Crude Drug

Source The inflorescence of *Celosia cristata* L. (Fam. Amaranthaceae).

Distribution In most regions of China, including Hong Kong.

Harvest & Processing Harvest inflorescences in August and September; cut off inflorescences with part of haulms; tie up in small bundles; dry under the sun or by airing; cut off haulms.

Description Spike mostly flattened and plump, cristate (crest-shaped); 8-25 cm long, 5-20 cm wide. Upper margin broad, corrugated (wrinkled or folded into alternating furrows and ridges), densely covered with linear (long and narrow) scales; tapering towards bottom end; remnants of flattened stem often still attached to bottom end. Outer surface red, purplish-red or yellowish-white; dense, numerous florets below the middle part; each floret with membranous bracts and tepals. Fruits dehiscent (splitting open at maturity) with the top separating like a lid. Seeds orbicular (round) and reniform (kidney-shaped), black, lustrous. Light in weight; soft and pliable. Odourless; taste: mild.

Indications 1. Epistaxis, haemoptysis, haematemesis, haemorrhoidal bleeding, haematuria, dysfunctional uterine bleeding 2. Diarrhoea 3. Leukorrhagia 4. Urinary tract infection.

Chemical Composition Mainly contains kaempferitrin and amaranthin.

Flos Chimonanthi Praecocis

Wintersweet Flower
Lameihua
蠟梅花

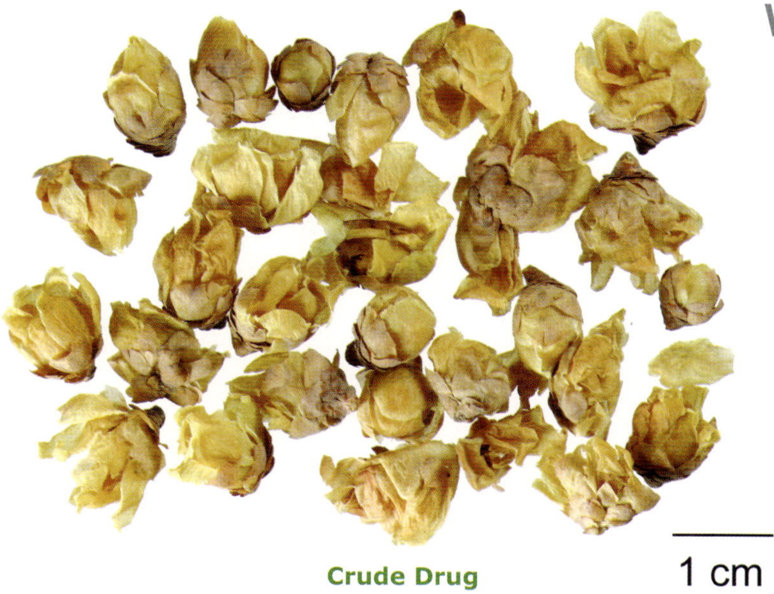

Crude Drug

Source The flower bud of *Chimonanthus praecox* (L.) Link (Fam. Calycanthaceae).

Distribution Mainly in Chinese provinces such as Jiangsu, Zhejiang, Sichuan and Guizhou.

Harvest & Processing Pick flowers in January and February when they start to bloom; dry under the sun or by heat.

Description Orbicular (round), or short and orbicular, or obovoid (inverse egg shaped); 1-1.5 cm long, 4-8 mm wide. Tepals overlapping, brownish-yellow; lower half covered with numerous membranous scales; scales dull yellowish-brown, triangular, with fine pubescence. Odour: fragrant; taste: slightly sweet and then bitter, slightly greasy.

Indications 1. Polydipsia 2. Dizziness, feeling of oppression in the chest, epigastric distension, globus hystericus 3. Sore throat, whooping cough, measles 4. Burn and scald

Chemical Composition Mainly contains essential oils with linalool and bornyl acetate as the main components.

Flos Chrysanthemi

Chrysanthemum Flower
Juhua

菊花

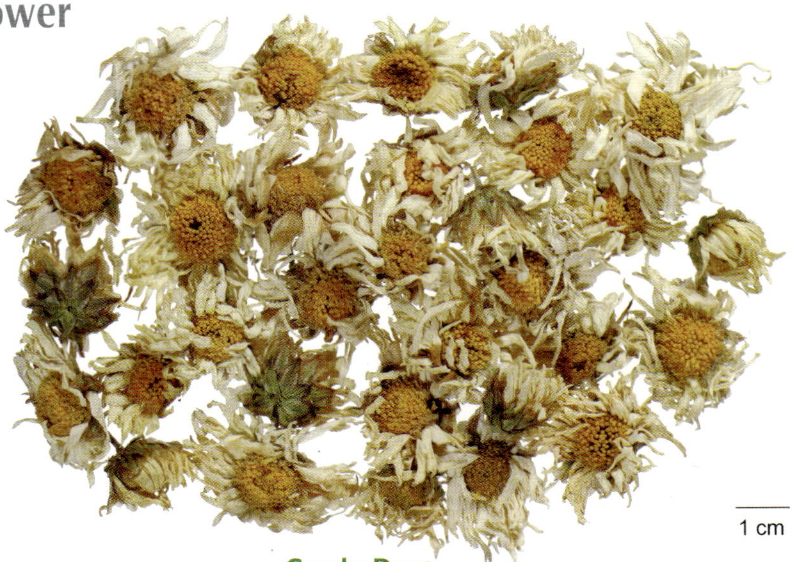

Crude Drug

Source The capitate inflorescence of *Chrysanthemum morifolium* Ramat. (Fam. Compositae).

Distribution Mainly in Zhejiang. Customarily called '*Hangju*' (Hangzhou Chrysanthemum Flower).

Harvest & Processing Collect capitula in batches from September to November when flowers are in full bloom; dry in shaded areas or by baking. Alternatively, steam and then dry under the sun.

Description Pateriform (saucer-shaped), or flattened and spherical, often sold as a mass consisting of several capitula clustered together; 2.5-4 cm in diameter. Phyllaries in many layers; outer surface green, pubescent (covered with short, soft hairs); margin membranous. Ligulate (strap-shaped) flowers off-white or yellow, smoothed out or slightly folded, joined together, usually without gland dots; tubular flowers numerous, exserted (protruding beyond the surrounding parts). Light in weight; soft and smooth; loose and brittle when dried. Odour: fresh and fragrant; taste: sweet, slightly bitter.

Indications 1. Vertigo 2. Red eyes, photophobia with lacrimation, conjunctivitis 3. Headache with fever.

Chemical Composition Mainly contains handelin chrysanthelide, chrysanthenmol and indicumenone.

Flos Chrysanthemi Indici

Wild Chrysanthemum Flower

Yejuhua

野菊花

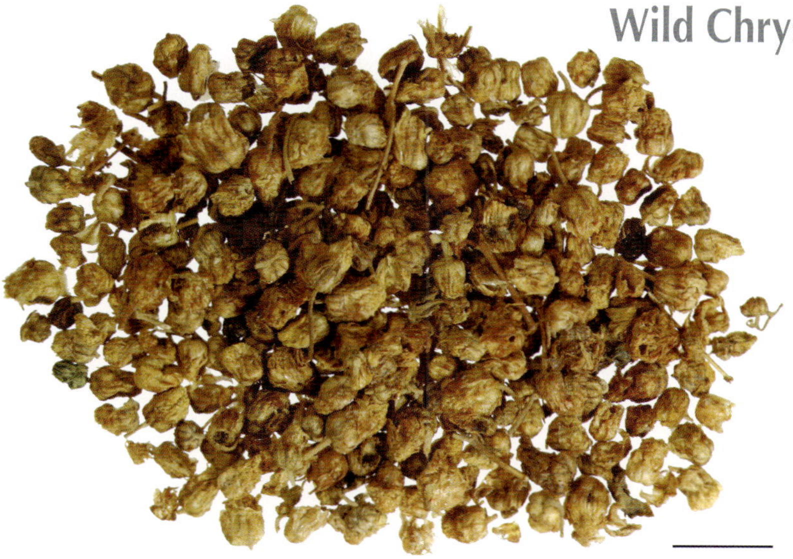

Crude Drug

Source The capitate inflorescences of *Chrysanthemum indicum* L. (Fam. Compositae).

Distribution In most regions of China, including Hong Kong.

Harvest & Processing Pick capitate inflorescences in autumn and winter when flowers start to bloom; dry under the sun, or steam and then dry under the sun.

Description Subspherical; 1-2.5 cm in diameter; brownish-yellow. Phyllaries in 4-5 layers. Outer bracts ovate (egg-shaped in outline and attached at the broad end) or linear (long and narrow); middle part of outer surface greyish-green or pale brown; outer surface usually covered with white pubescence; margin membranous. Inner bracts oblong and elliptical, membranous; outer surface glabrous (without hairs). Base of involucre sometimes with remnants of a common peduncle. Ligulate (strap-shaped) flowers in 1 whorl, yellow, shrivelled and curled; tubular flowers numerous, dark yellow. Light in weight. Odour: aromatic; taste: bitter.

Indications 1. Carbuncle, furuncle, skin nodules 2. Sore throat, influenza. 3. Red eyes, photophobia with lacrimation, conjunctivitis 4. Hypertension with headache, irritability, flushed face

Chemical Composition Mainly contains handelin chrysanthelide, chrysanthemol and acaciin.

Flos Citri Aurantii

Daidaihua Flower Bud
Daidaihua

玳玳花

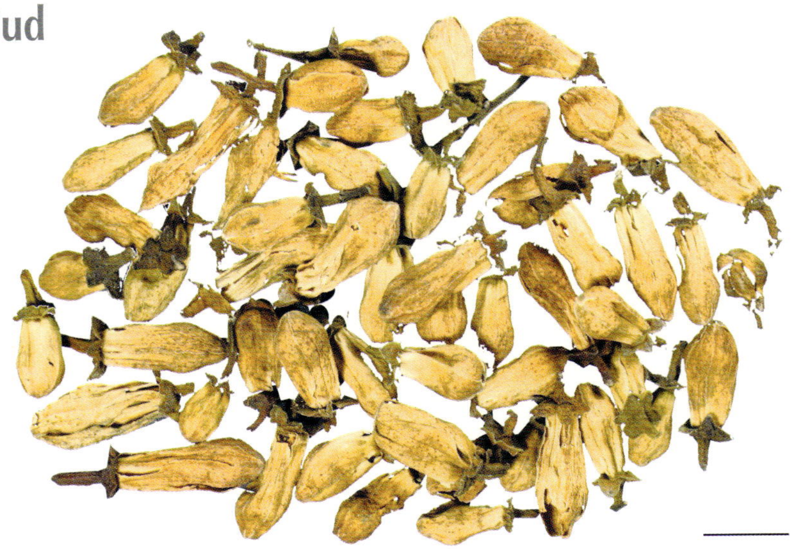

Crude Drug

Source The flower bud of *Citrus aurantium* L. var. *amara* Engl. (Fam. Rutaceae).

Distribution Mainly in Chinese provinces such as Jiangsu and Zhejiang; also in some regions in southeastern China.

Harvest & Processing On sunny mornings in mid-June, pick flower buds ready to burst; dry by the heat of a small fire.

Description Slightly oblong and ovoid (egg-shaped); apex slightly bulgy; 1-1.5 cm long, 6-8 mm in diameter; pedicellate (with a peticel). Calyx greyish-green, shrivelled and uneven; synobasic (with a united base); with 5 lobes; marked with dents of tiny oil dots. Petals 5, imbricate (overlapping like tiles on a roof), yellowish-white or light yellowish-brown; outer surface marked with brown oil dots and longitudinal striae. Stamens numerous, yellow; filaments synobasic and divided into several bundles. Pistils baculiform (rod-shaped); ovary obovoid (inverse egg shaped), dull green. Light in weight; brittle, breaks easily. Odour: fragrant; taste: slightly bitter.

Indications 1. Feeling of oppression in the chest 2. Abdominal distension and pain, anorexia, nausea and vomiting

Chemical Composition Mainly contains essential oils.

Flos Daturae

Datura Flower

Yangjinhua

洋金花

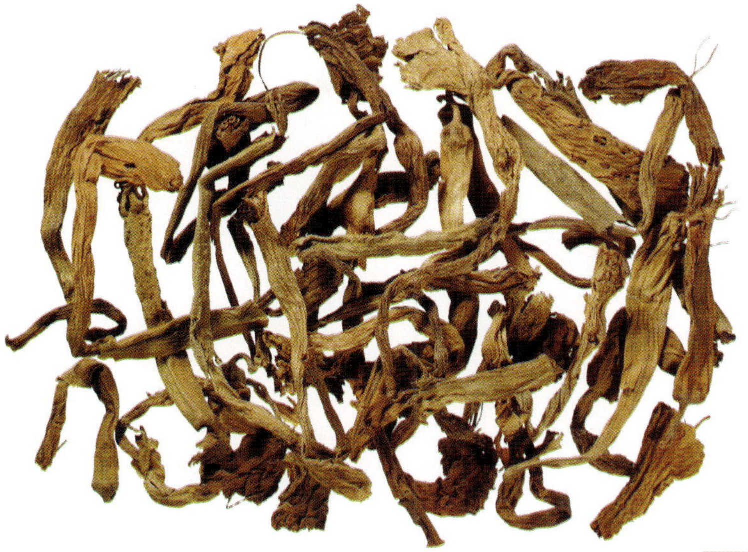

1 cm

Crude Drug

Source The flower of *Datura metel* L. (Fam. Solanaceae). Customarily called '*Nan yangjinhua*' (South Datura Flower).

Distribution Mainly in Chinese provinces such as Jiangsu, Zhejiang, Fujian and Guangdong. Mostly cultivated.

Harvest & Processing Collect flowers in batches when they start to bloom during efflorescence; dry under the sun or dry speedily by heat at low temperatures.

Description Mostly shrivelled and strip-shaped; when intact, 9-15 cm long. Calyx tubular, 2/5 the length of corolla, greyish-green or greyish-yellow; apex 5-lobed; base with 5 longitudinal venous (vein-like) striae; outer surface slightly pubescent (covered with short, soft hairs). Corolla trumpet-shaped, pale yellow or yellowish-brown; apex 5 lobed; each lobe mucronate (with a short straight point), with 3 prominent longitudinal venous striae on the underside near the tip; slightly notched between lobes. When cut open, 5 stamens exposed, filaments adnate (fused with an unlike organ) to corolla tube and 3/4 the length of corolla; pistil 1, stigma clavate (club-shaped, gradually widening towards the apex). Odour: distinctive. Those dried under the sun brittle; odour: faint; taste: slightly bitter.

Indications 1. Bronchial asthma, chronic bronchitis 2. Epigastric pain, toothache, rheumatic pain, post traumatic pain 3. Surgical anaesthesia.

Chemical Composition Mainly contains 0.12-0.82% alkaloids, such as scopolamine, hyoscyamine and atropine.

Note Listed in Hong Kong as Category I (Toxic/Potent) Chinese Materia Medica.

Flos Eriocauli

Pipewort Flower
Gujingcao

穀精草

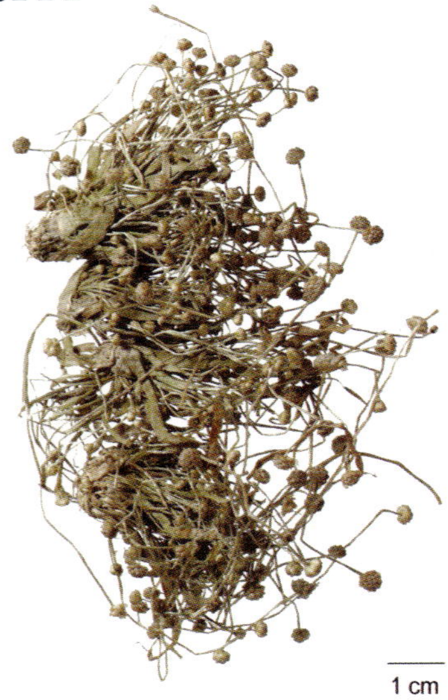

Crude Drug(Eriocaulon buergerianum)

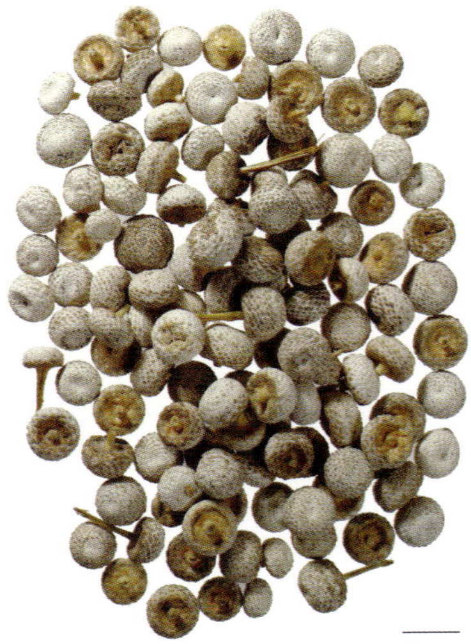

Crude Drug(Eriocaulon sexangulare)

Source The capitulum and the whole herb of *Eriocaulon buergerianum* Koern. (Fam. Eriocaulaceae).

Distribution Mainly in Chinese provinces such as Jiangsu, Zhejiang, Anhui and Jiangxi.

Harvest & Processing Pull up capitula together with peduncles in autumn; dry under the sun to produce '*Gujingcao*' (Pipewort Flower). The product with peduncles cut off is called '*Gujinzhu*' (Pipewort without Peduncles).

Description Capitulum hemispherical; 4-9 mm in diameter; base covered with dense layers of bracts; bracts pale yellowish-green, lustrous, upper margin covered densely with white pubescence; top part of capitulum greyish-white; when crumbled, numerous black anthers and tiny, green immature fruits exposed. Peduncle slender; varying in length, less than 1 mm in diameter; pale yellowish-green, with several twisting ridges. Soft. Odourless; taste: mild.

Indications 1. Conjunctivitis 2. Headache, toothache 3. Nebula

Chemical Composition Mainly contains flavonoid glycosides.

Note In Hong Kong, also used for medicinal purposes is the capitulum of *E. sexangulre* L.

Flos Farfarae

Common Coltsfoot Flower
Kuandonghua

款冬花

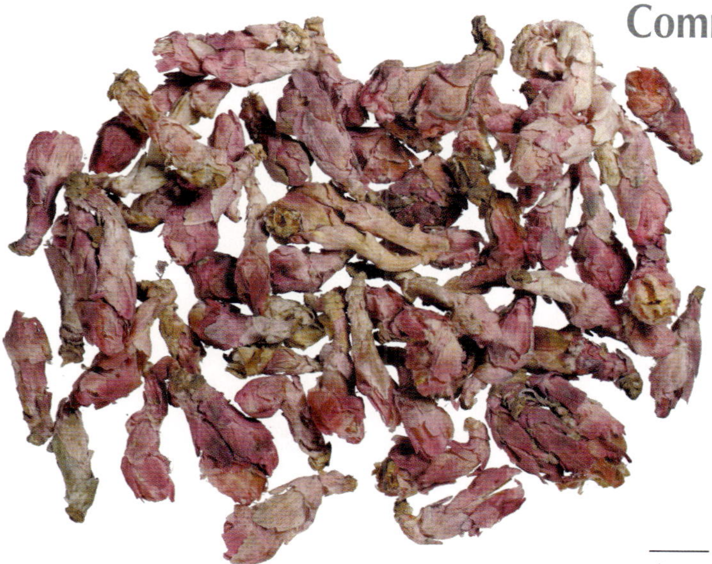

Crude Drug

1 cm

Source The flower bud of capitulum of *Tussilago farfara* L. (Fam. Compositae).

Distribution Mainly in Chinese provinces such as Henan, Gansu, Shanxi and Shaanxi.

Harvest & Processing Dig out flower buds in winter before they appear above the ground; dry in cool, well-ventilated places; when half-dry, sieve away soil and sand; remove pedicels; dry thoroughly by airing.

Description Irregular, orbicular (round) and clavate (club-shaped, gradually widening towards the apex). Solitary (occurring singly) or 2-3 flowers synobasic (with a united base); 1-2.5 cm long, 0.5-1 cm in diameter. Base with squamiform (scale-like) light purple leaves; capitate inflorescences covered with numerous squamiform bracts; outer surface of bracts purplish-red or pale red, inner surface with white tomenta. Ligulate (strap-shaped) flowers and tubular flowers small, about 2 mm long; ovary inferior (attached beneath). Light in weight; broken surface of capitate inflorescences with white filiform (thread-like) tomenta. Odour: fresh and fragrant; taste: slightly bitter, chewy; gossypine (cottony) when chewed.

Indications 1. Productive cough with dyspnoea, asthma

Chemical Composition Mainly contains alkaloids such as tussilagine, sesquiterpenes such as tussilagone, and triterpenes such as faradiol.

Flos Inulae

Inula Flower
Xuanfuhua

旋覆花

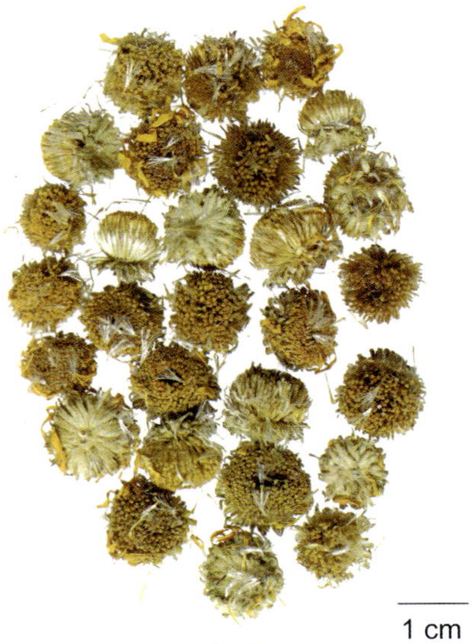

Crude Drug
(Inula japonica)

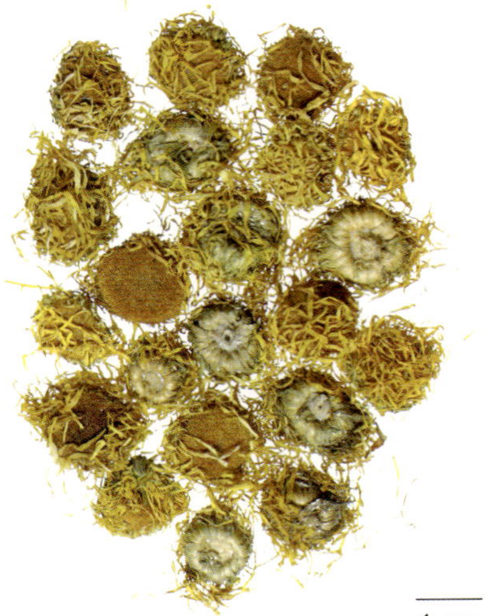

Crude Drug
(Inula britannica)

Source The capitate inflorescence of *Inula japonica* Thunb. (Fam. Compositae).

Distribution Mainly in Chinese provinces such as Henan, Hebei, Jiangsu and Zhejiang.

Harvest & Processing Collect capitate inplorescences in summer and autumn during efflorescence; remove foreign matter; dry under the sun or in shaded areas.

Description Flattened and spherical, or subspherical, mostly loose; 1-2 cm in diameter. Phyllaries in 5 layers, imbricate (overlapping like tiles on a roof), lanceolate (lance-head shaped) or linear (long and narrow), 4-11 mm long, greyish-yellow; involucre base sometimes with peduncle remnants; outer surface of phyllaries and peduncle covered with white pubescence. Ligulate (strap-shaped) flowers in 1 row, yellow, about 1 cm long; petals mostly curled, often fallen off; apex 3-toothed. Tubular flowers numerous, brownish-yellow, about 5 mm long; apex 5-toothed; top end of ovary with numerous white pappi about 5-6 mm long. Light in weight; brittle, breaks and scatters easily. Odour: faint; taste: slightly bitter.

Indications 1. Productive cough with thick sputum and difficult expectoration, feeling of oppression in the chest, dyspnoea 2. Vomiting and belching 3. Acute lumbar sprain.

Chemical Composition Mainly contains britannilactone, quercetin and tamarixetin.

Note According to *C.P.*, also used for medicinal purposes as Flos Inulae is the capitate inflorescence of *I. britannica* L.

Flos Jasmini

Largeflower Jasmine Flower

Suxinhua

素馨花

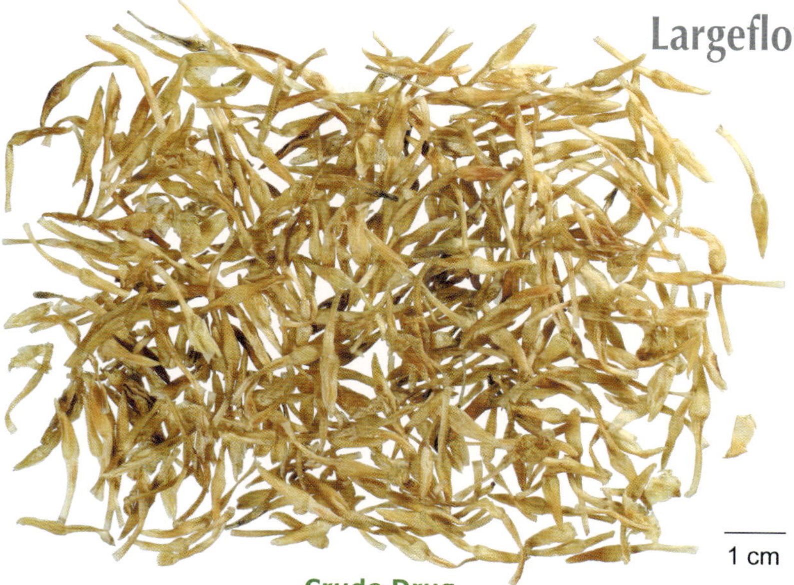

1 cm

Crude Drug

Source The flower bud or flower of *Jasminum officinale* var. *grandiflorum* (L.) Kobuski (Fam. Oleaceae).

Distribution Mainly in Chinese provinces such as Yunnan, Guangdong, Sichuan and Fujian.

Harvest & Processing Pick flower buds or flowers on sunny mornings in summer and autumn when flower buds are formed; steam for 15-20 minutes; take out when softened; dry under the sun.

Description Shaped like the head of a writing brush; 2-3 cm long. Outer surface golden-yellow or pale yellowish-brown; shrivelled. Corolla tube fine and fistular (hollow and cylindrical); 1-2 cm long, 1-1.5 mm in diameter. Corolla 5-lobed, imbricate (overlapping like tiles on a roof), 2-3 mm in diameter; when cut open, the two stamens on the upper part of corolla tube revealed; filaments short; anthers long, narrow and orbicular (round); centre often with style remnants. Relatively brittle; softens when moistened. Odour: fragrant; taste: slightly bitter-astringent.

Indications
1. Distension and pain over hypochondria and abdomen (due to peptic ulcer, dyspepsia, chronic hepatitis and cirrhosis etc.)
2. Dysentery with abdominal pain

Chemical Composition Mainly contains linalool, indole and jasmine lactone.

Flos Lonicerae

Honeysuckle Flower
Jinyinhua

金銀花

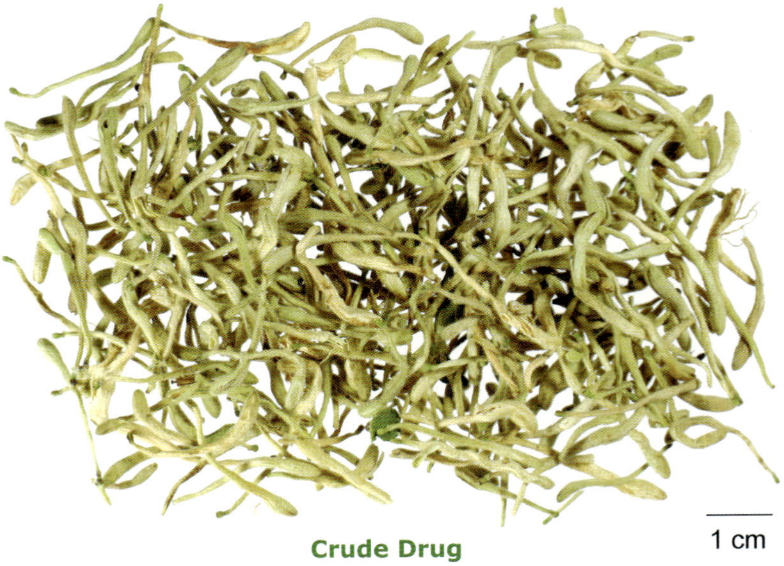

Crude Drug

Source The flower bud or newly-bloomed flower of *Lonicera japonica* Thunb. (Fam. Caprifoliaceae).

Distribution Mainly in Chinese provinces such as Shandong and Henan; also in most other regions of China.

Harvest & Processing Collect flower buds in May and June; dry in cool, well-ventilated places, or spread out and dry under the sun.

Description Small clavate (club-shaped, gradually widening towards the apex), thicker in the upper part and smaller in the lower part, slightly curved; 2-3 cm long; upper part about 3 mm in diameter, lower part about 1.5 mm in diameter. Outer surface yellowish-white or greenish-white, densely pubescent (covered with short, soft hairs), colour darkens when stored for a long time; occasionally with phylloid (leaf-like) bracts. Calyx green; apex 5-lobed, each lobe hairy and about 2 mm long. Corolla of opening flower buds tubular; apex bilabiate (two-lipped); stamens 5, yellow, adnate (fused with an unlike organ) to corolla tube wall; pistil 1, ovary glabrous (without hairs). Odour: fresh and fragrant; taste: mild, slightly bitter.

Indications 1. Influenza, upper respiratory infection, tonsillitis, acute conjunctivitis 2. Enteritis 3. Pyodermas, wound infections 4. Cervical erosion.

Chemical Composition Mainly contains chlorogenic acid, ginnol and essential oils.

Note According to *C.P.*, also used for medicinal purposes is the flower bud or newly-bloomed flower of *L. hypoglauca* Miq., of *L. confusa* DC. and of *L. dasystyla* Rehd.

Flos Magnoliae

Magnolia Flower Bud

Xinyi

辛夷

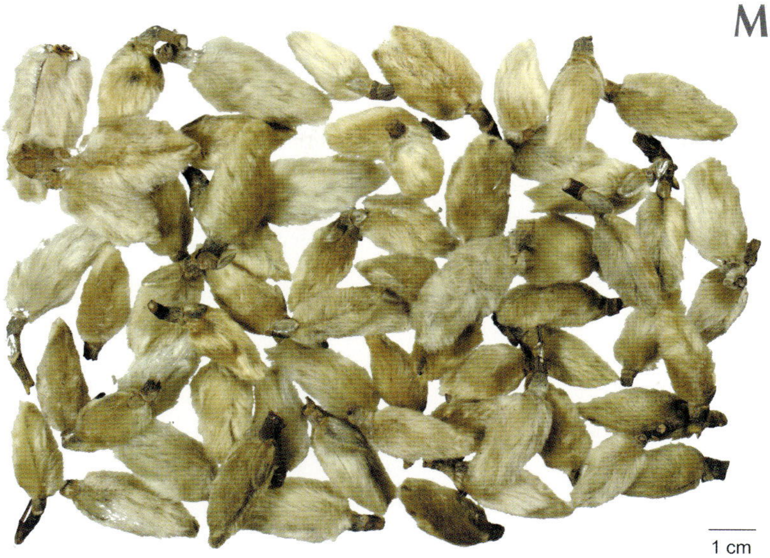

Crude Drug

Source The flower bud of *Magnolia biondii* Pamp. (Fam. Magnoliaceae).

Distribution Mainly in Chinese provinces such as Henan, Sichuan, Shaanxi and Hubei.

Harvest & Processing Collect flower buds from late winter to early spring and before efflorescence; remove foreign matter; dry in shaded areas.

Description Oblong and ovoid (egg-shaped), resembling the head of a writing brush; 1.2-2.5 cm long, 0.8-1.5 cm in diameter. Base mostly with a short pedicel marked with off-white punctiform (dot-like) lenticels. Bracts in 2-3 layers, 2 bracts in each layer, with a small scaly bud between layers; outer surface of bracts densely covered with long, lustrous, greyish-white or greyish-green pubescence; inner surface of bracts purplish-brown, glabrous (without hairs). Perianth in 9 brownish tepals; 3 tepals in outer whorl, linear (long and narrow), sepaloid (sepal-like in colour and texture); 6 tepals in 2 inner whorls, with 3 in each whorl. Numerous stamens and pistils arranged in a spiroid (spiral-like) pattern. Light in weight; brittle. Odour: aromatic; taste: acrid and slightly bitter, relieves blocked nose.

Indications 1. Headache 2. Nasal discharge, nasal congestion, acute and chronic rhinitis, sinusitis

Chemical Composition Mainly contains essential oils.

Note According to *C.P.*, also used for medicinal purposes is the flower bud of *M. denudata* Desr. and *M. sprengeri* Pamp.

Flos Magnoliae Cocinis

Chinese Magnolia Flower
Yehehua

夜合花

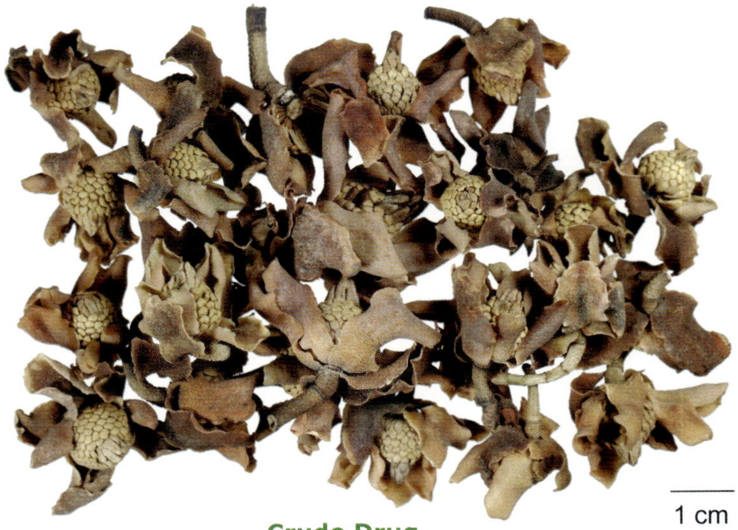

Crude Drug

Source The flower of *Magnolia coco* (Lour.) DC. (Fam. Magnoliaceae).

Distribution Mainly in Chinese provinces such as Guangdong, Guangxi, Fujian, Taiwan and Yunnan.

Harvest & Processing Collect flowers in May and June; remove foreign matter; dry under the sun.

Description Slightly umbelliform (umbrella-shaped), inverse campanulate (bell-shaped), or irregular and spherical; outer surface dull red to brownish-purple. Sepals 3, oblong and obovate (egg-shaped in outline and attached at the narrower end), with granular protuberances on both sides. Petals 6, obovate, curled and shrivelled; 3 outer pieces larger, about 2 cm long, about 1.2 cm wide; base of outer surface with granular protuberances; inner surface smooth; thick, hard and brittle. Stamens numerous, arranged in a spiroid (spiral-like) manner, rosulate (arranged in a dense radiating cluster). Pistil with 7-8 distinct (separate, not attached to like parts) carpels; carpels narrow, long and prismatic, dull purplish-brown or reddish-brown, strumulose (with small cushion-like protuberances). Odour: extremely aromatic; taste: mild.

Indications 1. Distension and pain in the hypochondrium and breast, hernia pain, trauma 2. Abdominal mass 3. Insomnia 4. Cough and dyspnoea 5. Leukorrhagia

Chemical Composition Mainly contains alkaloids and essential oils.

Note Commonly known as '*Hehuanhua*' (Silktree Albizia Flower) in Hong Kong.

Flos Magnoliae Officinalis

Officinal Magnolia Flower

Houpohua

厚樸花

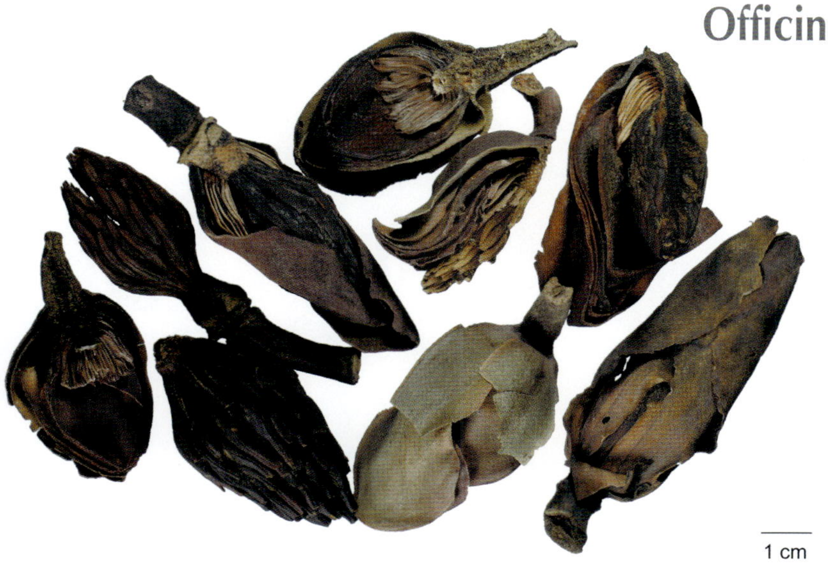

Crude Drug

Source The flower bud of *Magnolia officinalis* Rehd. et Wils. (Fam. Magnoliaceae).

Distribution Mainly in Chinese provinces such as Sichuan, Hubei, Zhejiang, Hunan, Jiangxi and Guizhou.

Harvest & Processing Harvest flower buds in late spring and early summer before efflorescence; place buds in a steamer; steam for 10 minutes or so after the steam starts to escape; take buds out; dry under the sun or over a gentle fire. Alternatively, dry buds over a gentle fire or under the sun without steaming.

Description Oblong and ellipsoid (elliptical in long-section and circular in cross-section); 4-8 cm long, 1.5-3 cm in diameter; brownish-red to reddish-brown. Pedicel 0.5-2 cm long, about 5 mm in diameter; densely covered with greyish-yellow villi. Tepals mostly 12, those of the outer whorl rectangular and obovate (egg-shaped in outline and attached at the narrower end), those of the inner whorl spatulate (spoon-shaped); fleshy; marked with numerous greyish-yellow punctiform (dot-like) warts. Stamens and pistils numerous, spirally arranged on an elongated receptacle; anthers linear (long and narrow), pale yellowish-brown; filaments thick and short. Brittle, breaks easily. Odour: fragrant; taste: mild and slightly hot.

Indications
1. Feeling of fullness in the chest and epigastrium distension
2. Anorexia

Chemical Composition Mainly contains lignans such as magnolol and honokiol; also contains camphor.

Note According to *C.P.*, also used for medicinal purposes is the flower bud of *M. officinalis* Rehd. et Wils. *var biloba* Rehd. et Wils.

Flos Plumeriae

Frangipani Flower
Jidanhua

雞蛋花

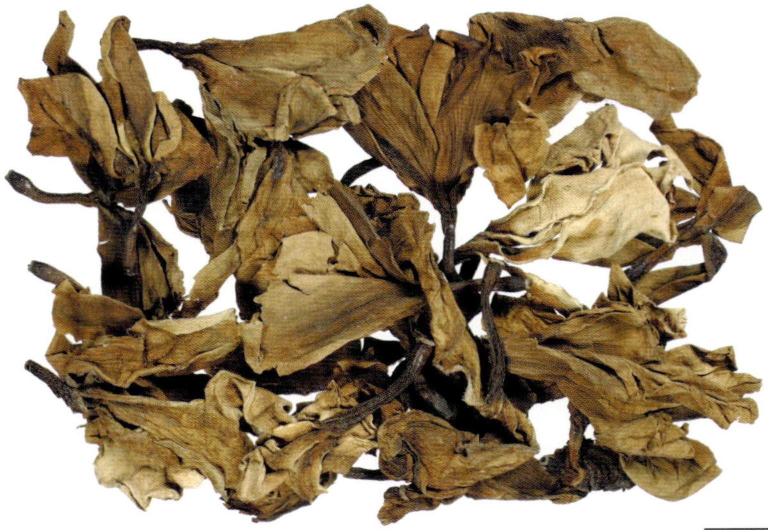

Crude Drug 1 cm

Source The flower of *Plumeria rubra* L. cv. acutifolia (Fam. Apocynaceae).

Distribution Mainly in Chinese provinces such as Fujian, Guangdong, Hainan, Taiwan, Guangxi and Yunnan; also in Hong Kong.

Harvest & Processing Pick flowers during efflorescence; dry under the sun or use while fresh.

Description Mostly shrivelled, long and narrow, or flat and triangular; pale brownish-yellow or dull yellowish-brown. When moistened and smoothed out, calyx relatively small. Corolla 5-lobed, obovate (egg-shaped in outline and attached at the narrower end); about 3 cm long, about 1.5 cm wide; arranged in spiroid (spiral-like) form; lower part accrete (grown or joined together), forming a fine tube about 1.5 cm long. Stamens 5; filaments extremely short. Sometimes ovoid (egg-shaped) ovary visible. Odour: fragrant; taste: slightly bitter.

Indications 1. Common cold with fever, cough with yellow sputum 2. Jaundice 3. Diarrhoea and dysentery 4. Renal stone 5. Heat stroke prevention

Chemical Composition Iridoids such as plumieride exist in the trunk bark and root.

Flos Rhododendri Mollis

Yellow Azalea Flower
Naoyanghua
鬧羊花

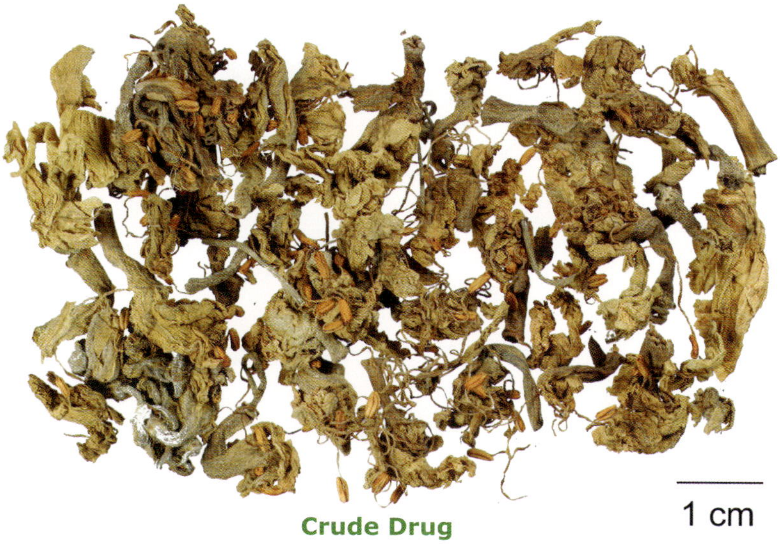

Crude Drug

Source The flower of *Rhododendron molle* G. Don (Fam. Ericaceae).

Distribution Mainly in Chinese provinces such as Henan, Jiangsu, Zhejiang and Jiangxi.

Harvest & Processing Collect flowers in April and May when they start to bloom; dry in shaded areas or under the sun.

Description Flowers already in bloom are mostly shrivelled and sometimes with pedicels; 6-12 flowers conglomerate (densely clustered) on 1 common pedicel. Pedicels 1-7cm long; reddish-brown; puberulent (covered with fine, short, soft hairs). Calyx small; 5-lobed; margin with longer fine hairs. Corolla tube about 3 cm long, curved at apex; yellowish-grey to dull yellowish-brown; outer surface sparsely pubescent (covered with short, soft hairs); 5-lobed, each lobe almost as long as corolla tube. Stamens relatively long, with filaments protruding beyond corolla; anthers reddish-brown, apex poricidal (opening by pores). Styles of pistils longer than stamens; stigmas capitate (head-shaped). Odour: slightly fragrant; taste: slightly numbing. Toxic.

Indications 1. Rheumatic arthralgia 2. Trauma 3. Ringworm infection.

Chemical Composition Contains ericolin and rhodomollein III.

Note Listed in Hong Kong as Category I (Toxic/Potent) Chinese Materia Medica.

Flos Rosae Chinensis

Chinese Rose Flower

Yuejihua

月季花

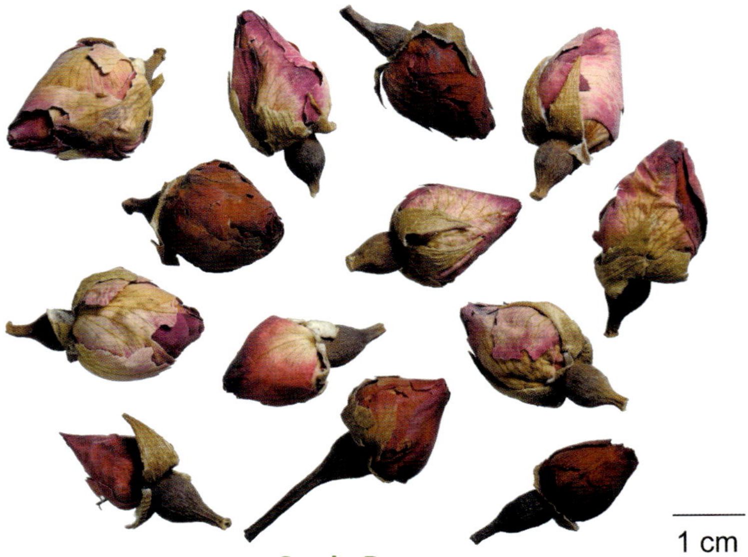

Crude Drug

Source The flower of *Rosa chinensis* Jacq. (Fam. Rosaceae).

Distribution Mainly in Chinese provinces such as Jiangsu, Hubei, Shandong, Hebei, Tianjin and Beijing; also in Hong Kong.

Harvest & Processing Collect flowers in half bloom in summer and autumn; dry by airing or over a gentle fire.

Description Flower bud usually ovoid (egg-shaped) or subspherical; 1-1.5 cm in diameter. Flower usually spherical. Receptacle obconical (inversely conical) or obovoid (inverse egg-shaped); 5-7 mm long, 3-5 mm in diameter; brownish-purple; base relatively pointed, often pedicellate (with a pedicel). Calyx in 5 sepals, apex pointed and usually curling downwards; outer surface sparsely pubescent (covered with short, soft hairs), inner surface covered with white tomenta. Petals 5, or double (with a larger number of petals than usual), with prominent veins. Stamens numerous, yellow; pistils numerous. Light in weight; brittle, breaks easily. Odour: fresh and fragrant; taste: slightly bitter and astringent.

Indications 1. Menstrual disorders, dysmenorrhoea 2. Trauma with ecchymosis and swellings, carbuncles, scrofula (not ruptured) (external use).

Chemical Composition Mainly contains essential oils.

Flos Sophorae

Pagodatree Flower
Huaihua
槐花

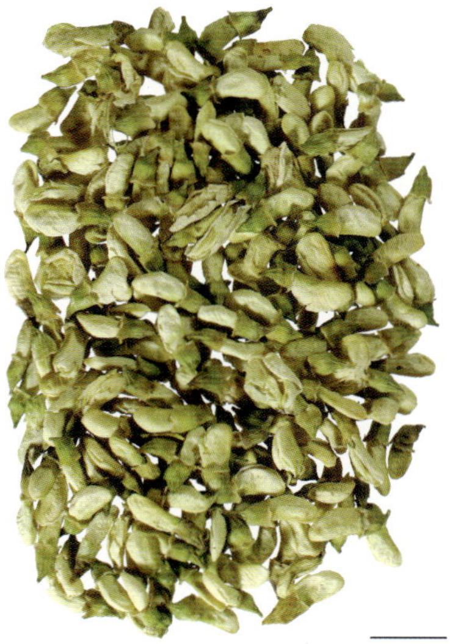

1 cm

Crude Drug(Huaihua)

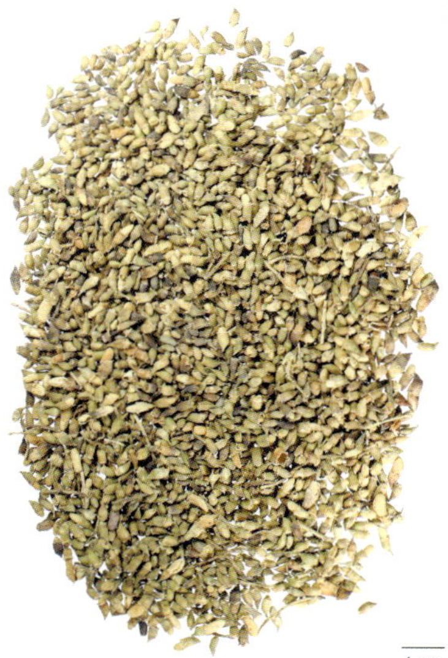

1 cm

Crude Drug(Huaimi)

Source The flower and flower bud of *Sophora japonica* L. (Fam. Leguminosae).

Distribution Mainly in Chinese provinces such as Liaoning, Hebei, Henan and Shandong.

Harvest & Processing In summer, collect flowers during efflorescence, and the flower buds when they are formed. Dry promptly; remove foreign matter. The flower is customarily known as '*Huaihua*' (Pagodatree Flower) and the bud as '*Huaimi*' (Pagodatree Rice).

Description *Huaihua*: Shrivelled and curled; petals mostly fallen off. When intact, calyx campanulate (bell-shaped), yellowish-green; apex 5-lobed. Petals 5, yellow or yellowish-white; 1 piece larger, suborbicular (almost round) and retuse (with a shallow notch in a round or blunt apex); the other 4 pieces oblong and orbicular (round). Stamens 10; 9 of them synobasic (with a united base); filaments slender. Pistil cylindrical and curved. Light in weight. Odourless; taste: slightly bitter.

Huaimi: Ovoid (egg-shaped) or ellipsoid (elliptical in long-section and circular in cross-section), like a grain of rice. Lower part of calyx with several longitudinal striae; above the calyx are yellowish-white petals not yet unfurled.

Indications 1. Bleeding such as haematochezia, haemorrhoidal bleeding, dysfunctional uterine bleeding 2. Diarrhoea.

Chemical Composition Mainly contains triterpene saponins such as kaikasaponins I, II, III, and flavonoids such as quercetin.

Folium Apocyni Veneti

Dogbane Leaf
Luobumaye

羅布麻葉

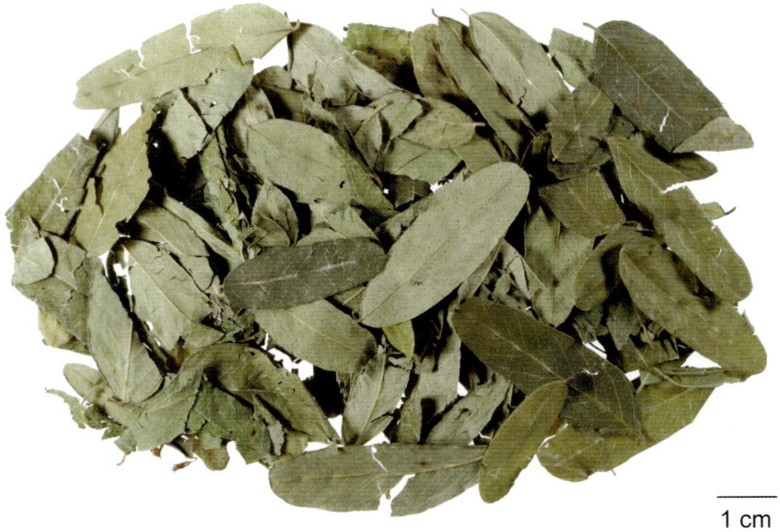

Crude Drug

Source The leaf of *Apocynum venetum* L. (Fam. Apocynaceae).

Distribution Mainly in northwestern, northeastern and northern China.

Harvest & Processing Collect leaves in summer; remove foreign matter; dry under the sun.

Description Mostly shrivelled and curled, some in fragments; when intact and smoothed out, blades elliptical and lanceolate (lance-head shaped), or ovate (egg-shaped in outline and attached at the broad end) and lanceolate; 2-5 cm long, 0.5-2 cm wide; dark green or greyish-green. Apex obtuse and mucronulate (with a very small, sharp tip), base obtuse or cuneate (wedge-shaped); margin serrulate (finely notched), often recurved (curved backwards); both sides glabrous (without hairs); main vein inconspicuous on upper surface but slightly protuberant on underside; lateral veins pinnate (feather-shaped), fine and dense, in 7-10 pairs or more. Petiole thin and short, about 4 mm long. Brittle. Odour: faint; taste: mild.

Indications 1. Headache, dizziness, irritability, insomnia, hypertension 2. Conjunctivitis 3. Cough, chronic cough, dyspnoea 4. Oedema, dysuria.

Chemical Composition Mainly contains flavonoids such as apocynin A, B, C , D.

Folium Artemisiae Argyi

Argy Wormwood Leaf

Aiye

艾葉

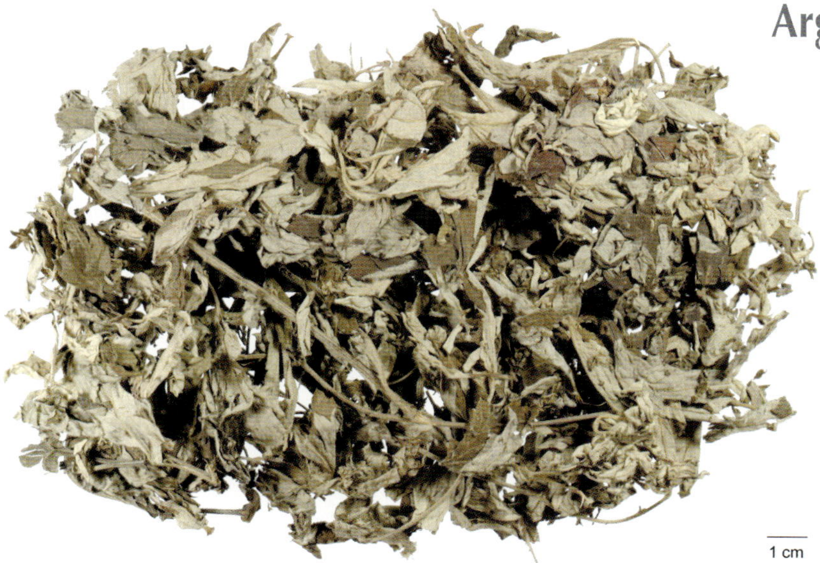

1 cm

Crude Drug

Source The leaf of *Artemisia argyi* Lévl. et Vant. (Fam. Compositae).

Distribution Mainly in Chinese provinces such as Shandong, Anhui, Hubei and Hebei; also in most regions of China.

Harvest & Processing Collect leaves before efflorescence in summer; remove foreign matter; dry under the sun.

Description Mostly shrivelled and in fragments, with a short petiole. When whole and smoothed out, blade ovate (egg-shaped in outline and attached at the broad end) and elliptical; pinnatipartite (parted in a feather-like manner); lobes elliptical and lanceolate (lance-head shaped); margin irregular and grossly serrate (with big saw-like teeth); upper surface greyish-green or dark green, with sparse short arachnoid (like a cobweb) tomenta and gland dots; underside densely covered with greyish-white villi. Texture soft. Odour: fresh and fragrant; taste: bitter.

Indications 1. Bleeding 2. Dysmenorrhoea, abdominal pain 3. Cough, asthma 4. Eczema, dermatitis 5. Recently used for chronic hepatitis and viral myocarditis (IVI).

Chemical Composition Mainly contains essential oils and flavonoids.

Folium Eriobotryae

Loquat Leaf
Pipaye

枇杷葉

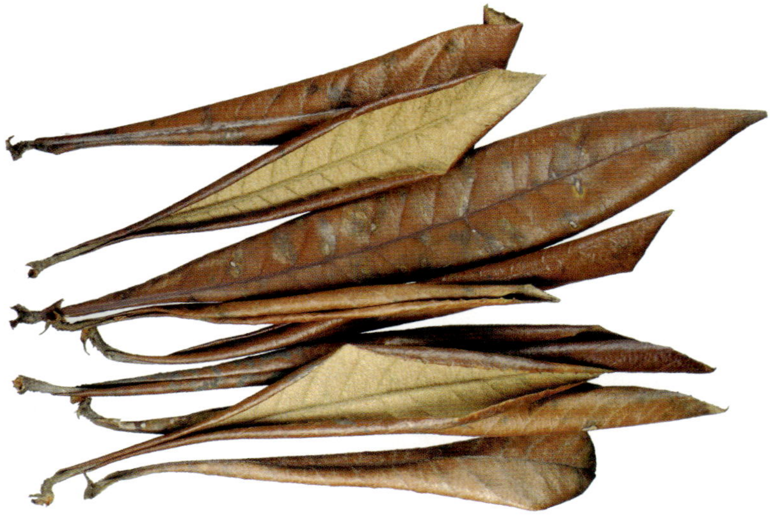

1 cm

Crude Drug

Source The leaf of *Eriobotrya japonica* (Thunb.) Lindl. (Fam. Rosaceae).

Distribution Mainly in regions south of Yangtze River valley in China; also in Hong Kong.

Harvest & Processing Collect leaves anytime during the year; dry under the sun.

Description Oblong and orbicular (round), or obovate (egg-shaped in outline and attached at the narrower end); 12-30 cm long, 3-9 cm wide. Apex pointed, base cuneate (wedge-shaped); margin sparsely serrate (saw-like) at upper part, entire (continuous and even) at base. Upper surface greyish-green, yellowish-brown or reddish-brown, relatively smooth; underside densely covered with yellow villi; main vein conspicuously protuberant on underside, lateral veins pinnate (feather-shaped). Petiole very short, covered with brownish-yellow villi. Coriaceous (leathery) but brittle, breaks easily. Odourless; taste: slightly bitter.

Indications 1. Bronchitis, cough 2. Vomiting.

Chemical Composition Mainly contains essential oils with nerolidol and farnesol as the main components; also contains amygdalin.

Folium et Cacumen Breyniae Fruticosae

Fruitcose Breyniae Leaf and Twig

Heimianshen

黑面神

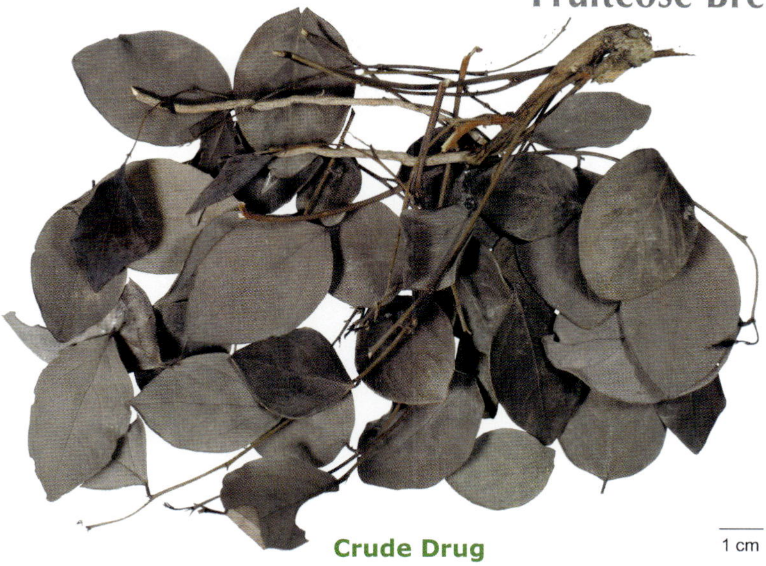

Crude Drug

Source The leaf-bearing twig of *Breynia fruticosa* (L.) Hook. f. (Fam. Euphorbiaceae).

Distribution Mainly in Chinese provinces such as Zhejiang, Fujian, Guangdong, Guangxi, Guizhou and Yunnan; also in Hong Kong.

Harvest & Processing Harvest leaf-bearing twigs anytime during the year; dry under the sun or use while fresh.

Description Twigs often purplish-red; young twigs greyish-green, glabrous (without hairs). Leaves alternate (borne singly at each node), simple (not separated into leaflets), with short petioles; blades coriaceous (leathery), ovate (egg-shaped in outline and attached at the broad end), or broad and ovate; 3-6 cm long, 2-3.5 cm wide; apex obtuse or acute; entire (with continuous, even margin); upper surface with vermiculate (worm-eaten like) markings, underside greyish-white; stipules triangular and lanceolate (lance-head shaped). Twigs and leaves turn black when dried. Odour: faint; taste: mild and slightly astringent.

Indications 1. Abdominal pain, diarrhoea, dysentery 2. Eczema, herpes zoster around waist and hypochondria, dermatitis, allergic dermatitis 3. Rheumatism 4. Galatostasis

Chemical Composition Tannins exist in the stems, roots and leaves; the leaves also contain pheonlics and triterpenes.

Folium et Cacumen Murrayae

Murraya Jasminorage Branch and Leaf
Jiulixiang

九里香

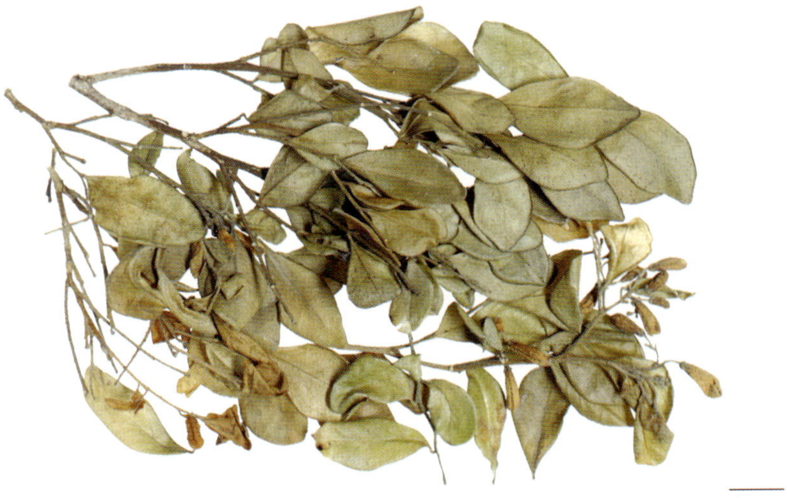

Crude Drug

Source The leaf and leaf-bearing young stem of *Murraya exotica* L. (Fam. Rutaceae).

Distribution Mainly in Chinese provinces such as Guangdong, Guangxi, Fujian and Yunnan; also in Hong Kong.

Harvest & Processing Collect young stems and leaves 1-2 times during peak growing season every year; dry under the sun or use while fresh.

Description Young stem cylindrical; 1-4 mm in diameter; outer surface dark green, pubescent (covered with fine, soft hairs); pliable, does not break easily; when broken, surface fibrous. Compound leaves pinnate (feather-shaped), each with 3-9 leaflets; leaflets ovate (egg-shaped in outline and attached at the broad end), elliptical or near-rhombic, with the widest part at the lower half. Apex mucronate (with a short straight point) or acuminate (tapering to a slender point); base cuneate (wedge-shaped) or slightly slanted; entire (with continuous, even margin); dark green when fresh, gradually turning yellow when dried; upper surface with transparent gland dots; petiolules short or nearly epetiolulate (without petiolules); brittle. Some with acrogenous (growing from the apex) or axillary (growing at axil) cyme; corolla about 4 cm in diameter. Odour: fragrant; taste: bitter, acrid and tongue-numbing.

Indications 1. Various kinds of pain such as stomachache, toothache, rheumatic arthralgia, post traumatic swelling and pain 2. Snakebite, insect bite (external use).

Chemical Composition Mainly contains coumarins.

Note According to *C.P.*, also used for medicinal purposes is the leaf and leaf-bearing young stem of *M. paniculata* (L.) Jack.

Folium Ginkgo

Ginkgo Leaf
Yinxingye

銀杏葉

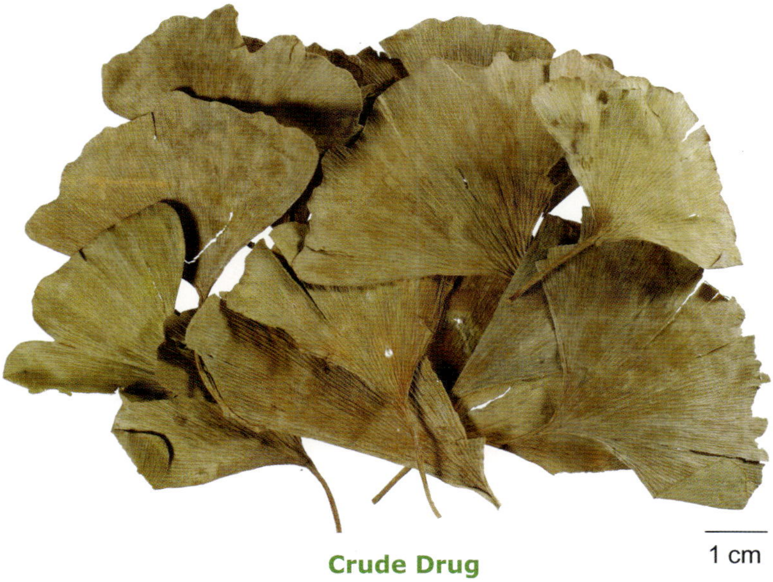

Crude Drug

Source The leaf of *Ginkgo biloba* L. (Fam. Ginkgoaceae).

Distribution Mainly in Chinese provinces such as Guangxi, Sichuan, Henan, Shandong, Hubei, Liaoning and Jiangsu; also cultivated in Hong Kong.

Harvest & Processing Collect leaves in autumn; remove foreign matter; wash leaves clean; dry under the sun.

Description Mostly shrivelled or in fragments, broad whole; 4-8 cm long, 5-10 cm wide; upper margin with irregular undulate (wavy) curves, sometimes notched at the centre; base cuneate (wedge-shaped); veins fine and dense, numerous, dichotomous (branched into two divisions) and parallel. Petiole 2-7 cm long. Papery in texture; tears easily longitudinally. Odour: faint; taste: slightly astringent.

Indications 1. Cough, asthma 2. Coronary heart diseases, angina pectoris, hyperlipidemia. 3. Forgetfulness

Chemical Composition Mainly contains flavonoids and diterpenes such as ginkgolide A, B, C.

Folium Glochidii Eriocarpi

Eriocarpous Glochidion Leaf
Qidagu

漆大姑

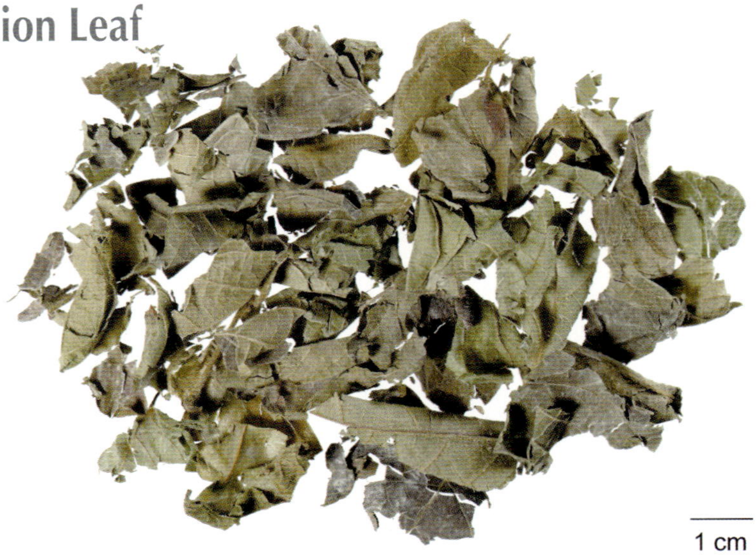

Crude Drug

Source The leaf of *Glochidion eriocarpum* Champ. *ex* Benth. (Fam. Euphorbiaceae).

Distribution Mainly in Chinese provinces such as Fujian, Taiwan, Guangxi, Guangdong, Guizhou and Yunnan; also in Hong Kong.

Harvest & Processing Harvest leaves in summer and autumn; use while fresh or dry under the sun.

Description Leaves simple (not separated into leaflets) and alternate (borne singly at each node); with short petioles. Blades oblong and ovate (egg-shaped in outline and attached at the broad end), or narrow and ovate; 4-8 cm long, 1.5-3.5 cm wide. Apex acuminate (tapering to a slender point); base obtuse or orbicular (round); entire (with continuous, even margin); both sides covered with villi, with those on the underside thicker; stipules subulate (awl-shaped). Papery. Odour: distinctive; taste: bitter-astringent.

Indications 1. Enteritis, dysentery 2. Sore throat, toothache 3. Mastitis 4. Leukorrhagia 5. Eczema, burn and scald

Chemical Composition Contains triterpenes such as gallic acid, glochidone and glochidonol.

Folium Isatidis

Dyers Woad Leaf

Daqingye

大青葉

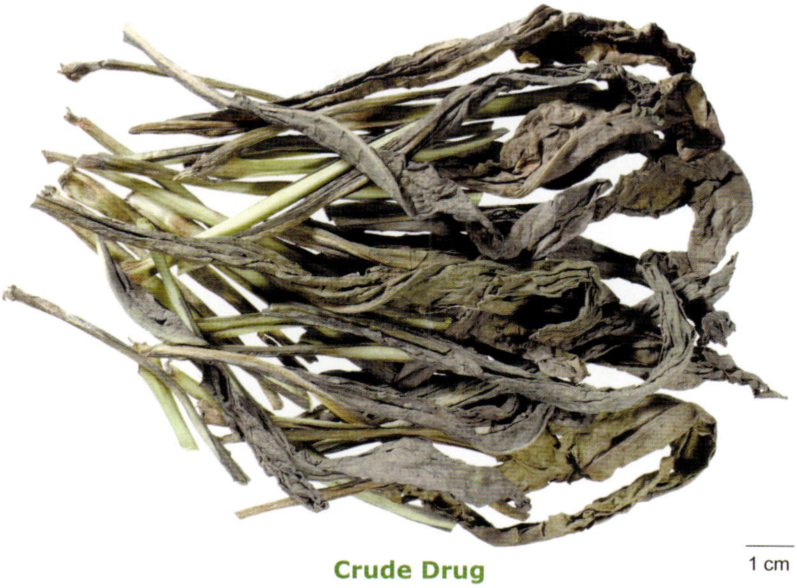

Crude Drug

Source The leaf of *Isatis indigotica* Fort. (Fam. Cruciferae).

Distribution Mainly in Chinese provinces such as Hebei, Shaanxi, Jiangsu and Anhui.

Harvest & Processing Collect leaves in different rounds in summer and autumn; remove foreign matter; dry under the sun.

Description Leaves mostly shrivelled and in fragments; when intact, blades oblong and elliptical to oblong, orbicular (round) and oblanceolate (inverse lance-head shaped); 4-16 cm long, 1-4 cm wide. Apex blunt but slightly pointed or obtuse; base attenuate (tapering gradually to a narrow tip or base) and decurrent (extending downwards), forming an aliform (wing-shaped) petiole; margin entire (continuous and even) or slightly undulate (wavy); upper surface and underside greyish-green or brownish-green, glabrous (without hairs), with pinnate (feather-shaped), reticulate (net-like) veins; main vein protuberant on underside. Brittle. Odour: faint; taste: slightly bitter.

Indications 1. Seasonal febrile diseases, pestilence 2. Influenza, epidemic meningitis, encephalitis B, viral pneumonia, mumps and other eruptive exanthem 3. Sore throat, aphthous ulcer

Chemical Composition Contains indigo, indigotin, isatan B and indirubin.

Folium Lantanae Camarae

Common Lantana Twig and Leaf

Mayingdan

馬纓丹

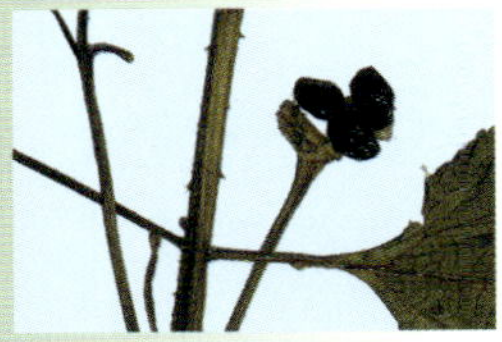

Common Lantana Twig and Leaf Magnified

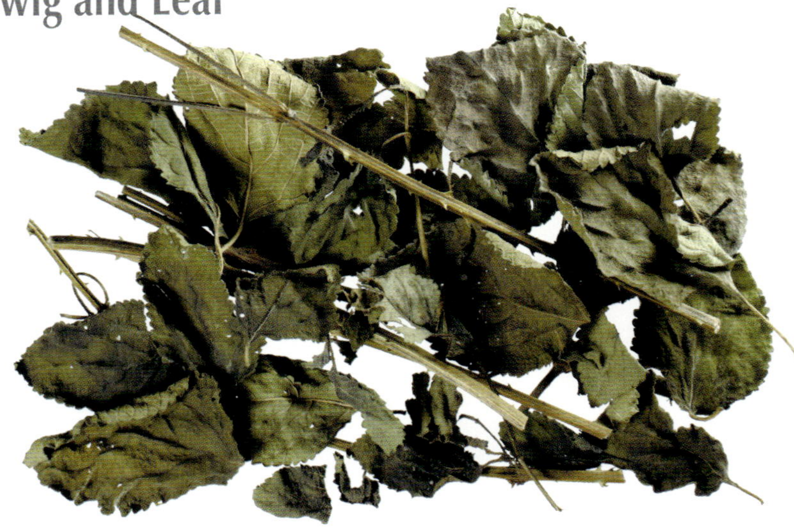

Crude Drug

1 cm

Source The young stem and leaf of *Lantana camara* L. (Fam. Verbenaceae).

Distribution Mainly in Chinese provinces such as Guangdong, Guangxi, Jiangxi, Hunan and Fujian; also in Hong Kong.

Harvest & Processing Harvest young stems and leaves in spring and summer; use while fresh or dry under the sun.

Description Stem quadrangular (four-angled); yellowish-green or greyish-green; usually with retrorse (directed downwards or backwards) barbs. Leaves opposite (borne in pairs at each node); blade yellowish-green, shrivelled; when smoothed out, ovate (egg-shaped in outline and attached at the broad end), or ovate, oblong and orbicular (round); 3-9 cm long, 1.5-5 cm wide. Apex acuminate (tapering to a slender point); base cuneate (wedge-shaped); margin blunt and crenate (with round-toothed edges); outer surface rough. Crumbles easily. Odour: bad.

Indications Flower: 1. Haemoptysis, pulmonary tuberculosis 2. Abdominal pain, vomiting and diarrhoea 3. Eczema, pruritus vulvae
Leaf: Carbuncle and sore, dermatitis, tinea and scabies, trauma

Chemical Composition Mainly contains oleanolic acid, salicyclic acid and lantadene A, B.

Folium Mori

Mulberry Leaf
Sangye
桑葉

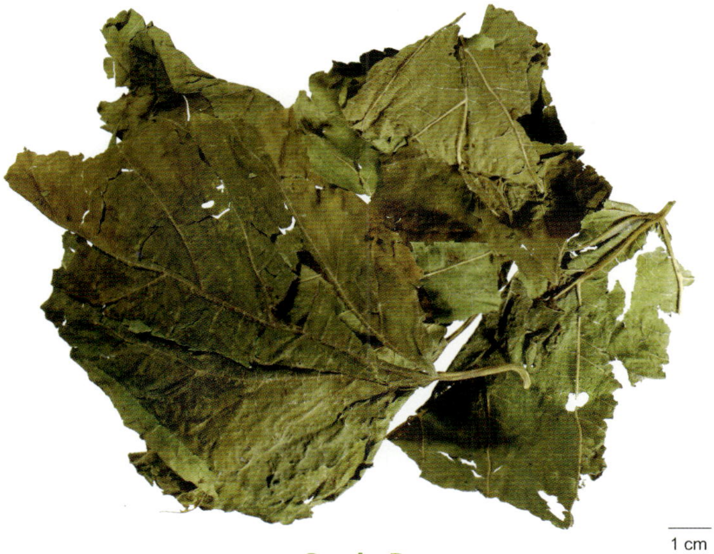

Crude Drug

Source ▶ The leaf of *Morus alba* L. (Fam. Moraceae).

Distribution ▶ Mainly in Chinese provinces such as Anhui, Zhejiang, Jiangsu, Sichuan and Hunan; also in Hong Kong.

Harvest & Processing ▶ Harvest leaves in October and November after frost; remove branchlets and foreign matter; dry under the sun.

Description ▶ Mostly shrivelled and in fragments. When whole, petiolate (with a petiole); petiole 1-2.5 cm long; when smoothed out, blade ovate (egg-shaped in outline and attached at the broad end), or broad and ovate, 8-15 cm long, 7-13 cm wide. Apex acuminate (tapering to a slender point); base truncate (squared as if cut off), orbicular (round) or cordate (heart-shaped); margin serrate (saw-like) or crenate (with round-toothed edges), in some cases irregular lobate (divided into lobes). Upper surface yellowish-green or light yellowish-brown, in some cases verruculose (with small wart-shaped protuberances); underside lighter in colour, with protuberant veins, veinlets reticulate (net-like); veins covered with sparse pubescence, vein base with tufted pubescence. Brittle. Odour: faint; taste: mild, slightly bitter-astringent.

Indications ▶ 1. Common cold, cough, sore throat 2. Red eyes, photophobia with lacrimation, conjunctivitis, blurring of vision 3. Haematemesis, haemoptysis 4. Night sweating.

Chemical Composition ▶ Mainly contains flavonoids such as kuwanon I, and coumarins such as bergapten.

Folium Perillae

Perilla Leaf
Zisuye
紫蘇葉

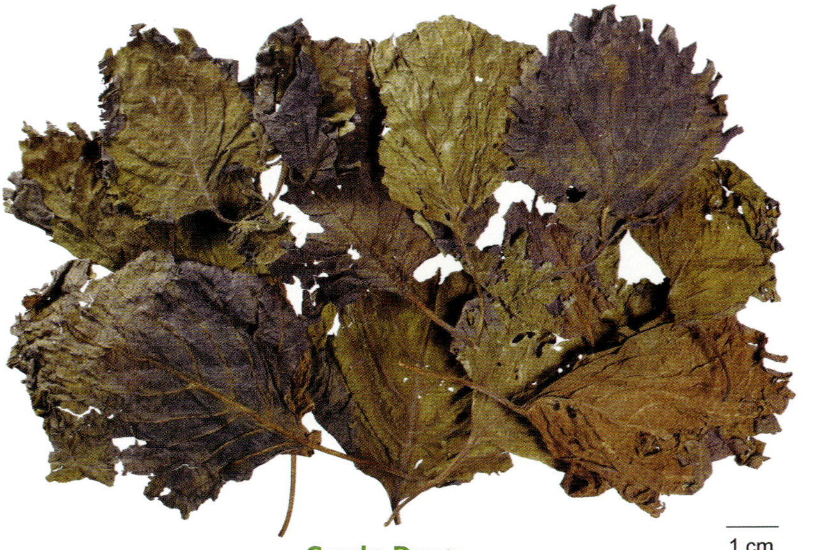

Crude Drug

1 cm

Source The leaf of *Perilla frutescens* (L.) Britt. (Fam. Labiatae).

Distribution Mainly in Chinese provinces such as Shaanxi and Gansu, and in the eastern, middle south and southwestern regions of China; also in Hong Kong.

Harvest & Processing Collect leaves in summer when branches and leaves are abundant; remove foreign matter; dry under the sun.

Description Blades mostly shrivelled, curled, and in fragments; ovate (egg-shaped in outline and attached at the broad end) when intact and smoothed out; 4-11 cm long, 2.5-9 cm wide. Apex acuminate (tapering to a slender point), or acute; base orbicular (round), or broad and cuneate (wedge-shaped). Margin grossly-serrate (with big saw-like teeth). Both sides purple, or upper surface green and underside purple; both sides sparsely covered with greyish-white hairs; underside with numerous dented punctiform (dot-like) glandular scales. Petiole 2-7 cm long, purple or purplish-green. Brittle. Odour: fresh and fragrant; taste: slightly acrid.

Indications 1. Common cold, headache, cough 2. Feeling of oppression in the chest, nausea, vomiting 3. Food poisoning from fish and crab.

Chemical Composition Mainly contains essential oils with perillaldehyde and α-bergamotene as the major components; also contains perilloside B, C.

Folium Photiniae

Chinese Photinia Leaf
Shinanye
石楠葉

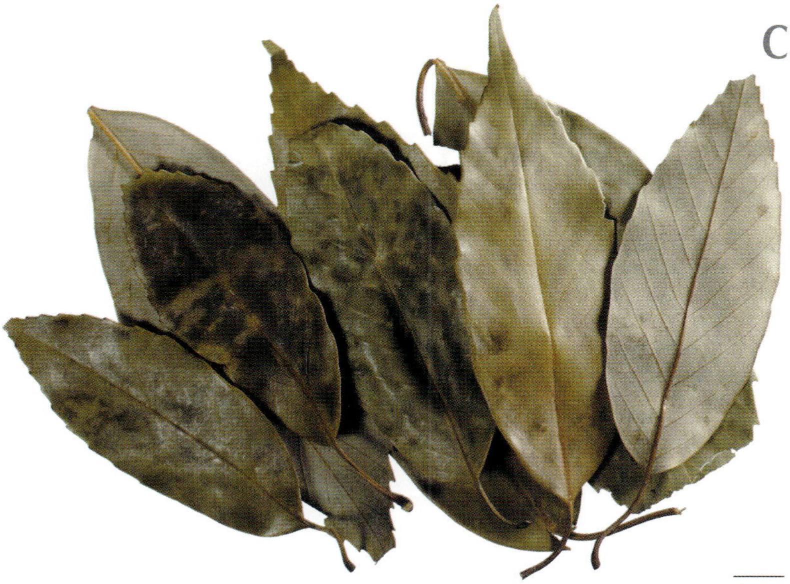

Crude Drug

1 cm

Source The leaf of *Photinia serrulata* Lindl. (Fam. Rosaceae).

Distribution Mainly in Chinese provinces such as Jiangsu.

Harvest & Processing Collect leaves anytime during the year, preferably in summer and autumn; dry under the sun.

Description Petiole 1-4 cm long, with a longitudinal groove on the upper surface; blade oblong and elliptical, or obovate (egg-shaped in outline and attached at the narrower end) and elliptical, 8-15 cm long, 2-6 cm wide. Apex pointed, base suborbicular (almost round) or cuneate (wedge-shaped); margin densely serrulate (finely notched); blade with aristiform (awn-like) tooth on margin when young and on sprout shoots; blade coriaceous (leathery) and brittle. Odour: faint; taste: slightly astringent.

Indications 1. Chronic rheumatic or rheumatoid diseases with back and loin ache, weakness of the extremities 2. Migraine 3. Impotence, emission, sterility 4. Menstrual disorders.

Chemical Composition Contains prunasin.

Folium Sauropi

Dragon's Tongue Leaf
Longliye

龍脷葉

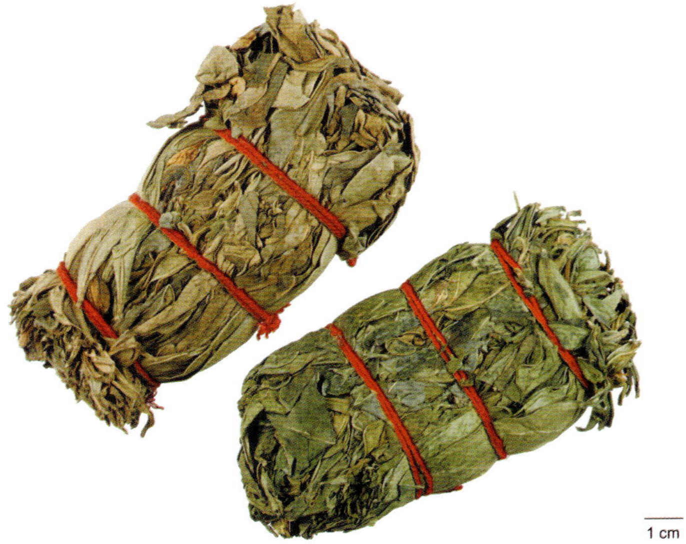

Crude Drug

Source The leaf of *Sauropus rostratus* Miq. (Fam. Euphorbiaceae).

Distribution Mainly in Chinese provinces such as Guangdong and Guangxi; also in Hong Kong.

Harvest & Processing Collect old leaves in May and June; dry under the sun; tie up in bundles. Usually each plant can yield 4-5 leaves each time; collect once every 15 days or so.

Description Ovate (egg-shaped in outline and attached at the broad end), or obovate (egg-shaped in outline and attached at the narrower end) and lanceolate (lance-head shaped), ligulate (strap-shaped). Apex blunt, or orbicular (round) and mucronulate (with a very small, sharp tip); base with a suborbicular (almost round) mucro. Entire (with continuous, even margin); withered-yellow or blackish-green; midrib on underside protuberant; lateral veins pinnate (feather-shaped); reticulate (net-like) veins joined near margin. Papery in texture, relatively thick. Odour: faint; taste: mild.

Indications 1. Cough and dyspnoea with copious yellow sputum, upper respiratory infection, acute bronchitis, bronchial asthma 2. Thirst 3. Constipation

Chemical Composition Mainly contains securinine.

Folium Sennae

Senna Leaf
Fanxieye
番瀉葉

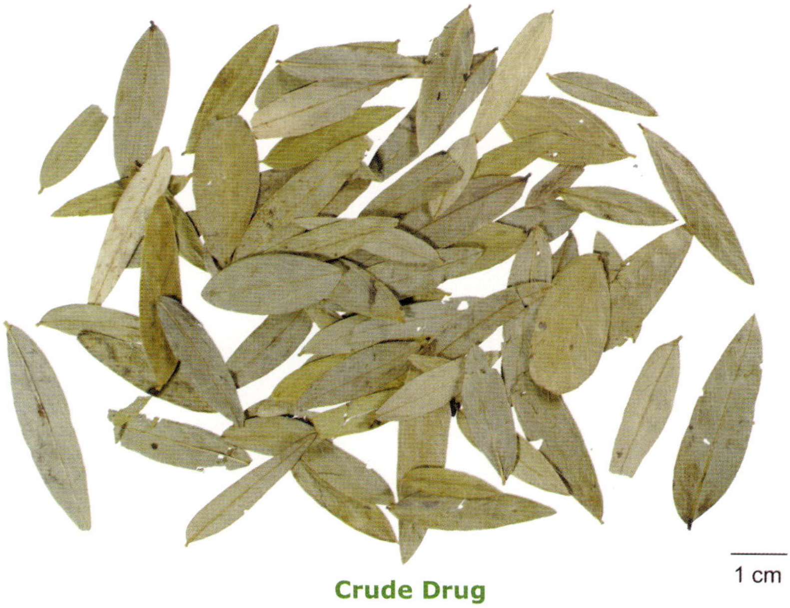

Crude Drug

Source The leaflet of *Cassia angustifolia* Vahl (Fam. Leguminosae).

Distribution Mainly in regions from the east of the Red Sea to India; nowadays widely cultivated in places like Tinnevelly in southern India. Commercial product is therefore called India Senna Leaf or Tinnevelly Senna Leaf. Introduced to and cultivated in Chinese provinces such as Guangdong, Hainan and Yunnan.

Harvest & Processing Pick blades before efflorescence; spread and dry under the sun promptly to avoid blades turning yellow; dry in shaded areas or at low temperatures; pack with a hydropress.

Description Oblong and ovate (egg-shaped in outline and attached at the broad end), or ovate and lanceolate (lance-head shaped); 1.5-5 cm long, 0.4-2 cm wide; entire (with continuous, even margin); apex acute, base slightly asymmetrical. Upper surface yellowish-green; underside light yellowish-green. Glabrous (without hairs) or nearly glabrous; leaf veins slightly protuberant; outer surface marked with markings of leaf veins formed by overlapping blades during the pressing process. Coriaceous (leathery). Odour: faint but distinctive; taste: slightly bitter. Slightly sticky. Tea-coloured when soaked in boiling water.

Indications 1. Constipation, simple intestinal obstruction, bowel preparation for gastrointestinal operation/procedure 2.Acute pancreatitis 3. Bacillary dysentery

Chemical Composition Mainly contains anthraquinone such as crysophanol, emodin and sennoside A, B, C, D.

Note According to *C.P.*, also used for medicinal purposes is the leaflet of *C. acutifolia* Delile.

Folium Viticis Negundo

Hempleaf Negundo Chastetree Leaf

Mujingye

牡荊葉

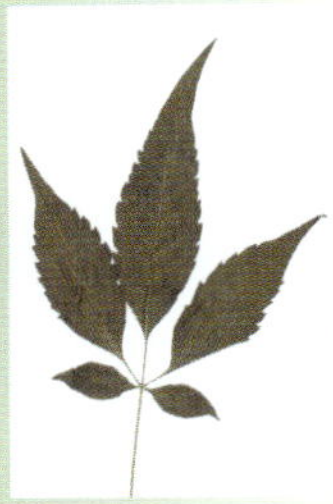

Hempleaf Negundo Chastetree Leaf Magnified

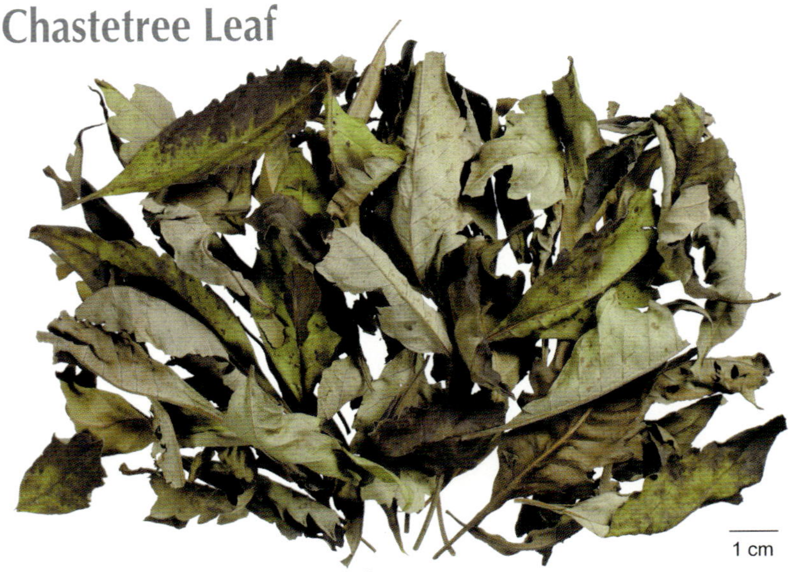

Crude Drug

Source: The leaf of *Vitex negundo* L. var. *cannabifolia* (Sieb. et Zucc.) Hand.-Mazz. (Fam. Verbenaceae).

Distribution: Mainly in Chinese provinces such as Jiangsu, Zhejiang, Anhui, Jiangxi, Fujian, Hunan, Guangxi and Guizhou.

Harvest & Processing: Collect leaves anytime during growing seasons; use while fresh or dry under the sun.

Description: Palmate (palm-shaped) compound leaf, mostly shrivelled and curled; with 3-5 leaflets when smoothed out; the three leaflets in the middle lanceolate (lance-head like) in shape, 6-10 cm long, 2-5 cm wide. Base cuneate (wedge-shaped), apex long and pointed, margin grossly serrate (with big saw-like teeth); leaflets on both sides smaller, ovate (egg-shaped in outline and attached at the broad end) and lanceolate. Upper surface dull greyish-brown or dull yellowish-brown, with sparse hairs; underside with protuberant pinnate (feather-shaped) veins. Primary petiole 3-8 cm long, densely covered with yellow pubescence. Odour: distinctive; taste: slightly bitter.

Indications: 1. Common cold, cough with thick sputum and difficult expectoration 2. Nausea, vomiting, diarrhoea and abdominal pain 3. Pruritus (external use).

Chemical Composition: Mainly contains essential oils and flavonoids.

Fructus Akebiae

Akebia Fruit
Yuzhizi
預知子

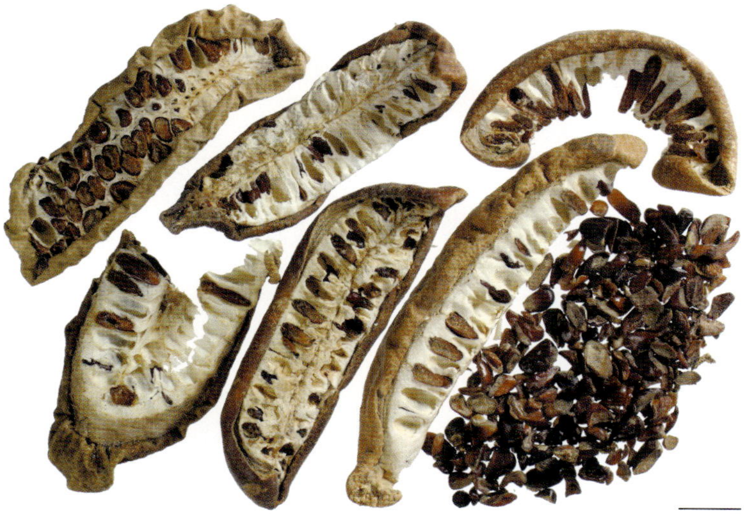

Crude Drug

Source The mature fruit of *Akebia quinata* (Thunb.) Decne. (Fam. Lardizabalaceae).

Distribution Mainly in Chinese provinces such as Jiangsu, Hubei, Hunan, Sichuan, Zhejiang and Anhui.

Harvest & Processing Pick mature fruits in August and September before dehiscence (splitting at maturity); string together with a rope and dry by airing (avoid piling as the heat produced will cause the fruits to rot), or soak thoroughly in boiling water and dry under the sun.

Description Reniform (kidney-shaped), or long and ellipsoid (elliptical in long-section and circular in cross-section), slightly curved; 3-9 cm long, 1.5-3.5 cm in diameter. Outer surface yellowish-brown or dull dark brown, marked with irregular reticulate (net-like) wrinkles; apex obtuse; base with a carpopodium scar. Hard, solid and heavy. When cut open, white starchy sarcocarp revealed; seeds numerous, triangular, purplish-red; seed surface fairly smooth. Odour: slightly fragrant; taste: bitter.

Indications 1. Epigastric and hypochondriac pain and distension
2. Amenorrhoea, dysmenorrhoea 3. Oliguria 4. Snake and insect bite.

Chemical Composition Mainly contains triterpene saponins.

Note According to *C.P.*, also used as Fructus Akebiae is the mature fruit of *A. trifoliata* (Thunb.) Koidz. and *A. trifoliata* (Thunb.) Koidz. *var. australis* (Diels) Rehd. Fructus Akebiae is commonly known as '*Bayue za*'(August Bundle) in Hong Kong.

Fructus Alpiniae Oxyphyllae

Sharpleaf Galangal Fruit
Yizhi

益智

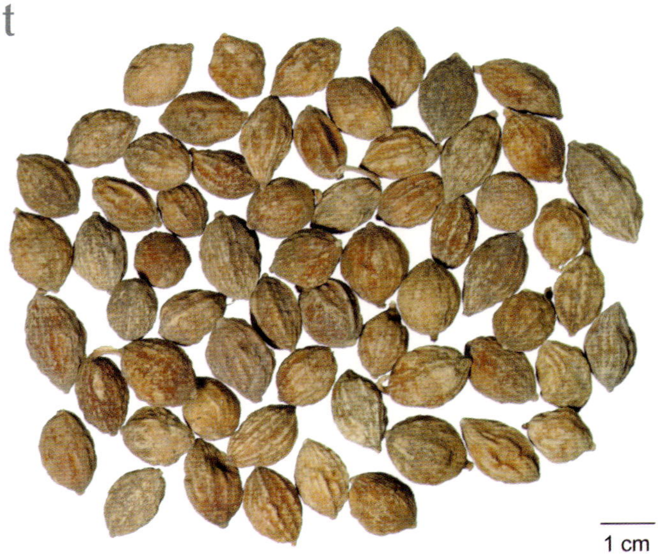

Crude Drug

Source The mature fruit of *Alpinia oxyphylla* Miq. (Fam. Zingiberaceae).

Distribution Mainly in Chinese provinces such as Hainan and Guangxi.

Harvest & Processing Harvest fruits between summer and autumn when they turn from green to red; dry under the sun or at low temperatures.

Description Ellipsoid (elliptical in long-section and circular in cross-section), slightly pointed at both ends; 1.2-2 cm long, 1-1.3 cm in diameter. Outer surface brown or greyish-brown, with 13-20 uneven, protuberant longitudinal ridges; apex with remnants of perianth base; base often with carpopodium remnants. Pericarp thin and fairly pliable, stuck fast with seeds. Seed cluster with septa in the middle dividing it into 3 cloves, each with 6-11 seeds. Seeds irregular and disc-like, each with shallow obtuse ridges; about 3 mm in diameter; outer surface dull greyish-brown or greyish-yellow, covered with pale brown membranous aril; hard; endosperms white. Odour: with a distinctive fragrance; taste: acrid and slightly bitter.

Indications 1. Stomachache, diarrhoea 2. Enuresis, urinary frequency 3. Spermatorrhoea, nocturnal emission.

Chemical Composition Mainly contains diarylheptanoids and essential oils with α-cyperone as the main component.

Fructus Amomi

Villous Amomum Fruit

Sharen

砂仁

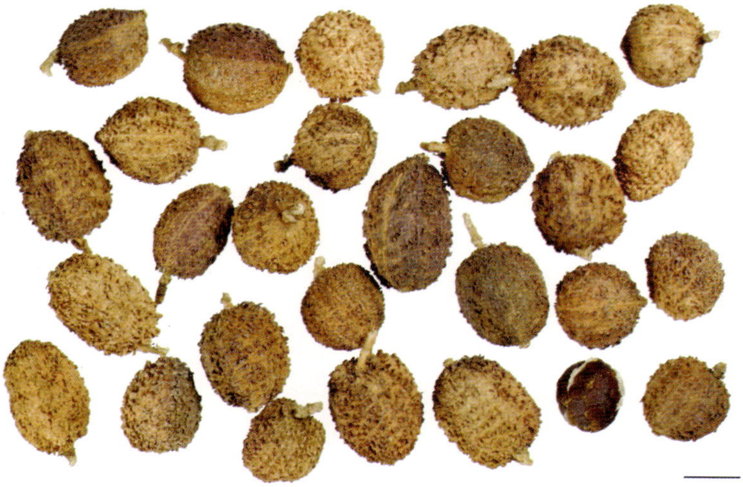

1 cm

Crude Drug

Source The mature fruit of *Amomum villosum* Lour. (Fam. Zingiberaceae).

Distribution Mainly in Chinese provinces such as Guangdong, with the ones from Yangchun and Yangjiang most famous.

Harvest & Processing Harvest fruits at maturation between summer and autumn; dry under the sun or at low temperatures to produce '*Kesha*' (Sand with a Shell). Alternatively, peel off pericarp and dry the seed clusters under the sun.

Description Ellipsoid or egg-shaped, with three indistinct ridges; 1.5-2 cm long, 1-1.5 cm in diameter. Outer surface reddish-brown, densely covered with spiniform protuberances; apex marked with remnants of perianth base; base often with a carpopodium. Pericarp thin and soft. Seeds in clusters; each cluster with three obtuse ridges, and with white septa in the middle dividing it into three cloves, each clove consisting of 5-26 seeds. Seeds in the form of irregular polyhedrons; 2-3 mm in diameter; outer surface reddish-brown or dull brown, marked with fine wrinkles and covered with pale brown membranous aril; hard; endosperms greyish-white. Odour: aromatic and strong; taste: acrid but fresh, slightly bitter.

Indications 1. Feeling of fullness and distending pain in the chest and upper abdomen, anorexia, nausea, vomiting, diarrhoea, abdominal pain 2. Threatened abortion.

Chemical Composition Contains essential oils with camphor and limonene as the main components.

Note According to *C.P.*, also used for medicinal purposes is the mature fruit of *A. villosum* Lour. *var. xanthioides* T. L. Wu et Senjen and *A. longiligulare* T. L. Wu.

Fructus Amomi Rotundus

Round Cardamon Fruit
Doukou

豆蔻

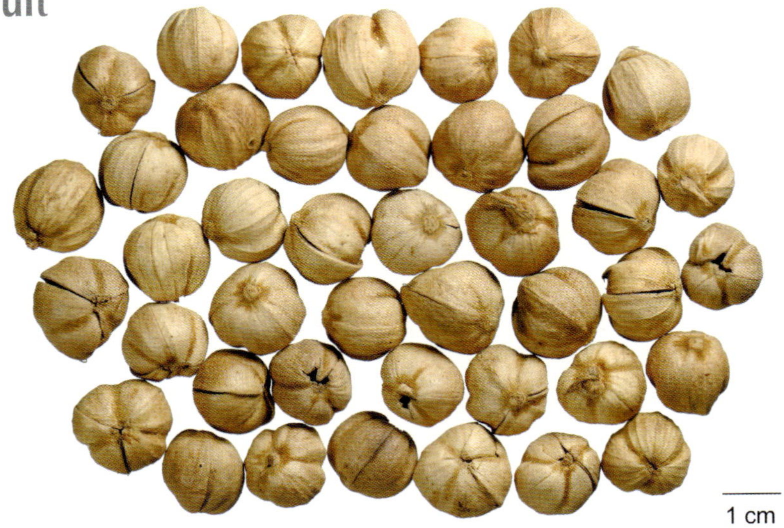

Crude Drug

Source The mature fruit of *Amomum kravanh* Pierre *ex* Gagnep. (Fam. Zingiberaceae).

Distribution Imported from countries like Cambodia, Thailand, Vietnam and Burma. Also cultivated in small amounts in Hainan province and southern Yunnan province in China.

Harvest & Processing Collect fruits between summer and autumn when they mature; dry under the sun or at low temperatures.

Description Subspherical; 1.2-1.8 cm in diameter. Outer surface yellowish-white to pale yellowish-brown, marked with 3 relatively deep longitudinal grooves; apex with a protuberant style base, base with a dented carpopodium scar; both ends covered with light brown villi. Pericarp thin; light in weight; brittle, breaks easily along the length. Divided into 3 locules, each containing about 10 seeds. Seeds in the form of irregular polyhedrons; dorsal side slightly bulgy; 3-4 mm in diameter; outer surface dull brown, marked with wrinkles and aril remnants. Odour: aromatic; taste: mint-like and acrid, slightly like camphor.

Indications 1. Anorexia, nausea, vomiting, dyspepsia 2. Feeling of oppression of chest, distension and pain in the chest and abdomen

Chemical Composition Mainly contains essential oils.

Note According to *C.P.*, also used for medicinal purposes is the mature fruit of *A. compactum* Soland *ex* Maton.

Fructus Anisi Stellati

Chinese Star Anise
Bajiaohuixiang

八角茴香

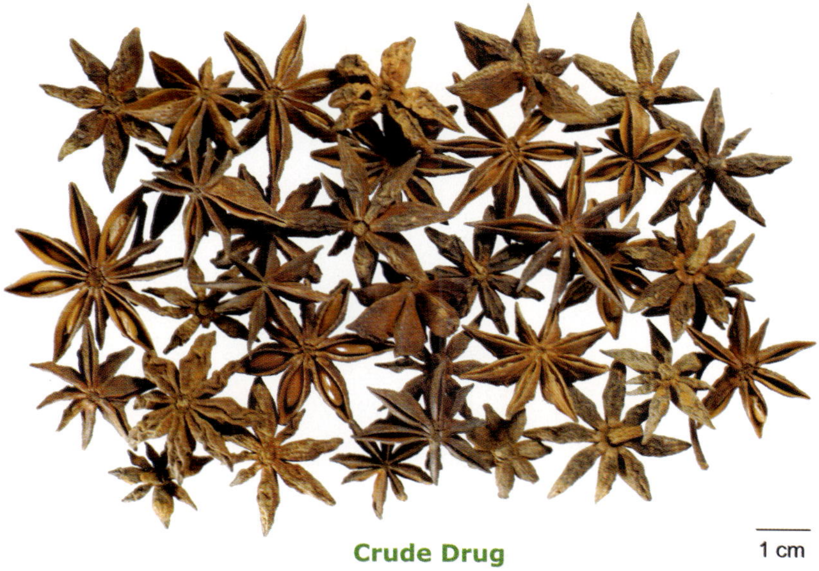

Crude Drug

Source The mature fruit of *Illicium verum* Hook. f. (Fam. Magnoliaceae).

Distribution Mainly in Chinese provinces such as Guangxi and Yunnan.

Harvest & Processing Collect spring fruits in April when they ripen and fall to the ground; dry under the sun. Collect autumn fruits from October to November; put in boiling water and stir for 5-10 minutes; dry under the sun or by heat.

Description Aggregate fruit consisting of about 5-13 (mostly 8) follicles of similar size radiating from central axis; follicles 1-2 cm long, 0.5-1 cm thick. Outer surface reddish-brown or dull reddish-brown, marked with irregular wrinkles; top end obtuse, or blunt but slightly pointed; pericarp relatively thick; upper side mostly dehisced, making follicles scaphoid (boat-shaped). Inner surface pale brown, lustrous. Each follicle with 1 seed; seed flattened and ovoid (egg-shaped), reddish-brown or greyish-brown, lustrous. Carpopodium 3-4 cm long; curved; usually fallen off. Odour: aromatic; taste: acrid and sweet.

Indications 1. Abdominal colic, vomiting, epigastric pain 2. Lumbago

Chemical Composition Contains 3-8% essential oils (50-60% anethole) and sesquiterpenes.

Fructus Arctii

Great Burdock Achene
Niubangzi

牛蒡子

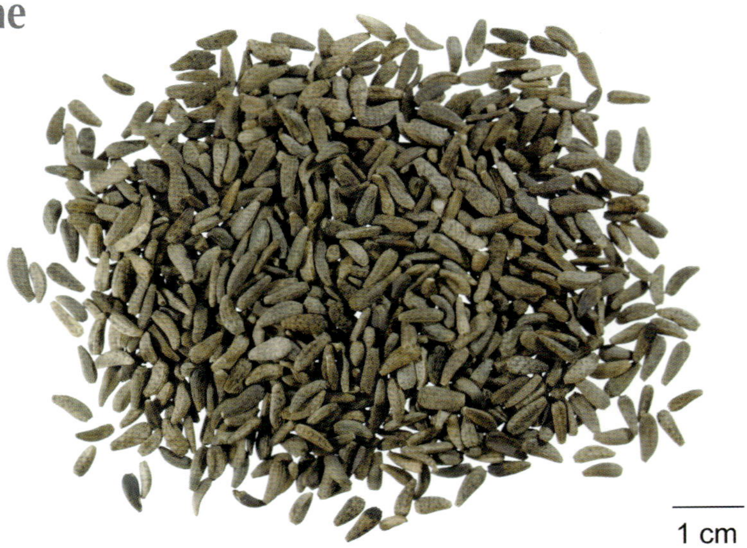

Crude Drug

Source The mature fruit of *Arctium lappa* L. (Fam. Compositae).

Distribution Mainly in Chinese provinces such as Zhejiang, Sichuan, Hubei, Hebei and Henan, and in northeastern China.

Harvest & Processing Harvest infructescences in autumn when fruits are ripe; dry under the sun; thresh to obtain fruits; remove foreign matter; dry under the sun again.

Description Oblong and obovoid (inverse egg shaped), slightly flattened and a little curved; 5-7 mm long, 2-3 mm wide. Outer surface dull greyish-brown; scattered purplish-black maculae visible under magnification; marked with several longitudinal ridges, usually with the middle 1-2 ridges more prominent. Apex obtuse, quite broad; apical side marked with a ring, with punctiform (dot-like) style scars in the centre. Base slightly narrow; areola relatively light in colour. Pericarp relatively hard; cotyledons 2, pale yellowish-white, highly oleaginous (oily). Odourless; taste: bitter, then slightly acrid and a little tongue-numbing.

Indications 1.Common cold, cough, headache 2. Sore throat 3. Inadequate measles eruption.

Chemical Composition Mainly contains arctin.

Fructus Anisi Stellati

Chinese Star Anise
Bajiaohuixiang

八角茴香

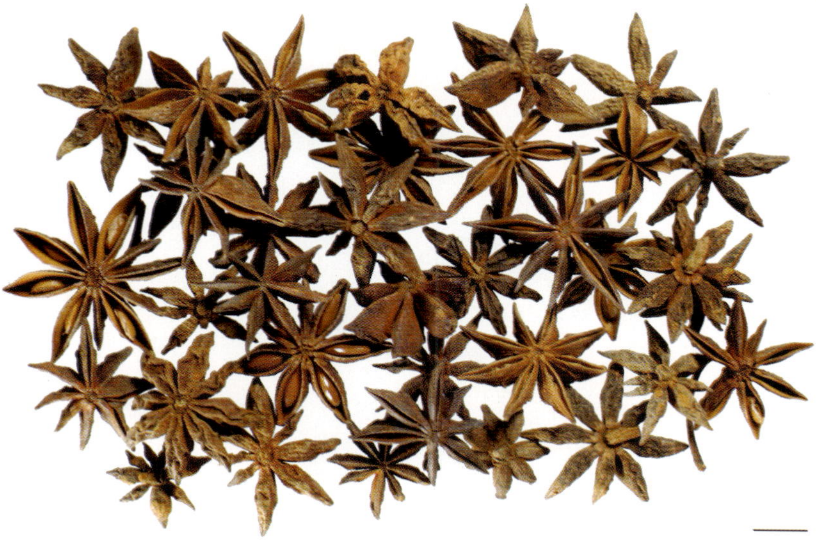

Crude Drug

1 cm

Source The mature fruit of *Illicium verum* Hook. f. (Fam. Magnoliaceae).

Distribution Mainly in Chinese provinces such as Guangxi and Yunnan.

Harvest & Processing Collect spring fruits in April when they ripen and fall to the ground; dry under the sun. Collect autumn fruits from October to November; put in boiling water and stir for 5-10 minutes; dry under the sun or by heat.

Description Aggregate fruit consisting of about 5-13 (mostly 8) follicles of similar size radiating from central axis; follicles 1-2 cm long, 0.5-1 cm thick. Outer surface reddish-brown or dull reddish-brown, marked with irregular wrinkles; top end obtuse, or blunt but slightly pointed; pericarp relatively thick; upper side mostly dehisced, making follicles scaphoid (boat-shaped). Inner surface pale brown, lustrous. Each follicle with 1 seed; seed flattened and ovoid (egg-shaped), reddish-brown or greyish-brown, lustrous. Carpopodium 3-4 cm long; curved; usually fallen off. Odour: aromatic; taste: acrid and sweet.

Indications 1. Abdominal colic, vomiting, epigastric pain 2. Lumbago

Chemical Composition Contains 3-8% essential oils (50-60% anethole) and sesquiterpenes.

Fructus Arctii

Great Burdock Achene
Niubangzi

牛蒡子

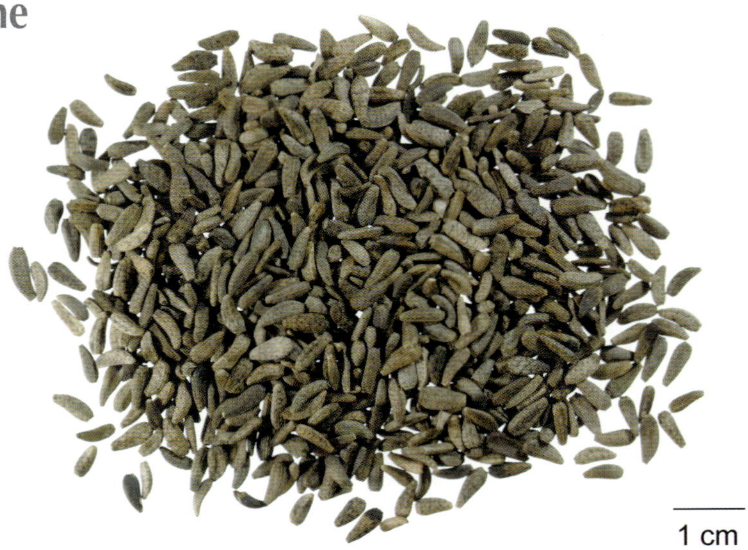

Crude Drug

Source The mature fruit of *Arctium lappa* L. (Fam. Compositae).

Distribution Mainly in Chinese provinces such as Zhejiang, Sichuan, Hubei, Hebei and Henan, and in northeastern China.

Harvest & Processing Harvest infructescences in autumn when fruits are ripe; dry under the sun; thresh to obtain fruits; remove foreign matter; dry under the sun again.

Description Oblong and obovoid (inverse egg shaped), slightly flattened and a little curved; 5-7 mm long, 2-3 mm wide. Outer surface dull greyish-brown; scattered purplish-black maculae visible under magnification; marked with several longitudinal ridges, usually with the middle 1-2 ridges more prominent. Apex obtuse, quite broad; apical side marked with a ring, with punctiform (dot-like) style scars in the centre. Base slightly narrow; areola relatively light in colour. Pericarp relatively hard; cotyledons 2, pale yellowish-white, highly oleaginous (oily). Odourless; taste: bitter, then slightly acrid and a little tongue-numbing.

Indications 1.Common cold, cough, headache 2. Sore throat 3. Inadequate measles eruption.

Chemical Composition Mainly contains arctin.

Fructus Aristolochiae

Dutohmanspipe Fruit
Madouling

馬兜鈴

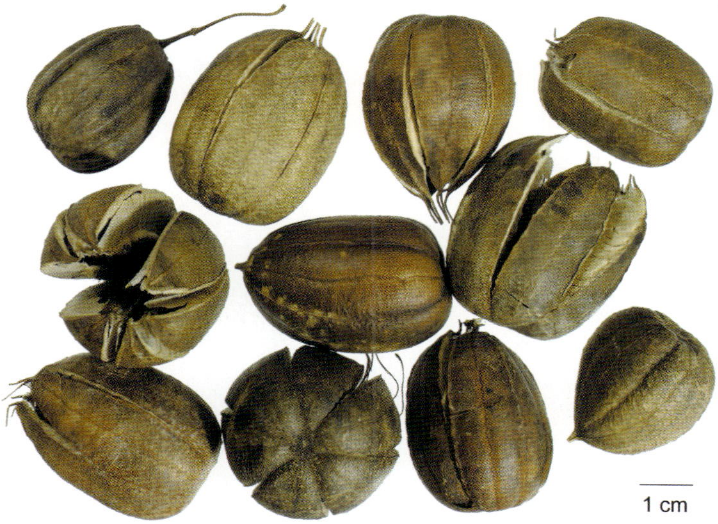

Crude Drug

Source The mature fruit of *Aristolochia contorta* Bge. (Fam. Aristolochiaceae).

Distribution Mainly in Chinese provinces such as Hebei, Shandong, Shaanxi and Shanxi, and in northeastern China.

Harvest & Processing Pick fruits together with carpopodiums in autumn when fruits turn from green to yellow; dry under the sun.

Description Ovoid (egg-shaped); 3-7 cm long, 2-4 cm in diameter. Outer surface yellowish-green, greyish-green or reddish-brown; marked with 12 longitudinal ridges branching out into numerous parallel transverse fine venous (vein-like) striae. Top end flat and blunt; base with a slender carpopodium. Pericarp light in weight and brittle, easily cracks into 6 segments, with carpopodium also split into 6 pieces. Inner surface of pericarp smooth and lustrous, marked with relatively dense transverse venous striae. Fruit divided into 6 locules, each with numerous seeds stacked in an orderly manner. Seeds flat and thin, each flabellate (fan-shaped) or the shape of an obtuse triangle; 6-10 mm long, 8-12 mm wide; margin with wings; pale brown in colour. Odour: distinctive; taste: slightly bitter.

Indications 1. Cough and dyspnoea 2. Dyspnoea with copious sputum and difficult expectoration

Chemical Composition Mainly contains alkaloids such as aristolochic acid A, C, D and magnoflorine.

Note According to *C.P.*, also used for medicinal purposes is the mature fruit of *A. debilis* Sieb. et Zucc.

Fructus Aurantii

Orange Fruit
Zhiqiao
枳殼

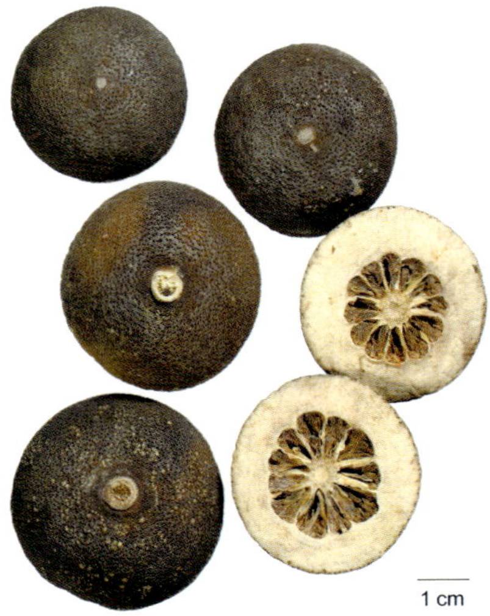

Crude Drug

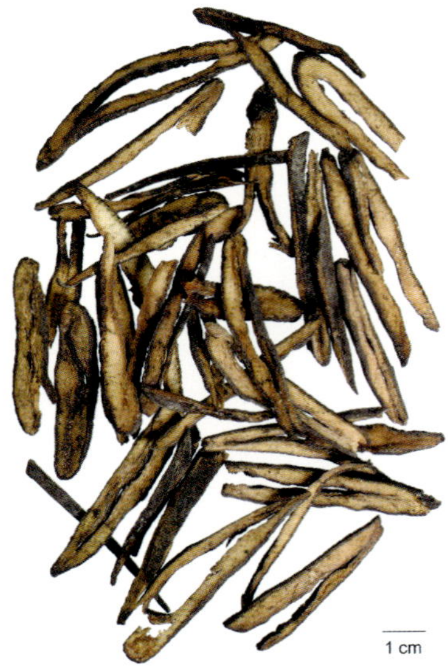

Decoction Pieces

Source The immature fruit of *Citrus aurantium* L. (Fam. Rutaceae) and its cultivated varieties.

Distribution Mainly in Chinese provinces such as Jiangxi, Sichuan and Hunan; hence the names '*Jiang zhiqiao*' (Jiangxi *Zhiqiao*), '*Chuan zhiqiao*' (Sichuan *Zhiqiao*) and '*Xiang zhiqiao*' (Hunan *Zhiqiao*) respectively. Mostly cultivated.

Harvest & Processing Collect immature fruits in July and August during the hottest weather and before maturation. Delay in harvest will affect quality as over-mature fruits have thin rind and copious pulp. Cross-cut into halves the fruits collected; dry under the sun. In Hong Kong, the dried fruits are pounded flat with a plane set-hammer before being cut into slices.

Description Hemispherical, with rolled-up edges like a pot; 3-5 cm in diameter. Outer surface reddish-brown to dull brown, marked with granular protuberances; top of protuberances with dented punctiform (dot-like) oil cavities. Apex marked with a conspicuous scar of the style base; base with a carpopodium scar. Hard, does not break easily. Cross-section slightly bulgy; mesocarp yellowish-white, with 7-12 dull brown pulp vesicles (occasionally up to 15); a few seeds in mesocarp; central axis 0.7-1.1 cm in diameter. Odour: faint; taste: bitter, then slightly sour.

Indications 1. Distension and pain in the chest and hypochondrium 2. Dyspepsia 3. Gastroptosis, rectal prolapse and uterine prolapse

Chemical Composition Pericarp Mainly contains naringin and lonicerin.

Fructus Aurantii Immaturus

Immature Orange Fruit
Zhishi
枳實

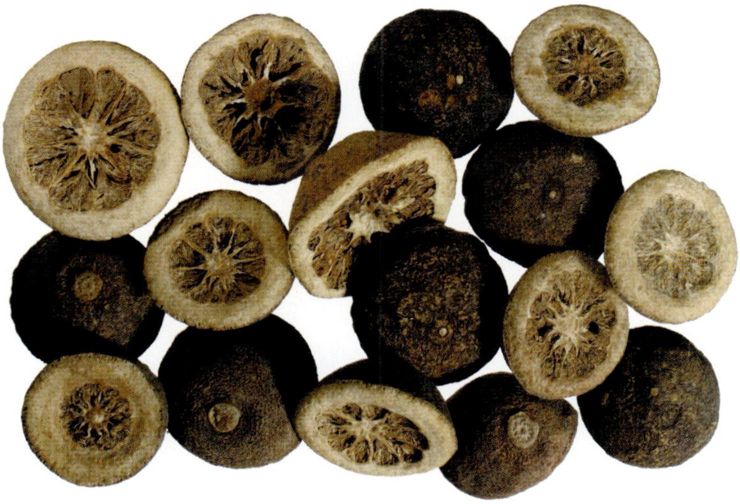

Crude Drug

1 cm

Source The young fruit of *Citrus aurantium* L. (Fam. Rutaceae).

Distribution Mainly in Chinese provinces such as Sichuan, Hunan and Jiangxi; hence the names '*Chuan zhishi*' (Sichuan *Zhishi*), '*Xiang zhishi*' (Hunan *Zhishi*) and '*Jiang zhishi*' (Jiangxi *Zhishi*) respectively.

Harvest & Processing Pick young fruits on the trees or collect fallen ones in May and June; cross-cut big ones into halves; dry under the sun.

Description Hemispherical, spherical or ovoid (egg-shaped); 0.5-2.5 cm in diameter. Outer surface dark green or dull brownish-green, marked with granular protuberances and wrinkles. Top part with a conspicuous scar of the style base; base with remnants of floral discs or a carpopodium scar. Cut surface shows slightly protuberant mesocarp yellowish-white or dull yellowish-brown in colour and 3-12 mm thick; margin scattered with 1-2 rows of oil cavities; pulp vesicles reddish-brown. Hard. Odour: fresh and fragrant; taste: bitter and slightly sour.

Indications 1. Feeling of fullness in the chest and upper abdomen, productive cough and chest pain 2. Diarrhoea, dysentery, constipation 3. Gastroptosis, rectal prolapse, uterine prolapse

Chemical Composition Mainly contains flavonoids.

Note According to *C.P.*, also used for medicinal purposes is the young fruit of *C. sinensis* (L) Osbeck.

Fructus Broussonetiae

Papermulberry Fruit
Chushizhi

楮實子

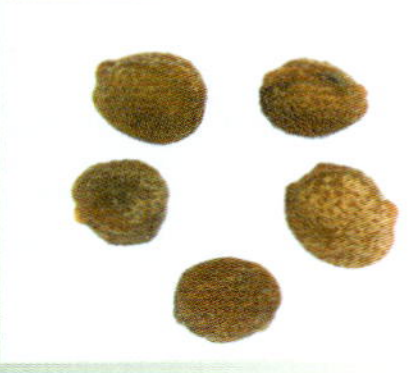

Papermulberry Fruit Magnified

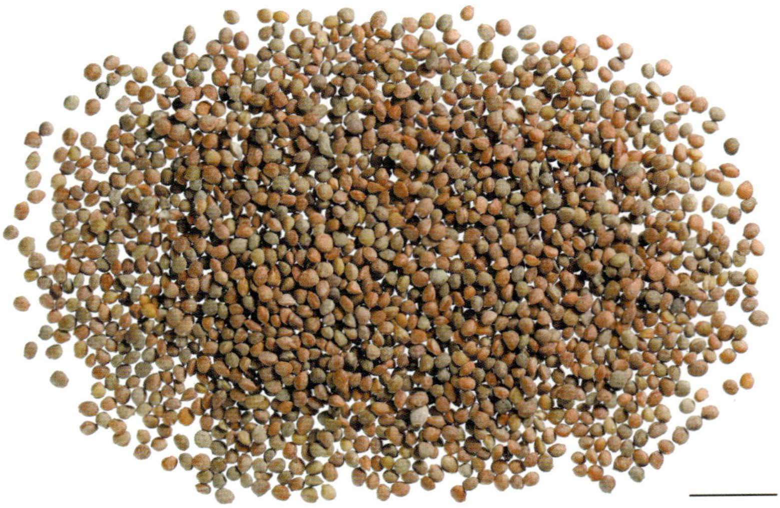

Crude Drug

Source The mature fruit of *Broussonetia papyrifera* (L.) Vent. (Fam. Moraceae).

Distribution Mainly in Chinese provinces such as Henan, Hubei, Hunan, Shanxi and Gansu; also in Hong Kong.

Harvest & Processing Pick fruits at maturation in autumn; wash clean; dry under the sun; remove greyish-white membranous perianth and foreign matter.

Description Flattened and spherical, or flattened and ovoid (egg-like); 2-2.5 mm long, 1.5-2 mm in diameter, up to 1 mm thick. Outer surface reddish-brown to brown, with reticulate (net-shaped) wrinkles or strumiform (cushion-like) protuberances; one side with longitudinal ridges, the other slightly flat or marked with grooves; usually with a carpopodium attached, occasionally with greyish-white membranous perianth still unremoved. Pericarp hard and brittle, crushed easily; membranous testa pressing tightly against the inside of pericarp; endosperms off-white, highly oleaginous (oily); embryo curved. Odourless; taste: mild.

Indications 1. Pain and weakness of the loins and knees 2. Consumptive fever 3. Dizziness and blurred vision 4. Nebula 5. Oedema.

Chemical Composition Mainly contains saponins, vitamin B and oils and fats.

Fructus Bruceae

Java Brucea Fruit
Yadanzi

鴉膽子

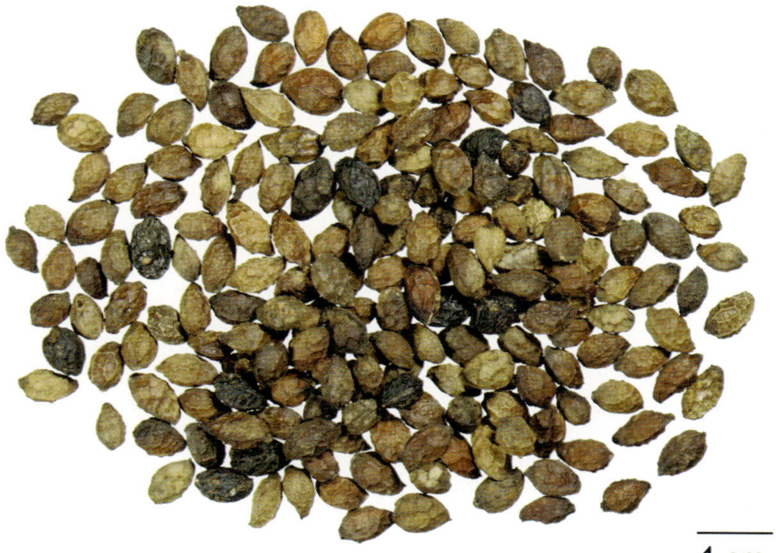

Crude Drug

Source The mature fruit of *Brucea javanica* (L.) Merr. (Fam. Simaroubaceae).

Distribution Mainly in Chinese provinces such as Guangxi, Guangdong and Yunnan; also in Hong Kong.

Harvest & Processing Harvest fruits at maturation in autumn; remove foreign matter; dry under the sun.

Description Ellipsoid (elliptical in long-section and circular in cross-section), both ends slightly pointed; 6-10 mm long, 4-7 mm in diameter. Outer surface black or brown, marked with raised, reticulate (net-like) wrinkles forming irregular polygonal meshes; apex acuminate (tapering to a slender point); both sides with prominent ridges; base with a dented carpopodium scar. Fruit shell hard and brittle. Seeds ovoid (egg-shaped), 5-6 mm long, 3-5 mm in diameter; outer surface off-white or yellowish-white, reticulate; the more pointed end coronoid (beak-shaped); testa thin; cotyledons milk-white, highly oleaginous (oily). Odourless; taste: extremely bitter, lasting.

Indications 1. Amoebic dysentery 2. Haemorrhoids 3. Warts, corns (external use).

Chemical Composition Contains quassinoids such as bruceine A, B, C, D.

Note Listed as slightly toxic in *C.P.*

Fructus Canarii

Chinese White Olive
Qingguo

青果

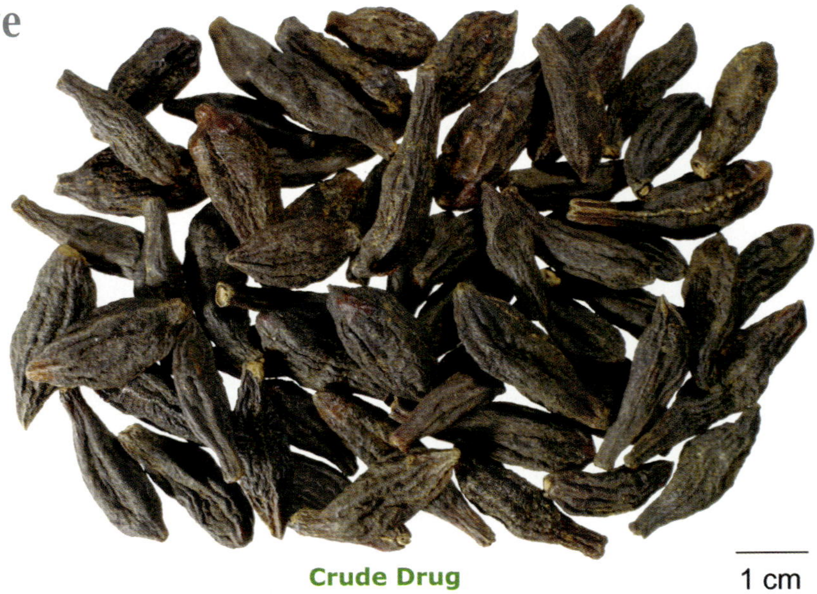

Crude Drug

Source The mature fruit of *Canarium album* (Lour.) Raeusch. (Fam. Burseraceae).

Distribution Mainly in Chinese provinces such as Fujian, Taiwan, Hainan, Guangdong and Guangxi.

Harvest & Processing Collect fruits in August and September when exocarp turns yellowish-green; wash clean; use while fresh or dry over gentle heat.

Description Spindle-shaped, both ends blunt but slightly pointed; 2.5-4 cm long, 1-1.5 cm in diameter. Outer surface brownish-yellow or dull blackish-brown, with irregular wrinkles. Sarcocarp thick; greyish-brown or reddish-brown. Endocarp spindle-shaped; dull reddish-brown; outer surface marked with 3 longitudinal ridges, each pair of ridges with two curved, arch-like grooves in between. Hard; when cut open, mostly with 3 locules inside, each containing 1 seed. Exotesta yellow, often pressing against endocarp; endotesta reddish-brown, membranous; endosperms extremely thin; cotyledons 2. Odourless; taste of sarcocarp: astringent, slightly sweet after chewing for some time.

Indications 1. Sore throat, cough 2. Polydipsia 3. Allergic to fish and crab.

Chemical Composition Mainly contains essential oils with β -caryophyllene and camphene as the main components.

Fructus Cannabis

Hemp Fruit
Huomaren

火麻仁

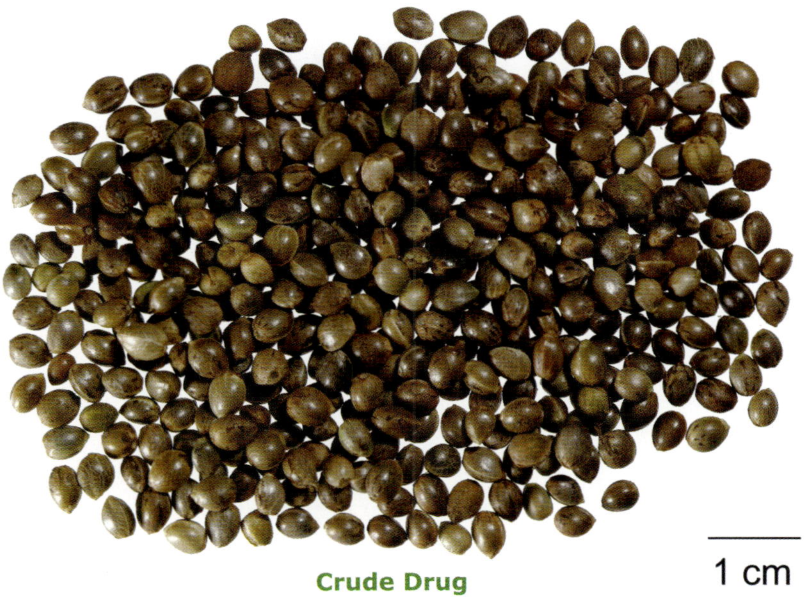

Crude Drug

Source The mature fruit of *Cannabis sativa* L. (Fam. Moraceae).

Distribution Cultivated in all parts of China.

Harvest & Processing Pick fruits at maturation in autumn; remove foreign matter; dry under the sun.

Description Ovoid (egg-shaped); 4-5 mm long, 3-4 mm in diameter. Outer surface greyish-green to grey, slightly lustrous, marked with light-coloured reticulate (net-like) striae; the edge on either side ridged; base with an orbicular (round) carpopodium scar. Pericarp thin and brittle. Seed 1, subspherical in shape; testa thin and dull green, often firmly attached to endocarp. Endosperms greyish-white, encircling the curled embryo; cotyledons 2, plump, highly oleaginous (oily). Odourless; taste: mild.

Indications 1. Constipation 2. Postpartum anaemia

Chemical Composition Contains trigonelline and fatty acids.

Fructus Carotae

Wild Carrot Fruit
Nanheshi

南鶴虱

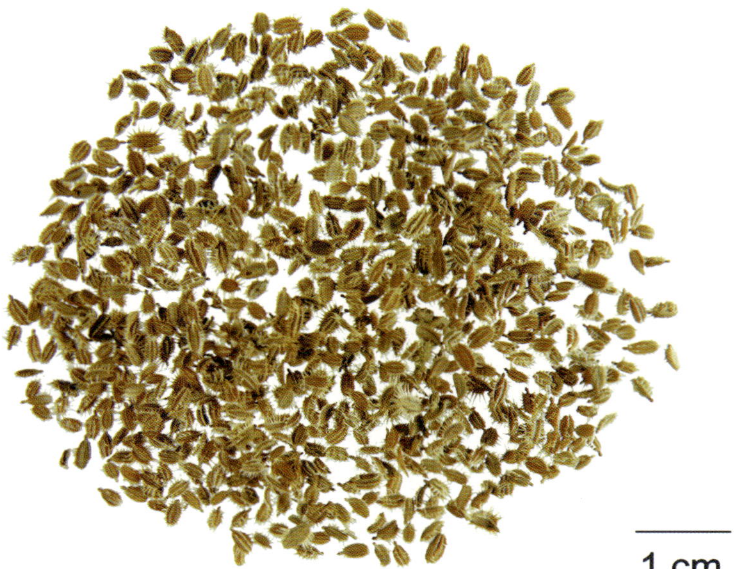
1 cm

Crude Drug

Source The mature fruit of *Daucus carota* L. (Fam. Umbelliferae).

Distribution Mainly in Chinese provinces such as Jiangsu, Zhejiang, Anhui and Hubei.

Harvest & Processing Cut off fruit spurs in autumn when fruits are ripe; dry under the sun; thresh to get fruits; remove foreign matter.

Description Cremocarp ellipsoid (elliptical in long-section and circular in cross-section), mostly divided into mericarps. Mericarps 3-4 mm long, 1.5-2.5 mm wide. Outer surface pale greenish-brown or brownish-yellow; base obtuse; dorsal side raised, with 4 narrow aliform (wing-shaped) subribs densely covered with yellowish-white hooked thorns about 1.5 mm long; at indentations between subribs lie indistinct main ribs covered with sparse pubescence; commissure even, with 3 venous (vein-like) striae covered with pubescence. Kernel off-white, oleaginous (oily). Light in weight. Odour: with a distinctive fragrance when crumbled; taste: slightly acrid, bitter.

Indications 1. Ascariasis, oxyuriasis, taeniasis, abdominal pain caused by intestinal parasitosis 2. Malnutrition and dyspepsia due to improper ingestion.

Chemical Composition Contains essential oils with asarone, biasabolene and asarylaldehyde; also contains flavonoids.

Note Listed as slightly toxic in *C.P.*

Fructus Chaenomelis

Common Floweringqince Fruit
Mugua
木瓜

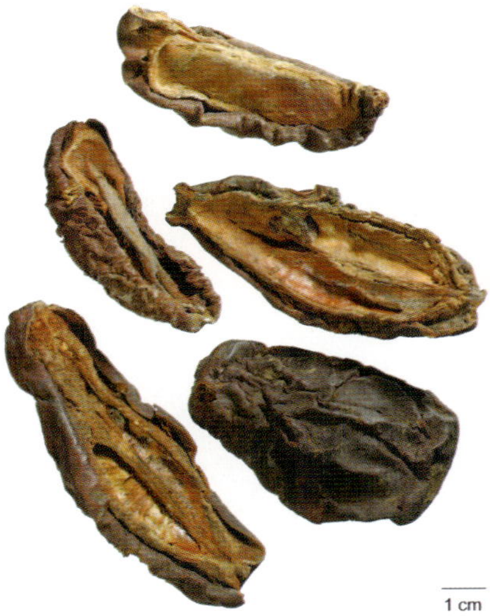

Crude Drug

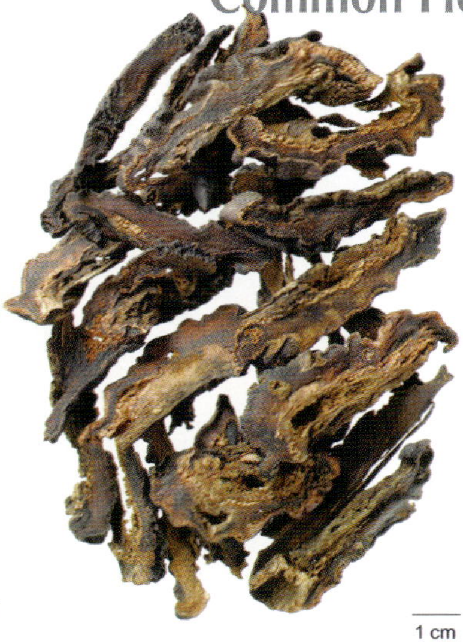

Decoction Pieces

Source The near-mature fruit of *Chaenomeles speciosa* (Sweet) Nakai (Fam. Rosaceae).

Distribution Mainly in Chinese provinces such as Anhui, Hubei, Sichuan and Zhejiang. Mostly cultivated nowadays.

Harvest & Processing Harvest fruits in summer and autumn when they turn greenish-yellow; cut length-wise into halves or 4 segments; dry under the sun. Alternatively, boil in water until exocarp changes colour; cut length-wise; dry under the sun.

Description Length-wise cut pieces oblong and orbicular (round) in shape; 4-8 cm long, 2-5 cm wide; length-wise cut slices linear (long and narrow) in shape. Outer surface purplish-red or brownish-red; marked with numerous irregular deep wrinkles; rim of cut surface curled inwards. Sarcocarp reddish-brown; with a dented brownish-yellow ovary locule in the centre. Seeds often fallen off, leaving a smooth and shiny surface. Seeds shaped like tangerine pits but slightly larger and flat; outer surface reddish-brown, wrinkled. Hard and solid. Odour of sarcocarp: slightly fresh and fragrant; taste: sour, slightly astringent.

Indications
1. Numbness and weakness of the lower part of the body
2. Vomiting and diarrhoea, abdominal pain.

Chemical Composition Contains malic acid, tartaric acid, citric acid and saponins.

Fructus Chebulae

Medicine Terminalia Fruit
Hezi

訶子

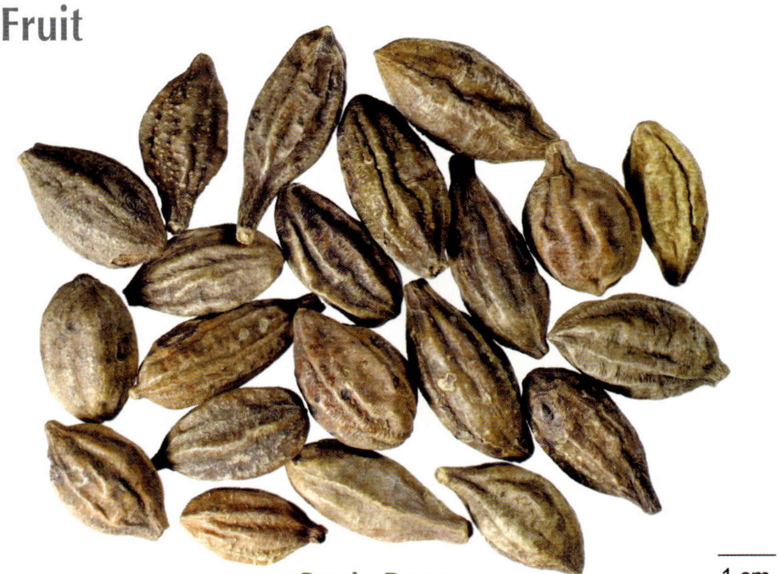

Crude Drug

Source The mature fruit of *Terminalia chebula* Retz. (Fam. Combretaceae).

Distribution Mainly in Yunnan province in China.

Harvest & Processing Harvest fruits at maturation on sunny days in late autumn and early winter; dry under the sun or by heat.

Description Oblong and spherical, or ovoid (egg-shaped); 2-4 cm long, 2-2.5 cm in diameter. Outer surface yellowish-brown or dull brown, slightly lustrous, marked with 5-6 longitudinal ridges and irregular wrinkles; base with an orbicular (round) carpopodium scar. Hard. Sarcocarp 2-4 mm thick, yellowish-brown or dull yellowish-brown. Pit 1.5-2.5 cm long, 1-1.5 cm in diameter; light yellow in colour; rough and hard. Seeds oblong and spindle-shaped, about 1 cm long, 2-4 mm in diameter; testa yellowish-brown; cotyledons 2, white, overlapping and interwined. Odourless; taste: sour-astringent and then sweet.

Indications 1. Diarrhoea, enterorrhagia 2. Dysfunctional uterine bleeding, metritis, morbid leukorrhoea.

Chemical Composition Mainly contains tannin such as chebulinic acid; also contains triterpenes.

Note According to *C.P.*, also used for medicinal purposes is the mature fruit of *T. chebula* Retz. var. *tomentella* Kurt.

Fructus Citri

Citron Fruit
Xiangyuan

香櫞

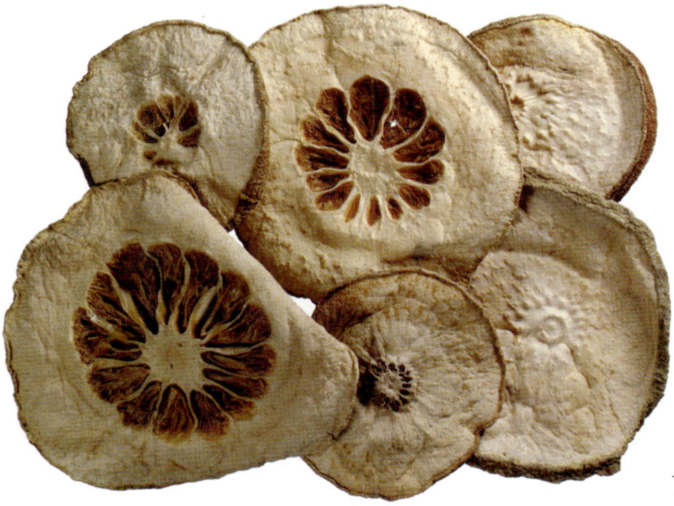

1 cm

Decoction Pieces

Source The mature fruit of *Citrus medica* L. (Fam. Rutaceae).

Distribution Mainly in Chinese provinces such as Yunnan, Sichuan and Fujian.

Harvest & Processing Harvest fruits in September and October when they turn yellow at maturation; put in a heap of husks for a week to let the fruits turn golden yellow; cut into slices 1 cm thick; spread out and dry under the sun, or dry by heat during rainy days.

Description Slices orbicular (round), or oblong and orbicular; 4-10 cm in diameter, 2-5 mm thick. Cross-cut slices with yellow or yellowish-green exocarp, margin undulate (wavy) and scattered with dented oil dots; mesocarp 1-3 cm thick, yellowish-white, marked with irregular, reticulate (net-like) and protuberant vascular bundles, divided into 10-17 pulp vesicles. Length-wise cut slices with relatively thick central axis. Pliable. Odour: fresh and fragrant; taste: slightly sweet, bitter and acrid.

Indications 1. Distending pain in the chest and hypochondria 2. Epigastric distension, vomiting and belching 3. Cough with copious expectoration.

Chemical Composition Mainly contains hesperidin and citric acid.

Note According to *C.P.*, also used for medicinal purposes is the mature fruit of *C. wilsonii* Tanaka.

Fructus Citri Sarcodactylis

Finger Citron
Foshou

佛手

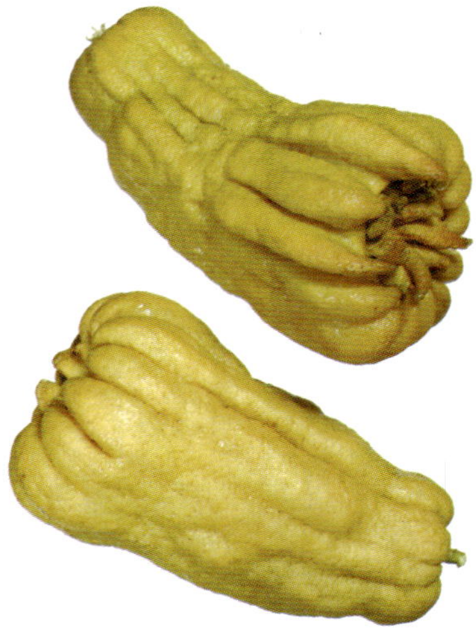

1 cm

Crude Drug

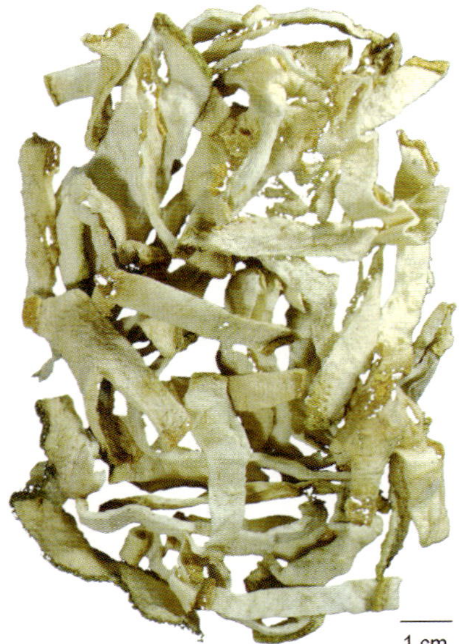

1 cm

Decoction Pieces

Source The fruit of *Citrus medica* L. var. *sarcodactylis* Swingle (Fam. Rutaceae).

Distribution Mainly in Chinese provinces such as Guangdong and Guangxi.

Harvest & Processing Harvest fruits in autumn before or when they turn yellow; cut length-wise into thin slices; dry under the sun or at low temperatures.

Description Subelliptical or ovate (egg-shaped in outline) slices, often shrivelled or curled up; 6-10 cm long, 3-7 cm wide, 2-4 mm thick. Top part broader, often with 3-5 digitiform (finger-shaped) petals; base narrower, occasionally with a carpopodium scar. Exocarp yellowish-green or orange-yellow, marked with wrinkles and oil dots. Sarcocarp light yellowish-white, scattered with uneven linear (long and narrow) or punctiform (dot-like) vascular bundles. Hard and brittle; turns pliable when moistened. Odour: fragrant; taste: slightly sweet and then bitter.

Indications 1. Distension and pain of the hypochondria and breast 2. Dysmenorrhoea, menstrual disorders 3. Epigastric pain and distension 4. Productive cough and dyspnoea

Chemical Composition Mainly contains limettin, nomillin, 6, 7-dimethoxycoumarin and diosmin.

Fructus Cnidii

Common Cnidium Fruit
Shechuangzi

蛇床子

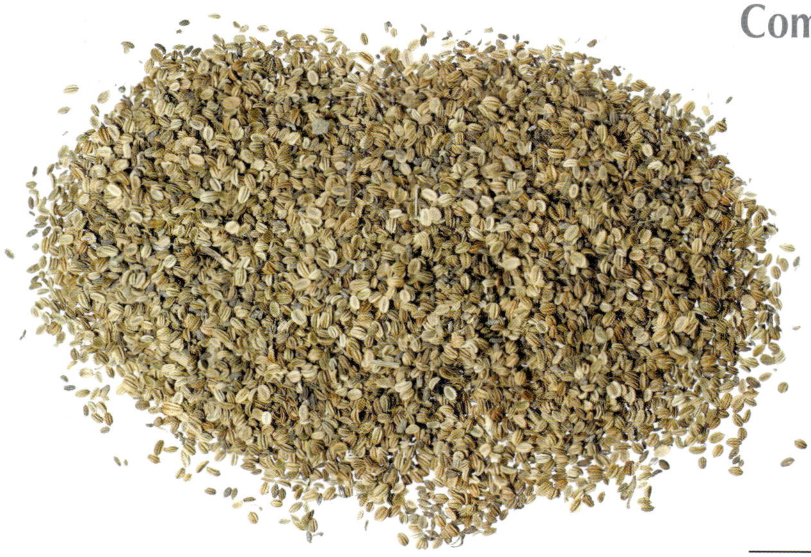

Crude Drug

1 cm

Source The mature fruit of *Cnidium monnieri* (L.) Cusson (Fam. Umbelliferae).

Distribution Mainly in Chinese provinces such as Hebei, Shandong, Guangxi and Zhejiang.

Harvest & Processing Harvest fruits at maturation in summer and autumn; remove foreign matter; dry under the sun.

Description Ellipsoid (elliptical in long-section and circular in cross-section) cremocarp, formed by two mericarps attached to each other; 2-4 mm long, 2 mm in diameter. Outer surface greyish-yellow or dull greyish-brown; top end with 2 stylopodiums curled outwards; base occasionally with a small carpopodium. Dorsal side of mericarps marked with 5 thin, protuberant, longitudinal ridges; commissure fairly flat, with 2 brown, slightly protuberant, longitudinal ridges. Testa loose, brittle, falls off easily when rubbed. Seeds small, greyish-brown, oleaginous (oily). Odour: fragrant; taste: acrid, cool and tongue-numbing.

Indications 1. Impotence, sterility 2. Enuresis, urinary frequency 3. Loin and knees ache 4. Tinea, scasbies, eczema, leukorrhagia with pruritus vulvae, tricomonas vaginitis (as pessaries)

Chemical Composition Mainly contains essential oils; also contains coumarins such as osthol and isopimpinellin.

Fructus Coriandri

Coriander Fruit
Yuansuizi

芫荽子

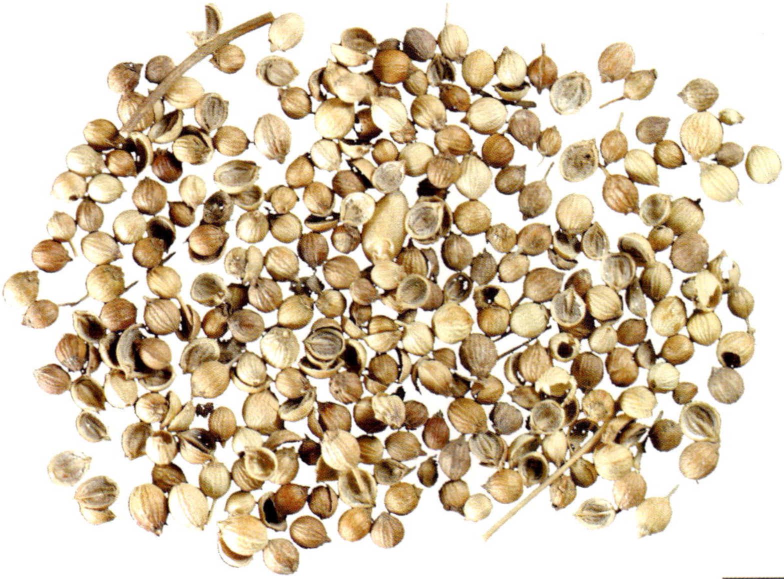

Crude Drug

Source The fruit of *Coriandrum sativum* L. (Fam. Umbelliferae).

Distribution Mainly in Chinese provinces such as Jiangsu, Anhui and Hubei.

Harvest & Processing Harvest fruits at maturation in August and September; remove foreign matter; dry under the sun.

Description Schizocarp spherical, formed by 2 mericarps. Pale yellowish-brown to earthy yellowish-brown; apex with extremely short remnants of stylopodium; mostly parted in two; surrounded by 5 sepals of persistent calyx. Outer surface relatively rough, with 10 fairly faint undulate (wavy), longitudinal ridges arranged alternately with 10 prominent, straight, longitudinal ridges. Base obtuse, occasionally with a small carpopodium. Mericarps protuberant on dorsal side; dented in the centre on ventral side, with 3 longitudinal ridges - the middle one fairly straight while the two lateral ones crescent-like; occasionally with a carpopodium. Fairly hard. Odour: fragrant, releases a heavy and distinctive aroma when crumbled by hand; taste: slightly hot.

Indications 1. Common cold with nasal congestion 2. Eruptive exanthem 3. Anorexia 4. Toothache.

Chemical Composition Mainly contains essential oils and flavonoids.

Fructus Corni

Asiatic Cornelian Cherry Fruit

Shanzhuyu

山茱萸

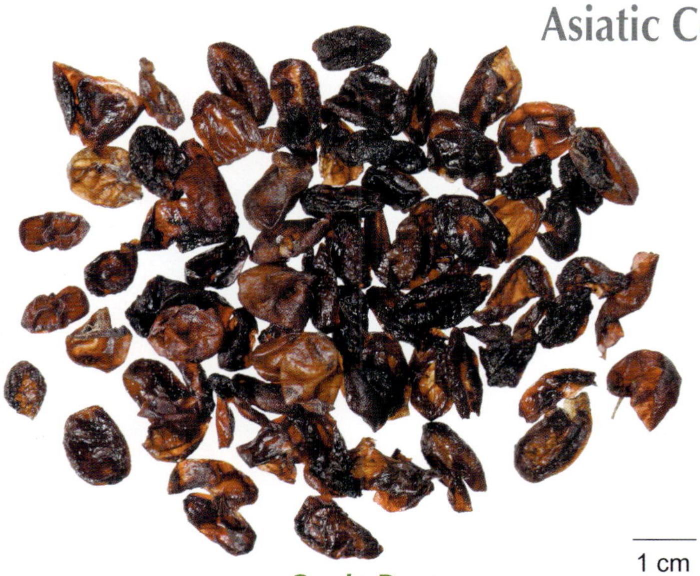

Crude Drug

Source The mature sarcocarp of *Cornus officinalis* Sieb. et Zucc. (Fam. Cornaceae).

Distribution Mainly in Chinese provinces such as Zhejiang, Henan, Anhui and Shaanxi.

Harvest & Processing Harvest fruits in late autumn and early winter when exocarp turns red; dry over gentle heat or blanch in boiling water; remove pits promptly; dry sarcocarp.

Description Irregular pieces or irregular and sacciform (sac-like) pieces; 1-1.5 cm long, 0.5-1 cm wide. Pericarp cracked and shrivelled, irregular in shape. Sarcocarp purplish-red when fresh, purplish-black after long storage. Outer surface shrivelled and lustrous. Top end occasionally with an orbicular (round) scar of persistent calyx; base with a carpopodium scar. Soft. Odour: faint; taste: sour, astringent and slightly bitter.

Indications 1. Weakness of the lower part of body and lower limbs, nocturnal emissions, impotence, urinary frequency 2. General weakness, spontaneous sweating 3. Dizziness, deafness.

Chemical Composition A variety of tannins and glycosides exist in the pulp.

Fructus Crataegi

Hawthorn Fruit
Shanzha

山楂

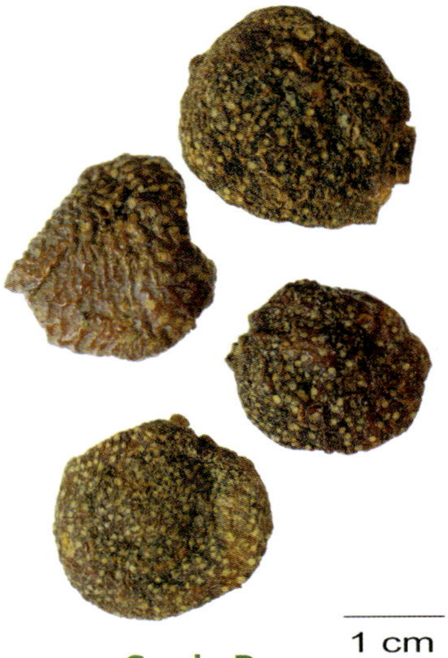

Crude Drug

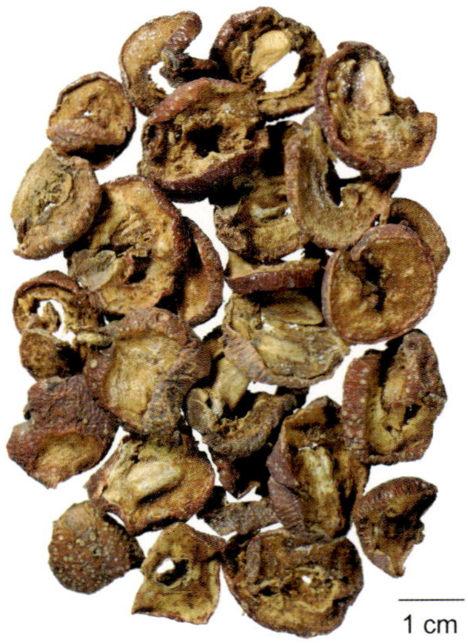

Decoction Pieces

Source The mature fruit of *Crataegus pinnatifida* Bunge *var. major* N. E. Br. (Fam. Rosaceae).

Distribution Mainly in Chinese provinces such as Shandong, Hebei, Henan and Liaoning.

Harvest & Processing Harvest fruits promptly after maturation; cut into slices while fresh; dry under the sun.

Description Cross-cut slices orbicular (round) in shape; mostly with curled edges; shrivelled and uneven. Exocarp red; marked with fine wrinkles and greyish-white dots. Sarcocarp dark yellow to light brown. Cross-section shows 5 light yellow pits; pits sometimes fallen off, leaving annular (ring-like) cavities. Some slices with short and fine carpopodiums or dented calyx scars. Odour: slightly fresh and fragrant; taste: sour, slightly sweet.

Indications 1. Dyspepsia, diarrhoea and dysentery 2. Amenorrhoea, postpartum abdominal pain with lochiostasis, 3. Hernia pain 4. Angina pectoris, hypertension and hyperlipidemia.

Chemical Composition Contains epicatechin, quercetin and citric acid.

Note According to *C.P.*, also used for medicinal purposes is the mature fruit of *C. pinnatifida* Bge.

Fructus Crotonis

Croton Seed
Badou
巴豆

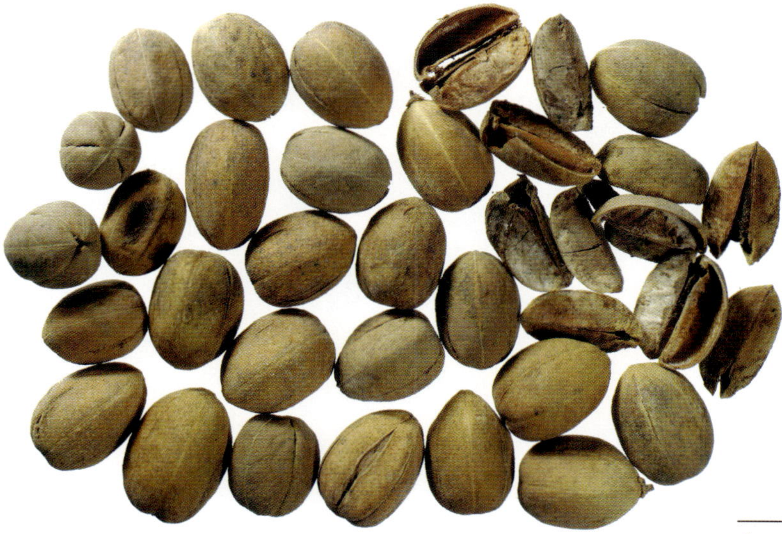

Crude Drug

1 cm

Source The mature fruit or seed of *Croton tiglium* L. (Fam. Euphorbiaceae).

Distribution Mainly in Chinese provinces such as Sichuan, Yunnan, Guangxi, Guizhou and Hubei, with Sichuan as the largest producer.

Harvest & Processing Harvest mature fruits in autumn; spread out for 2-3 days; dry under the sun or by heat; alternatively remove fruit shells and dry under the sun.

Description Ovoid (egg-shaped), usually with 3 ridges. Outer surface greyish-yellow or a little darker, rough, with 6 longitudinal striae; top part truncate (squared as if cut off), base with a carpopodium scar. When cracked open, fruit shell marked with 3 locules, each containing 1 seed. Seed ellipsoid (elliptical in long-section and circular in cross-section), slightly flattened; outer surface brown or greyish-brown; one end with a small punctiform (dot-like) hilum and caruncle scar, the other with a slightly dented chalaza, in between lies a protuberant raphe; exotesta thin and brittle, endotesta white and membranous; kernel yellowish-white, oleaginous (oily). Odourless; taste: pungent.

Indications 1. Ascites 2. Copious expectoration 3. Ileus (external use).

Chemical Composition Contains crotonic acid, tiglic acid and phorbol. Crotin I, II also exist in the kernd.

Note According to *C.P.*, also used for medicinal purposes is a processed Fructus Crotonis called '*Badou shuang*' (Defatted Croton Seed Powder). Fructus Crotonis is listed in Hong Kong as Category I (Toxic/Potent) Chinese Materia Medica, and the processed Fructus Crotonis, Category II.

Fructus Evodiae

Medicinal Evodia Fruit

Wuzhuyu

吴茱萸

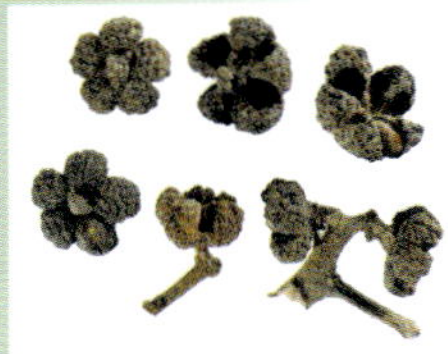

Medicinal Evodia Fruit Magnified

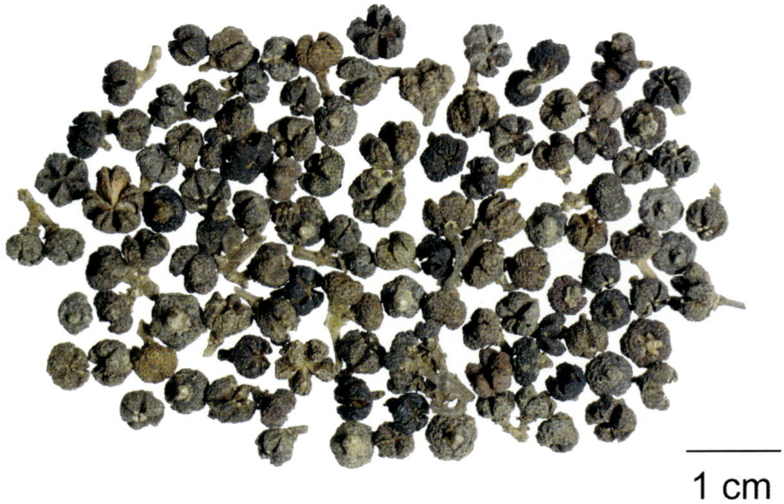

Crude Drug

Source The near-mature fruit of *Evodia rutaecarpa* (Juss.) Benth. (Fam. Rutaceae).

Distribution Mainly in Chinese provinces such as Guizhou, Guangxi, Hunan and Yunnan.

Harvest & Processing Collect fruit spurs in August and September when fruits are tea-green in colour and have not yet dehisced (split open at maturity); dry under the sun or at low temperatures; remove foreign matter.

Description Spherical, or roughly the shape of a flattened, pentagonal sphere; 2-5 mm in diameter. Outer surface dull yellowish-green to dull brown; rough; marked with numerous punctiform (dot-like) protuberances or dented oil dots. Top part with a suture the shape of a five-pointed star; base with remnants of carpopodium covered with yellow pubescences. Hard and brittle. When cracked open, black interior revealed; under magnification, oil cavities in the form of black oleaginous (oily) specks visible along the edge. Cross-section shows 5-loculed ovary; each locule with 1 light yellow seed. Odour: heavily aromatic; taste: pungent and bitter. Oozes mucilage when soaked in water.

Indications 1. Nausea, vomiting, abdominal pain, belching, diarrhoea 2. Headache

Chemical Composition Mainly contains alkaloids such as evodiamine.

Note According to *C.P.*, also used for medicinal purposes and listed as slightly toxic is the near-mature fruit of *E. rutaecarpa* (Juss.) Benth. var. *officinalis* (Dode) Huang and *E. rutaecarpa* (Juss.) Benth. var. *bodinieri* (Dode) Huang.

Fructus Foeniculi

Fennel
Xiaohuixiang
小茴香

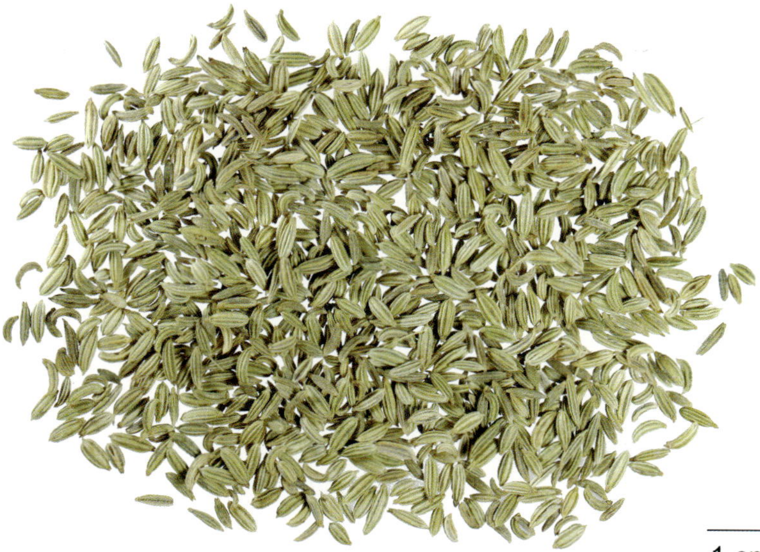

1 cm

Crude Drug

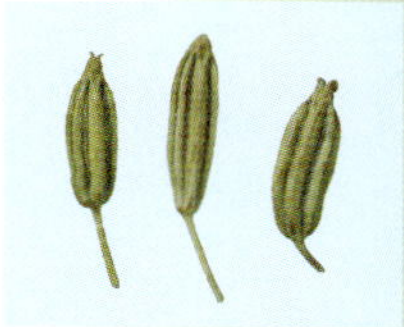

Fennel Magnified

Source The mature fruit of *Foeniculum vulgare* Mill. (Fam. Umbelliferae).

Distribution Originated in Europe. Cultivated in all parts of China.

Harvest & Processing Harvest plants in autumn when fruits begin to ripen; dry under the sun; thresh to get fruits; remove foreign matter.

Description Cylindrical cremocarp, occasionally slightly curved; 4-8 mm long, 1.5-2.5 mm in diameter. Outer surface yellowish-green or pale yellow, both ends somewhat pointed; top end with protuberant yellowish-brown stylopodium remnants; base occasionally with a small carpopodium. Mericarps oblong and ellipsoid (elliptical in long-section and circular in cross-section), with 5 longitudinal ridges at the back; commissure flat and fairly broad. Cross-section slightly pentagonal, with the four sides at the back about the same length. Odour: with a distinctive fragrance; taste: slightly sweet and acrid.

Indications 1. Feeling of cold and pains in stomach and lower abdomen.
2. Dysmenorrhoea 3. Hernia pain.

Chemical Composition Mainly contains essential oils with 50-60% of anethole.

Fructus Forsythiae

Weeping Forsythia Capsule
Lianqiao

連翹

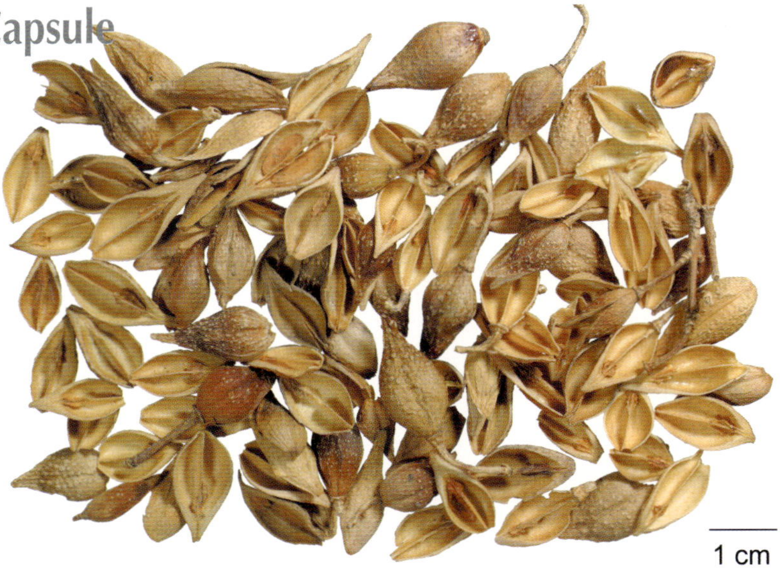

1 cm

Crude Drug

Source The fruit of *Forsythia suspense* (Thunb.) Vahl (Fam. Oleaceae).

Distribution Mainly in Chinese provinces such as Shanxi, Shaanxi and Henan.

Harvest & Processing Harvest fruits in autumn when they first mature and still look greenish; remove foreign matter; dry under the sun.

Description Ovoid (egg-shaped), or oblong and ovoid, slightly flattened. Outer surface marked with irregular longitudinal wrinkles and numerous small protuberant maculae; with 1 conspicuous longitudinal groove on either side; top end acute; a small carpopodium at base or just a scar. Fruit acrocidal (split on top) or split into two cloves; outer surface yellowish-brown or reddish-brown, inner surface mostly light yellowish-brown, smooth and with 1 longitudinal septum; brittle; seeds brown, mostly fallen off. Odour: slightly fragrant; taste: bitter.

Indications 1. Common cold 2. Pharyngitis 3. Dermatitis 4. Scrofula, carbuncle and sores

Chemical Composition Mainly contains lignans such as arctiin.

Fructus Galangae

Galanga Galangal Fruit
Hongdoukou

紅豆蔻

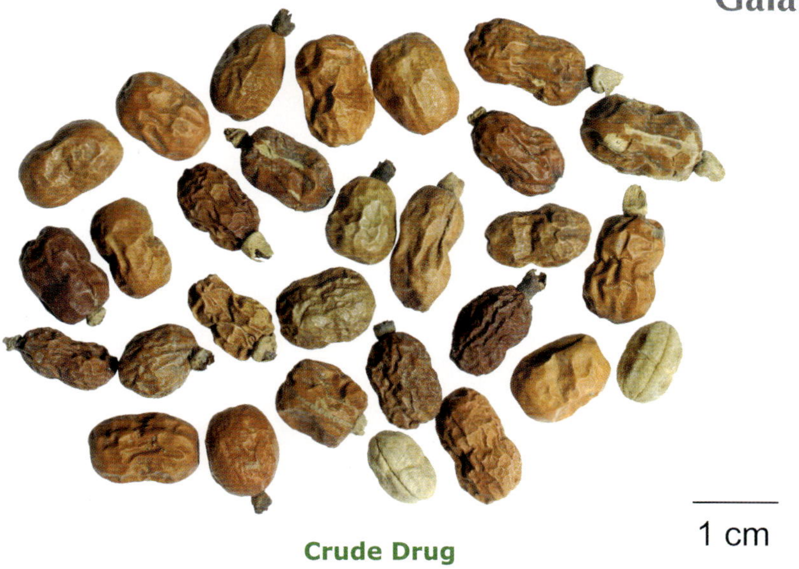

Crude Drug

Source The mature fruit of *Alpinia galanga* Willd. (Fam. Zingiberaceae).

Distribution Mainly in Chinese provinces such as Guangdong, Guangxi, Hainan and Yunnan; also in Hong Kong.

Harvest & Processing Harvest fruits in autumn when they turn red; remove foreign matter; dry in shaded areas.

Description Oblong and spherical, slightly shrunken in the middle; 0.7-1.2 cm long, 5-7 mm in diameter. Outer surface reddish-brown or dull red, slightly shrivelled; apex with remnants of yellowish-white fistular (hollow and cylindrical) persistent calyx; base with carpopodium scars. Pericarp thin, breaks easily. 3 locules, each with 2 seeds. Seeds disc-like or in the form of triangular polyhedrons; blackish-brown or reddish-brown; covered with yellowish-white membranous aril; endosperms greyish-white. Odour: fragrant; taste: pungent.

Indications 1. Epigastric pain with cold sensation 2. Dyspepsia with abdominal distension 3. Vomiting and diarrhoea 4. Excessive alcohol drinking.

Chemical Composition Mainly contains essential oils with (+) 2-terpinyl acetate as the main component.

Fructus Gardeniae

Cape Jasmine Fruit
Zhizi

梔子

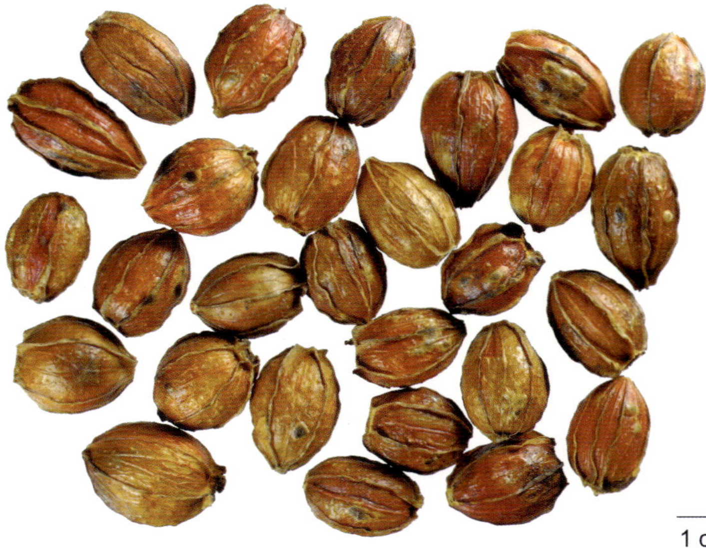

Crude Drug

Source The mature fruit of *Gardenia jasminoides* Ellis (Fam. Rubiaceae).

Distribution Mainly in Chinese provinces such as Hunan, Jiangxi, Hubei and Zhejiang; also in Hong Kong.

Harvest & Processing Harvest reddish-yellow mature fruits between September and November; blanch in boiling water; scoop up almost immediately and dry under the sun, or steam and then dry under the sun.

Description Oblong and ovoid (egg-shaped), or ellipsoid (elliptical in long-section and circular in cross-section); 1.5-3.5 cm long, 1-1.5 cm in diameter. Outer surface reddish-yellow or brownish-red, marked with 6 aliform (wing-shaped) longitudinal ridges; 1 prominent, rameous (branched) longitudinal vein usually lying between the ridges. Top end with sepal remnants; base relatively pointed, with carpopodium remnants. Pericarp thin and brittle, slightly lustrous; inner surface paler in colour, lustrous, with 2-3 raised pseudoseptums. Seeds numerous, flattened and ovoid, packed in clusters, dark red or reddish-yellow; outer surface densely verruculose (with small wart-shaped protuberances). Odour: faint; taste: slightly sour, bitter.

Indications 1. Jaundice, infectious hepatitis, aphthous ulcer, toothache 2. Common cold, fever 3. Red eyes, photophobia with lacrimation 4. Insomnia 5. Bleeding, trauma

Chemical Composition Mainly contains iridoids such as gardenoside; also contains pigment crocin.

Fructus Gleditsiae Abnormalis

Chinese Honeylocust Abnormal Fruit

Zhuyazao

豬牙皂

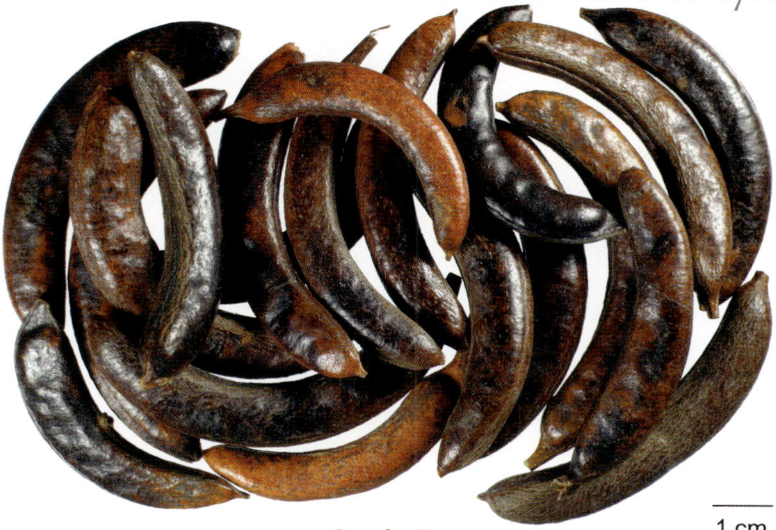

Crude Drug

Source The sterile fruit of *Gleditsia sinensis* Lam. (Fam. Leguminosae).

Distribution Mainly in Chinese provinces such as Shandong, Hubei and Sichuan.

Harvest & Processing The plants bear fruits after 5-6 years of cultivation. Collect fruits in autumn when they turn black at maturation; dry under the sun.

Description Fruit long and sheath-like, slightly flattened and curved; 15-20 cm long, 2-3.5 cm wide; 0.8-1.5 cm thick. Outer surface dark purplish-brown to blackish-brown, covered with grey powder; bulgy where seeds are; tapering and slightly curving towards the base; base with a short carpopodium or carpopodium scar; both sides with conspicuous longitudinal ridges. Rattles when shaken. Hard; when cut open, surface of pericarp yellow and fibrous. Seeds numerous, flattened and elliptical, yellowish-brown, smooth. Odour: distinctive, heavily pungent; powder sternutatory (inducing sneezing) when sniffed; taste: pungent.

Indications 1. Impairment of consciousness in stroke and epilepsy 2. Sore throat, dyspnoea, cough with thick sputum and difficult expectoration 3. Constipation 4. Pyogenic skin infection.

Chemical Composition Mainly contains triterpene saponins such as gleditsioside and gleditsia saponins.

Note Listed as slightly toxic in *C.P.*

Fructus Hordei Germinatus

Germinated Barley
Maiya

麥芽

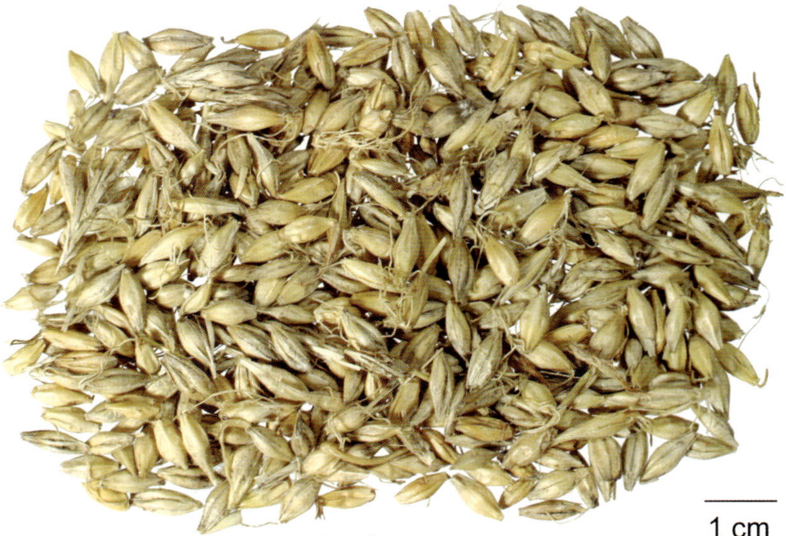

Crude Drug

Source The germinated mature grain of *Hordeum vulgare* L. (Fam. Gramineae).

Distribution In all regions of northern China.

Harvest & Processing Germinate barley grains anytime during the year, preferably in winter and spring. Get barley grains with foreign matter removed; soak in clean water for 3-4 hours; scoop up and put in a drainable container; cover up; water 2-3 times a day; keep moist until buds grow to 2-3 mm long; take out the grains and dry under the sun.

Description Narrow and pointed at both ends, slightly spindle-shaped; 8-15 mm long, 2.5-4.5 mm in diameter. Outer surface pale yellow; dorsal side enveloped by lemma and marked with 5 veins, long arista at apex broken off; ventral side enveloped by palea and marked with a longitudinal groove. Plumule and fibrous roots can be seen growing at radicle base when palea and lemma are removed; plumule oblong, lanceolate (lance-head shaped) and linear (long and narrow), yellowish-white; fibrous roots several, slender and curved. Hard; broken surface white and starchy. Odourless; taste: slightly sweet.

Indications 1. Dyspepsia, anorexia 2. As lactifuge for breast-feeding women.

Chemical Composition Mainly contains hordenin and hordatine A, B.

Fructus Jujubae

Chinese Date

Dazao

大棗

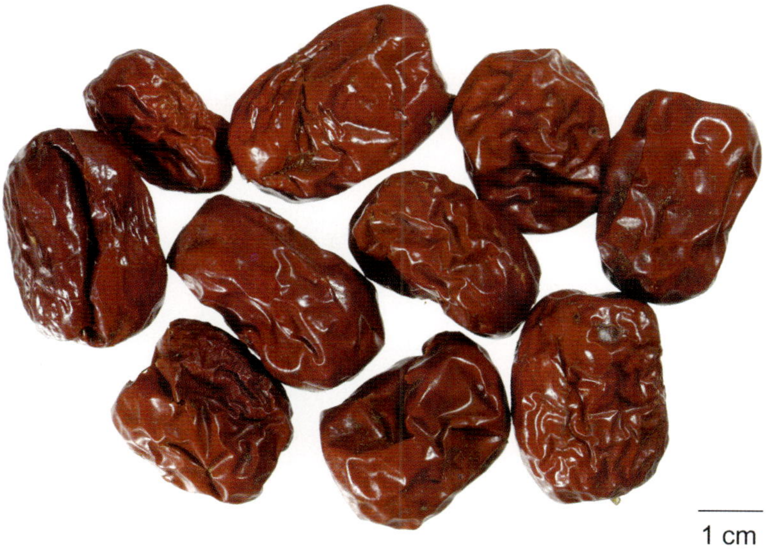

1 cm

Crude Drug

Source
The mature fruit of *Ziziphus jujuba Mill.* (Fam. Rhamnaceae). Customarily called '*Hongzao*' (Red Chinese Date) in Hong Kong.

Distribution
Mainly in Chinese provinces such as Henan and Shandong, also in provinces such as Hebei, Shanxi, Sichuan and Guizhou.

Harvest & Processing
Collect fruits at maturation in autumn; dry under the sun.

Description
Ellipsoid (elliptical in long-section and circular in cross-section) or spherical; 2.5-3 cm long; 1.5-2.5 cm in diameter. Outer surface dull red, slightly lustrous. Base dented, with a short carpopodium. Exocarp thin; mesocarp brownish-yellow or pale dull brown; fleshy; soft; highly sugary, oily and soft. Pit spindle-shaped, both ends acute; hard. Odour: slightly fragrant; taste: sweet.

Indications
1. Anorexia, fatigue, loose stool 2. Insomnia, vexation and restlessness. 3. Counteracting the toxicity or side effects of potent drugs 4. Anaphylactoid purpura and bronchial asthma.

Chemical Composition
Mainly contains triterpene saponins such as zizyphus saponins I, II, IV.

Fructus Kochiae

Belvedere Fruit
Difuzi

地膚子

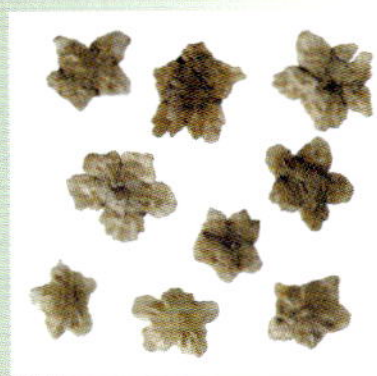

Belvedere Fruit Magnified

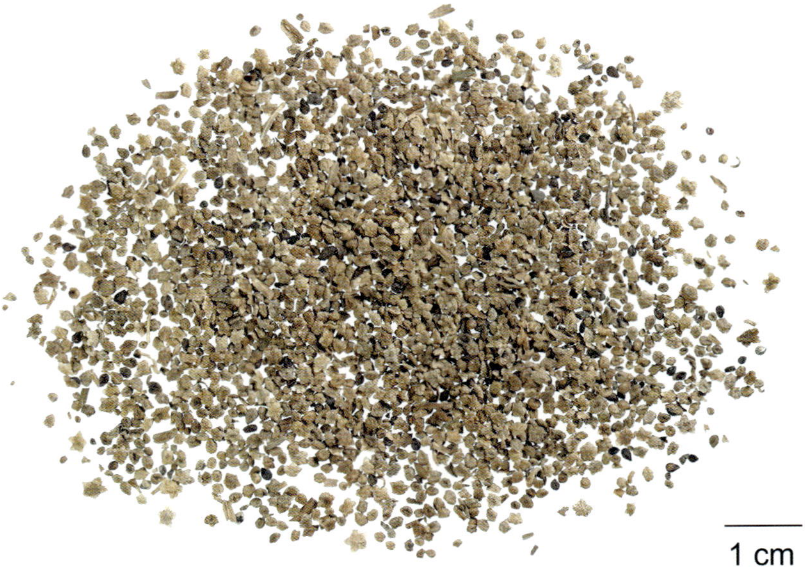

Crude Drug

Source The mature fruit of *Kochia scoparia* (L.) Schrad. (Fam. Chenopodiaceae).

Distribution Mainly in Chinese provinces such as Shandong, Jiangsu, Henan and Hebei.

Harvest & Processing Harvest whole herbs in autumn when fruits ripen; dry under the sun; thresh to get fruits; remove foreign matter.

Description Flattened, spherical, and five-pointed star in shape; 1-3 mm in diameter, covered with persistent perianth. Outer surface greyish-green or light brown, surrounded by 5 membranous winglets; centre of the dorsal side marked with a slightly protuberant, punctiform (dot-like) carpopodium scar and 5-10 radial venous (vein-like) striae; pericarp translucent and membranous. Seeds flattened and ovoid (egg-shaped), about 1 mm long, black; embryo curved and hippocrepiform (horseshoe-shaped), pale yellow. Odour: faint; taste: slightly bitter.

Indications 1. Urinary tract infection 2. Urticaria, eczema, pruritus.

Chemical Composition Mainly contains oleanolic acid and its glycosides.

Fructus Leonuri

Motherwort Fruit
Chongweizi

茺蔚子

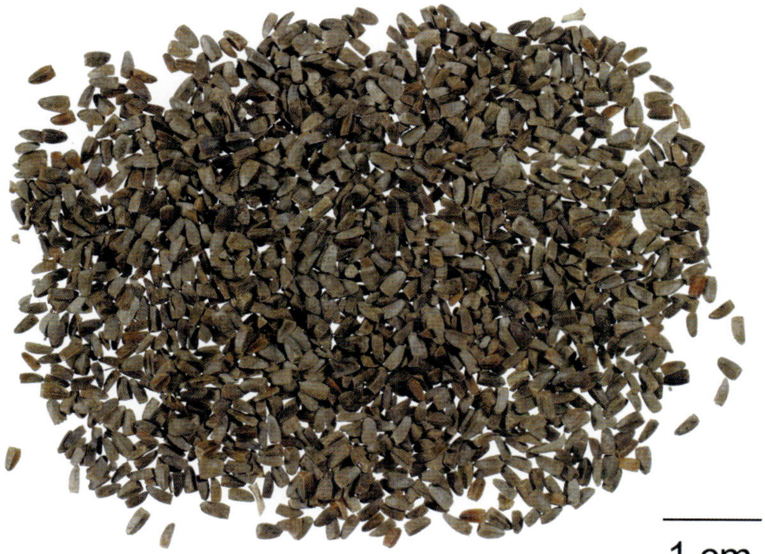

1 cm

Crude Drug

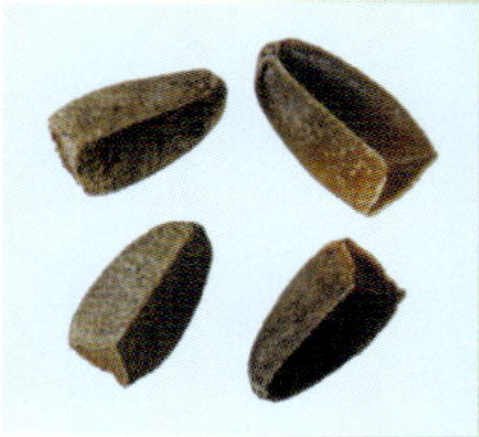

Motherwort Fruit Magnified

Source The mature fruit of *Leonurus japonicus* Houtt. (Fam. Labiatae).

Distribution In all parts of China, including Hong Kong.

Harvest & Processing Collect above-ground parts in autumn when fruits are ripe; dry under the sun; thresh to get fruits; remove foreign matter.

Description Oblong and spherical, with 3 ridges; 2-3 mm long; 1-1.5 mm in diameter; one end truncate (squared as if cut off), tapering to the other end; with a dented carpopodium scar. Outer surface dull greyish-brown or dull brown; sparsely marked with dark-coloured maculae; no lustre, or slightly rough. Cross-cut surface triangular under a microscope; pericarp dull brown; endosperms and cotyledons white; cotyledons highly oleaginous (oily). Odourless; taste: bitter.

Indications 1. Menstrual disorders, amenorrhoea and dysmenorrhoea 2. Inflammation of the eyes with formation of nebula 3. Dizziness, headache.

Chemical Composition Mainly contains alkaloids such as leonurinine and stachydrine.

Fructus Ligustri Lucidi

Glossy Privet Fruit
Nüzhenzi

女貞子

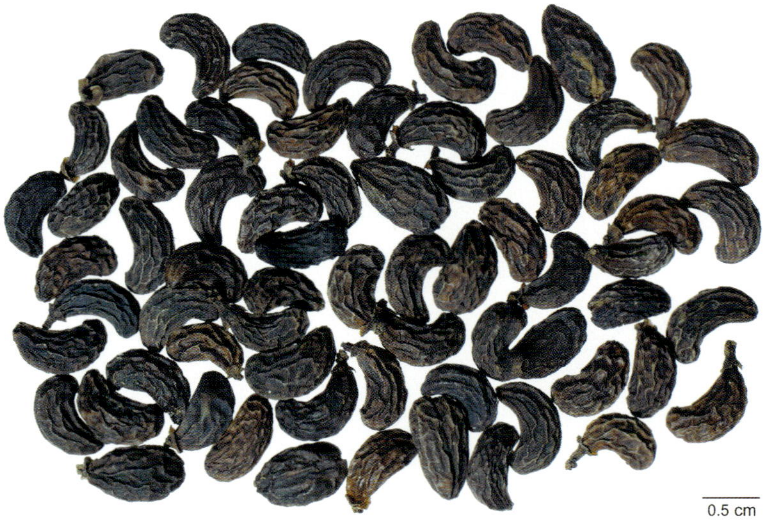

Crude Drug

Source The mature fruit of *Ligustrum lucidum* Ait. (Fam. Oleaceae).

Distribution Mainly in Chinese provinces such as Zhejiang, Jiangsu, Fujian and Hunan.

Harvest & Processing Harvest fruits at maturation in winter; remove branches and leaves; steam for a little while or blanch in boiling water and then dry; alternatively dry without steaming or blanching.

Description Ovoid (egg-shaped), ellipsoid (elliptical in long-section and circular in cross-section) or reniform (kidney-shaped); 6-8.5 mm long, 3.5-5.5 mm in diameter. Outer surface dark purple or greyish-black; shrivelled and uneven; base with a carpopodium scar, or with a persistent calyx and a short carpopodium. Light in weight. Exocarp thin; mesocarp relatively loose and soft, easily peeled off; endocarp ligneous (woody), yellowish-brown, marked with a longitudinal ridge. When broken open, usually 1 seed revealed; seed reniform, purplish-black, oleaginous (oily). Odourless; taste: sweet and slightly bitter-astringent.

Indications 1. Dizziness, vertigo and tinnitus 2. Weakness of the loin and knees, hectic fever, nocturnal emission 3. Poliosis, alopecia 4. Blurring of vision, central retinitis and early cataract

Chemical Composition Mainly contains triterpenes such as oleanolic acid and ursolic acid.

Fructus Liquidambaris

Beautiful Sweetgum Fruit
Lulutong

路路通

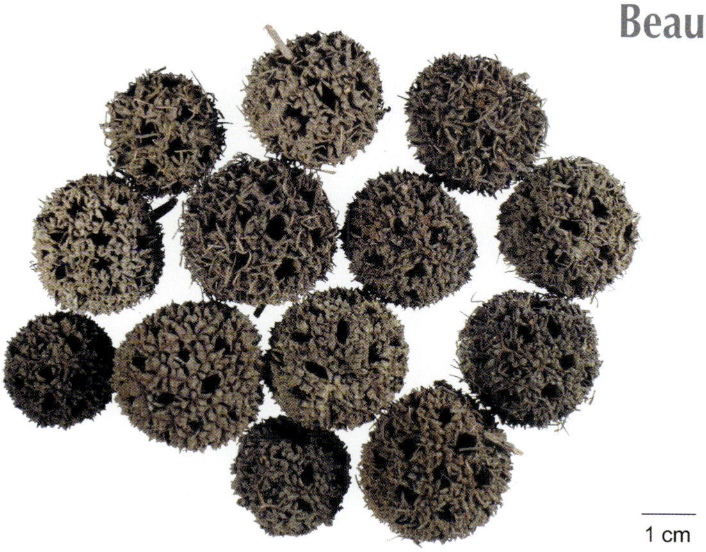

Crude Drug

Source The mature infructescence of *Liquidambar formosana* Hance (Fam. Hamaelidaceae).

Distribution Mainly in Chinese provinces such as Jiangsu, Zhejiang, Anhui, Fujian, Hubei, Hunan and Shaanxi; also in Hong Kong.

Harvest & Processing Pick mature infrustescences in winter; remove foreign matter; wash clean; dry under the sun.

Description Globose (spherical), composed of small scales enclosing the ovary; 2-3 cm in diameter. Outer surface greyish-brown to reddish-brown; with numerous spiniform (spine-shaped) persistent calyx teeth and coronoid (beak-shaped) styles, often broken or bended; numerous honeycomb-like holes revealed at removal of calyx teeth and styles; cylindrical carpopodium at base, 3-4.5 cm long, often broken or with just the scar remaining. Small capsules acrocidal (split on top), forming cavities. Numerous seeds visible within cavities; incompletely developed ones small, polygonal, around 1 mm in diameter; the few fully developed ones yellowish-brown to reddish-brown, flattened, oblong and orbicular (round), winged, dull brown. Light in weight; hard, not easily cracked. Odour: slightly fragrant; taste: mild.

Indications 1. Insufficient lactation, galactostasis 2. Menstrual disorders 3. Rheumatic arthralgia, lumbago 4. Dysuria 5. Urticaria.

Chemical Composition Mainly contains flavonoids and triterpenes.

Fructus Litseae

Mountain Spicy Fruit

Bichengqie

蓽澄茄

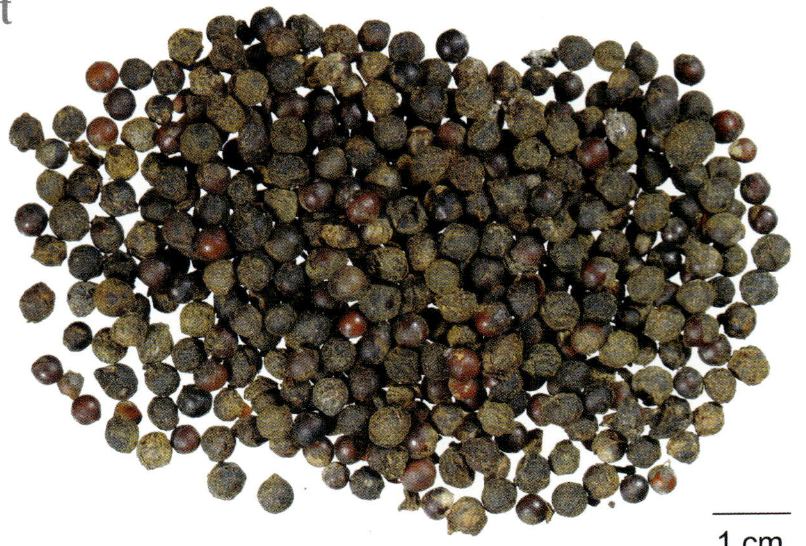

Crude Drug

Source The mature fruit of *Litsea cubeba* (Lour.) Pers. (Fam. Lauraceae).

Distribution Mainly in Chinese provinces such as Jiangsu, Zhejiang, Sichuan and Fujian; also in Hong Kong.

Harvest & Processing Harvest mature fruits in autumn; remove foreign matter; dry under the sun.

Description Subspherical; 4-6 mm in diameter. Outer surface reddish-brown to brownish-black, marked with reticulate (net-like) wrinkles; base often marked with a carpopodium scar. Mesocarp can be peeled off easily; endocarp dull brown, pericarp hard and brittle; seed 1, containing 2 plump, highly oleaginous (oily) cotyledons. Odour: with a distinctive, penetrating aroma; taste: acrid, mint-like.

Indications 1. Epigastric and abdominal pain, abdominal colic 2. Vomiting, hiccup, diarrhoea.

Chemical Composition The fresh fruit contains 1.6% - 3% essential oils with citral, geranial and neral as the main components.

Fructus Lycii

Barbary Wolfberry Fruit

Gouqizi

枸杞子

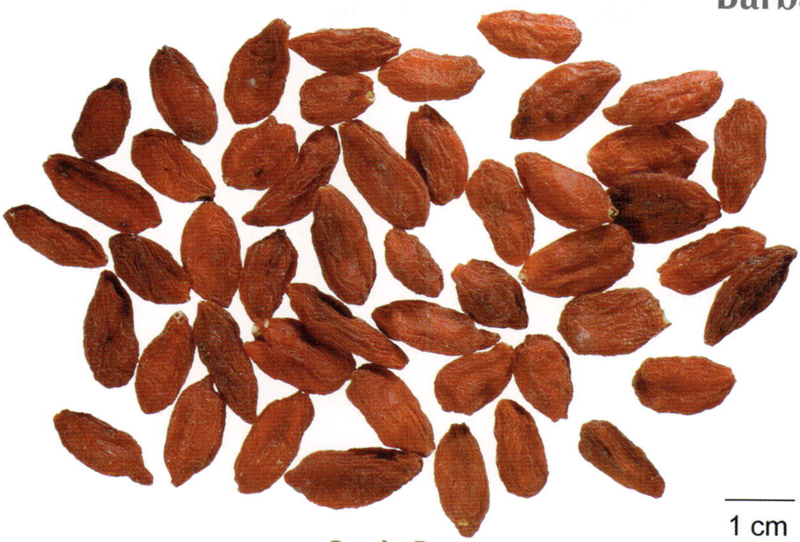

Crude Drug

Source The mature fruit of *Lycium barbarum* L. (Fam. Solanaceae).

Distribution Mainly in Chinese provinces such as Gansu and Qinghai, and in Ningxia and Xinjiang.

Harvest & Processing Harvest fruits in summer and autumn when they turn red; air until wrinkled; dry under the sun until exocarp is dry and hard and sarcocarp soft; remove carpopodiums.

Description Roughly spindle-shaped, or ellipsoid (elliptical in long-section and circular in cross-section); 6-20 mm long, 3-10 mm in diameter. Outer surface red or dull red; top end with a slightly protuberant style scar, base with a white carpopodium scar. Pericarp wrinkled, soft and pliable; sarcocarp fleshy, soft and smooth. Seeds 20-50, roughly reniform (kidney-shaped), flattened but curved; 1.5-1.9 mm long, 1-1.7 mm wide; outer surface light yellow or brownish-yellow. Odour: faint; taste: sweet; chewing it turns saliva reddish-yellow.

Indications 1. Seminal emissions 2. Ache of the lower part of the body 3. Vertigo, amblyopia.

Chemical Composition Mainly contains polysaccharides and carotenoids such as β-carotene.

Fructus Momordicae

Grosvener Momordica Fruit
Luohanguo

羅漢果

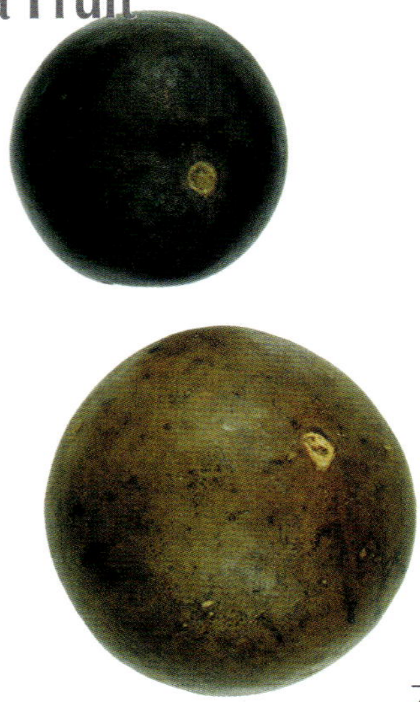

1 cm

Crude Drug

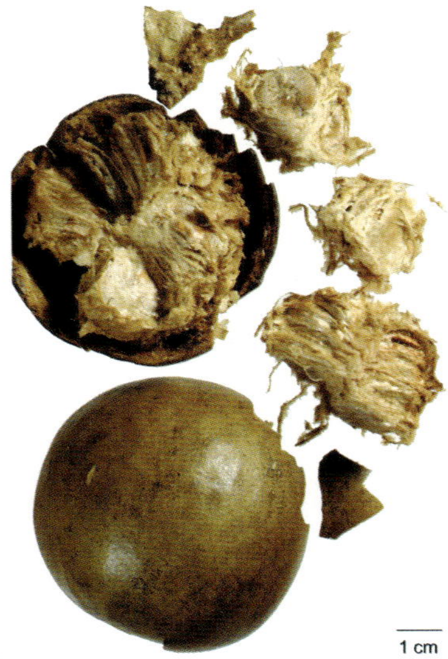

1 cm

Cracked Crude Drug

Source The fruit of *Momordica grosvenori* Swingle (Fam. Cucurbitaceae).

Distribution Mainly in Guangxi provinces in China.

Harvest & Processing Collect mature fruits between September and October; dry by heat; store in dry places.

Description Ovoid (egg-shaped), ellipsoid (elliptical in long-section and circular in cross-section) or spherical; 5-8 cm in diameter. Outer surface dull brown, dull yellowish-brown or dull greenish-brown; covered with dark-coloured maculae and yellow pubescence. Apex marked with a style scar; base with a carpopodium scar. Light in weight; brittle; pericarp thin; breaks easily. Sarcocarp (mesocarp and endocarp) spongilliform (spongy) and light brown. Seeds disc-like, numerous; about 1.5 cm long, about 1.2 cm wide; light red to brownish-red; slightly dented in the middle on both surfaces; indentations surrounded by radial furrows; margin with a groove. Odour: faint; taste: sweet.

Indications 1.Dry cough, sore throat, hoarseness of voice 2. Constipation.

Chemical Composition Mainly contains triterpenes, triterpene saponins and flavonoids.

Fructus Mori

Mulberry Fruit
Sangshen

桑椹

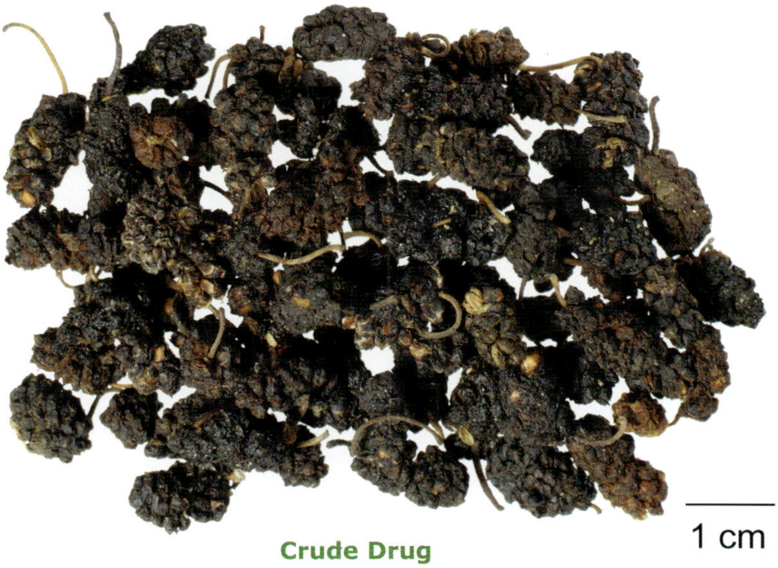

Crude Drug

Source The fruit spike of *Morus alba* L. (Fam. Moraceae).

Distribution Mainly in Chinese provinces such as Jiangsu, Zhejiang, Hunan, Sichuan, Hebei, Shandong, Anhui, Liaoning, Henan and Shanxi; also in Hong Kong.

Harvest & Processing Collect fruit spikes from April to June when they turn red; dry under the sun, or steam and dry under the sun.

Description Aggregate fruit consisting of numerous small achenes, oblong and spherical; 1-2 cm long, 5-8 mm in diameter. Yellowish-brown, brownish-red to dull purple; with a short infructescence stalk. Small achenes ovoid (egg-shaped), slightly flat; about 2 mm long, about 1 mm wide; with 4 fleshy tepals on the outside. Odour: faint; taste: slightly sour, sweet.

Indications 1. Dizziness, tinnitus, vexation, insomnia, neurasthenia 2. Diabetes mellitus 3. Constipation 4. Anaemia 5. Hypertension.

Chemical Composition Contains essential oils with cineole and linalool as the main components; also contains cyanidin and chrysanthemin.

Fructus Mume

Smoked Plum

Wumei

烏梅

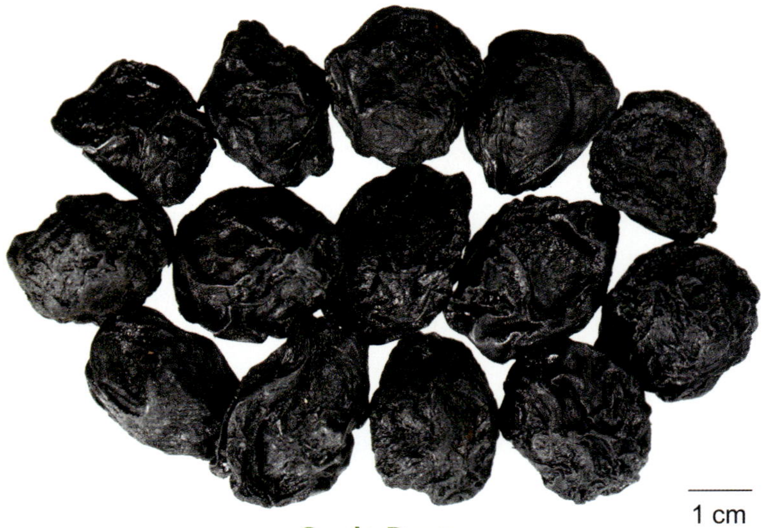

Crude Drug

Source The near-mature fruit of *Prunus mume* (Sieb.) Sieb. et Zucc. (Fam. Rosaceae).

Distribution Mainly in Chinese provinces such as Sichuan, Zhejiang, Fujian and Guangdong.

Harvest & Processing Harvest near-mature fruits in summer; dry by heat at low temperatures; keep in tightly closed containers for 2-3 days to let blacken.

Description Flattened and spherical, or irregular and spherical; 1.5-3 cm in diameter. Outer surface brownish-black to jet black; shrivelled and uneven; one end with a conspicuous orbicular (round) hilum. Sarcocarp soft; can be peeled off. Pit hard, ellipsoid (elliptical in long-section and circular in cross-section), brownish-yellow; outer surface uneven, marked with numerous pores and reticulate (net-like) markings; containing a pale yellow kernel. Odour of sarcocarp: with a light but distinctive sour and smoky smell; taste: extremely sour.

Indications 1. Chronic diarrhoea, abdominal pain caused by ascarides 2. Chronic cough 3. Thirst, diabetes 4. Haematochezia, dysfunctional uterine bleeding 5. Callus, corns (topically).

Chemical Composition Contains essential oils and a variety of organic acid.

Fructus Oryzae Germinatus

Rice-grain Sprout
Daoya
稻芽

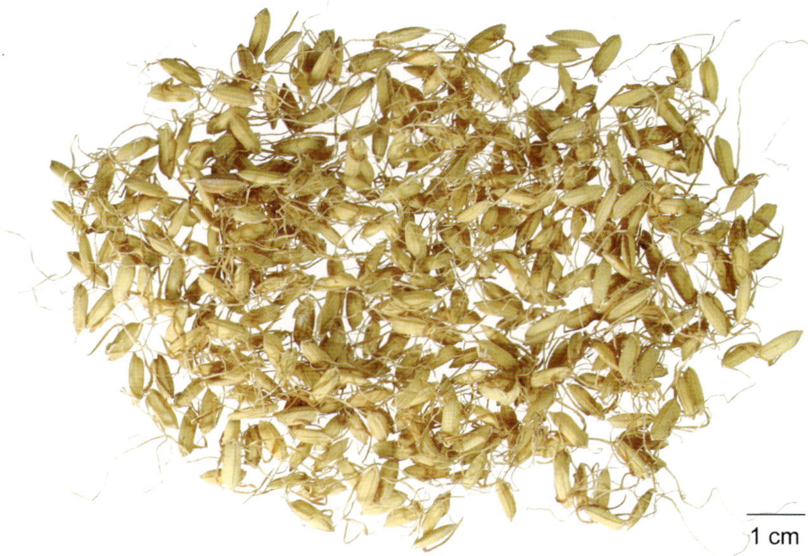

Crude Drug

Source The germinated mature grain of *Oryza sativa* L. (Fam. Gramineae).

Distribution In all rice-producing regions of China; mostly in southern China.

Harvest & Processing Process mature grains, mostly in spring and autumn. Pick rice-grains with foreign matter removed; soak in water for 1-2 days; scoop up; put in drainable containers; cover up; water once daily; keep moist; let grains germinate until fibrous roots grow to about 3.3-7 mm long; take out and dry under the sun.

Description Slightly flattened, oblong and ellipsoid (elliptical in long section and circular in cross section), both ends slightly pointed; 6-9 mm long, about 3 mm wide. Lemma hard; outer surface yellow, puberulent (covered with fine, short, soft hairs); with 5 veins. 2 white linear (long and narrow) lodicules at base, about 2 mm long, waxy; curved, pale yellow primary roots jutting out from the inner side of one lodicule. Palea membranous, smooth, yellowish-white, containing the grain. Hard; broken surface white and starchy. Odourless; taste: slightly sweet.

Indications Dyspepsia with abdominal distension and foul breath, anorexia

Chemical Composition Mainly contains proteins and amino acids.

Fructus Perillae

Perilla Fruit

Zisuzi

紫蘇子

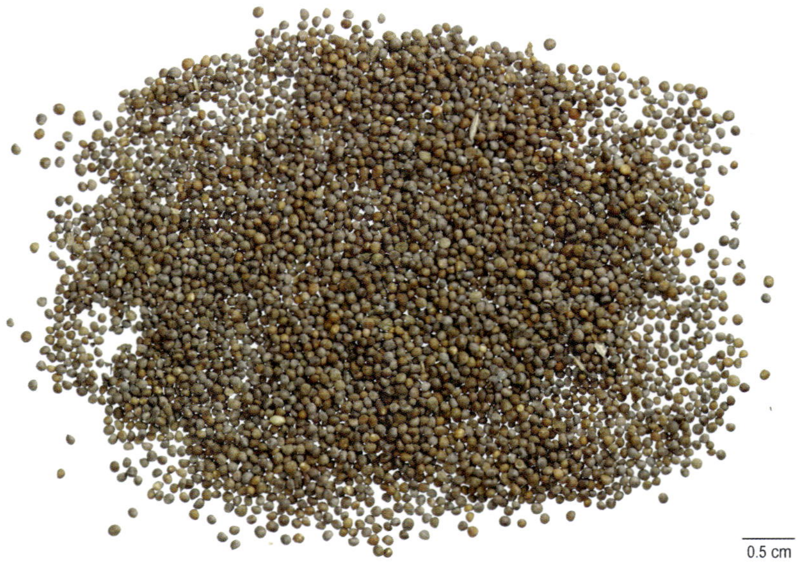

Crude Drug

Source The mature fruit of *Perilla frutescens* (L.) Britt. (Fam. Labiatae).

Distribution Mainly in Chinese provinces such as Jiangsu, Zhejiang and Hebei. Mostly cultivated.

Harvest & Processing Cut off whole herbs or fruit spikes in autumn when fruits ripen; dry in shaded areas; thresh to get fruits; remove foreign matter; dry under the sun.

Description Ovoid (egg-shaped) or subspherical; about 1.5 mm in diameter. Outer surface greyish-brown or dull greyish-brown; slightly protuberant, dull purple reticulate (net-like) striae visible under magnification; base slightly pointed, with a greyish-white punctiform (dot-like) carpopodium scar. Pericarp thin and brittle, easy to crush. Seeds yellowish-white; testa membranous; cotyledons 2, off-white, oleaginous (oily). Odour: fragrant when crushed; taste: slightly acrid.

Indications Productive cough, dyspnoea, asthma.

Chemical Composition The seed oil contains egomaketone.

Fructus Phyllanthi

Emblic Leafflower Fruit
Yuganzi

餘甘子

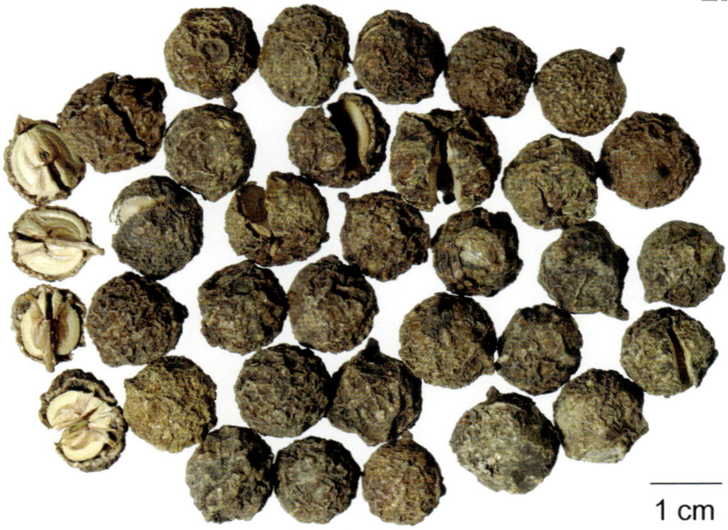

Crude Drug

Source The mature fruit of *Phyllanthus emblica* L. (Fam. Euphorbiaceae).

Distribution Mainly in Chinese provinces such as Yunnan, Sichuan, Guangdong, Guangxi, Fujian and Guizhou; also in Hong Kong.

Harvest & Processing Gather mature fruits in September and October; boil thoroughly, or soak in salt water; dry under the sun.

Description Spherical, or flattened and spherical; 1.2-2 cm in diameter. Outer surface brownish-green to dark green, marked with pale yellow granular protuberances, wrinkles, and 6 indistinct ridges; carpopodium about 1 mm long; mesocarp about 1-4 mm thick; hard and brittle. Endocarp yellowish-white, pit-like; outer surface with 6 faint ridges; upper part of dorsal suture with several vascular bundles; cracked into 6 segments when dried. Seeds 6, roughly triangulate (three-angled), brown. Odour: faint; taste: sour-astringent, then sweet.

Indications 1. Dyspepsia, abdominal pain 2. Cough, sore throat, dryness of mouth.

Chemical Composition Mainly contains tannins.

Fructus Piperis Longi

Long Pepper
Bibo

蓽茇

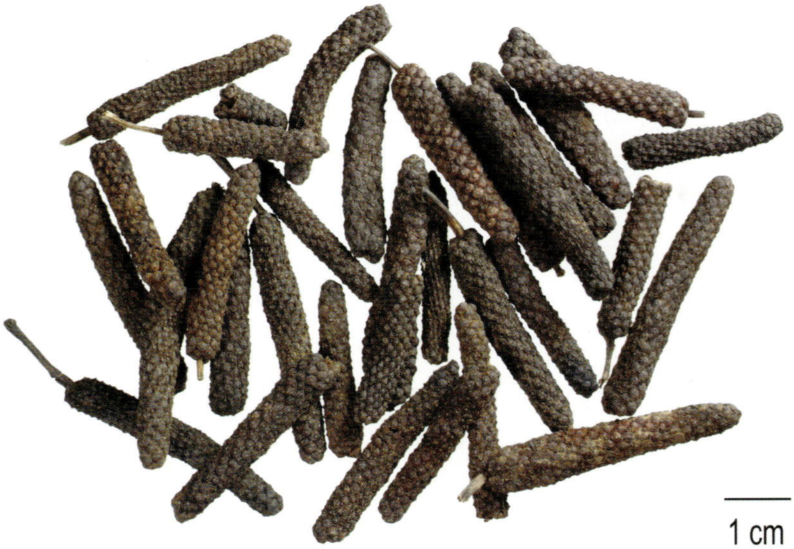

Crude Drug

Source The near-mature or mature fruit spike of *Piper longum* L. (Fam. Piperaceae).

Distribution Originated in Sumatra of Indonesia, and the Philippines and Vietnam. Cultivated in Yunnan and Hainan provinces in China.

Harvest & Processing Pick fruit spikes between September and October when fruits turn from yellow to black; dry under the sun.

Description Roughly cylindrical, sometimes slightly curved, the common carpopodium usually fallen off; fruit spike about 1.5-3 cm long, about 3-5 mm in diameter. Outer surface dull blackish-brown or brown; an aggregate of numerous small, immature berries partly embedded into and combined with rachis, forming a dense and orderly pattern of interlaced small protuberances; berries roughly spherical, bracteate (with bracts), about 1 mm in diameter. Hard; when cracked open, white endosperms revealed. Odour: with a peppery fragrance; taste: pungent.

Indications 1. Vomiting, hiccup, epigastric and abdominal pain, diarrhoea 2. Epilepsy 3. Toothache due to dental caries (external use).

Chemical Composition Piperine exists mainly in the fruit; sylvatine and diaeudesmin exist in the seeds.

Fructus Polygoni Orientalis

Prince's-Feather Fruit
Shuihonghuazi

水紅花子

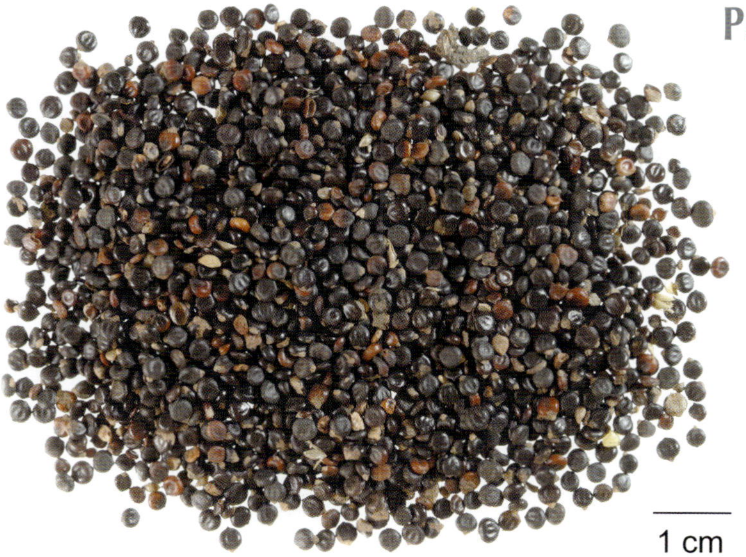

Crude Drug

Source The mature fruit of *Polygonum orientale* L. (Fam. Polygonaceae).

Distribution Mainly in Chinese provinces such as Heilongjiang, Jilin, Liaoning, Hebei and Shanxi, and in Inner Mongolia; also in Hong Kong.

Harvest & Processing Cut off mature fruit spikes after autumn; dry under the sun, rub away perianths covering fruits; remove foreign matter.

Description Flattened and spherical; 2-3.5 mm in diameter; 1-1.5 mm thick. Immature ones yellowish-brown, mature ones blackish-brown. Lustrous; slightly dented on both sides; one side marked with 2 shallow longitudinal grooves in the centre; apex with remnants of style base; base suborbicular (almost round), with a yellowish-white carpopodium scar; surface occasionally with remnants of yellowish-white membranous perianth. Hard; containing 1 seed, seed yellowish-white, flattened and spherical; apex of the seed protuberant, the other end with an orbicular (round) brown hilum. Endosperms white, starchy. Odour: faint; taste: slightly acrid.

Indications Distension and pain of abdomen and stomach.

Chemical Composition Contains quercetin and taxifolin.

Fructus Psoraleae

Malaytea Scurfpea Fruit
Buguzhi

補骨脂

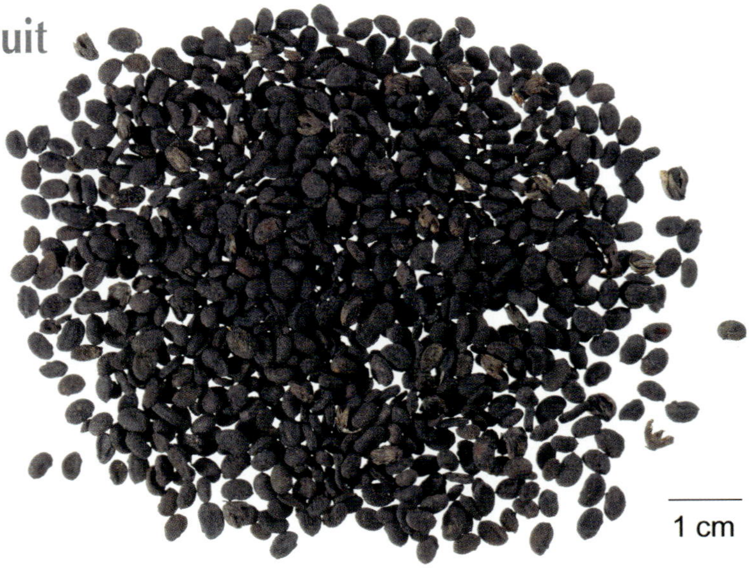

Crude Drug

Source The mature fruit of *Psoralea corylifolia* L. (Fam. Leguminosae).

Distribution In most regions of China.

Harvest & Processing Collect infructescences in autumn when fruits are ripe; dry under the sun; rub out fruits; remove foreign matter.

Description Reniform (kidney-shaped), slightly flattened; 3-5 mm long, 2-4 mm wide, about 1 mm thick. Pericarp black, dull dark brown or dull greyish-brown, marked with fine reticulate (net-like) wrinkles. Fruit surface uneven under magnification. Occasionally attached with green membranous persistent calyx marked with brown gland dots. Seed 1, smooth, yellowish-brown; hilum at one end of the dented side, in the form of a punctiform (dot-like) protuberance; the other side with a slightly protruding chalaza. Hard. Cotyledons yellowish-white, highly oleaginous (oily). Odour: slightly fragrant; taste: acrid and slightly bitter.

Indications 1. Diarrhoea due to poor health 2. Enuresis in old men 3. Urinary frequency 4. Seminal emissions, impotence 7.Vitiligo, psoriasis, tinea capitis, corns (external use).

Chemical Composition Mainly contains coumarin such as psoralen.

Fructus Quisqualis

Rangooncreeper Fruit
Shijunzi
使君子

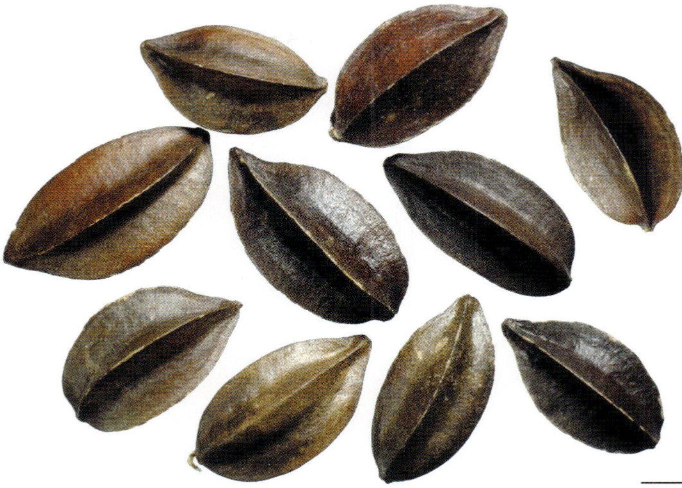

1 cm

Crude Drug

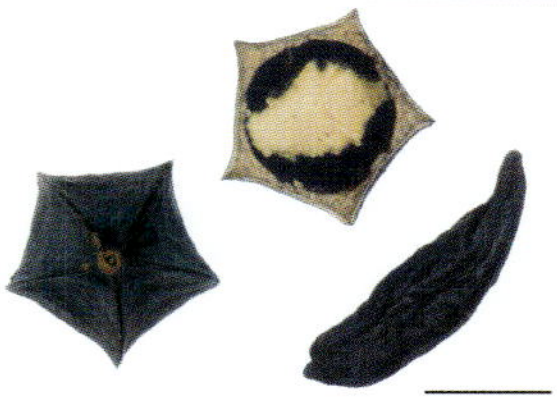

1 cm

Fruit cross-cut and seed

Source The mature fruit of *Quisqualis indica* L. (Fam. Combretaceae).

Distribution Mainly in Chinese provinces such as Sichuan, Guangdong and Guangxi; also in Hong Kong.

Harvest & Processing Harvest mature fruits from September to November when seeds ripen and exocarp turns purplish-black; dry under the sun or over gentle heat.

Description Ellipsoid (elliptical in long-section and circular in cross-section) or ovoid (egg-shaped), with 5 longitudinal ridges (occasionally 4-9); 2.5-4 cm long, about 2 cm in diameter. Outer surface dull dark brown to purplish-black, smooth, slightly lustrous. Top end narrow and pointed; base obtuse, with a prominent orbicular (round) carpopodium scar. Hard; cross-section mostly in the shape of a five-pointed star; fruit shell thicker at ridges, with a suborbicular (almost round) cavity in the centre. Seeds oblong and elliptical, or spindle-shaped. Odour: slightly fragrant; taste: slightly sweet.

Indications 1. Ascariasis 2. Ringworm infection 3. Infant malnutrition.

Chemical Composition Contains quisqualic acid, D-mannitol and fatty acids.

Fructus Rosae Laevigatae

Cherokee Rose Fruit
Jinyingzi

金樱子

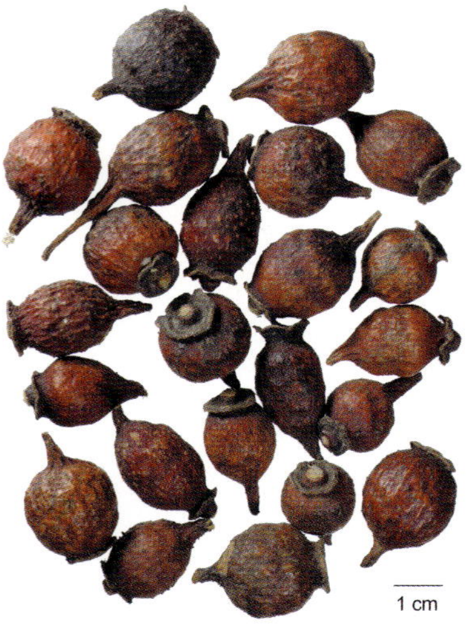

Crude Drug

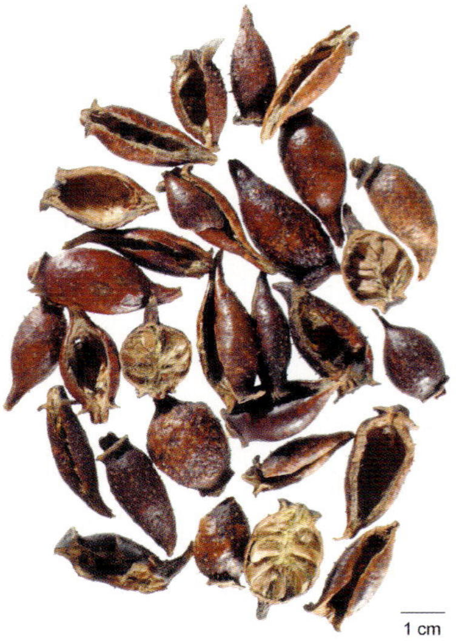

Cherokee Rose Sarcocarp

Source The mature fruit of *Rosa laevigata* Michx. (Fam. Rosaceae).

Distribution Mainly in Chinese provinces such as Zhejiang, Jiangxi, Guangdong and Guangxi; also in Hong Kong.

Harvest & Processing Harvest pseudocarps in October and November when they turn red at maturation; dry under the sun; remove bristles to produce '*Jinyingzi*' (Cherokee Rose Fruit). Cut open longitudinally; put in water and dig out small achenes and remove villi; dry under the sun again to produce '*Jinyingzi rou*' (Cherokee Rose Sarcocarp).

Description Obovoid (inverse egg-shaped), slightly resembling a vase; 2-3.5 cm long, 1-2 cm in diameter. Outer surface reddish-yellow or reddish-brown; with small protuberant spiniform (spine-shaped) dots all over. Carpopodium relatively fine, bulgy in the middle. Tip of persistent calyx campanulate (bell-shaped); remnants of calyx base mostly broken, disciform (disc-like), slightly protuberant in the centre; when receptacle stripped off, pale reddish-yellow inner wall is exposed, with 30-40 small achenes inside; achenes enveloped by pale yellow villi. Odourless; taste: sweet-sour, slightly astringent.

Indications 1. Malabsorption and diarrhoea 2. Chronic cough 3. Spontaneous sweating, night sweating 4. Enuresis, urinary frequency, nocturnal emission 5. Leukorrhagia

Chemical Composition Mainly contains citric acid and malic acid. Tannins exists in the pericarp.

Fructus Rubi

Palmleaf Raspberry Fruit
Fupenzi
覆盆子

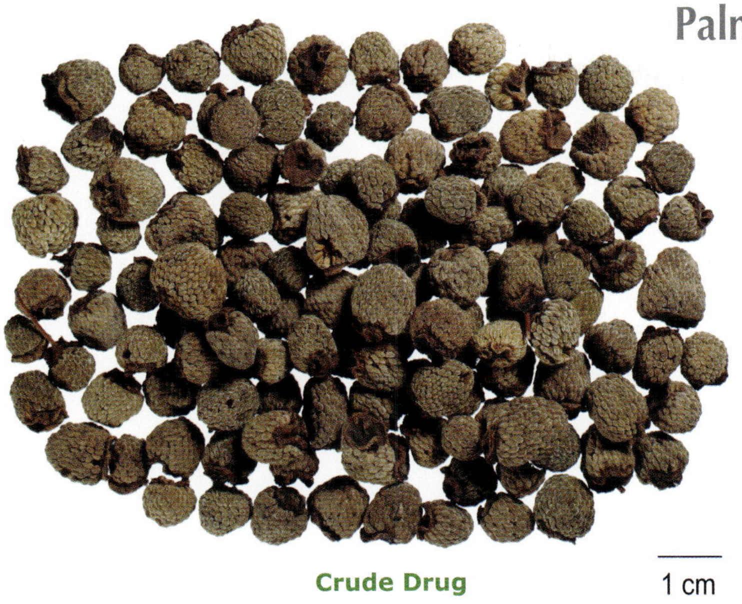

Crude Drug

Source The fruit of *Rubus chingii* Hu (Fam. Rosaceae).

Distribution Mainly in Chinese provinces such as Zhejiang, Hubei, Jiangxi and Fujian.

Harvest & Processing Harvest fruits in early summer when they turn from green to greenish-yellow; remove carpopodiums and leaves; blanch in boiling water or steam briefly; take out and dry.

Description Conical, or spherical, or flattened and conical aggregate fruit consisting of numerous drupelets; 0.6-1.3 cm thick, 0.5-1.2 cm in diameter. Outer surface yellowish-green or pale brown, covered with greyish-white pubescence with silky lustre; upper part obtuse; bottom flat, with dull brown persistent calyx; persistent calyx sometimes with brown hairs, and often with a slender carpopodium underneath. Drupelet triangulate (three-angled), lunate (crescent-shaped); ventral side covered densely with greyish-white pubescence; lateral sides with conspicuous reticulate (net-like) striae; containing 1 brown seed. Odourless; taste: sweet, slightly sour.

Indications
1. Nocturnal emission, impotence, enuresis, urinary frequency
2. Blurring of vision.

Chemical Composition Mainly contains fupenzic acid.

Fructus Schisandrae Chinensis

Chinese Magnoliavine Fruit
Wuweizi

五味子

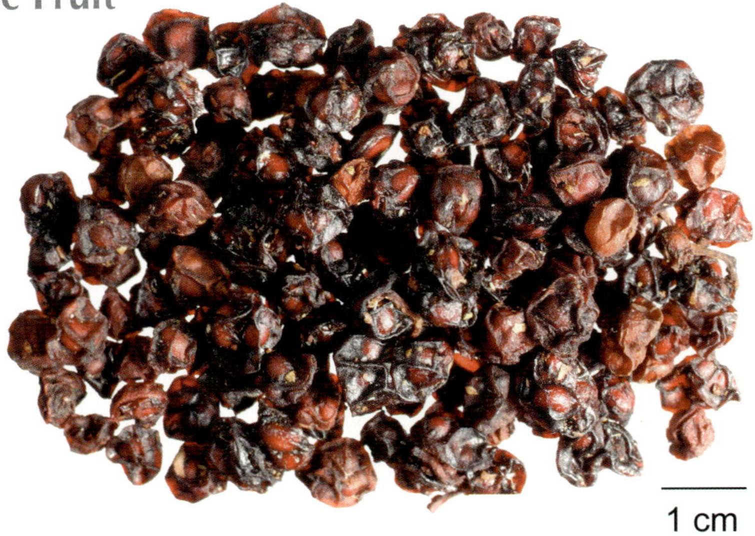

Crude Drug

Source The mature fruit of *Schisandra chinensis* (Turcz.) Baill. (Fam. Magnoliaceae).

Distribution Mainly in Chinese provinces such as Jilin, Liaoning and Heilongjiang. Customarily called "*Bei wuweizi*"(North Chinese Magnoliavine Fruit).

Harvest & Processing Collect fully-matured fruits in autumn; remove foreign matter; dry under the sun.

Description Somewhat spherical, or flattened and spherical; 5-8 mm in diameter. Outer surface purplish-red or dull red, shrivelled, oily; sarcocarp soft; surface sometimes blackish-red or glaucous (covered with white powder). Seeds 1-2, reniform (kidney-shaped); outer surface brownish-yellow, lustrous. Testa thin and brittle, breaks quite easily. Kernel hook-shaped; yellowish-white; translucent; highly oleaginous (oily). Odour of sarcocarp: faint; taste: sour. Odour of seeds: fragrant when broken; taste: acrid, slightly bitter.

Indications 1. Neurasthenia 2. Spontaneous sweating, night sweating, seminal emissions 3. General fatigue

Chemical Composition Mainly contains lignans such as schizandrin.

Fructus seu Herba Physalis Peruvianae

Peruvian Groundcherry Fruit or Herb

Denglongcao

燈籠草

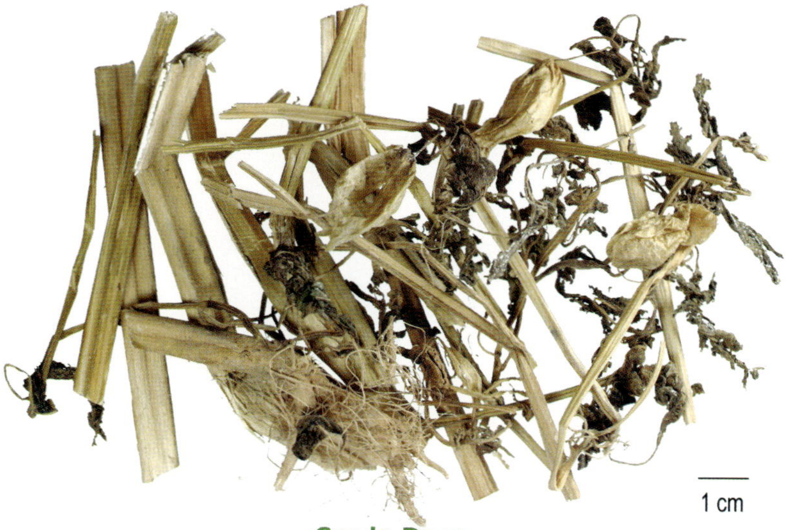

Crude Drug

Source The calyx-bearing fruit or whole herb of *Physalis peruviana* L. (Fam. Solanaceae).

Distribution Mainly in Chinese provinces such as Guangdong, Guangxi and Hainan.

Harvest & Processing Collect calyx-bearing fruits or whole herbs in summer and autumn; wash clean; use while fresh or dry under the sun.

Description Whole herb 25-60 cm long. Stem slightly flattened, quadrangular (four-angled); outer surface dull yellowish-white or greyish-green, densely covered with white pubescence. Leaves shrivelled and curled; when smoothed out, blades ovate (egg-shaped in outline and attached at the broad end). Apex pointed, base cuneate (wedge-shaped) or slightly cordate (heart-shaped); margin nearly entire (continuous, even), or with irregular and sparse big teeth; leaves dull green or yellowish-green; both sides covered with white pubescence; with long petioles. Calyx at leaf axil lantern-shaped and bulgy, sometimes compressed; about 2.5 cm long, about 2 cm wide; pale yellowish-green; papery; translucent; covered with pubescence; containing dull yellowish-green berries subspherical in shape and about 1 cm in diameter. Odour: faint; taste: sweet, bitter.

Indications 1. Common cold, cough, sore throat, mumps 2. Pemphigus

Chemical Composition Contains alkaloids such as hygrine.

Fructus Sophorae

Japanese Pagodatree Pod
Huaijiao

槐角

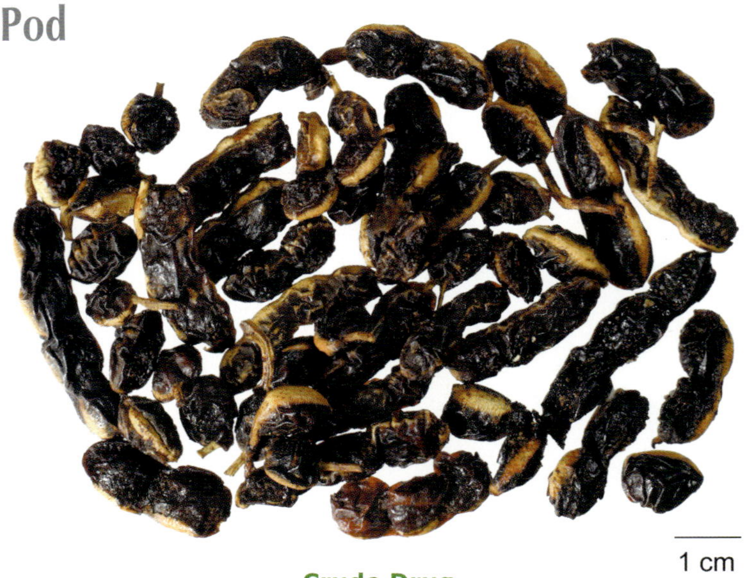

Crude Drug

Source The mature fruit of *Sophora japonica* L. (Fam. Leguminosae).

Distribution Mainly in northern China.

Harvest & Processing Harvest fruits at maturation, mostly in November and December; spread them out on mattresses and dry thoroughly under the sun until they turn yellowish-green; remove carpopodiums and foreign matter. Alternatively, blanch fruits in boiling water and then dry thoroughly under the sun.

Description Torose (cylindrical with alternate swellings and constrictions), occasionally curved; 1-6 cm long, 0.6-1 cm in diameter. Outer surface yellowish-green or dull yellowish-brown, shrivelled and rough, slightly lustrous; yellow belt on dorsal suture; apex with protuberant remnants of style base, base often with remnants of carpopodium. Soft and smooth, breaks easily at points of constriction. When broken, sarcocarp yellowish-green, viscid, translucent and cuticular. Seeds 1-6. Odour: faint; taste: slightly bitter, bean-like when chewed.

Indications 1. Haematochezia, haemorrhoidal bleeding 2. Headache, dizziness and conjunctivitis.

Chemical Composition Mainly contains flavonoids such as genistein; alkaloids such as cystisine exist in the seeds.

Fructus Toosendan

Szechwan Chinaberry Fruit
Chuanlianzi

川楝子

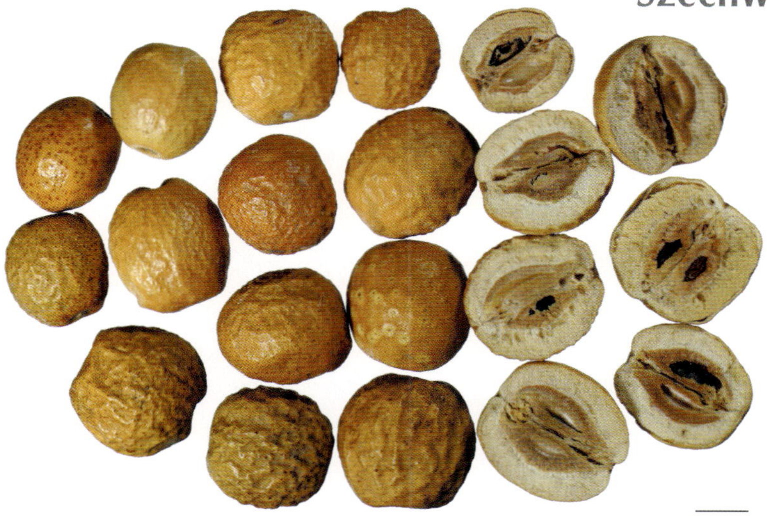

Crude Drug

Source The mature fruit of *Melia toosendan* Sieb. et Zucc. (Fam. Meliaceae).

Distribution Mainly in Chinese provinces such as Sichuan, Gansu and Yunnan.

Harvest & Processing Harvest fruits in winter when they are yellow in colour, or collect yellow fruits fallen after a frost; dry under the sun or by heat.

Description Subspherical; 2-3.2 cm in diameter. Outer surface golden-yellow to brownish-yellow, slightly lustrous. Top part with remnants of a style scar; base dented, with a carpopodium scar. Exocarp coriaceous (leathery), often separated from sarcocarp by narrow gaps; sarcocarp loose and soft, pale yellow in colour, viscid upon contact with water. Pit spherical or ovoid (egg-shaped); hard; both ends truncate (squared as if cut off); with 6-8 longitudinal ridges; divided into 6-8 locules, each containing 1 dark brown, oblong and spherical seed. Kernels milky-white, oblong and spherical, highly oleaginous (oily). Odour: distinctive; taste: sour and bitter.

Indications 1. Distending pain in the chest, hypochondrium and epigastrium 2. Colic in the lower abdomen 3. Abdominal pain due to intestinal parasitosis.

Chemical Composition Mainly contains toosendanin and melianone.

Note Listed as slightly toxic in *C.P.*

Fructus Tribuli

Puncturevine Caltrop Fruit

Jili

蒺藜

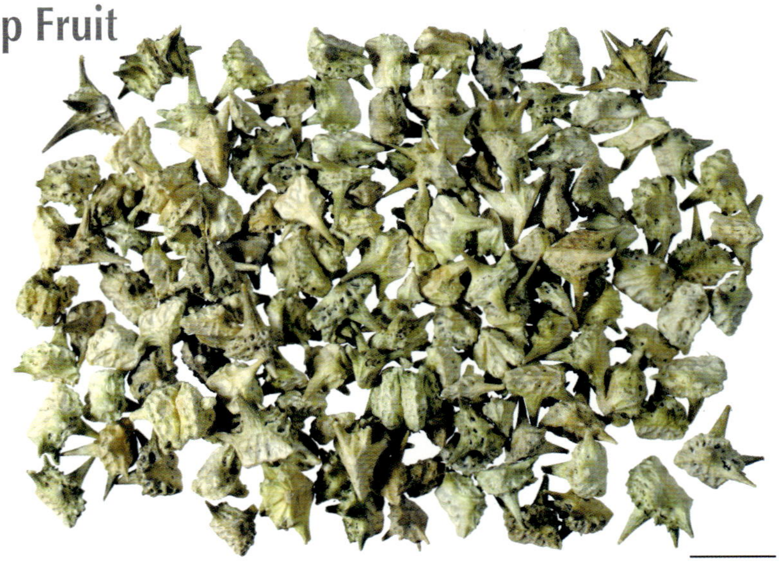

Crude Drug 1 cm

Source The fruit of *Tribulus terrestris* L. (Fam. Zygophyllaceae).

Distribution Mainly in Chinese provinces such as Henan, Hebei, Shandong, Anhui, Jiangsu, Sichuan and Shaanxi.

Harvest & Processing Cut off whole plants in autumn when fruits ripen; dry under the sun for several days; thresh to get fruits; dry under the sun again.

Description Formed by 5 mericarps arranged in a radial pattern, pentagonal and spherical in shape; 7-12 mm in diameter; often split into single mericarps dolabriform (axe-shaped) and triangular in shape. Mericarps 3-6 mm long; pale yellowish-green; dorsal side bulgy, with longitudinal ridges, numerous spinules, 1 pair of long spines and 1 pair of short spines, with each pair splaying out symmetrically; the two lateral sides rough, marked with reticulate (net-like) striae, greyish-white. Pericarp hard, ligneous (woody), containing 3-4 seeds; seeds ovoid (egg-shaped), quite flat, oleaginous (oily). Odour: faint; taste: bitter.

Indications 1. Headache, dizziness, hypertension 2. Red eyes, photophobia with lacrimation 3. Feeling of oppression and fullness in the chest and hypochondria, irritability 4. Galactostasis 5.Urticaria

Chemical Composition Mainly contains alkaloids and steroidal saponins.

Fructus Trichosanthis

Snakegourd Fruit
Gualou
瓜蔞

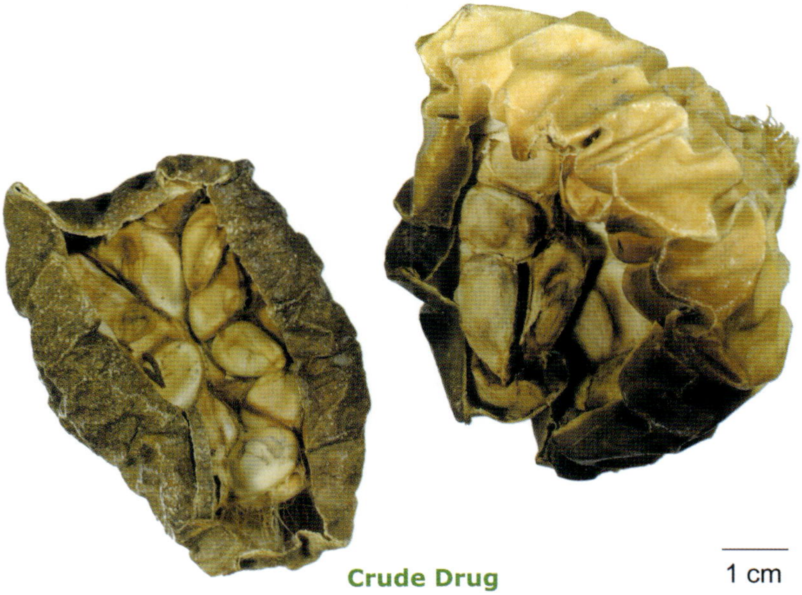

Crude Drug

Source The mature fruit of *Trichosanthes kirilowii* Maxim. (Fam. Cucurbitaceae).

Distribution Mainly in Shandong province in China; also in provinces such as Hebei, Shanxi and Shaanxi.

Harvest & Processing Cut off fruits together with carpopodiums in late September when fruits are ripe but still green in colour; dry in shaded areas.

Description Subspherical or oval; 7-15 cm long, 6-10 cm in diameter. Outer surface orange-red or orange-yellow, shrivelled or relatively smooth; apex with orbicular (round) remnants of style base; base slightly pointed, with carpopodium remnants. Varying in weight; brittle. Commercially sold products often cut open; inner surface yellowish-white, marked with reddish-yellow veins; sarcocarp orange-yellow, sticky, forming clusters with numerous seeds. Odour: caramel-like; taste: slightly sour, sweet.

Indications 1. Cough with sticky sputum, feeling of oppression in the chest 2. Constipation 3. Abscess.

Chemical Composition Contains triterpene saponins.

Note According to *C.P.*, also used for medicinal purposes is the mature fruit of *T rosthornii* Harms, whose pericarp is also used as Pericarpium Trichosanthis for medicinal purposes.

Fructus Tritici Levis

Blighted Wheat
Fuxiaomai

浮小麥

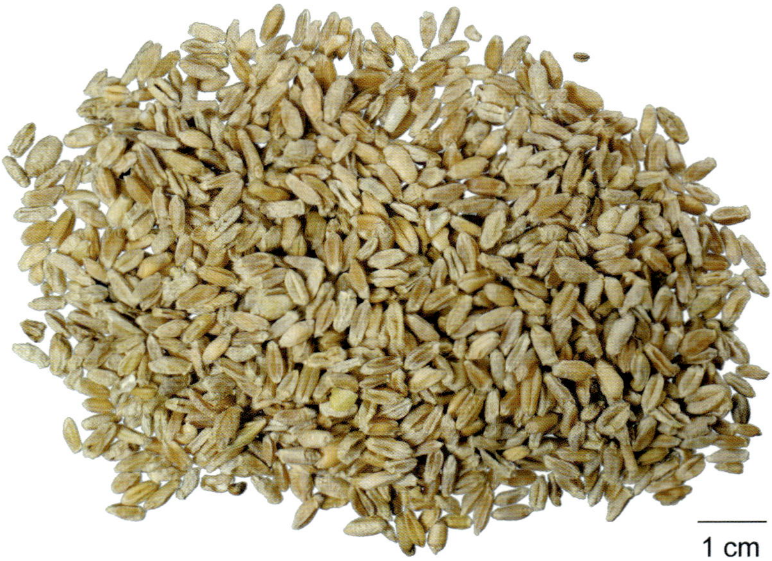

Crude Drug

Source The light, shrivelled grain of *Triticum aestivum* L. (Fam. Gramineae).

Distribution In all wheat-producing regions of China.

Harvest & Processing Harvest ripe grains in late June; pick out light, shrivelled grains, lemmas and paleae still attached; sieve away foreign matter; wash grains with water; dry under the sun.

Description Oblong and spherical, slightly pointed at both ends; about 7 mm long, about 3 mm in diameter. Outer surface yellowish-white, shrivelled; occasionally with bits of lemmas and paleae still attached. Ventral side with a deep longitudinal groove; apex obtuse, covered with light yellowish-brown pubescence; the other end slanted and pointed, with a hilum. Hard and brittle, breaks easily; broken surface white, mildly starchy. Odourless; taste: mild.

Indications 1. Spontaneous sweating, night sweating 2. Hysteria, forgetfulness, palpitation, insomnia, excessive dreams

Chemical Composition Mainly contains sitosterols and a variety of polysaccharides.

Fructus Tsaoko

Tsaoko Amomum Fruit

Caoguo

草果

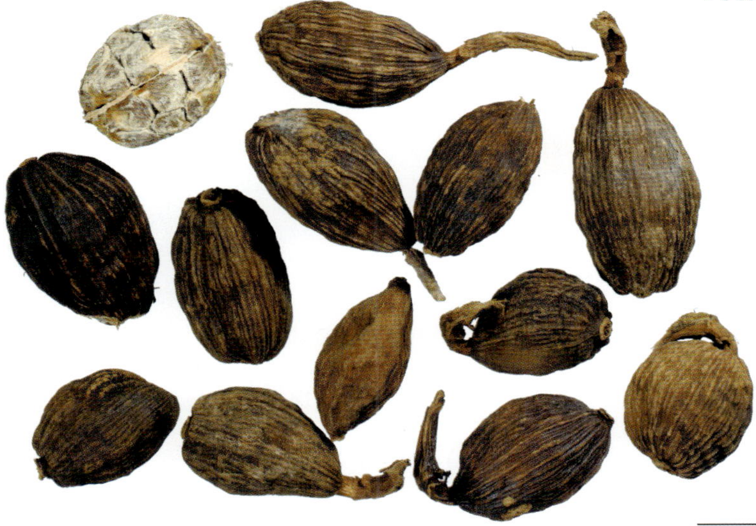

Crude Drug

1 cm

Source The mature fruit of *Amomum tsao-ko* Crevost et Lemaire (Fam. Zingiberaceae).

Distribution Mainly in Chinese provinces such as Yunnan, Guangxi and Guizhou.

Harvest & Processing Harvest fruits at maturation in autumn; remove foreign matter; dry under the sun or at low temperatures.

Description Oblong and ellipsoid (elliptical in long-section and circular in cross-section), with three obtuse ridges; 2-4 cm long, 1-2.5 cm in diameter. Outer surface greyish-brown to reddish-brown, marked with longitudinal grooves and ridges; apex with orbicular (round) protuberant style base; base with a carpopodium or carpopodium scars. Pericarp strong and pliable, can be torn off length-wise easily. Seeds cluster in 3 cloves, with yellowish-brown septa in the middle; each clove bearing 8-11 seeds. Seeds in the form of conical polyhedrons; about 5 mm in diameter; outer surface reddish-brown, covered with greyish-white membranous aril; raphe in the form of a longitudinal groove; apex with a dented hilum; hard; endosperms greyish-white. Odour: with a distinctive fragrance; taste: acrid and slightly bitter.

Indications 1. Feeling of fullness, oppression, distending pain in the abdomen, anorexia 2. Malaria with feeling of oppression in the chest

Chemical Composition Contains essential oils with linalool and nerolidol as the main components.

Fructus Viticis

Simpleleaf Shrub Chastetree Fruit
Manjingzi

蔓荊子

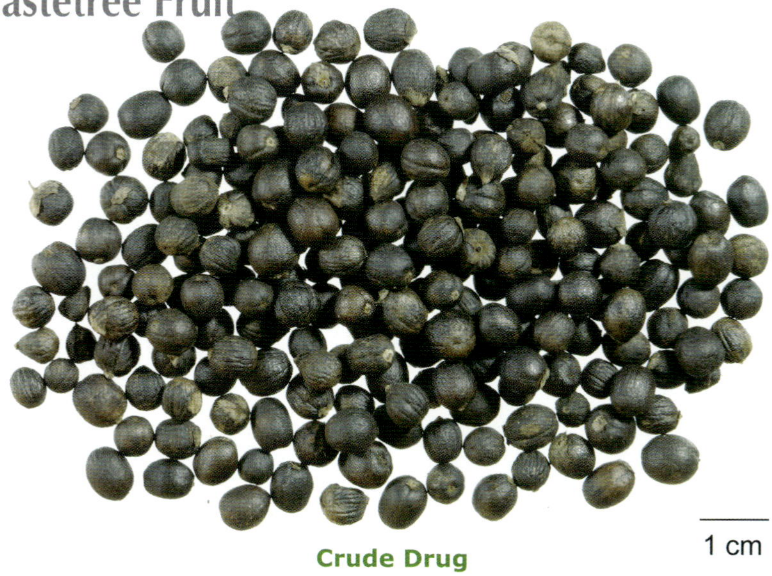

Crude Drug

Source The mature fruit of *Vitex trifolia* L. *var. simplicifolia* Cham. (Fam. Verbenaceae).

Distribution Mainly in Chinese provinces such as Shandong, Jiangxi and Zhejiang; also in Hong Kong.

Harvest & Processing Harvest fruits at maturation in autumn; remove foreign matter; dry under the sun.

Description Spherical; 4-6 mm in diameter. Outer surface greyish-black or dull blackish-brown, covered with pulverulent (powdery) greyish-white pubescence, marked with 4 shallow longitudinal grooves; top part slightly dented; base with greyish-white persistent calyx and a short carpopodium. Calyx 1/3-2/3 the length of fruit; densely pubescent; margin with 5 teeth, 2 of them deeper. Light in weight; pliable but strong, does not break easily.

Indications 1. Headache 2. Gingivitis 3. Conjunctivitis, blurring of vision and dizziness

Chemical Composition Mainly contains essential oils and flavonoids such as vitexicarpin.

Note According to *C.P.*, also used for medicinal purposes is the mature fruit of *V. trifolia* L.

Fructus Xanthii

Siberian Cocklebur Fruit
Cang'erzi
蒼耳子

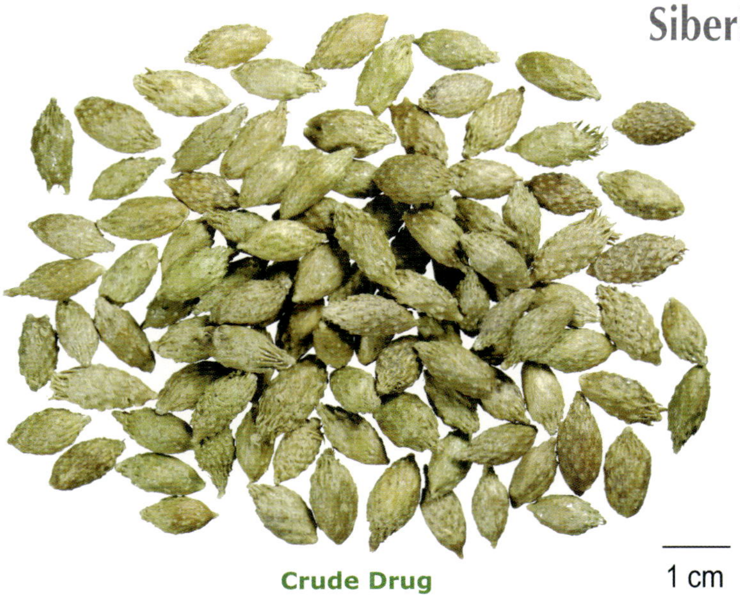

Crude Drug

Source The mature fruit of *Xanthium sibiricum* Patr. (Fam. Compositae).

Distribution In most regions of China, including Hong Kong.

Harvest & Processing Harvest fruits at maturation in autumn; dry under the sun; remove foreign matter.

Description Spindle-shaped or ovoid (egg-shaped); 1-1.5 cm long, 4-7 mm in diameter. Outer surface yellowish-brown or yellowish-green, with hooked spines on all sides; apex with 2 thicker spines, separated or joined; base with carpopodium scars. Hard but pliable. Cross-section marked with a longitudinal septum in the centre, dividing the fruit into 2 locules, each with 1 achene. Achenes spindle-shaped, with one side more even; apex with 1 protuberant style base; pericarp thin, greyish-black, marked with fine longitudinal striae. Testa membranous, light grey; cotyledons 2, oleaginous (oily). Odour: faint; taste: slightly bitter.

Indications 1. Common cold 2. Nasal discharge 3. Fever 4. Arthralgia
5. Urticaria, pruritus (external use).

Chemical Composition Contains 9.2% fatty oils; also contains 1,3,5-tri-O-caffeoylquinic acid and 3,5-di-O-caffeoylquinic acid.

Note Listed as toxic in *C.P.*

Herba Abri

Canton Love-Pea Vine

Jigucao

雞骨草

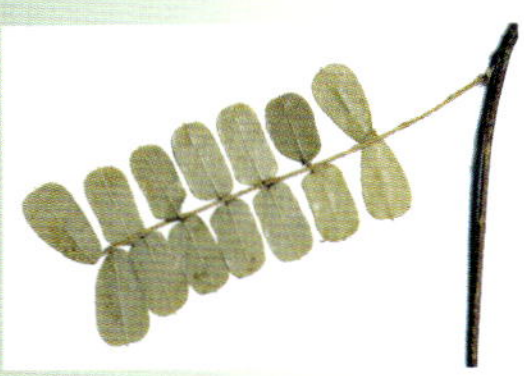

Canton Love-Pea Vine Magnified

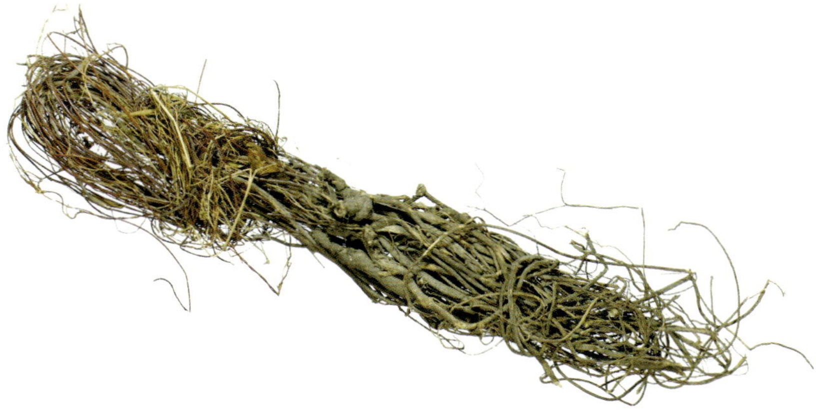

5 cm

Crude Drug

Source The whole herb of *Abrus cantoniensis* Hance (Fam. Leguminosae).

Distribution Mainly in Chinese provinces such as Guangdong and Guangxi; also in Hong Kong.

Harvest & Processing Harvest whole herbs anytime during the year; remove legumes (toxic) and foreign matter; dry under the sun.

Description Mostly intertwined into a bundle. Root cylindrical or conical, rameous (branched); varying in length and thickness, 3-15 mm in diameter; outer surface greyish-brown, marked with fine longitudinal striae; hard. Rhizome short; nodular. Stems caespitose (growing in tufts), vine-shaped; up to 1 m long, 1.5-2.5 mm in diameter; outer surface dull greyish-brown; branchlets brownish-red, sparsely puberulent (covered with fine, short, soft hairs). Leaves even-pinnate (compound in a feather-like manner with an even number of leaflets); leaflet oblong and orbicular (round): 8-12 mm long; underside covered with strigae. Odour: faint; taste: slightly bitter.

Indications 1. Hepatitis, hepatochirrhosis 2. Stomachache, stranguria, rheumatic arthralgia, trauma 3. Snakebite 4. Mastitis (external use).

Chemical Composition Mainly contains abrines such as abrisaponins.

Fructus Xanthii

Siberian Cocklebur Fruit

Cang'erzi

蒼耳子

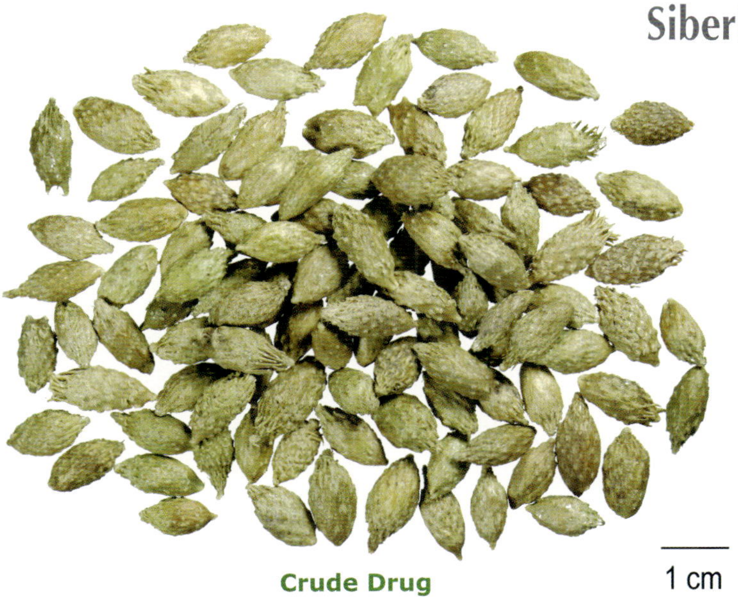

Crude Drug

Source The mature fruit of *Xanthium sibiricum* Patr. (Fam. Compositae).

Distribution In most regions of China, including Hong Kong.

Harvest & Processing Harvest fruits at maturation in autumn; dry under the sun; remove foreign matter.

Description Spindle-shaped or ovoid (egg-shaped); 1-1.5 cm long, 4-7 mm in diameter. Outer surface yellowish-brown or yellowish-green, with hooked spines on all sides; apex with 2 thicker spines, separated or joined; base with carpopodium scars. Hard but pliable. Cross-section marked with a longitudinal septum in the centre, dividing the fruit into 2 locules, each with 1 achene. Achenes spindle-shaped, with one side more even; apex with 1 protuberant style base; pericarp thin, greyish-black, marked with fine longitudinal striae. Testa membranous, light grey; cotyledons 2, oleaginous (oily). Odour: faint; taste: slightly bitter.

Indications 1. Common cold 2. Nasal discharge 3. Fever 4. Arthralgia 5. Urticaria, pruritus (external use).

Chemical Composition Contains 9.2% fatty oils; also contains 1,3,5-tri-O-caffeoylquinic acid and 3,5-di-O-caffeoylquinic acid.

Note Listed as toxic in *C.P.*

Galla Chinensis

Chinese Gall
Wubeizi

五倍子

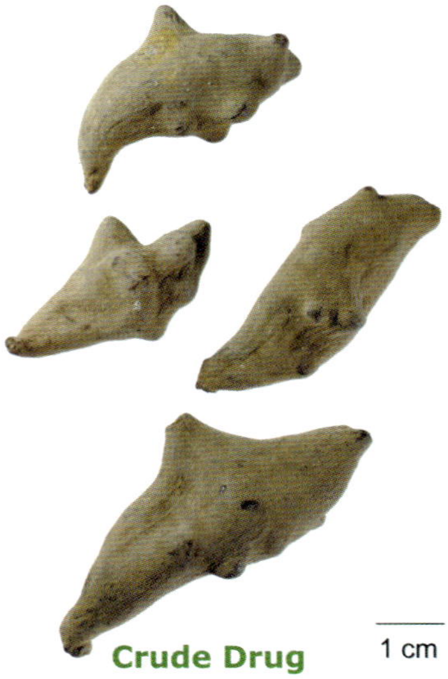

Crude Drug
(Knobbly Gall)

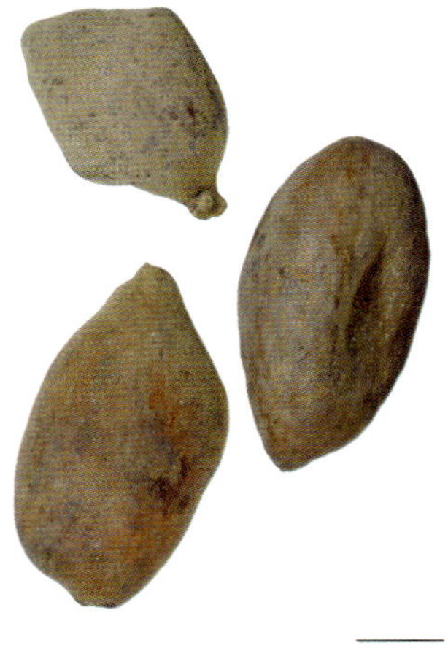

Crude Drug
(Rounded Gall)

Source The gall formed mainly by the parasitic *Melaphis chinensis* (Bell) Baker on the leaves of *Rhus chinensis* Mill. (Fam. Anacardiaceae).

Distribution Mainly in Chinese provinces such as Sichuan, Guizhou, Yunnan and Shaanxi; also in Hong Kong.

Harvest & Processing Collect galls from early August to early September when they turn from green to dull yellowish-brown; blanch in boiling water or steam until they turn grey to make sure the aphids inside are killed; take out the galls and dry them under the sun. Commercial products are classified according to shape.

Description *Dubei* (Rounded Gall): Long and orbicular (round) or spindle-shaped and sacciform (sac-like); 2.5-9 cm long, 1.5-4 cm in diameter. Outer surface dull greyish-brown or greyish-brown, pubescent (covered with short, soft hairs). Hard and brittle, breaks easily. When broken, surface cuticular and lustrous; gall wall 2-3 mm thick, with smooth inner surface; inside the gall are dull, dark brown dead aphids and powdery grey excreta. Odour: distinctive; taste: astringent.
Jiaobei (Knobbly Gall): Rhombic, irregular and knobbly; pubescence more conspicuous.

Indications 1. Chronic cough and asthma 2. Protracted diarrhoea 3. Sweating 4. Seminal emission 5. Dysfunctional uterine bleeding, haematochezia and haemorrhoidal bleeding

Chemical Composition Mainly contains Chinese gallotannin.

Note According to *C.P.*, also used for medicinal purposes is the gall on the leaves of *R. potaninii* Maxim. and *R. punjabensis* Stew. *var. sinica* (Diels) Rehd. et Wils.

Ganoderma

Glossy Ganoderma

Lingzhi

靈芝

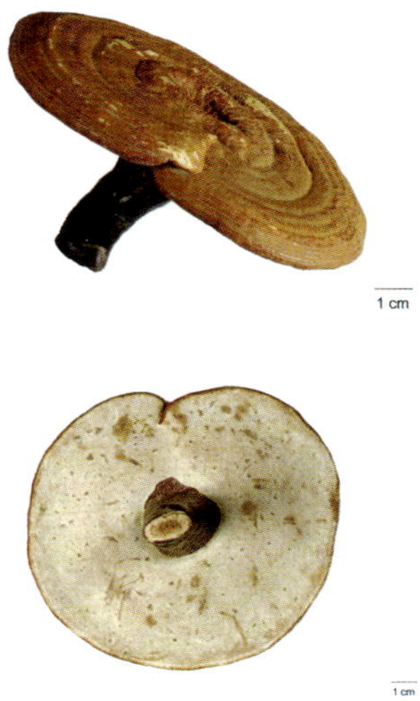

Crude Drug

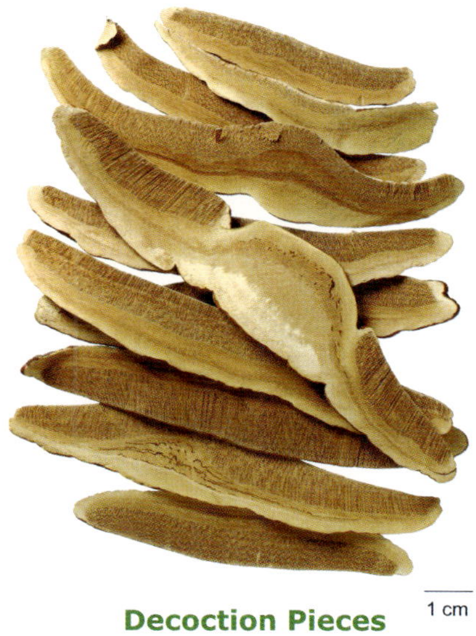

Decoction Pieces

Source The fruiting body of *Ganoderma lucidum* (Leyss. ex Fr.) Karst. (Fam. Poloporaceae). Commonly known as '*Chizhi*' (Red Glossy Ganoderma).

Distribution Mainly in Chinese provinces such as Hebei, Shanxi, Jiangxi and Guangxi, and in eastern and southwestern China. Mostly cultivated.

Harvest & Processing Collect fruiting bodies in autumn; remove soil, sand and other foreign matter; dry in shaded areas or under the sun.

Description Umbrella-shaped, with a semicircular, reniform (kidney-shaped) or suborbicular (almost round) pileus 10-18 cm wide and 1-2 cm thick. Epicutis hard, dull yellowish-brown to dull reddish-brown, lustrous, marked with annular (ring-like) ridges and radial wrinkles; margin thin and truncate (squared as if cut off), often slightly involute (with margin rolling inwards). Gills on the underside of pileus white to light brown, consisting of innumerable tubules. Stipe lateral (borne on or at the side); 7-15 cm long, 1-3.5 cm in diameter; dull reddish-brown to dull purplish-brown; lustrous. Numerous minute, dull yellowish-brown spores in tubules. Odour: slightly fragrant; taste: bitter-astringent.

Indications 1. Dizziness, insomnia, palpitation 2. Dyspnoea, consumptive cough, asthma.

Chemical Composition Mainly contains polysaccharides and triterpenes such as ganoderic acid.

Note According to *C.P.*, also used for medicinal purposes, and commonly known as '*Zizhi*' (Purple Glossy Ganoderma), is the fruiting body of *G. sinense* Zhao, Xu et Zhang.

Herba Abri

Canton Love-Pea Vine
Jigucao

雞骨草

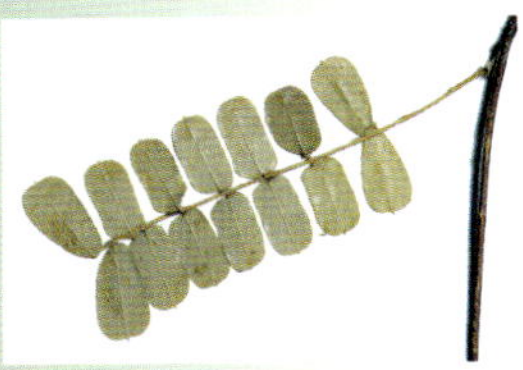

Canton Love-Pea Vine Magnified

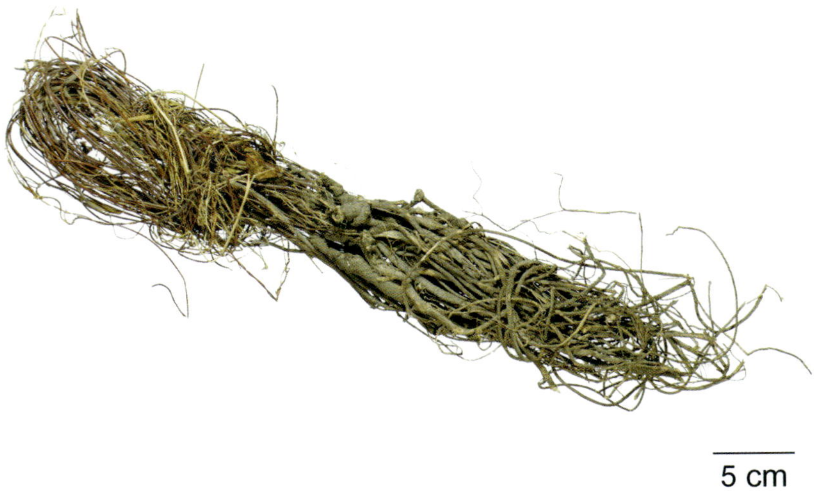

Crude Drug

Source The whole herb of *Abrus cantoniensis* Hance (Fam. Leguminosae).

Distribution Mainly in Chinese provinces such as Guangdong and Guangxi; also in Hong Kong.

Harvest & Processing Harvest whole herbs anytime during the year; remove legumes (toxic) and foreign matter; dry under the sun.

Description Mostly intertwined into a bundle. Root cylindrical or conical, rameous (branched); varying in length and thickness, 3-15 mm in diameter; outer surface greyish-brown, marked with fine longitudinal striae; hard. Rhizome short; nodular. Stems caespitose (growing in tufts), vine-shaped; up to 1 m long, 1.5-2.5 mm in diameter; outer surface dull greyish-brown; branchlets brownish-red, sparsely puberulent (covered with fine, short, soft hairs). Leaves even-pinnate (compound in a feather-like manner with an even number of leaflets); leaflet oblong and orbicular (round): 8-12 mm long; underside covered with strigae. Odour: faint; taste: slightly bitter.

Indications 1. Hepatitis, hepatochirrhosis 2. Stomachache, stranguria, rheumatic arthralgia, trauma 3. Snakebite 4. Mastitis (external use).

Chemical Composition Mainly contains abrines such as abrisaponins.

Herba Agrimoniae

Hairyvein Agrimonia Herb
Xianhecao

仙鶴草

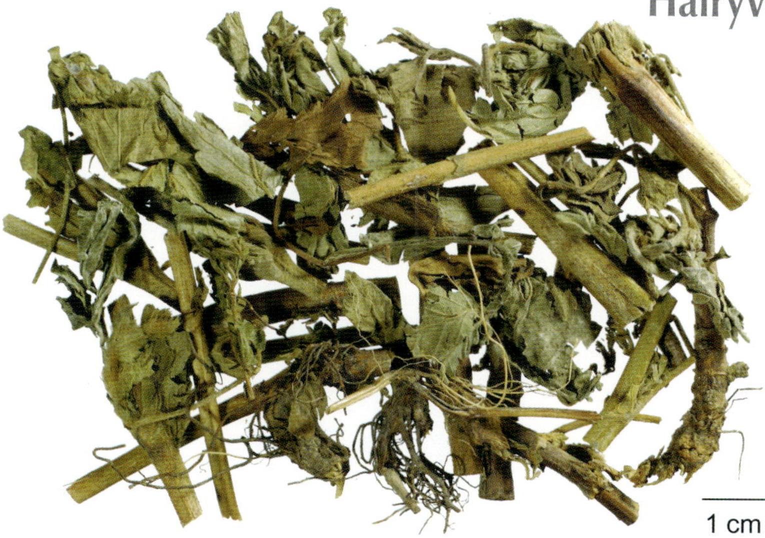

Crude Drug

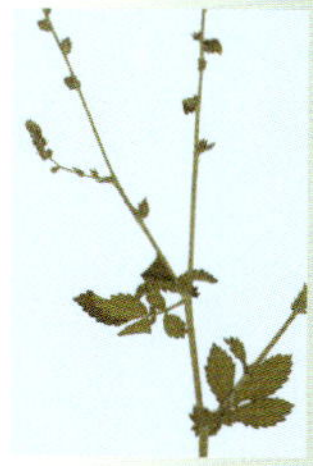

Hairyvein Agrimonia Herb Magnified

Source The whole herb of *Agrimonia pilosa* Ledeb. (Fam. Rosaceae).

Distribution Mainly in Chinese provinces such as Zhejiang and Jiangsu; also in Hong Kong.

Harvest & Processing Cut off whole herbs in summer and autumn when leaves flourish; remove foreign matter; dry under the sun.

Description Whole herb covered with white pubescence; 50-100 cm long. Lower part of stem cylindrical, 4-6 mm in diameter; upper part quadrangular (four-angled), slightly dented on four sides, marked with longitudinal grooves and ridges; nodes conspicuous. Light in weight; hard, breaks easily; broken surface hollow in the centre. Leaves odd-pinnate (compound in a feather-like manner with an odd number of leaflets), alternate (borne singly at each node); some blades big and some small, big ones and small ones alternating with each other on rachis. Terminal leaflet larger; when intact and smoothed out, leaflets ovate (egg-shaped in outline and attached at the broad end), or oblong and elliptical. Apex pointed, base cuneate (wedge-shaped); margin serrate (saw-like). Stipules 2, amplexicaul (surrounding the stem), oblique-ovate. Raceme slender; lower part of calyx tubular; upper part of calyx tube with hooked spines. Odour: faint; taste: slightly bitter.

Indications 1. Various kinds of bleeding such as epistaxis, gastrointestinal bleeding, haematuria, dysfunctional uterine bleeding 2. Diarrhoea 3. Fatique 4. Vaginal trichomoniasis (external use).

Chemical Composition Mainly contains flavonoids, trpterpenes and tannins.

Herba Andrographis

Common Andrographis Herb
Chuanxinlian

穿心蓮

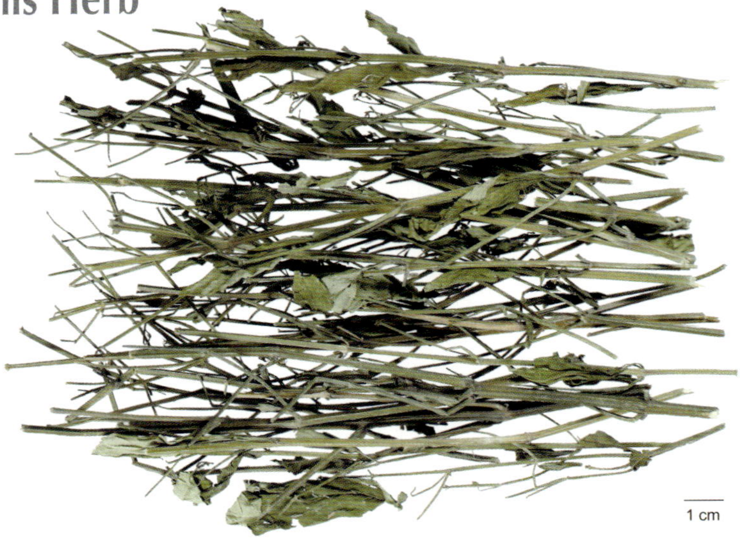

Crude Drug

Source The above-ground part of *Andrographis paniculata* (Burm. f.) Nees (Fam. Acanthaceae).

Distribution Mainly cultivated in Chinese provinces such as Guangdong, Guangxi, Fujian, Yunnan, Sichuan, Jiangxi and Jiangsu.

Harvest & Processing Cut off above-ground parts in early autumn when leaves flourish; remove foreign matter; dry under the sun.

Description Stem quadrangular (four-angled), ramose (with many branches); 50-70 cm long; nodes slightly bulgy; brittle, breaks easily. Leaves simple (not separated into leaflets) and opposite (borne in pairs at each node), with short petioles or nearly epetiolate (without a petiole); blades shrivelled, crumble easily; when whole and smoothed out, blades lanceolate (lance-head shaped), or ovate (egg-shaped in outline and attached at the broad end) and lanceolate, 3-12 cm long, 2-5 cm wide. Apex acuminate (tapering to a slender point); base cuneate (wedge-shaped) and decurrent (extending downwards); margin entire (continuous and even) or undulate (wavy); upper surface green, underside greyish-green; both sides smooth. Odour: faint; taste: extremely bitter.

Indications 1. Gastroenteritis 2. Common cold, tonsillitis 3. Boils, wound infection 4. Snakebite.

Chemical Composition Mainly contains diterpenes such as andrographolide, and flavonoids such as oroxylin A.

Herba Ardisiae Japonicae

Japanese Ardisia Herb
Aidicha
矮地茶

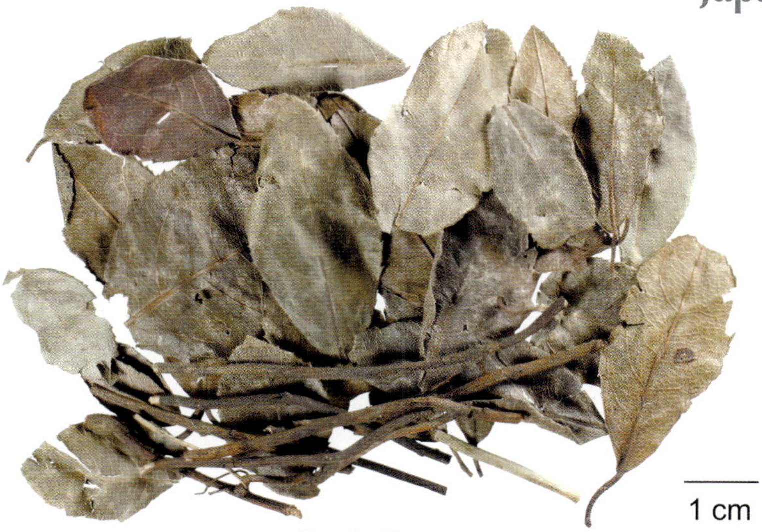

Crude Drug

Source The whole herb of *Ardisia japonica* (Thunb.) Bl. (Fam. Myrsinaceae).

Distribution In regions south of the Yangtze River in China.

Harvest & Processing Harvest whole herbs in autumn; remove foreign matter; wash clean; dry under the sun.

Description Whole plant 15-25 cm long. Stem cylindrical or slightly flattened; 2-5 mm in diameter. Outer surface dull reddish-brown, marked with fine longitudinal striae and protuberant leaf scars; base with sparse growth of beard-like adventitious roots; apex occasionally with pedicels or small, shrivelled, spherical, dull red fruits. Brittle, breaks easily; with white pith in the centre. Leaves often 3-5, acrogenous (growing from the apex); blades slightly curled or in fragments, elliptical when smoothed out; outer surface greyish-green to dull reddish-brown. Odour: faint; taste: slightly astringent.

Indications 1. Chronic cough, haemoptysis, pulmonary tuberculosis, tuberculous pleuritis, Chronic bronchitis 2. Jaundice, oedema 3. Amenorrhoea, trauma, rheumatism, haematemesis.

Chemical Composition Mainly contains 0.1%-0.2% essential oils; also contains bergenin and ardisinol.

Note In *Zhonghua Bencao* (Chinese Materia Medica), the official name adopted is '*Pingdimu*' (Level-Ground Wood).

Herba Artemisiae Annuae

Sweet Wormwood Herb
Qinghao
青蒿

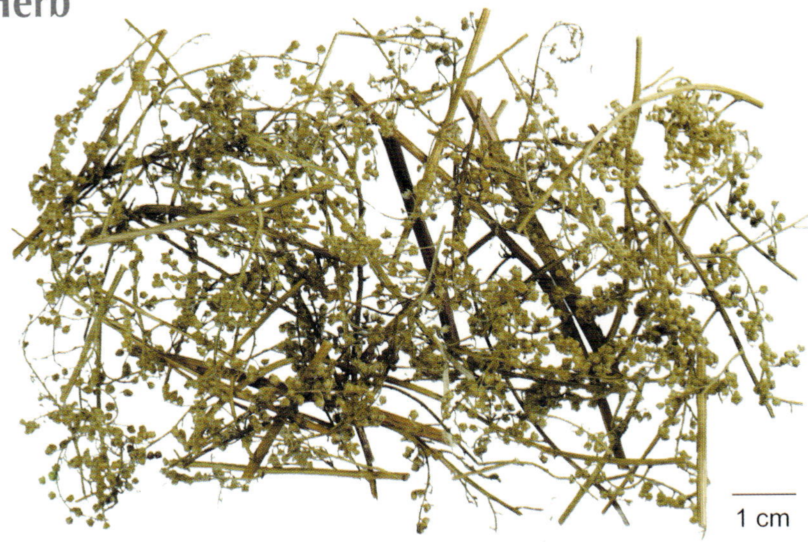

Crude Drug

Source The above-ground part of *Artemisia annua* L. (Fam. Compositae).

Distribution In all parts of China.

Harvest & Processing Collect above-ground parts in summer and autumn when flowers are in full bloom; remove old stems; dry in shaded areas.

Description Stem cylindrical, upper part ramose (with many branches); 30-80 cm long, 2-6 mm in diameter. Outer surface yellowish-green or brownish-yellow, marked with longitudinal ridges. Fairly hard, breaks easily; broken surface yellowish-white, with pith in the centre. Leaves opposite (borne in pairs at each node), dull green or brownish-green, curled and shrivelled, crumble easily; when whole and smoothed out, tripinnatipartite (parted three times in a feather-like manner); lobes and lobules oblong and orbicular (round), or oblong and elliptical, pubescent (covered with short, soft hairs) on both sides. Odour: fragrant and distinctive; taste: slightly bitter.

Indications 1. Fever due to summer heat, low-grade fever without sweating 2. Intermittent fever due to tuberculosis 3. Malaria

Chemical Composition Mainly contains sesquiterpene and artemisinin; also contains coumarins, essential oils and flavonoids.

Note In Hong Kong, commonly used for medicinal purposes is the inflorescence of *Artemisia annua* L.

Herba Artemisiae Scopariae

Virgate Wormwood Herb

Yinchen

茵陳

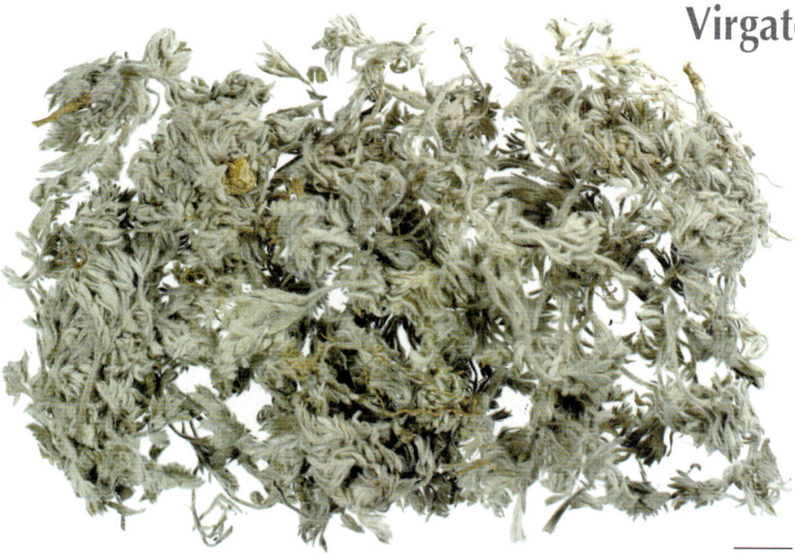

1 cm

Crude Drug (Mianyinchen)

Source ▶ The above-ground part of *Artemisia scoparia* Waldst. et Kit. (Fam. Compositae).

Distribution ▶ Mainly in Chinese provinces such as Hebei and Shandong, and in northeastern China; also in Hong Kong.

Harvest & Processing ▶ Collect above-ground parts in spring or in autumn when flower buds mature; remove foreign matter and old stems; dry under the sun. The ones collected in spring are customarily called "*Mian yinchen*" (Soft Virgate Wormwood Herb), and those collected in autumn, "*Yinchen hao*"(Capillary Wormwood Herb).

Description ▶ Mostly curled into a leafy mass; greyish-white or greyish-green. Stem small; 1.5-2.5 cm long, 1-2 mm in diameter; conspicuous longitudinal striae visible upon removal of white villi on outer surface; brittle, breaks easily. Leaves petiolate (with a petiole); when smoothed out, pinnatisect (divided in a feather-like manner) to tripinnatisect (divided three times in a feather-like manner); blades 1-3 cm long, about 1 cm wide; lobules ovate (egg-shaped in outline and attached at the broad end), slightly oblanceolate (inverse lance-head shaped), or slightly linear (long and narrow); apex acute. Odour: fresh and fragrant; taste: slightly bitter.

Indications ▶ 1. Jaundice, infectious hepatitis, cholelithiasis, cholecystitis, haemolytic jaundice 2. Hypercholesteremia 3. Prurigo, urticaria, tinea (both orally and external use).

Chemical Composition ▶ Mainly contains essential oils and flavonoids.

Note ▶ According to *C.P.*, also used for medicinal purposes is the above-ground part of *A. capillaris* Thunb.

Herba Asari

Manchurian Wildginger
Xixin

細辛

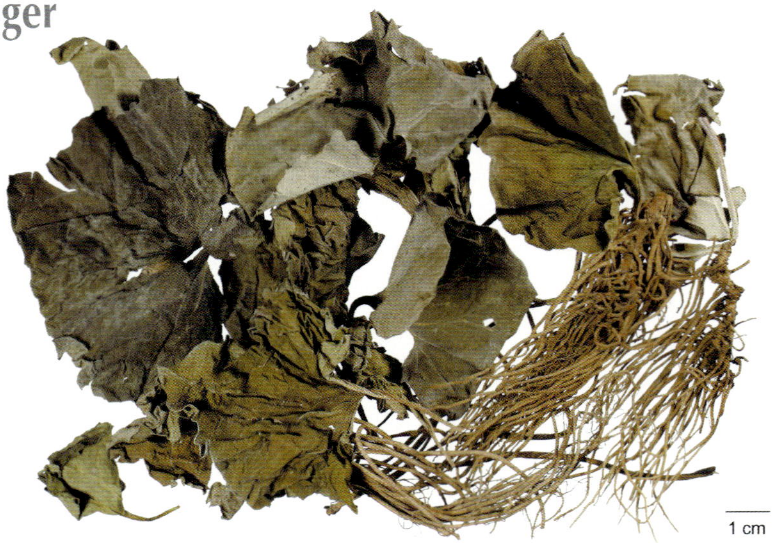

Crude Drug

Source The whole herb of *Asarum heterotropoides* Fr. Schmidt *var. mandshuricum* (Maxim.) Kitag. (Fam. Aristolochiaceae).

Distribution Mainly in northeastern China. Customarily called '*Liao xixin*' (Northeast-Region Manchurian Wildginger).

Harvest & Processing Dig out whole herbs in summer during fructescence or in early autumn; remove soil and sand; dry in shaded areas.

Description Whole herb often curled into a leafy mass. Rhizome growing transversely, irregular and cylindrical in shape; with short branches; outer surface greyish-brown, rough; branch tip with a bowl-shaped stem scar. Roots slender, growing densely on nodes; outer surface greyish-yellow, smooth or with longitudinal wrinkles, marked with fibrous roots and scars of fibrous roots. Basal leaves 1-3, with long petioles; outer surface pale green, smooth; blades cordate (heart-shaped) to reniform (kidney-shaped) and cordate; entire (with continuous, even margin). Apex acute; base cordate with a deep notch in the centre. Fruits hemispherical. Odour: acrid and fragrant; taste: pungent and tongue-numbing.

Indications 1. Common cold with severe headache and generalized pain, headache, toothache, arthralgia 2. Cough and dyspnoea with thin and whitish sputum 3. Collapse (as nasal spray)

Chemical Composition Mainly contains essential oils with camphene and asaricin as the components.

Note According to *C.P.*, also used for medicinal purposes is the whole herb of *A. sieboldii* Miq. var. *seoulense* Nakai and *A. sieboldii* Miq.

Herba Catharanthi Rosei

Madagascar Periwinkle Herb
Changchunhua

長春花

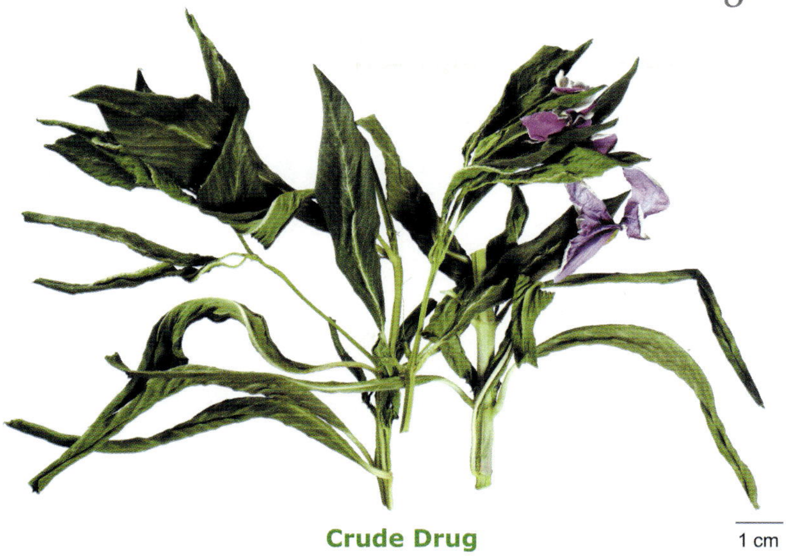

Crude Drug

Source The whole plant of *Catharanthus roseus* (L.) G. Don (Fam. Apocynaceae).

Distribution Mainly in Chinese provinces such as Shandong, Jiangsu, Fujian, Guangdong, Guangxi, Hainan and Yunnan; widely cultivated in Hong Kong for display.

Harvest & Processing Harvest above-ground parts on sunny days in autumn; remove lignified parts of stems; cut the rest into sections 6 cm long; dry under the sun or use while fresh.

Description Whole plant 30-50 cm long. Stem and branches green or dull reddish-brown, subcylindrical, angulate (with ridges); broken surface fibrous; pith hollow. Leaves opposite (borne in pairs at each node), shrivelled; when smoothed out, blades obovate (egg-shaped in outline and attached at the narrower end), or oblong and round, 3-6 cm long, 1.5-2.5 cm wide; apex obtuse, mucronate (with a short straight point); base cuneate (wedge-shaped), dark green or dull greenish-brown; pinnate (feather-shaped) veins prominent; petioles very short. Flowers at shoot tips or leaf axils; corolla salverform (with a slender tube and an abruptly spreading, flattened limb), about 3 cm long, pale red or purplish-red. Odour: faint; taste: slightly sweet, bitter.

Indications 1. Leukemia, lymphosarcoma 2. Hypertension, diabetes mellitus 3. Primary thrombocytopenic purpura.

Chemical Composition Mainly contains alkaloids such as vinblastine, vincristine and lewosine.

Herba Centipedae

Small Centipeda Herb
Ebushicao

鵝不食草

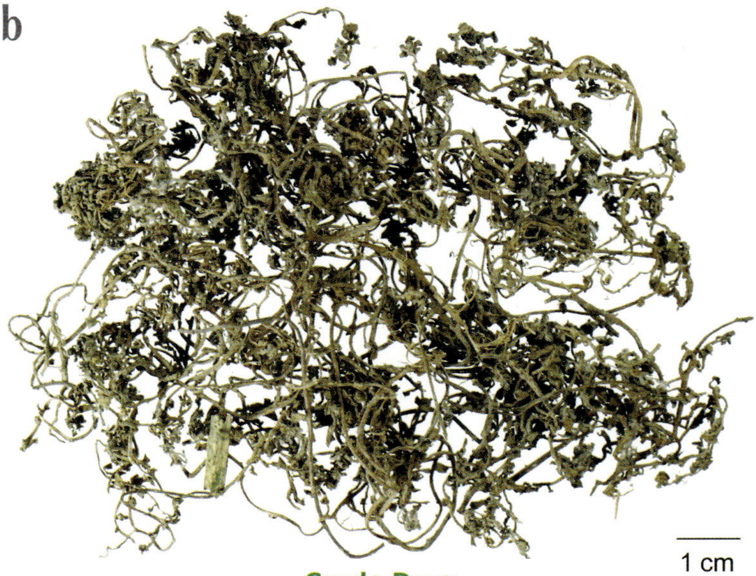

Crude Drug

Source

The whole herb of *Centipeda minima* (L.) A. Br. et Aschers. (Fam. Compositae).

Distribution

In most regions of China, including Hong Kong.

Harvest & Processing

Harvest whole herbs in summer during efflorescence; wash away soil; dry under the sun.

Description

Intertwined into masses. Fibrous roots fine and slender, pale yellow. Stem slender; brittle; broken surface yellowish-white. Leaves small; mostly shrivelled or in fragments; when smoothed out, intact ones spatulate (spoon-shaped); outer surface greyish-green or reddish-brown; margin with 3-5 teeth. Capitate inflorescences yellow or dull yellowish-brown. Odour: slightly fragrant, pungent on prolonged inhalation; taste: bitter and slightly acrid.

Indications

1. Common cold with headache, cough with sputum and nasal congestion 2. Sinusitis with nasal discharge.

Chemical Composition

Mainly contains sesquiterpene lactones such as 6-O-methylacrylylplenolin.

Herba Cirsii

Field Thistle Herb

Xiaoji

小薊

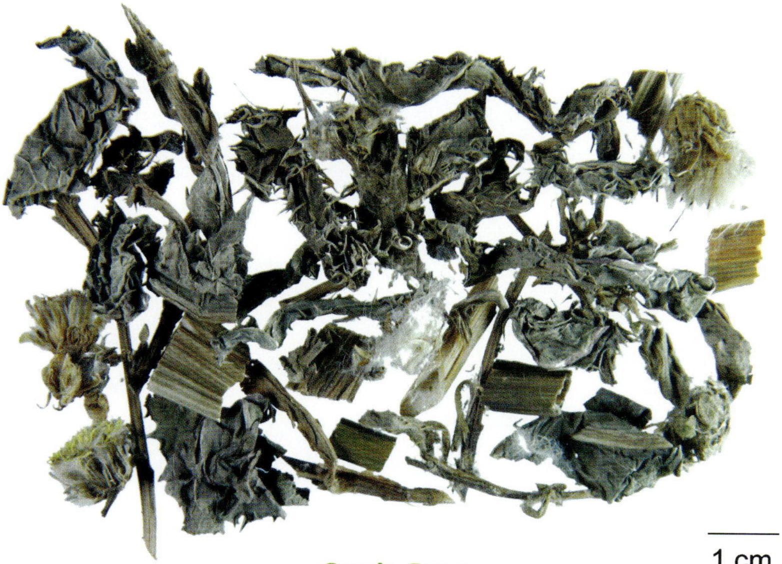

Crude Drug

Source The whole herb of *Cirsium setosum* (Willd.) MB. (Fam. Compositae).

Distribution In most regions of China.

Harvest & Processing Cut off whole herbs during efflorescence in May and June; dry under the sun or use while fresh.

Description Stem cylindrical; outer surface greyish-green or purplish, with longitudinal ridges and white pubescence; brittle, breaks easily; broken surface hollow in the centre. Leaves alternate (borne singly at each node), epetiolate (without a petiole) or with short petioles; blades shrivelled or in fragments; blades oblong and elliptical, or oblong, orbicular (round) and lanceolate (lance-head shaped); entire (with continuous, even margin), or pinnatilobate (lobed in a feather-like manner), pinnatifid (cleft in a feather-like manner) or pinnatipartite (parted in a feather-like manner), with the lobes or divisions serrate (saw-like); upper surface dull greenish-brown, underside greyish-green, both sides with white pubescence. Capitate inflorescence single or several, acrogenous (growing from the apex); involucre campanulate (bell-shaped), bracts in 5-8 layers, yellowish-green; florets purplish-red. Odour: faint; taste: slightly bitter.

Indications 1. Various kinds of bleeding such as epistaxis and haematuria. 2. Pyogenic condition.

Chemical Composition Mainly contains acaciin, acacetin, chlorogenic acid, taratxasterol etc.

Note Customarily, Herba Cirsii and Herba Cirsii *Japonici* are interchangeably used in Hong Kong.

Herba Cirsii Japonici

Japanese Thistle Herb
Daji
大薊

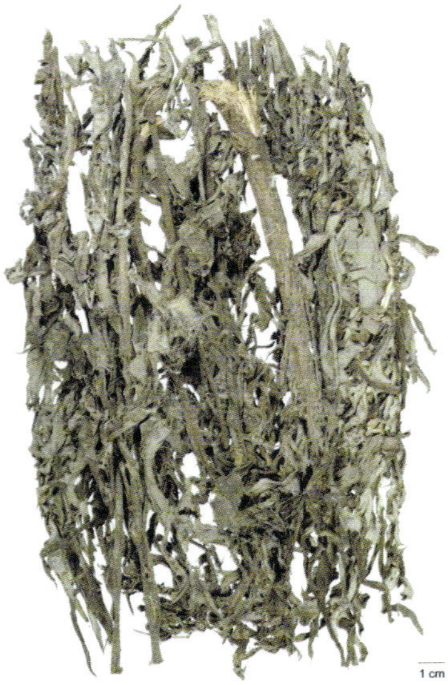

Crude Drug (above-ground part)

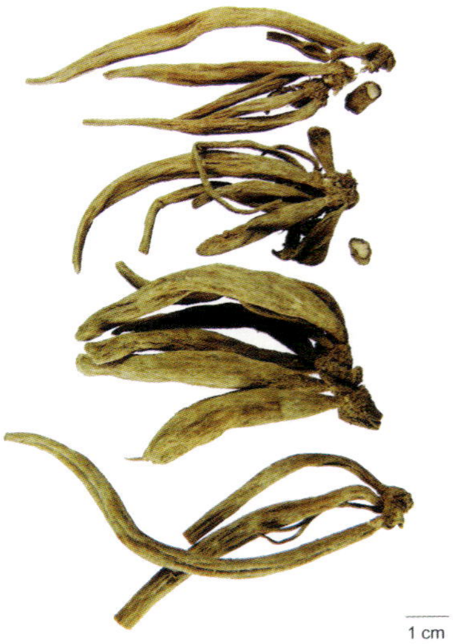

Crude Drug (Root)

Source The above-ground part of *Cirsium japonicum* DC. (Fam. Compositae).

Distribution Mainly in Chinese provinces such as Jiangsu, Zhejiang and Sichuan; also in Hong Kong.

Harvest & Processing Collect above-ground parts when flowers bloom in summer and autumn; dry under the sun.

Description Herbaceous stem cylindrical, stem base up to 1.2 cm in diameter; outer surface dull greenish-brown or reddish-brown, marked with several longitudinal ridges and covered with silky hair; broken surface greyish-white, pith loose and porous. Leaves shrivelled; mostly in fragments; when whole and smoothed out, blades oblanceolate (inverse lance-head shaped), or obovate (egg-shaped in outline and attached at the narrower end) and elliptical; pinnatipartite (parted in a feather-like manner); rim with spikes of irregular lengths; both sides covered with silky greyish-white hair. Capitate inflorescences acrogenous (growing from the apex), spherical; involucre dull yellowish-brown; pinnate (feather-shaped) pappi greyish-white. Odour: faint; taste: mild.

Indications 1. Various kinds of bleeding such as haematuria, haemoptysis, epistaxis, haematochezia, dysfunctional uterine bleeding and traumatic bleeding 2. Carbuncles and sores.

Chemical Composition Contains dotriacontanol, stigmasterol, β -sitosterol. Essential oils exist in the roots.

Note Both Herba Cirsii Japoni ci and Herba Cirsii are interchangeably used in Hong Kong.

Herba Cistanches

Desertliving Cistanche
Roucongrong
肉蓯蓉

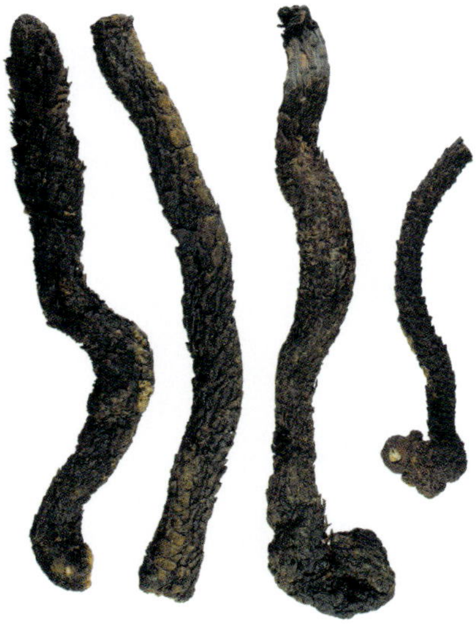

Crude Drug

1 cm

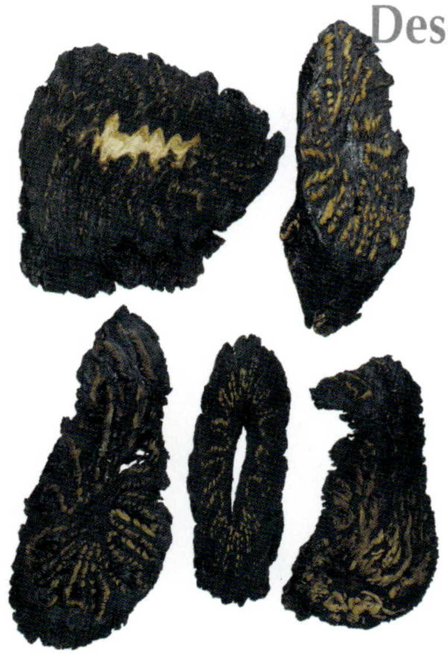

Decoction Pieces

1 cm

Source The scale-leaf-bearing fleshy stem of *Cistanche deserticola* Y. C. Ma (Fam. Orobanchaceae).

Distribution Mainly in Chinese provinces such as Shaanxi and Gansu, and in Ningxia Inner Mongolia and Xinjiang.

Harvest & Processing Dig out and collect stems, usually in spring, before or when shoots just begin to come up above the ground; remove inflorescences; cut stems into sections; dry under the sun.

Description Stem flattened and cylindrical, slightly curved; usually 3-15 cm long, 2-8 cm in diameter. Outer surface reddish-brown or greyish-brown, densely covered with imbricate (overlapping like tiles on a roof) fleshy scales; apex of scales usually broken. Heavy; hard, fairly pliable, does not break easily; when broken, surface reddish-brown, with pale brown punctiform (dot-like) vascular bundles arranged in undulate (wavy) annulations. Odour: faint; taste: sweet and slightly bitter.

Indications 1. Impotence, seminal emission, infertility and generalised weakness with loin and knee ache 2. Constipation.

Chemical Composition Mainly contains iridoids such as cistanosides A, B, C, D, E.

Herba Cynomorii

Songaria Cynomorium Herb

Suoyang

鎖陽

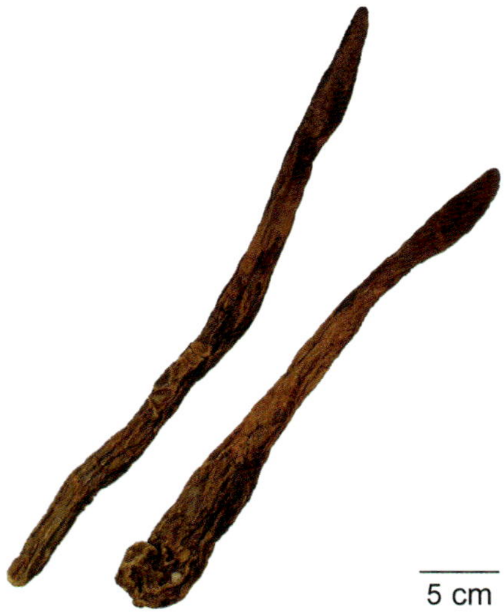

5 cm

Crude Drug

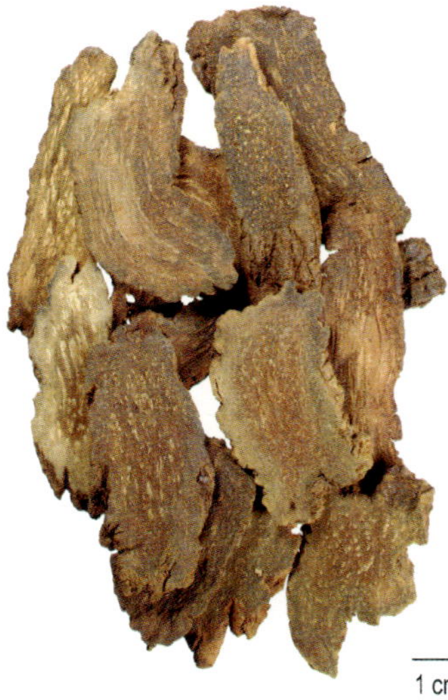

1 cm

Decoction Pieces

Source The fleshy stem of *Cynomorium songaricum* Rupr. (Fam. Cynomoriaceae).

Distribution Mainly in Chinese provinces such as Gansu, and in Inner Mongolia, Ningxia and Xinjiang.

Harvest & Processing Dig out whole herbs in summer; remove inflorescences; cut fleshy stems into sections; dry under the sun.

Description Stem flattened and cylindrical, with one end thinner and slightly curved; 5-15 cm long, 1.5-5 cm in diameter. Outer surface brown to reddish-brown; rough; marked with conspicuous longitudinal grooves and irregular indentations, in some cases with remnants of triangular, blackish-brown scales. Heavy; hard, difficult to break; broken surface light brown or reddish-brown, with triangular, yellow vascular bundles. Odour: faint; taste: sweet and astringent.

Indications 1. Impotence, emission 2. Weakness and paralysis of extremities, pain and cold feeling of the loin and knee 3. Constipation of elderly.

Chemical Composition Mainly contains acetylursolic acid and tannins.

Herba Dendrobii

Dendrobium

Shihu

石斛

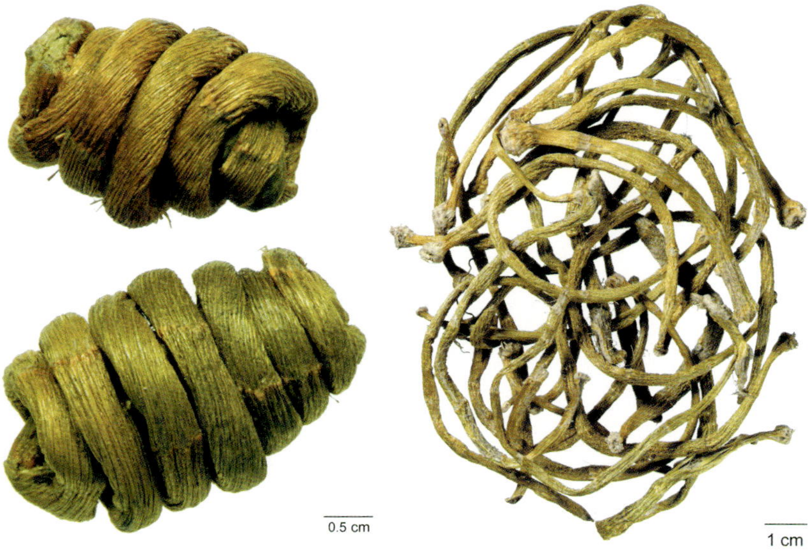

Different forms of Dendrobium in the market

Source The stem of *Dendrobium chrysanthum* Wall. (Fam. Orchiadaceae).

Distribution Mainly in Chinese provinces such as Guangxi, Guizhou, Guangdong and Yunnan; also in Hong Kong.

Harvest & Processing Harvest anytime during the year. Remove roots, soil and sand; use while fresh. Alternatively, remove foreign matter; blanch in boiling water or soften by heat; rub and dry under the sun repeatedly to remove leaf sheaths; dry.

Description Stem slender and cylindrical, with the upper and middle parts irregular and curved; 30-80 cm long, 3-5 mm in diameter; internodes 2-3.5 cm long. Outer surface golden-yellow to pale yellowish-brown, marked with longitudinal grooves. Light in weight; solid, breaks easily; broken surface slightly fibrous. Odour: faint; taste: slightly bitter; sticky when chewed.

Indications 1. Thirst and dryness of the tongue 2. Debility and fever during convalescence 3. Retching.

Chemical Composition Mainly contains a variety of alkaloids.

Note In Hong Kong, commonly used for medicinal purposes is the stem of *D. fimbriatum* (BL.) Lindl.

Herba Desmodii Styracifolii

Snowbellleaf Tickclover Herb

Guangjinqiancao

廣金錢草

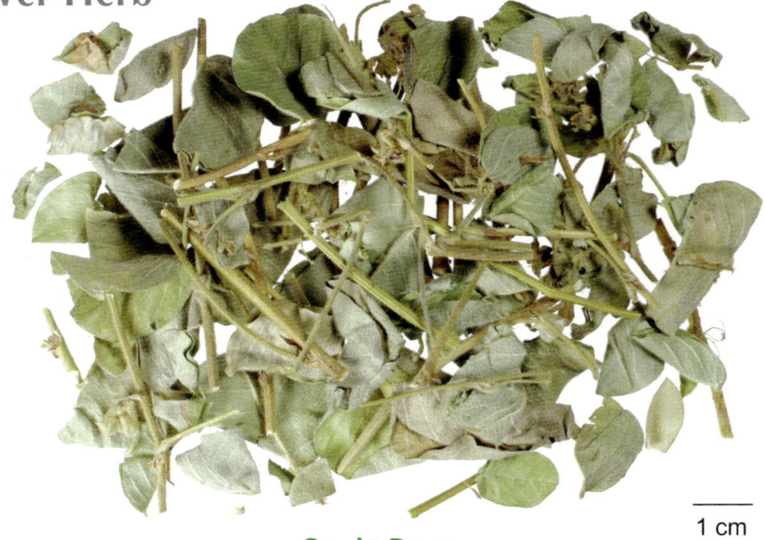

Crude Drug

Source The above-ground part of *Desmodium styracifolium* (Osb.) Merr. (Fam. Leguminosae).

Distribution Mainly in Chinese provinces such as Guangdong, Guangxi, Fujian and Hunan; also in Hong Kong.

Harvest & Processing Cut off above-ground parts in summer and autumn; remove foreign matter; dry under the sun.

Description Stem and branches cylindrical, usually up to 60 cm long. Stem 2-5 mm thick; outer surface pale brownish-yellow, densely covered with yellow pubescence; fairly brittle; broken surface with pith in the centre. Leaves alternate (borne singly at each node); leaflets 1-3, orbicular (round), or oblong and orbicular, 2-4 cm in diameter. Apex slightly notched; base cordate (heart-shaped); entire (with continuous, even margin). Upper surface of leaves yellowish-green or greyish-green, glabrous (without hairs); underside covered with greyish-white appressed (pressed close or flat against another surface or organ) silky hairs. Lateral veins pinnate (feather-shaped); petioles 1-2 cm long; stipules in 1 pair, lanceolate (lance-head shaped), about 8 mm long. Odour: slightly fragrant; taste: slightly sweet.

Indications 1. Stranguria 2. Infectious hepatitis, cholelithiasis, cholecystitis 3. Coronary heart diseases

Chemical Composition Mainly contains triterpene saponins such as soyasaponins I.

Herba Dianthi

Lilac Pink Herb

Qumai

瞿麥

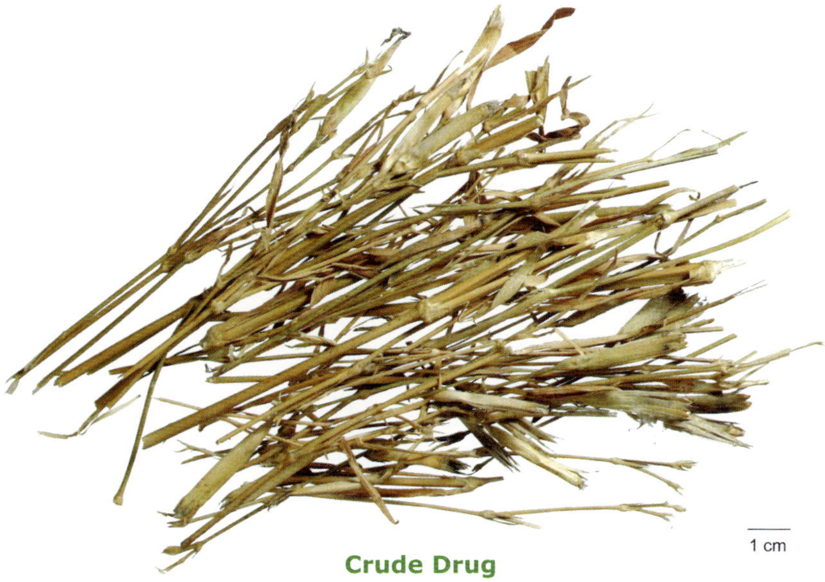

1 cm

Crude Drug

Source The flower-and-fruit-bearing whole herb of *Dianthus superbus* L. (Fam. Caryophyllaceae).

Distribution Mainly in Chinese provinces such as Hebei, Henan, Shaanxi, Shandong, Sichuan, Hubei, Hunan, Zhejiang and Jiangsu.

Harvest & Processing Cut off flower-and-fruit-bearing whole herbs during efflorescence and fructescence in summer and autumn; remove weeds and soil; cut into sections or leave as whole herbs; dry under the sun.

Description Stem cylindrical, upper part rameous (branched); 30-60 cm long; outer surface pale green or yellowish-green, smooth and glabrous (without hairs); nodes conspicuous, slightly bulgy; broken surface hollow. Leaves opposite (borne in pairs at each node), mostly shrivelled, yellowish-green; when smoothed out, blade linear (long and narrow) to lanceolate (lance-head shaped). Top part of branches with flowers and fruits; calyx tubular, 2.7-3.7 cm long; bracts 4-6, broad and ovate (egg-shaped in outline and attached at the broad end), about 1/4 the length of calyx tube; petals brownish-purple or brownish-yellow, curled, apex parted into filiform (thread-like) divisions. Capsules long and tubular, same length as persistent calyx. Seeds small, numerous. Odourless; taste: mild.

Indications 1. Genito-urinary infection, gravel, oliguria 2. Haematuria 3. Amenorrhoea 4. Eczema.

Chemical Composition Contains flavonoids; also contains pinitol.

Note According to *C.P.*, also used for medicinal purposes is the flower-and-fruit-bearing whole herb of *D. chinensis* L.

Herba Duchesneae Indicae

Indian Mock Strawberry Herb

Shemei

蛇莓

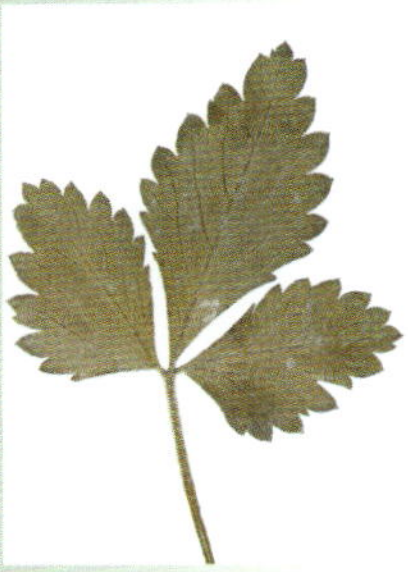

Indian Mock Strawberry Herb Magnified

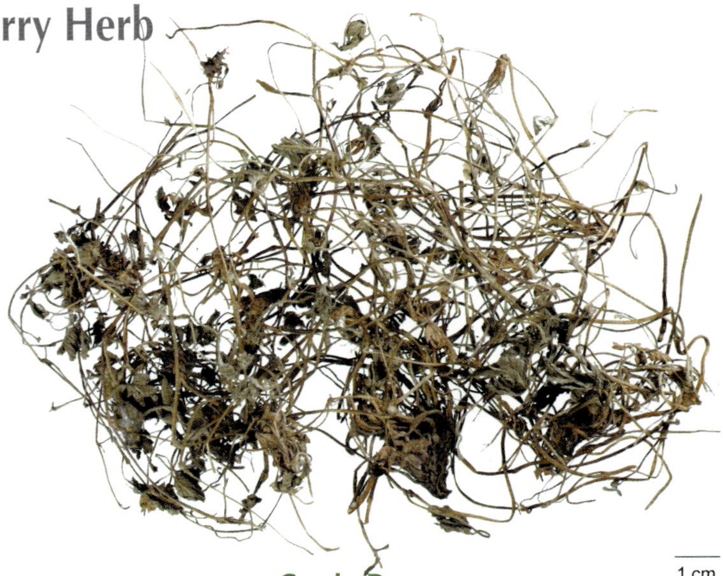

Crude Drug

Source The whole herb of *Duchesnea indica* (Andr.) Focke (Fam. Rosaceae).

Distribution In most regions of China, including Hong Kong.

Harvest & Processing Harvest whole herbs from June to November; wash clean; dry under the sun or use while fresh.

Description Mostly intertwined into masses, covered with fine, white pubescence, with stolons. Leaves alternate (borne singly at each node); compound leaves ternate (in threes); petioles of basal leaves 6-10 cm long. Leaflets mostly shrivelled; when whole, obovate (egg-shaped in outline and attached at the narrower end), 1.5-4 cm long, 1-3 cm wide; base oblique (with unequal sides); crenate (with round-toothed edges); outer surface yellowish-green, upper surface nearly glabrous (without hairs), underside with sparse pubescence. Flowers solitary (occurring singly) at leaf axil; with long pedicels. Aggregate fruits reddish-brown; achenes small, with persistent calyx. Odour: faint; taste: slightly astringent.

Indications 1. Common cold, febrile disease, convulsion 2. Dysentery, jaundice 3. Aphtha, sore throat, mumps 4. Boils, trauma, burn and scald, snakebite 5. Bleeding, menstrual disorders

Chemical Composition Mainly contains condensed tannins and ellagitannins.

Herba Ecliptae

Yerbadetajo Herb
Mohanlian

墨旱蓮

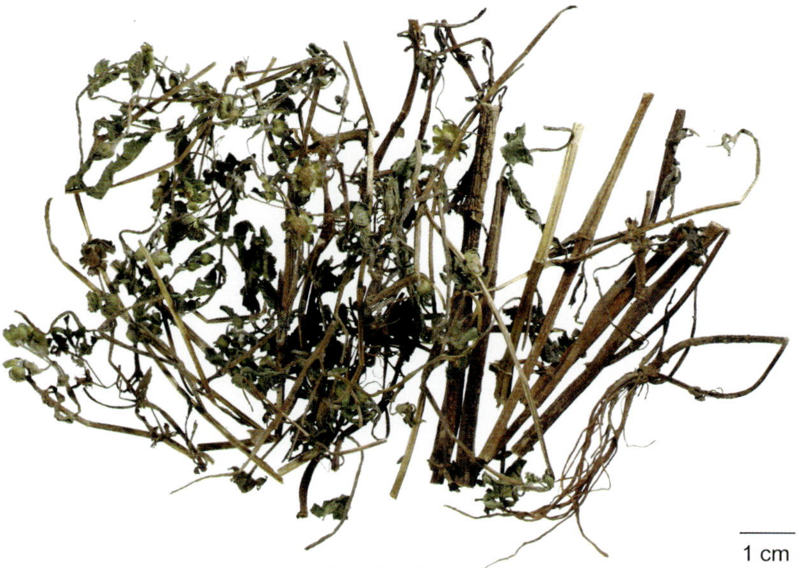

1 cm

Crude Drug

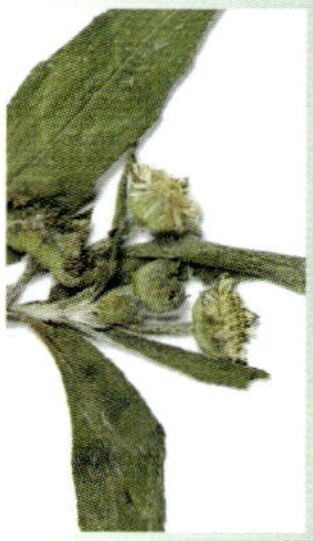

Yerbadetajo Herb Magnified

Source The whole herb of *Eclipta prostrata* L. (Fam. Compositae).

Distribution Mainly in Chinese provinces such as Jiangsu, Zhejiang, Jiangxi and Hubei; also in Hong Kong.

Harvest & Processing Harvest whole herbs in summer and autumn during efflorescence; remove foreign matter; dry in shaded areas or under the sun. Can be used immediately after picking.

Description Whole herb covered with thick white hairs. Stem cylindrical, ramose (with many branches); outer surface greyish-green or purplish, marked with longitudinal ridges; brittle, breaks easily; broken surface yellowish-white, with white porous pith or sometimes a cavity in the centre. Leaves opposite (borne in pairs at each node); mostly shrivelled or in fragments; dark green; when smoothed out, intact blades lanceolate (lance-head shaped); margin entire (continuous, even), or slightly serrulate (finely notched); petioles almost undetectable. Capitate inflorescences solitary (occurring singly) at shoot tips; common peduncle slender; phyllaries 5-6, yellowish-green or reddish-brown; corolla mostly fallen off. Achenes flattened and ellipsoid (elliptical in long-section and circular in cross-section); brown; outer surface strumulose (with small cushion-like protuberances). Odour: slightly fragrant; taste: mild and slightly salty-astringent.

Indications 1. Bleeding 2. Diarrhoea, infant malnutrition 3. Tinnitus, neurasthenia 4. Premature greying of hair 5. Tinea pedis, eczema, ulcers, rice-field dermatitis.

Chemical Composition Contains alkaloids such as nicotine, flavonoids such as apigenin, and coumarin such as wedelolactone.

Herba Elephantopi Scaberis

Scabrous Elephant-foot Herb

Didantou

地膽頭

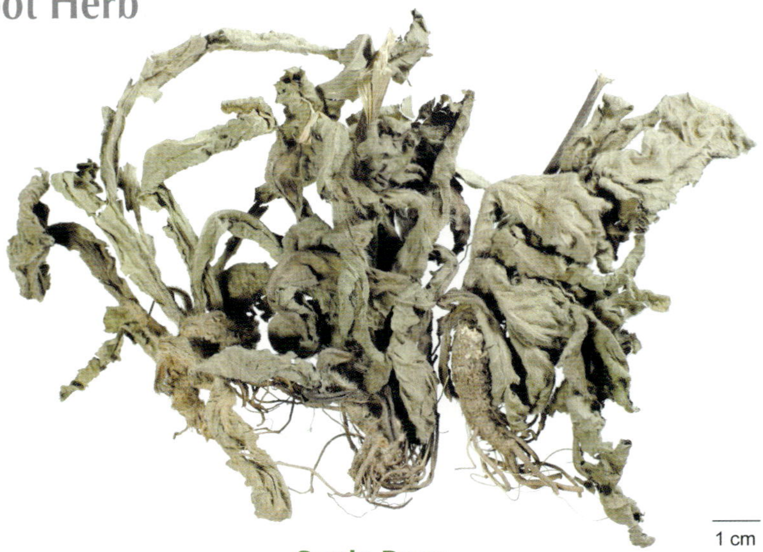

1 cm

Crude Drug

Source The whole herb of *Elephantopus scaber* L. (Fam. Compositae).

Distribution Mainly in Chinese provinces such as Guangdong, Guangxi, Fujian and Jiangxi; also in Hong Kong.

Harvest & Processing Collect whole herbs in late summer; wash clean; use while fresh or dry under the sun.

Description Whole herb 15-40 cm long. Rhizome with annular (ring-like) nodes, densely covered with appressed (pressed close or flat against another surface or organ) greyish-white coarse hairs; hard, does not break easily; when broken, surface yellowish-white. Numerous shrivelled reddish-brown fibrous roots conglomerate (densely clustered) beneath rhizome. Stem cylindrical, often dichotomous (branched into two divisions); densely covered with appressed greyish-white coarse hairs. Leaves mostly basal; when intact and smoothed out, leaves spatulate (spoon-shaped) or oblanceolate (inverse lance-head shaped); with relatively numerous gland dots. Apex obtuse or acute, base attenuate (tapering gradually to a narrow tip or base); margin slightly crenate (with round-toothed edges); both sides, especially those of younger leaves, densely covered with appressed greyish-white coarse hairs; petioles short, roughly sheath-shaped, amplexicaul (surrounding the stem); cauline (grown on stems) leaves few and small. Odour: faint; taste: slightly bitter.

Indications 1. Influenza, sore throat, tonsillitis 2. Red eyes, photophobia with lacrimation 3. Jaundice, oedema 4. Menstrual disorders, leukorrhoea 5. Boils and sores, eczema, snake and insect bites

Chemical Composition Contains triterpenes such as epifriedelinol, lupeol and lupeol acetate.

Herba Emiliae

Sowthistle Tasselflower Herb
Yidianhong

一點紅

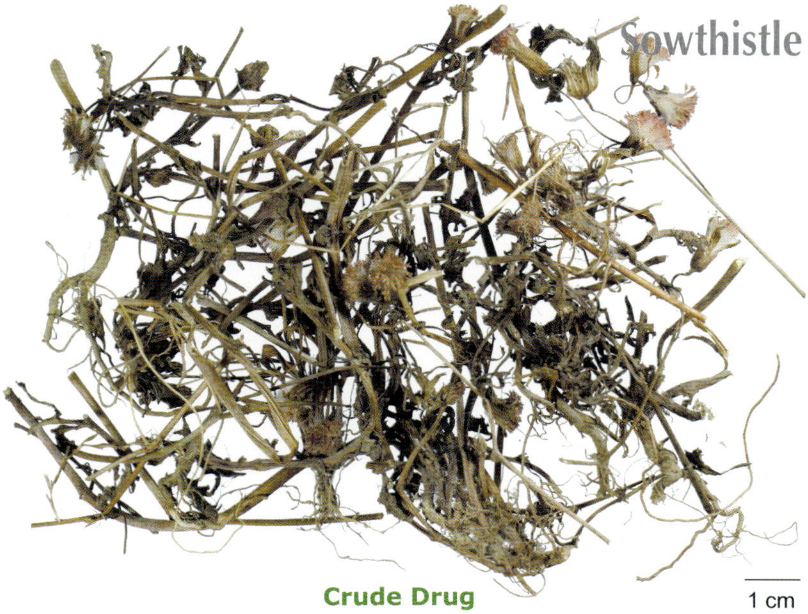

Crude Drug

Source The whole herb of *Emilia sonchifolia* (L.) DC. (Fam. Compositae).

Distribution Mainly in Chinese provinces such as Jiangxi, Guangdong, Guangxi, Fujian, Hunan and Guizhou; also in Hong Kong.

Harvest & Processing Collect whole herbs anytime during the year; wash clean; use while fresh or dry under the sun.

Description Whole herb about 30 cm long. Rhizome slender and cylindrical; light brownish-yellow. Stem with few branches; fine and cylindrical; marked with longitudinal striae; greyish-green or dull yellowish-brown. Leaves mostly shrivelled, greyish-green; basal leaves ovate (egg-shaped in outline and attached at the broad end), or lyriform (lyre-shaped); leaves at upper part relatively small, base slightly amplexicaul (surrounding the stem); papery. Capitate inflorescences withered; corolla fallen off at an early stage; receptacle and involucre persistent; bracts tea-brown, membranous; achenes light yellowish-brown; pappi numerous, white. Odour: faint; taste: mild, slightly salty.

Indications 1. Diarrhoea, dysentery 2. Conjunctivitis 3. Leukorrhagia, urinary tract infection 4. Skin infection 5. Herpes zoster, eczema and insect bite (external use).

Chemical Composition Alkaloids such as senkirkine, and flavonoids such as hyperoside exist in the upper part.

Herba Ephedrae

Ephedra
Mahuang

麻黄

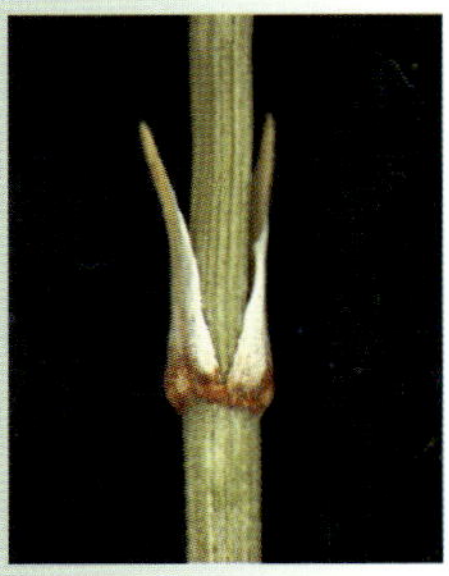

Ephedra Magnified

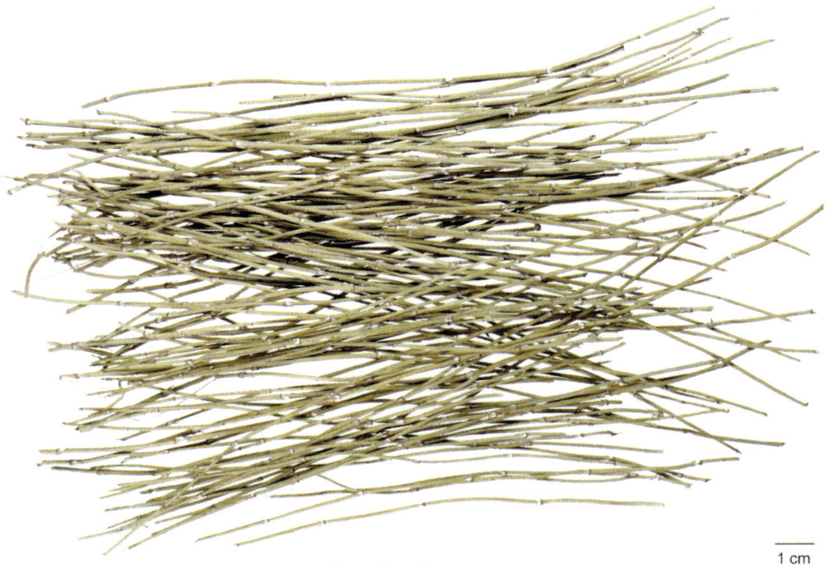

Crude Drug

Source The herbaceous stem of *Ephedra sinica* Stapf (Fam. Ephedraceae).

Distribution Mainly in Chinese provinces such as Shanxi and Shaanxi, and in Xinjiang, Inner Mongolia and Ningxia.

Harvest & Processing Collect green herbaceous stems in autumn and dry under the sun.

Description Stem slender and cylindrical, with few branches; 1-2mm in diameter. Outer surface pale green to yellowish-green, marked with fine, slightly rough longitudinal ridges. Nodes prominent, internodes 2-6 cm long. On the nodes are membranous scale leaves 3-4 mm long and with 2 lobes (very occasionally 3), each lobe the shape of an acute triangle, with greyish-white apex curling downwards and tubular reddish-brown base. Light in weight; brittle, breaks easily. When broken, surface slightly fibrous, with a yellowish-green rim and suborbicular (almost round) reddish-brown pith. Odour: slightly fragrant; taste: astringent and slightly bitter.

Indications 1. Common cold, fever with anhidrosis 2. Cough and dyspnoea 3. Oedema.

Chemical Composition Mainly contains alkaloids such as ephedrine and pseudoephedrine.

Note According to *C.P.*, also used for medicinal purposes is the herbaceous stem of *E. intermedia* Schrenk et C.A.Mey. and *E. equisetina* Bge.

Herba Epimedii

Epimedium Herb

Yinyanghuo

淫羊藿

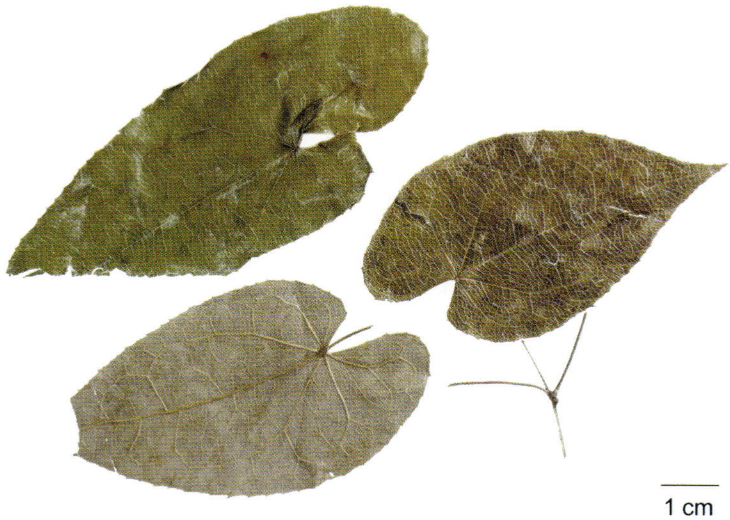

1 cm

Crude Drug

Source The above-ground part of *Epimedium brevicornum* Maxim. (Fam. Berberidaceae).

Distribution Mainly in Chinese provinces such as Shaanxi, Hubei, Zhejiang and Anhui.

Harvest & Processing Cut off above-ground parts in summer and autumn when leaves flourish; remove foreign matter; dry under the sun or in shaded areas.

Description Stem fine and cylindrical; about 20 cm long; outer surface yellowish-green or pale yellow, slightly lustrous. Cauline leaves opposite; compound leaves biternate; leaflet ovate, 3-8 cm long, 2-6 cm wide. Apex slightly pointed. Terminal leaflet with a cordate base; leaflets on both sides smaller, cordate but slanted, with the outer side of leaflet blade larger, forming the shape of an ear. Leaflets with fine, setiform, yellow teeth at margin; upper surface yellowish-green, underside greyish-green; both sides with 7-9 main veins, sparsely covered with long, fine hairs at base; veinlets protuberant on both sides, reticulate and prominent; petiolule 1-5 cm long. Blade nearly coriaceous. Odourless; taste: slightly bitter.

Indications 1. Impotence, premature ejaculation, incontinence of urine
2. Rheumatic arthritis, pain and cold feeling in the lower body and legs 3. Climacterium hypertension, chronic tracheitis.

Chemical Composition Contains glycosides such as icariin.

Note According to *C.P.*, also used for medicinal purposes is the above-ground part of *E. sagittatum* (Sieb. et Zucc.) Maxim., of *E. pubescens* Maxim., of *E. wushanense* T.S. Ying and of *E. koreanum* Nakai.

Herba Equiseti Hiemalis

Common Scouring Rush Herb

Muzei

木賊

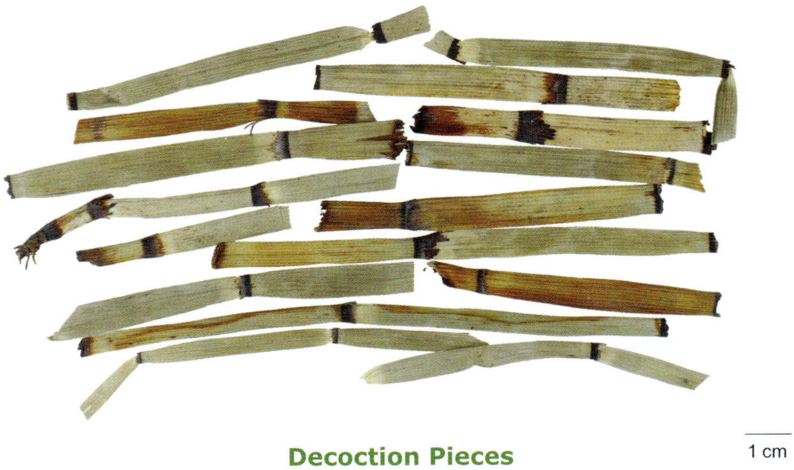

Decoction Pieces

Source The whole herb of *Equisetum hiemale* (L.) Borner (Fam. Equisetaceae).

Distribution Mainly in Chinese provinces such as Liaoning, Jilin, Heilongjiang, Shaanxi and Hubei.

Harvest & Processing Cut off whole herbs in summer and autumn; wash clean; dry under the sun.

Description Stem long and fistular (hollow and cylindrical), straight; 20-60 cm long; 2-6 mm in diameter; nodes conspicuous; internodes 2.5-9 cm long, not rameous (branched). Outer surface greyish-green or yellowish-green, rough, with 20-30 ridges; ridges marked with numerous small, lustrous verruciform (wart-shaped) protuberances. Nodes with sheath-shaped leaves; sheath brownish-black at base and at the tooth, pale yellow in the middle part. Light in weight; brittle, breaks easily; when broken, surface hollow in the centre, with numerous orbicular (round) cavities at the rim. Odour: faint; taste: sweet, mild, astringent. Gritty when chewed.

Indications 1. Nebula, sore eye, sore throat 2. Carbuncles 3. Haematochezia and haemorrhoidal bleeding 4. Rectal prolapse 5. Malaria

Chemical Composition Mainly contains flavonoids and essential oils.

Herba Eupatorii

Fortune Eupatorium Herb

Peilan

佩蘭

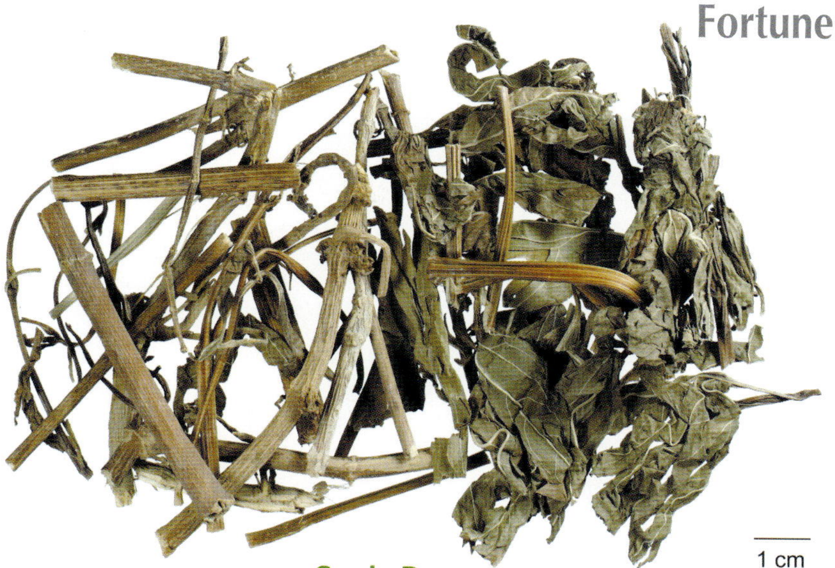

1 cm

Crude Drug

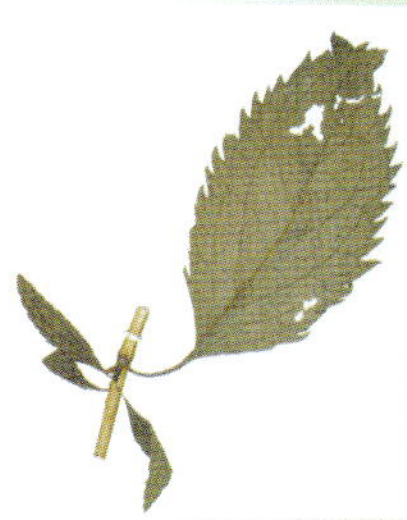

Fortune Eupatorium Herb Magnified

Source The above-ground part of *Eupatorium fortunei* Turcz. (Fam. Compositae).

Distribution Mainly in Chinese provinces such as Hebei, Shandong, Jiangsu and Zhejiang.

Harvest & Processing Cut off above-ground parts in two rounds in summer and autumn; remove foreign matter; dry under the sun.

Description Stem cylindrical; 30-100 cm long, 2-5 mm in diameter; outer surface yellowish-brown or yellowish-green, in some cases purplish; with conspicuous nodes and longitudinal ridges; brittle; broken surface with white pith or hollow in the centre. Leaves opposite (borne in pairs at each node), petiolate (with a petiole); blades mostly shrivelled and in fragments, dull greenish-brown; when intact, blades not lobed, or 3-lobed with the middle lobe larger; lobes lanceolate (lance-head shaped), or oblong, orbicular (round) and lanceolate, base narrow, margin serrate (saw-like); non-lobed blades ovate (egg-shaped in outline and attached at the broad end), or ovate and lanceolate, or elliptical. Odour: aromatic; taste: slightly bitter.

Indications 1. Feeling of fullness and oppression in the chest and abdominal distension, anorexia, nausea, vomiting, diarrhoea 2. Aversion to cold, fever, fullness in the head

Chemical Composition Mainly contains essential oils. Taraxasterol and palmitic acid exist in the flowers and leaves. Stems contain fumaric acid and succinic acid.

Herba Gendarussae

Common Gendarussa Herb
Xiaobogu

小駁骨

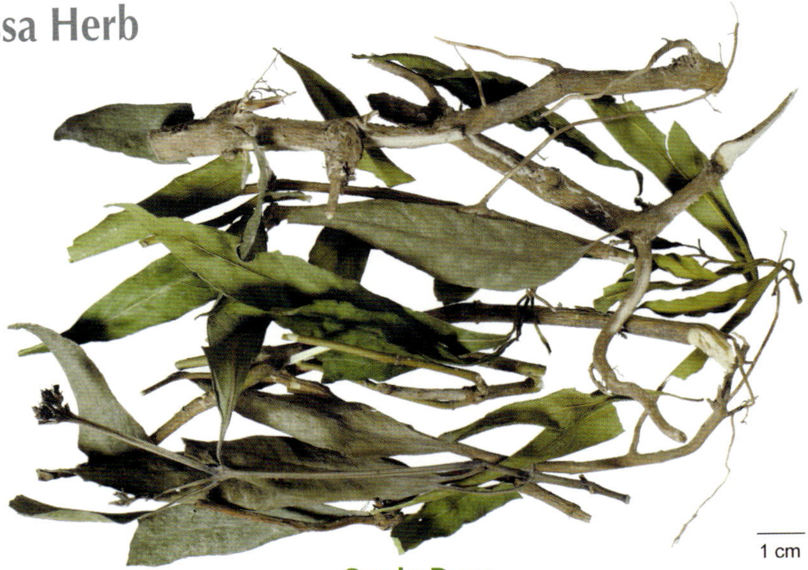

Crude Drug

Source The whole herb of *Gendarussa valgaris* Nees (Fam. Acanthaceae).

Distribution Mainly in Chinese provinces such as Guangdong and Guangxi; also in Hong Kong.

Harvest & Processing Harvest whole plants anytime during the year; wash clean; cut into sections; dry under the sun or use while fresh.

Description Stem cylindrical, ramose (with many branches); twigs with bulgy, quadrangular (four-angled) nodes; young branches green. Leaves mostly shrivelled; when whole, blades narrow and lanceolate (lance-head shaped) or linear (long and narrow) and lanceolate; 4-14 cm long, 1-2 cm wide; apex acuminate (tapering to a slender point), base cuneate (wedge-shaped); entire (with continuous, even margin); upper surface emerald-green, underside yellowish-green and shiny; midrib thick, dark purple in colour as lateral veins; in some cases, lateral veins translucent. Odour: faint; taste: mild.

Indications 1. Rheumatism 2. Trauma, fracture 3. Menstrual disorders, post-partum abdominal pain

Chemical Composition Mainly contains justicin and essential oils.

Herba Geranii

Carolina Cranesbill Herb

Laoguancao

老鸛草

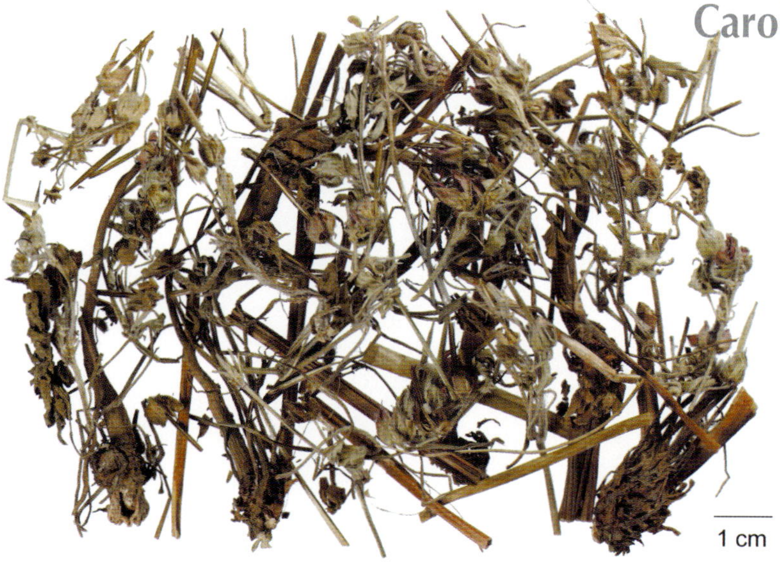

Crude Drug

Source The above-ground part of *Geranium carolinianum* L. (Fam. Geraniaceae).

Distribution Mainly in Chinese provinces such as Tianjin, Hebei and Shandong.

Harvest & Processing Cut off above-ground parts or pull up whole plants in autumn when fruits are nearly mature; remove soil and foreign matter; dry under the sun.

Description Stem 20-45 cm long, 2-4 mm in diameter, often flattened. Nodes bulgy, ramose (with many branches); outer surface light brown, marked with longitudinal grooves and sparse pubescence; brittle, breaks easily; broken surface often hollowed. Leaves opposite (borne in pairs at each node); petioles thin, 3-8 cm long; blade shrivelled, brittle and breaks easily; when whole and smoothed out, reniform (kidney-shaped) or cordate (heart-shaped); with 5-7 lobes, each lobe with 3-5 lobules; lobules linear (long and narrow), pointed at apex, with pubescence on both sides. Capsules subspherical; with 5 locules; surface covered with villi; apex with long rostrums, 1-1.5 cm long; each locule containing 1 seed. Odourless; taste: mild.

Indications 1. Rheumatic or rheumatoid arthralgia, numbness and limitation of movement of limbs 2. Diarrhoea, dysentery.

Chemical Composition Mainly contains essential oils, geraniin and flavonoids.

Note According to *C.P.*, also used for medicinal purposes is the above-ground part of *Erodium stephanianum* Willd. and *G. wilfordii* Maxim., both of which belong to the same family as *G. carolinianum* L.

Herba Glechomae

Longtube Ground Ivy Herb
Lianqiancao

連錢草

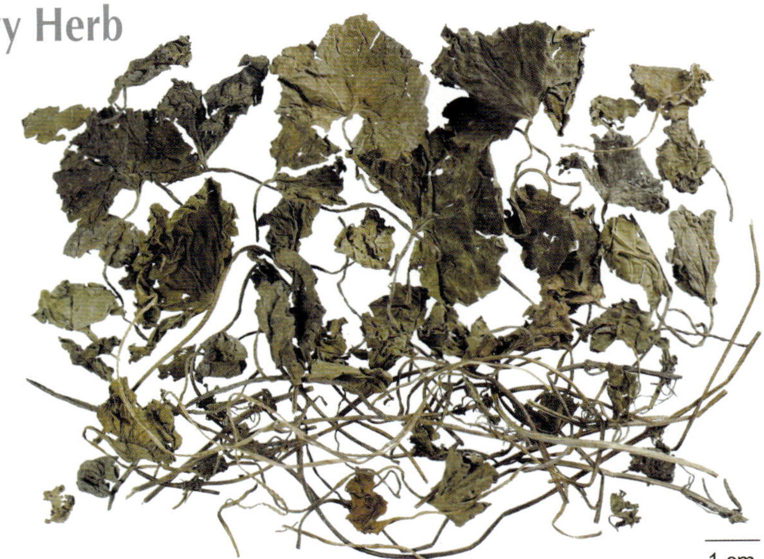

Crude Drug

Source The above-ground part of *Glechoma longituba* (Nakai) Kupr. (Fam. Labiatae).

Distribution In most regions of China, including Hong Kong.

Harvest & Processing Harvest above-ground parts from spring to autumn; remove foreign matter; dry in shaded areas.

Description Above-ground part 10-20 cm long; sparsely pubescent (covered with short, soft hairs). Stem quadrangular (four-angled), 1-2 mm in diameter; outer surface yellowish-green or purplish-red, with adventitious roots on nodes; brittle, breaks easily; broken surface often hollowed. Leaves opposite (borne in pairs at each node); blades usually shrivelled; when smoothed out, reniform (kidney-shaped) or subcordate (almost heart-shaped), 1-3 cm long, 1.5-3 cm wide; greyish-green or dull greenish-brown; crenate (with round-toothed edges); petioles 4-7 cm long. Verticillaster axillary (growing at axil); corolla pale blue or purple, bilabiate (two-lipped), with length up to 2 cm. Odour: aromatic when rubbed on the palms; taste: slightly bitter.

Indications 1. Acute urinary infection, urolithiasis 2. Acute jaundice 3. Painful swelling in sores and carbuncles 4. Trauma

Chemical Composition Mainly contains essential oils, ursolic acid and choline.

Herba Gynostemmatis

Fiveleaf Gynostemma Herb

Jiaogulan

絞股藍

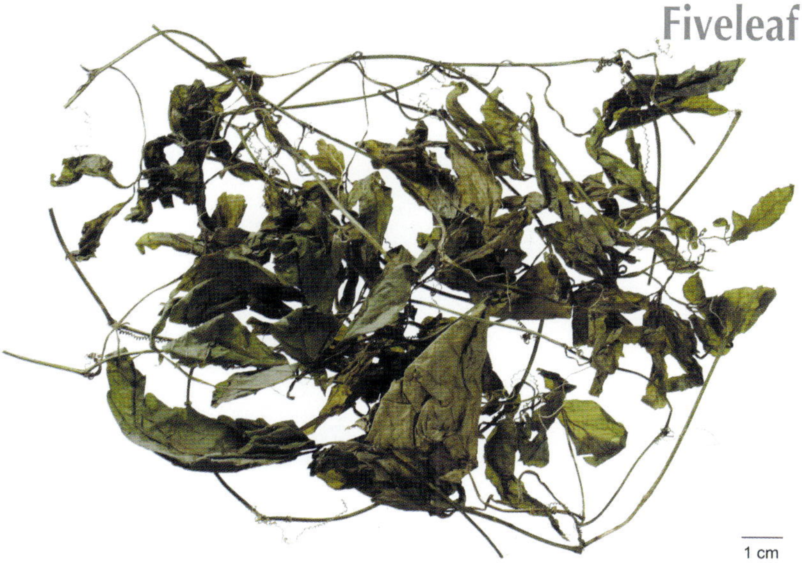

Crude Drug

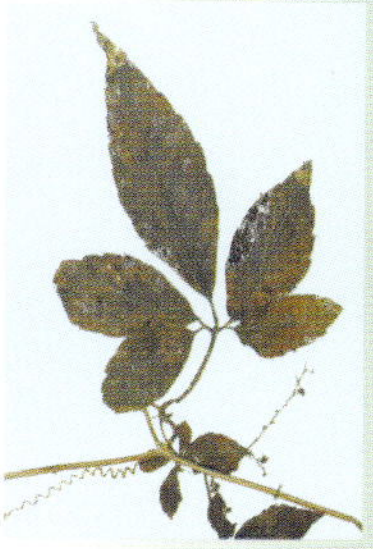

Fiveleaf Gynostemma Herb Magnified

Source The whole herb of *Gynostemma pentaphyllum* (Thunb.) Makino (Fam. Cucurbitaceae).

Distribution Mainly in regions south of the Yangtze River in China; also in Hong Kong.

Harvest & Processing Harvest whole herbs 3-4 times in summer and autumn; wash clean; dry under the sun.

Description Whole herb dry and shrivelled. Stem slender; greyish-brown or dull brown; outer surface marked with longitudinal grooves; covered with sparse fine pubescence, which extends when moistened. Compound leaves; leaflets membranous, usually 5-7 pieces; petioles 2-4 cm long, covered with strigae. Lateral leaflets ovate (egg-shaped in outline and attached at the broad end), oblong and orbicular (round), or oblong, orbicular and lanceolate (lance-head shaped). Central leaflet larger, 4-12 cm long, 1-3.5 cm wide; apex acuminate (tapering to a slender point), base cuneate (wedge-shaped); both sides covered with thick hairs; margin serrate (saw-like), with aristae on apex of teeth. Fruit spherical, about 5 mm in diameter; carpopodium 3-5 mm long. Taste: bitter; odour: grassy.

Indications 1. Debility, seminal emission due to wasting disease
2. Leukocyctopenia, hyperlipidemia 3. Viral hepatitis 4. Chronic gastritis 5. Chronic bronchitis

Chemical Composition Mainly contains gypenosides.

Herba Hedyotidis Diffusae

Spreading Hedyotis Herb
Baihuasheshecao

白花蛇舌草

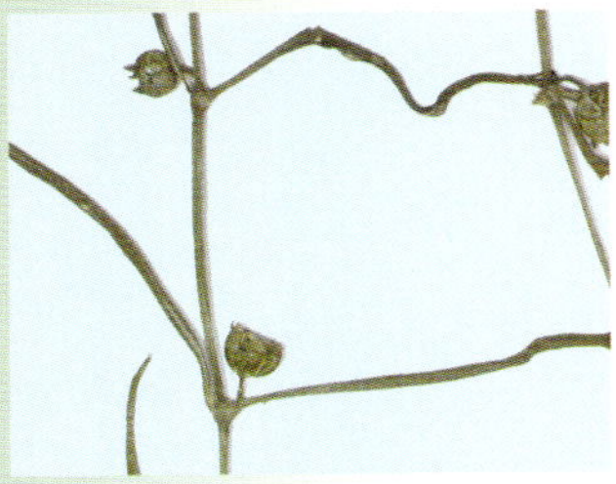

Spreading Hedyotis Herb Magnified

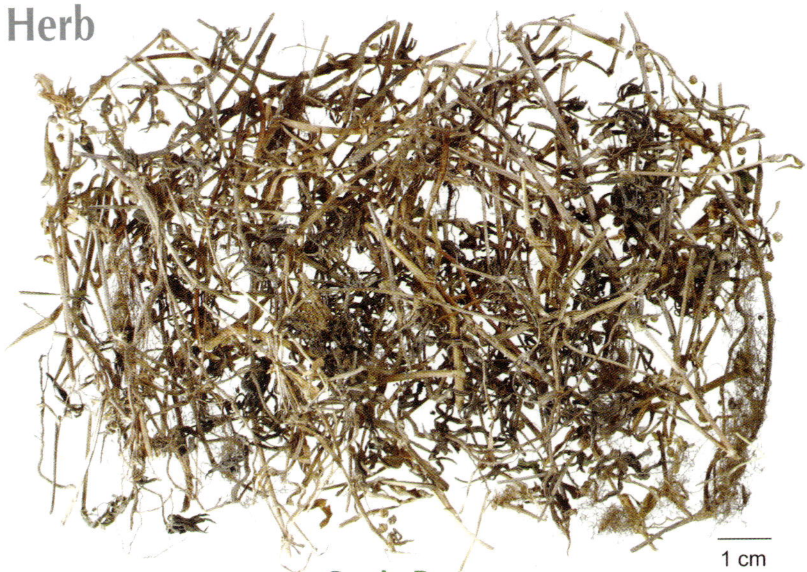

Crude Drug

Source The whole herb of *Hedyotis diffusa* Willd. (Fam. Rubiaceae).

Distribution Mainly in Chinese provinces such as Fujian, Guangdong and Guangxi; also in Hong Kong.

Harvest & Processing Harvest whole herbs in summer and autumn; dry under the sun or use while fresh.

Description Intertwined into a loose mass; greyish-green or greyish-brown; 1 axial root; rootlets fine. Stem fine and curled; marked with longitudinal ridges. Leaves opposite (borne in pairs at each node), mostly in fragments, extremely shrivelled, fall off easily; when intact, blades linear (long and narrow); with stipules, 1-2 mm long, membranous, lower part accrete (grown or joined together), top end serrulate (finely notched). Flowers usually solitary (occurring singly) and axillary (grown at axil); mostly pedicellate (with a pedicel). Capsules flattened and spherical; top end with 4-toothed persistent calyx. Odour: faint; taste: mild.

Indications 1. Carbuncles and sores, appendicitis, sore throat 2. Snakebite 3. Fibroid, lymphoma, cancer of digestive tract, liver, pancreas and urinary bladder 4. Dysuria, oedema

Chemical Composition Mainly contains iridoid glycosides such as asperuloside.

Herba Houttuyniae

Heartleaf Houttuynia Herb

Yuxingcao

魚腥草

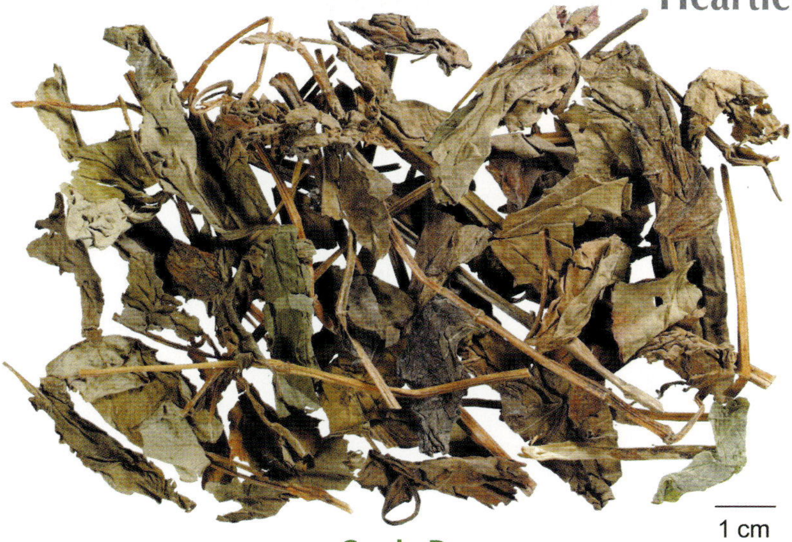

1 cm

Crude Drug

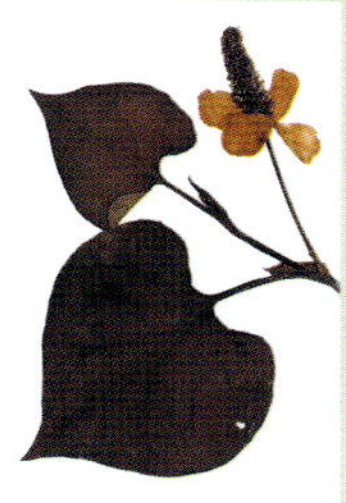

Heartleaf Houttuynia Herb Magnified

Source The whole herb of *Houttuynia cordata* Thunb. (Fam. Saururaceae).

Distribution Mainly in provinces south of the Yangtze River in China; also in Hong Kong.

Harvest & Processing Cut off whole herbs in summer when leaves and spikes flourish; remove foreign matter; dry under the sun.

Description Stem flattened and cylindrical, twisted; 20-35 cm long, 2-3 mm in diameter; outer surface brownish-yellow, marked with several longitudinal ridges; nodes prominent; lower part with remnants of rootlets on nodes; brittle, breaks easily. Leaves alternate (borne singly at each node); blades curled and shrivelled, cordate (heart-shaped) when smoothed out, 3-5 cm long, 3-4.5 cm wide. Apex acuminate (tapering to a slender point); entire (with continuous, even margin); upper surface dull yellowish-green to dull brown, underside dull yellowish-green or greyish-brown; petioles 1-3 cm long, base and stipules accrete (grown or joined together), forming the shape of a sheath. Spike acrogenous (growing from the apex), yellowish-brown. Odour: fishy when rubbed; taste: slightly astringent.

Indications 1. Lung abscess, cough, pneumonia, diarrhoea, stranguria 2. Rhinitis, sinusitis, chronic pyogenic otitis media. 3. Pelvic inflammatory diseases, chronic adnexitis, endometritis

Chemical Composition Mainly contains essential oils and hyperin.

Herba Hyperici Japonici

Japanese St. John's Swort Herb
Tianjihuang

田基黃

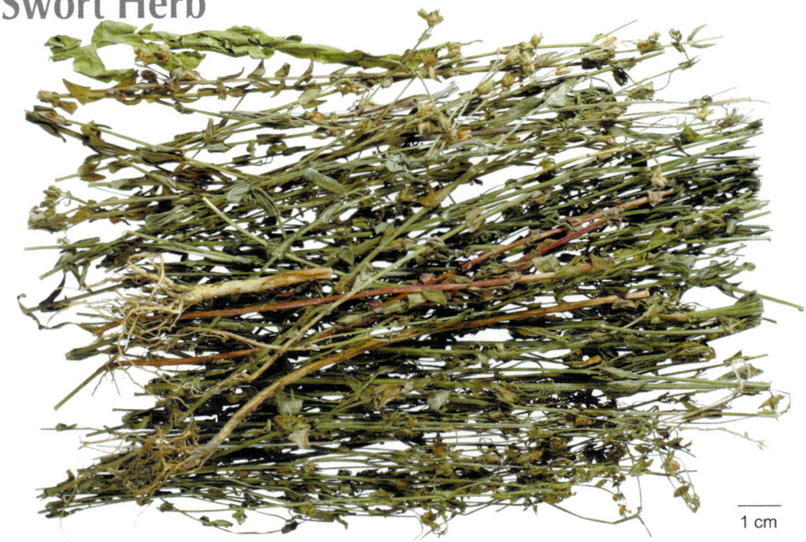

Crude Drug

Source The whole herb of *Hypericum japonicum* Thunb. ex Murray (Fam. Guttiferae).

Distribution Mainly in Chinese provinces such as Jiangxi, Fujian, Hunan, Guangdong, Guangxi, Sichuan and Guizhou; also in Hong Kong.

Harvest & Processing Harvest whole herbs in spring and summer during efflorescence; dry under the sun or use while fresh.

Description Whole plant 10-40 cm long. Roots beard-like, dull yellowish-brown. Stem solitary (occurring singly), base rameous (branched), smooth, quadrangular (four-angled); outer surface yellowish-green or yellowish-brown; brittle; breaks easily; broken surface hollowed. Leaves opposite (borne in pairs at each node), epetiolate (without a petiole); when whole, blades ovate (egg-shaped in outline and attached at the broad end), entire (with continuous, even margin), with tiny transparent gland dots and 3-5 basal veins. Cyme acrogenous (growing from the apex); flowers small, orange-yellow. Odourless; taste: slightly bitter.

Indications 1. Jaundice, diarrhoea, dysentery, 2. Aphthous ulcer, tonsillitis, lung abscess, appendicitis, conjunctivitis 3. Venomous-snake bite 4. Trauma.

Chemical Composition Mainly contains quercitrin, isoquercitrin and filixic acid BBB.

Herba Leonuri

Motherwort Herb
Yimucao

益母草

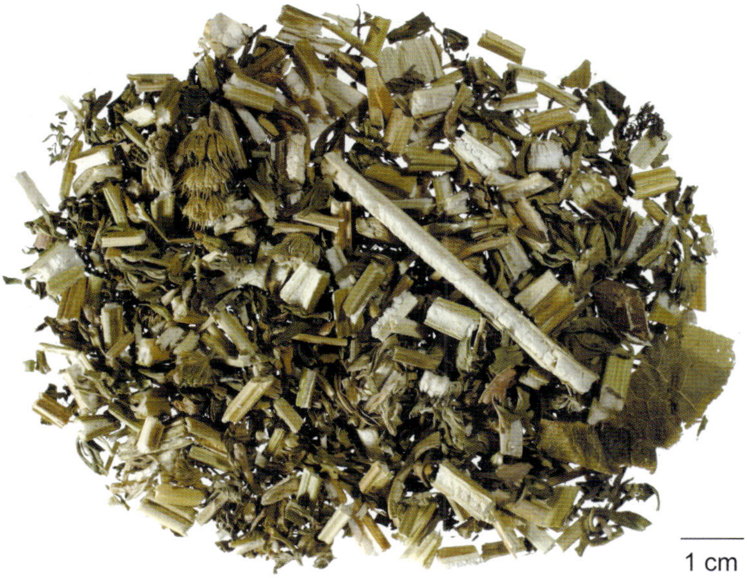

Decoction Pieces

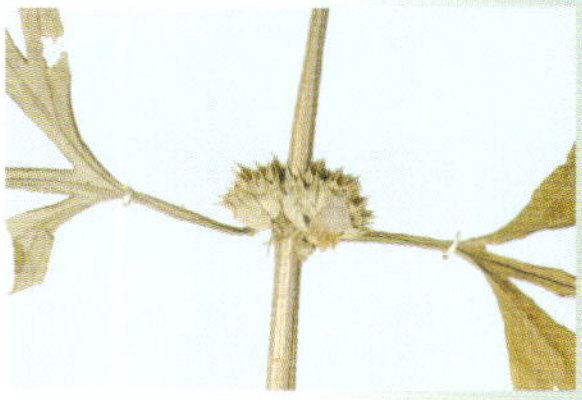

Motherwort Herb Magnified

Source The above-ground part of *Leonurus japonicus* Houtt. (Fam. Labiatae).

Distribution In all parts of China, including Hong Kong.

Harvest & Processing Cut off upper part of stems in summer when leaves flourish and before or when flowers start to bloom; dry in shaded areas or under the sun.

Description Stem quadrangular (four-angled); outer surface greyish-green or yellowish-green, upper part ramose (with many branches); surface with longitudinal grooves, densely pubescent (covered with short, soft hairs), especially on ridges and nodes; 30-60 cm long, 2-5 mm in diameter. Light in weight; pliable; broken surface with pith in the centre. Leaves opposite (borne in pairs at each node), petiolate (with a petiole); blades greyish-green, mostly shrivelled and in fragments, fall off easily. Verticillaster axillary (growing at axil); calyx tubular; corolla bilabiate (two-lipped). Odour: faint; taste: slightly bitter.

Indications 1. Menstrual disorders 2. Postpartum abdominal pain, lochiorrhagia 3. Nephritic oedema, oliguria, haematuria 4. Trauma 5. Carbuncles and sores, prurigo (external use).

Chemical Composition Mainly contains alkaloids such as leonurine, and diterpenes such as galeopsin and leoheterin.

Note In Hong Kong, commonly used for medicinal purposes is the young shoot of *Leonurus japonicus* Houtt.

Herba Lobeliae Chinensis

Chinese Lobelia Herb
Banbianlian

半邊蓮

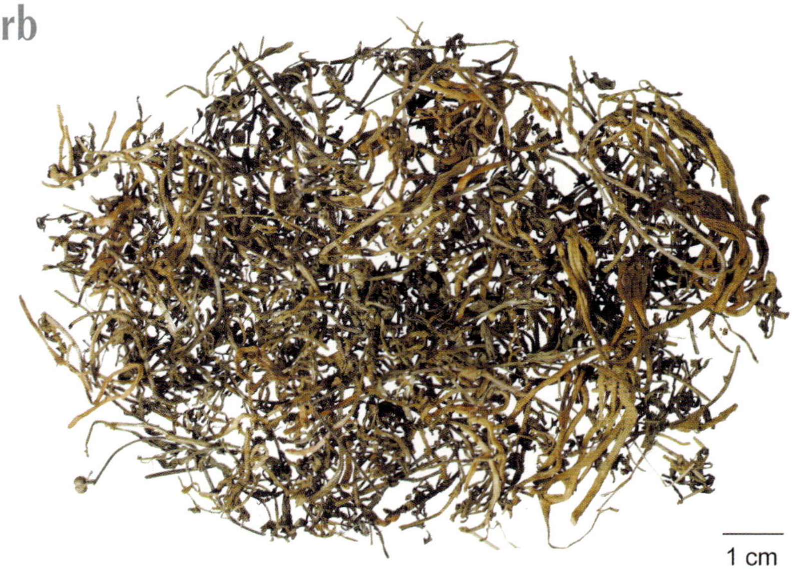

Crude Drug

Source The whole herb of *Lobelia chinensis* Lour. (Fam. Campanulaceae).

Distribution Mainly in Chinese provinces such as Anhui, Jiangsu and Zhejiang; also in Hong Kong.

Harvest & Processing Pull out whole herbs, together with roots, on sunny days in summer and autumn when plants flourish; wash clean; dry under the sun or use while fresh.

Description Whole herb 15-35 cm long. Root small, with slender, lateral (borne on or at the side) fibrous roots. Rhizome slender, 1-2 mm in diameter; outer surface pale yellow or yellowish-brown, with fine longitudinal striae. Stem slender, rameous (branched); outer surface greyish-green; nodes prominent. Leaves alternate (borne singly at each node) and epetiolate (without a petiole); blades mostly shrivelled, dull greenish-brown; when smoothed out, blades narrow and lanceolate (lance-head shaped), or ovate (egg-shaped in outline and attached at the broad end) and orbicular (round), 1-2.5 cm long, 2-5 mm wide; margin sparsely serrate (saw-like). Pedicels slender; flowers small, solitary (occurring singly) at leaf axil; corolla light purplish-red, synobasic (with a united base), upper part 5-lobed. Odour: faint; taste: slightly sweet, acrid.

Indications
1. Snake and insect bites, carbuncles and boils, breast abcess
2. Jaudice, oedema and ascites from cirrhosis, late schistosomiasis and cancer in digestive tract

Chemical Composition Mainly contains alkaloids such as lobeline.

Herba Lophatheri

Lophatherum Herb

Danzhuye

淡竹葉

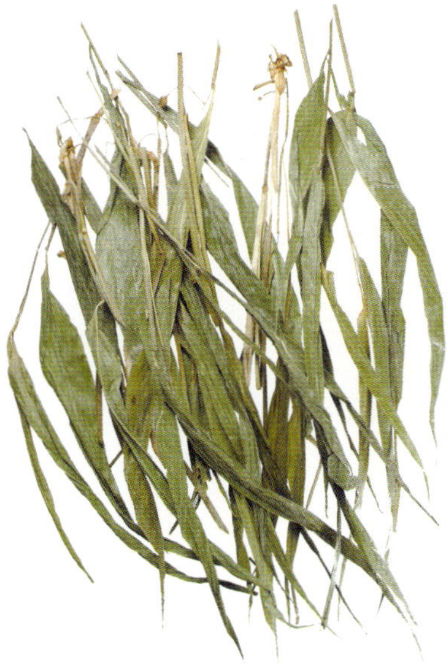

Crude Drug

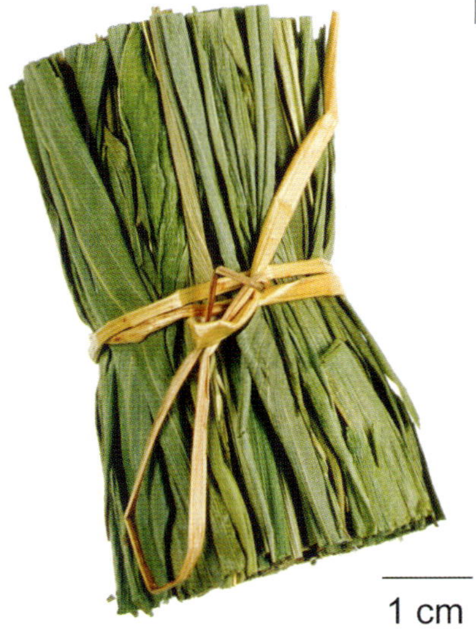

Decoction Pieces

Source The stem and leaf of *Lophatherum gracile* Brongn. (Fam. Gramineae).

Distribution Mainly in Chinese provinces such as Zhejiang, Jiangsu, Hunan and Hubei; also in Hong Kong.

Harvest & Processing Collect stems and leaves in summer before plants put forth spikes; dry under the sun.

Description Stem and leaf together 25-75 cm long. Stem cylindrical, nodose (with nodes); outer surface pale yellowish-green; broken surface hollow in the centre. Leaf sheath with clefts. Leaf blades lanceolate (lance-head shaped), occasionally shrivelled and curled; 5-20 cm long, 1-3.5 cm wide; upper surface yellowish-green, underside light green or light purple. Leaf veins parallel, with transverse veinlets, forming rectangular meshes; those on the underside especially conspicuous. Light in weight; pliable. Odour: faint; taste: mild.

Indications 1. Hyperpyrexia, anxiety, thirst 2. Aphthous ulcer, gingivitis 3. Urethritis, ardour urinae, deep yellow or reddish urine.

Chemical Composition Mainly contains triterpenes such as atundoin and cylindrin.

Herba Lycopi

Hirsute Shiny Bugleweed Herb

Zelan

澤蘭

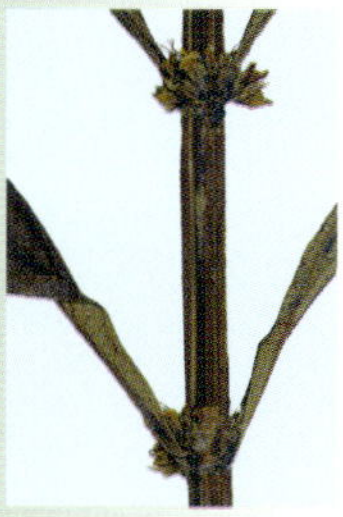

Hirsute Shiny Bugleweed Herb Magnified

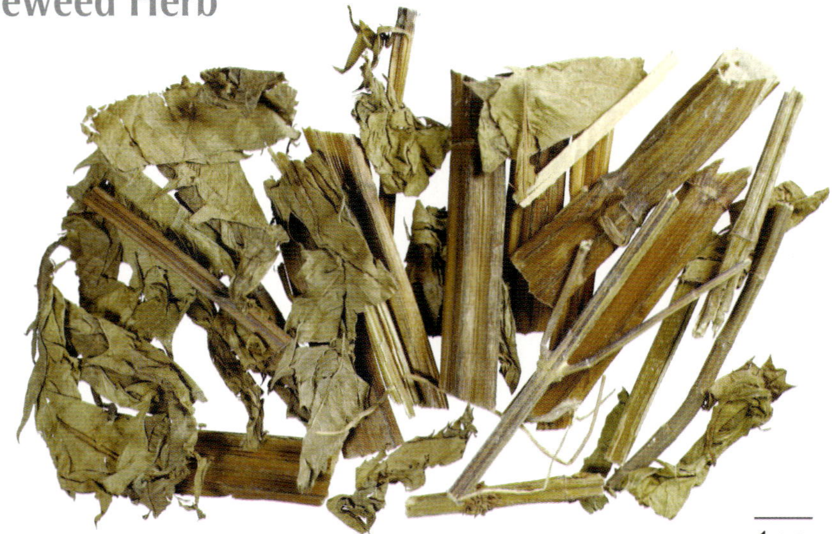

Crude Drug

Source The above-ground part of *Lycopus lucidus* Turcz. *var. hirtus* Regel (Fam. Labiatae).

Distribution In most regions of China.

Harvest & Processing Cut off above-ground parts in summer and autumn when leaves flourish; dry under the sun.

Description Stem quadrangular (four-angled), seldom rameous (branched), marked with shallow longitudinal grooves on all sides; 50-100 cm long, 2-6 mm in diameter. Outer surface yellowish-green or purplish in colour; purple prominent at nodes; nodes covered with sparse white pubescence; brittle; broken surface yellowish-white, with hollow pith. Leaves opposite (borne in pairs at each node), with short petioles; blades mostly shrivelled; when smoothed out, blades lanceolate (lance-head shaped), or oblong and orbicular (round), 5-10 cm long; upper surface dark green, with dense gland dots; both sides pubescent (covered with short, soft hairs). Apex pointed; margin serrate (saw-like). Flowers axillary (growing at axil) and conglomerate (densely clustered), verticillate (arranged in whorls); corolla mostly fallen off; bracts and calyx persistent, dull yellowish-brown in colour. Odourless; taste: mild.

Indications 1. Amenorrhoea, menstrual disorders 2. Postpartum haematoma 3. Oedema 4. Trauma.

Chemical Composition Contains lacceroic acid and betulinic acid.

Herba Lycopodii

Common Clubmoss Herb
Shenjincao

伸筋草

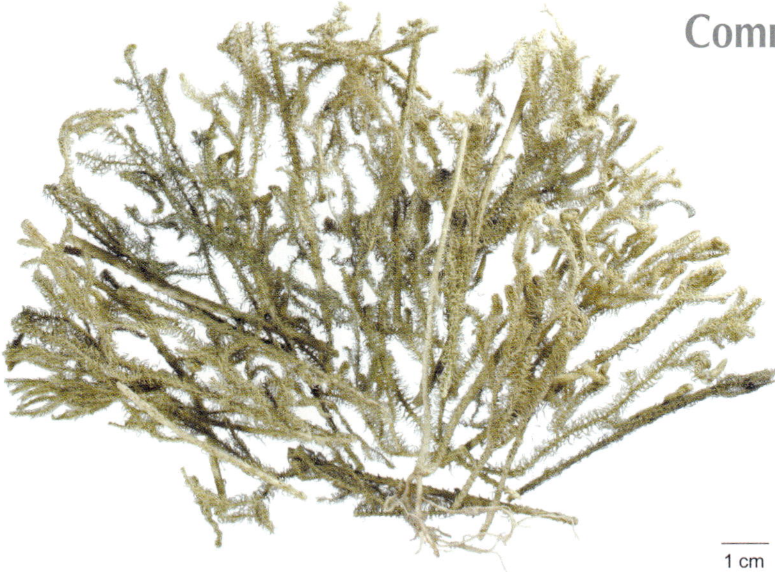

1 cm

Crude Drug

Source The whole herb of *Lycopodium japonicum* Thunb. (Fam. Lycopodiaceae).

Distribution Mainly in Chinese provinces such as Zhejiang, Hubei and Jiangsu; also in Hong Kong.

Harvest & Processing Collect whole herbs in summer and autumn when leaves are in luxuriance; remove foreign matter; dry under the sun.

Description Stolons cylindrical, slender and curved; up to 2 m long, 1-3 mm in diameter. Outer surface yellowish-green; with fibrous roots. Stem mostly bifurcate (forked into two divisions); young stem densely covered with small yellowish-green scale leaves arranged in a spiroid (spiral-like) form. Apex of leaves acuminate (tapering to a slender point), aristiform (awn-like). Soft and pliable, does not break easily; when broken, outer layer of surface made up of light yellowish-green and relatively thin cortex, inner layer made up of yellowish-white woody core. Bark of roots mostly fallen off, exposing yellow woody core. Odourless; taste: mild.

Indications Arthralgia with joint stiffness.

Chemical Composition Mainly contains alkaloids such as lycopodine.

Herba Lysimachiae

Christina Loosestrife
Jinqiancao

金錢草

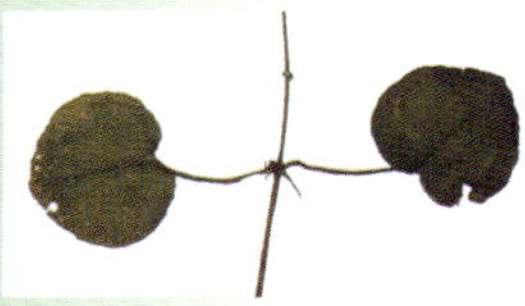

Christina Loosestrife Magnified

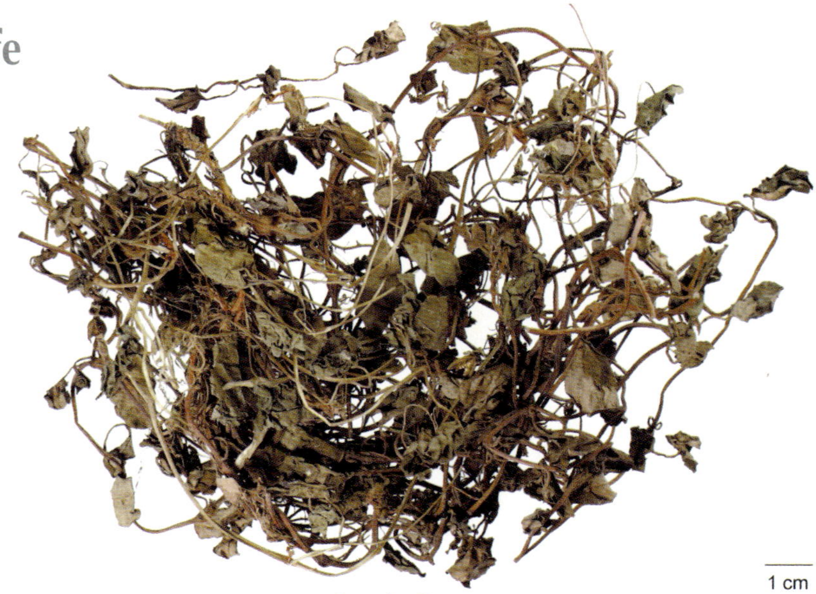

Crude Drug

Source The whole herb of *Lysimachia christinae* Hance (Fam. Primulaceae).

Distribution Mainly in Chinese provinces such as Sichuan, Yunnan and Guizhou.

Harvest & Processing Harvest whole herbs in summer and autumn; remove foreign matter; dry under the sun.

Description Whole herb usually intertwined into a bundle; glabrous (without hairs) or sparsely pubescent (covered with short, soft hairs). Stem twisted; outer surface brown or dull brownish-red, marked with longitudinal striae; broken surface solid. Leaves opposite (borne in pairs at each node), mostly shrivelled; when smoothed out, broad and ovate (egg-shaped in outline and attached at the broad end), or cordate (heart-shaped), 1-4 cm long, 1-5 cm wide; base slightly notched; entire (with continuous, even margin); upper surface greyish-green or reddish-brown, underside lighter in colour; main vein protuberant and conspicuous; after being soaked in water, black or dull brown striae visible when seen against the light; petioles 1-4 cm long. Flowers solitary (occurring singly) at leaf axil and with long pedicels; capsules spherical. Whole herb breaks easily. Odour: faint; taste: mild.

Indications 1. Jaundice, cholelithiasis, infectious hepatitis 2. Stranguria, renal stone, oedema 3. Skin infection.

Chemical Composition Mainly contains flavonoids.

Herba Menthae

Peppermint
Bohe
薄荷

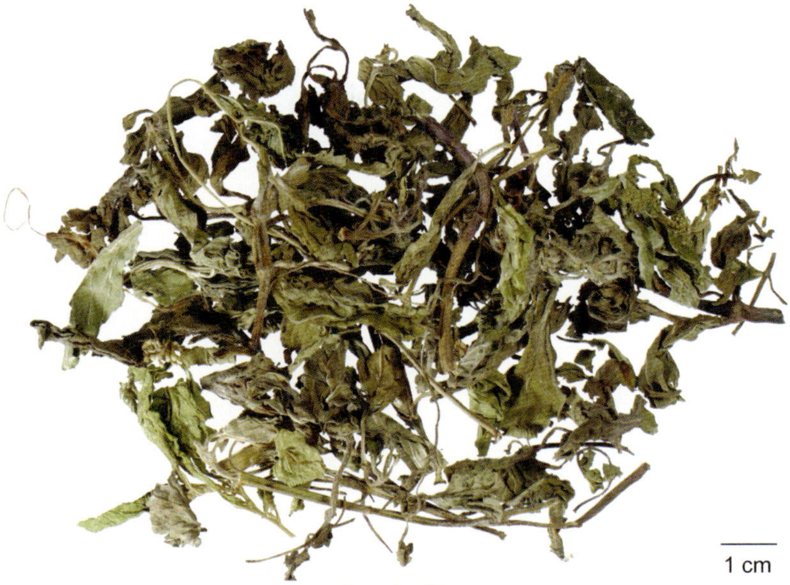

1 cm

Crude Drug

Source The above-ground part of *Mentha haplocalyx* Briq. (Fam. Labiatae).

Distribution Mainly in Chinese provinces such as Jiangsu, Zhejiang, Hunan and Jiangxi.

Harvest & Processing Cut off above-ground parts on sunny days in summer and autumn when leaves or flowers flourish; dry under the sun or in shaded areas.

Description Stem quadrangular (four-angled), with opposite (borne in pairs at each node) branches; outer surface purplish-brown or pale green; pubescent (covered with short, soft hairs) at the angled edges; internodes 2-5 cm long; brittle; broken surface white, with hollow pith. Leaves opposite, with short petioles; blades shrivelled and curled; when intact and smoothed out, blades broad and lanceolate (lance-head shaped), oblong and elliptical, or ovate (egg-shaped in outline and attached at the broad end), 2-7 cm long, 1-3 cm wide; upper surface dark green, underside greyish-green; both sides sparsely pubescent; underside marked with dented gland dots. Verticillasters axillary (growing at axil); calyx campanulate (bell-shaped), apex 5-toothed; corolla pale purple. Odour: with a distinctive fresh fragrance after being rubbed; taste: mint-like and acrid.

Indications 1. Colds and fever, sore throat, pharyngitis, cough 2. Early stages of measles 3. Dyspepsia, abdominal distension 4. Pruritus.

Chemical Composition Contains 1% - 2% essential oils, in which 65% - 90% is (-) - menthol.

Herba Moslae

Chinese Mosla
Xiangru

香薷

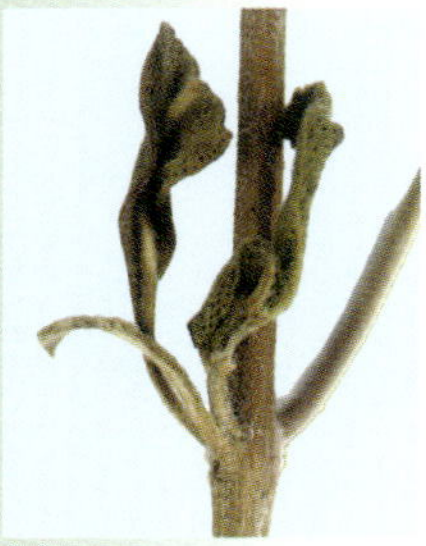

Chinese Mosla Magnified

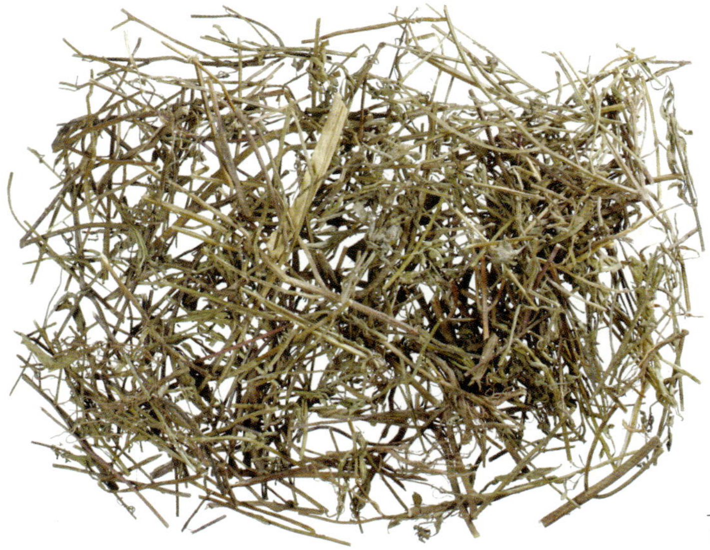

Crude Drug

Source

The above-ground part of *Mosla chinensis* Maxim. (Fam. Labiatae). The naturally grown ones are customarily called '*Qing xiangru*' (Green Chinese Mosla) and the cultivated ones, '*Jiang xiangru*' (Jiangxi Chinese Mosla).

Distribution

Qing xiangru: mainly in Chinese provinces such as Guangdong, Guangxi, Fujian and Hunan; *Jiang xiangru*: mainly in Jiangxi and Zhejiang provinces.

Harvest & Processing

Cut off above-ground parts in summer and autumn when leaves flourish and fruits ripen; remove foreign matter; dry under the sun.

Description

Base purplish-red. Stem quadrangular (four-angled), nodes prominent; brittle, breaks easily. Leaves opposite (borne in pairs at each node), mostly shrivelled or fallen off; blades oblong and ovate (egg-shaped in outline and attached at the broad end), or lanceolate (lance-head shaped) when smoothed out; margin sparsely serrate (saw-like). Spike acrogenous (growing from the apex) and axillary (growing at axil); calyx persistent, apex 5-lobed. Nutlets 4, subspherical, marked with reticulate (net-like) striae; sutures between nets slightly dented. Odour: fresh, fragrant and strong; taste: slightly acrid, mint-like.

Indications

1. Common cold manifested as aversion to cold, fever, headache and anhidrosis or vomiting, diarrhoea, and abdominal pain
2. Oedema, dysuria.

Chemical Composition

Contains approximately 0.1% of essential oils with carvacrol and β-carypohyllene as the main components.

Herba Paederiae

Chinese Fevervine Herb

Jishiteng

雞屎藤

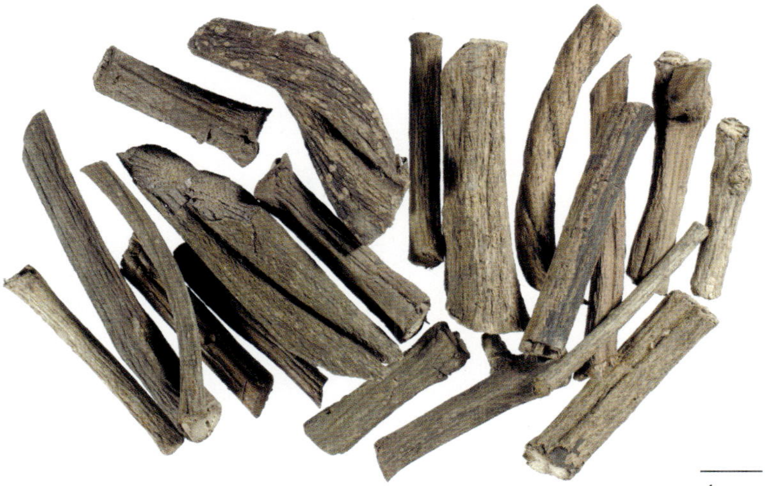

Crude Drug

Source The stem or above-ground part of *Paederia scandens* (Lour.) Merr. (Fam. Rubiaceae).

Distribution Mainly in Yangtze River valley and regions south of the valley in China; also in Hong Kong.

Harvest & Processing Cut off above-ground parts in summer; dry under the sun or by airing.

Description Stem flattened and cylindrical, slightly twisted; outer surface marked with longitudinal wrinkles and scars of broken petioles; breaks easily; broken surface even, greyish-yellow. Leaves opposite (borne in pairs at each node), mostly shrivelled or in fragments; when whole and smoothed out, blade broad and ovate (egg-shaped in outline and attached at the broad end), or lanceolate (lance-head shaped). Apex pointed; base cuneate (wedge-shaped), orbicular (round), or cordate (heart-shape) with a shallow notch; entire (with continuous, even margin); dull greenish-brown; both sides glabrous (without hairs) or almost glabrous; petioles glabrous or with hairs. Odour: distinctive; taste: slightly bitter, astringent.

Indications 1. Dyspepsia, anorexia, abdominal distension and pain, infantile malnutrition 2. Cough 3. Pain due to gynaecopathy and obstetrics, trauma, rheumatism, neuralgia, biliary or renal colic

Chemical Composition Iridoid glycosides such as paederoside exist in the whole plant.

Herba Patriniae

Dahurian Partinia Herb

Baijiangcao

敗醬草

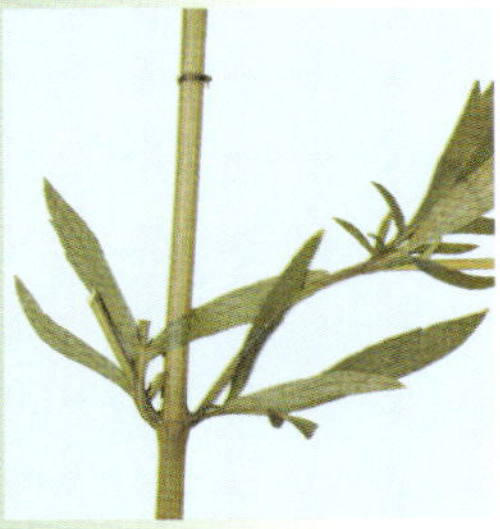

Dahurian Partinia Herb Magnified

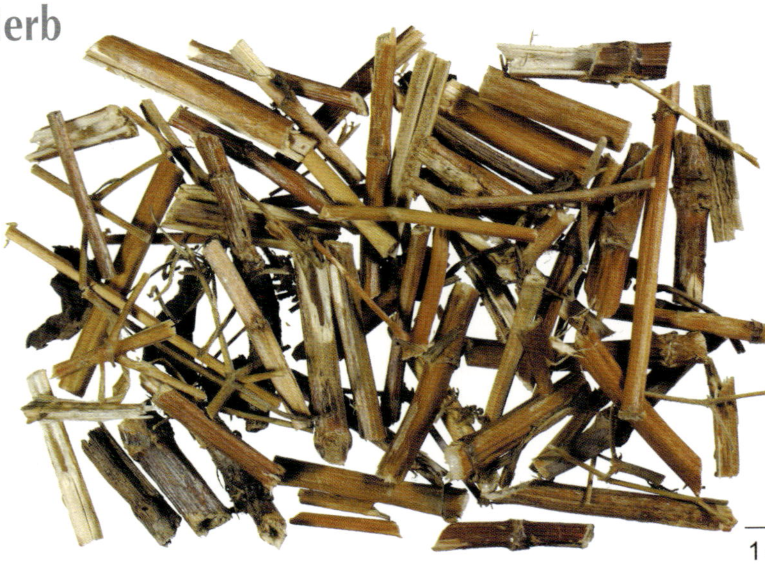

Crude Drug

Source The whole herb of *Patrinia scabiosaefolia* Fisch. ex Trev. (Fam. Valerianaceae).

Distribution Mainly in Chinese provinces such as Liaoning, Jilin, Heilongjiang Hebei, Shandong, Jiangxi, Henan, Hunan and Yunnan, and in Inner Mongolia.

Harvest & Processing Dig up whole herbs in summer and autumn; cultivated herbs can be harvested before efflorescence. Wash clean; dry under the sun.

Description Stems cylindrical, 2-10 mm in diameter. Outer surface yellowish-green or yellowish-brown, marked with longitudinal ridges and fine grain markings; with retrorse (directed downwards or backwards) strigae. Cauline (grown on stems) leaves mostly shrivelled or in fragments, with diffuse white pubescence on both sides; when whole, blades multi-pinnatipartite (parted into many lobes in a feather-like manner) , with 5-11 lobes, margin serrate (saw-like); leaves on upper part of stems relatively small, often trifid (cleft into three divisions). Some stems carry inflorescences or infructescences at apex. Odour: distinctive; taste: slightly bitter.

Indications 1. Fever 2. Abscesses.

Chemical Composition Triterpene saponins such as patrinoside A_1, B_1, C_1, D_1 exist in the roots and stems.

Herba Phyllanthi Urinariae

Common Leafflower Herb
Yexiazhu

葉下珠

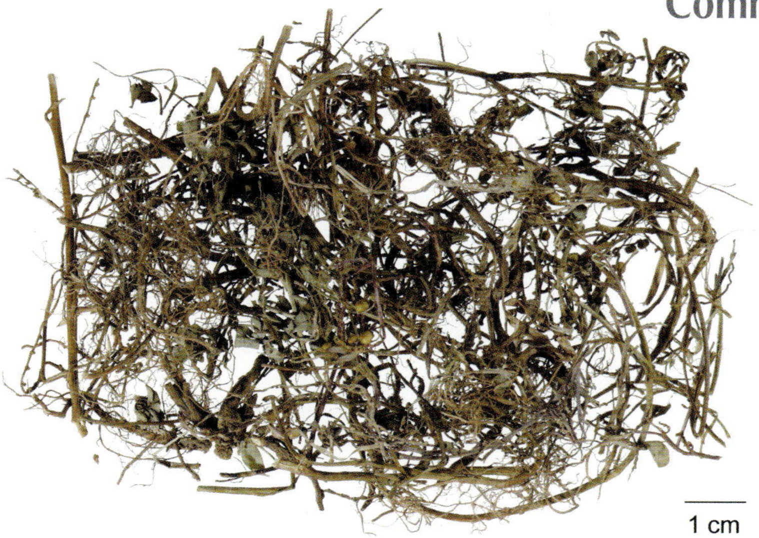

Crude Drug

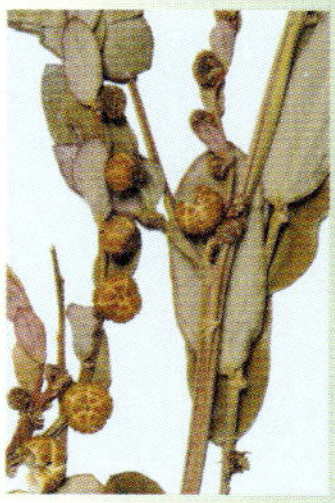

Common Leafflower Herb Magnified

Source The whole herb of *Phyllanthus urinaria* L. (Fam. Euphorbiaceae).

Distribution Mainly in regions south of Yangtze River valley in China; also in Hong Kong.

Harvest & Processing Harvest whole herbs in summer and autumn; remove foreign matter; use while fresh or dry under the sun.

Description Herbs vary in length. Outer surface of rhizome light brown; axial root not well-developed, with numerous light greyish-brown fine roots. Old stem dull greyish-brown at base. Twigs marked with longitudinal wrinkles; greyish-brown; brittle, break easily; broken surface hollow. Branches with indistinct membranous aliform (wing-shaped) ridges. Leaf blades thin and small; oblong and elliptical; greyish-green; shrivelled. Apex mucronate (with a short straight point), base orbicular (round) or oblique (with unequal sides); margin with white pubescence. Flowers small, axillary (growing at axil) at underside of leaves, mostly dried and shrivelled. Some herbs with triangulate (three-angled), flattened and spherical yellowish-brown fruits marked with squamiform (scale-like) protuberances and often with 6 longitudinal sutures on outer surface. Odour: slightly fragrant; taste: slightly bitter.

Indications 1. Diarrhoea, dysentery, jaundice 2. Oedema, stranguria due to urinary tract infection and renal stone 3. Red eyes, night blindness

Chemical Composition Contains ellagic acid and ferulic acid.

Herba Plantaginis

Plantain Herb
Cheqiancao

車前草

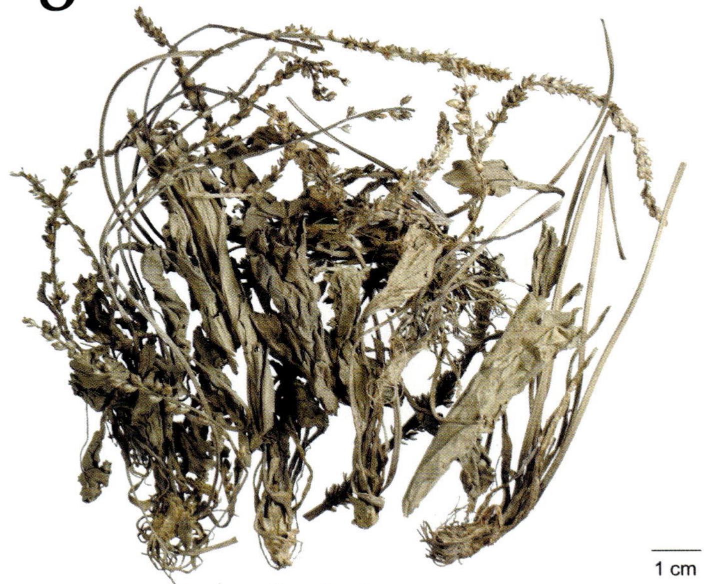

Crude Drug

Source The whole herb of *Plantago asiatica* L. (Fam. Plantaginaceae).

Distribution In all parts of China, including Hong Kong.

Harvest & Processing Collect whole herbs in summer; remove soil and sand; dry under the sun.

Description Roots caespitose (growing in tufts). Leaves basal, with long petioles; blades shrivelled; when smoothed out, blades ovate (egg-shaped in outline and attached at the broad end) and elliptical, or broad and ovate; 6-13 cm long, 2.5-8 cm wide; outer surface greyish-green or blackish-green, marked with 5-7 prominent arch-like veins. Apex obtuse or mucronate (with a short straight point), base broad and cuneate (wedge-shaped); margin entire (continuous and even) or with irregular shallow teeth. Spikes several; scapes long. Capsules dehiscent (splitting open at maturity) with the top separating like a lid, each capsule with a persistent calyx. Odour: slightly fragrant; taste: slightly bitter.

Indications 1. Urinary stones and infections, nephritic oedema 2. Diarrhoea 3. Cold, cough, bronchitis 4. Acute conjunctivitis 5. Dermatitis and boils (external use).

Chemical Composition Mainly contains iridoid glycosides such as plantaginin and aucubin.

Note According to *C.P.*, also used for medicinal purposes is the whole herb of *P. depressa* Willd.

Herba Pogostemonis

Cablin Patchouli Herb

Guanghuoxiang

廣藿香

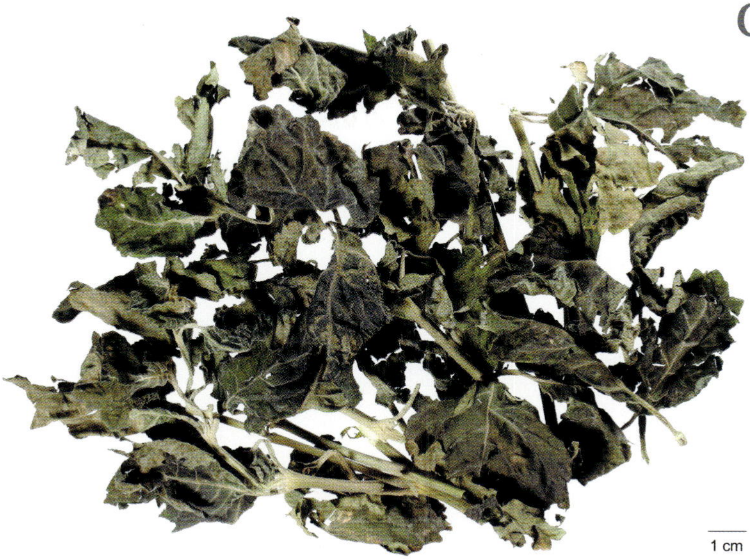

Crude Drug

Source The above-ground part of *Pogostemon cablin* (Blanco) Benth. (Fam. Labiatae).

Distribution Mainly in Guangdong province China; also cultivated in other Chinese provinces such as Hainan, Taiwan, Guangxi and Yunnan. According to origins, classified into '*Shipai Guanghuoxiang*' and '*Hainan Guanghuoxiang*'.

Harvest & Processing Cut off above-ground parts in summer and autumn when branches and leaves are abundant; dry under the sun during the day and put in closed places at night, repeat the process until completely dry.

Description Stem slightly quadrangular (four-angled), ramose (with many branches), with branches slightly curved; 30-60 cm long, 2-7 mm in diameter. Outer surface pubescent (covered with short, soft hairs); brittle, breaks easily; broken surface with pith. Leaves opposite (borne in pairs at each node), curled into a papery mass; when smoothed out, blades ovate (egg-shaped in outline and attached at the broad end) or elliptical; both sides covered with greyish-white pubescence. Apex mucronate (with a short straight point) or obtuse, base cuneate (wedge-shaped) or obtuse; margin uneven and crenate (with round-toothed edges); petioles fine, pubescent. Odour: with a distinctive fragrance; taste: slightly bitter.

Indications 1. Fever caused by heat stroke, headache 2. Anorexia, nausea, vomiting 3. Diarrhoea.

Chemical Composition The stems contain essential oils with patchouli alcohol (31.9%) as the main component; also contain flavonoids.

Herba Polygalae Japonicae

Japanese Milkwort Herb

Guazijin

瓜子金

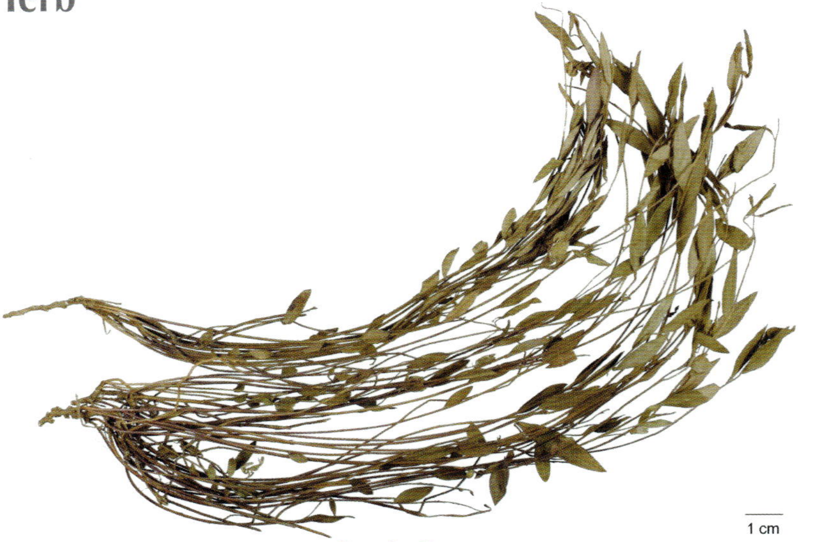

1 cm

Crude Drug

Source The whole herb of *Polygala japonica* Houtt. (Fam. Polygalaceae).

Distribution Mainly in Chinese provinces such as Anhui, Zhejiang and Jiangsu.

Harvest & Processing Collect whole herbs in autumn; wash clean; dry under the sun.

Description Root cylindrical, slightly curved; up to 4 mm in diameter; outer surface dull yellowish-brown, marked with longitudinal wrinkles; hard; when broken, surface yellowish-white. Stem with few branches; puberulent (covered with fine, short, soft hairs). Leaves shrivelled; when smoothed out, ovate (egg-shaped in outline and attached at the broad end), or ovate and lanceolate (lance-head shaped); lateral veins conspicuous. Apex mucronate (with a short straight point), base orbicular (round) or cuneate (wedge-shaped); entire (with continuous, even margin); puberulent. Racemes axillary (growing at axil); the uppermost inflorescence growing lower than stem apex. Capsules flattened and spherical; about 7 mm long; with relatively wide wings, wings not ciliate (with a marginal fringe of hairs); with persistent sepals. Seeds flattened and ovoid (egg-shaped); dull brown; densely pubescent (covered with short, soft hairs). Odour: faint; taste: slightly acrid-bitter.

Indications 1. Sore throat, cough with copious sputum 2. Rheumatism 3. Gastrointestinal bleeding 4. Palpitation, insomnia 5. Carbuncles and sores, venomous-snake bite, trauma

Chemical Composition Mainly contains triterpene saponins.

Herba Polygoni Avicularis

Common Knotgrass Herb

Bianxu

萹蓄

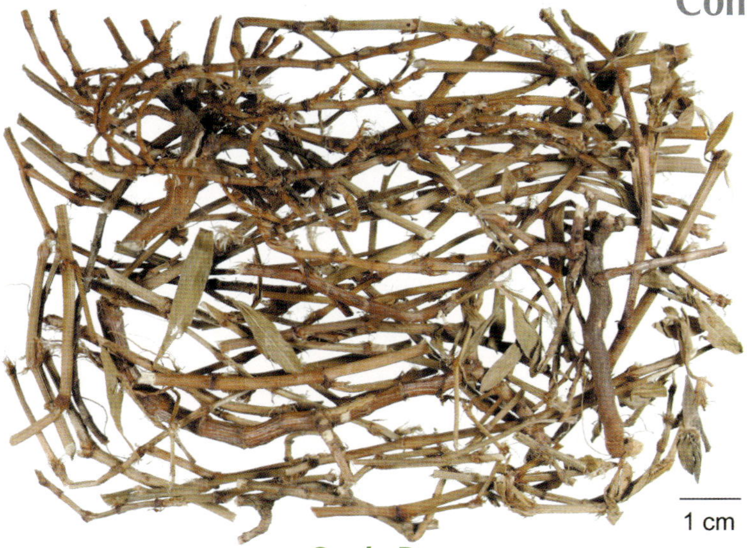

Crude Drug

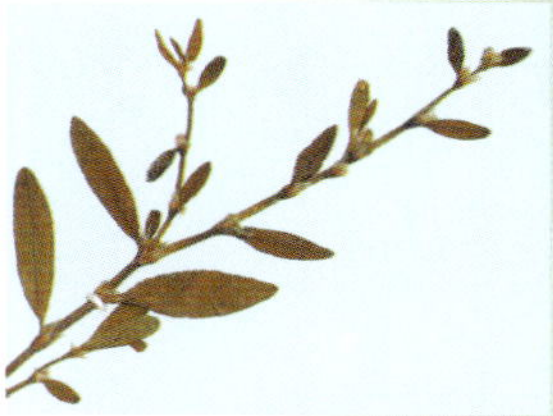

Common Knotgrass Herb Magnified

Source The whole herb of *Polygonum aviculare* L. (Fam. Polygonaceae).

Distribution Mainly in Chinese provinces such as Hebei, Henan, Shanxi and Hubei, and in northeastern China.

Harvest & Processing Harvest whole herbs during the period of luxuriant growth in summer; remove foreign matter and roots; dry under the sun.

Description Stem cylindrical and slightly flattened, rameous (branched); 15-40 cm long, 1.5-3 mm in diameter. Outer surface greyish-green or brownish-red, marked with dense and slightly protuberant longitudinal striae; nodes slightly bulgy, with light brown membranous ocreae; internodes varying in length. Hard, breaks easily; broken surface shows white pith. Leaves alternate (borne singly at each node); blades mostly fallen off, or shrivelled and in fragments; those intact oblong and elliptical, or lanceolate (lance-head shaped), 1-4 cm long, about 5 mm wide; entire (with continuous, even margin); greyish-green or brownish-green. Some herbs with small, ovoid (egg-shaped) and triangulate (three-angled), dull blackish-brown achenes bearing persistent perianth. Odour: faint; taste: slightly bitter.

Indications 1. Stranguria caused by renal stone 2. Diarrhoea, jaundice 3. Haematuria, dysfunctional uterine bleeding 4. Eczema, trichomonas vaginitis, pruritus valvae.

Chemical Composition Mainly contains flavonoids such as quercetin, and coumarin such as umbelliferone.

Herba Polygoni Chinensis

Chinese Knotweed Herb
Huotanmu

火炭母

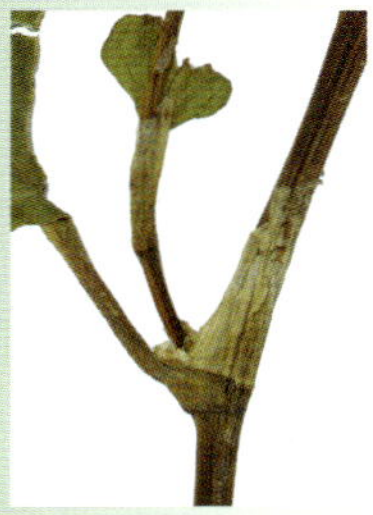

Chinese Knot-weed Herb Magnified

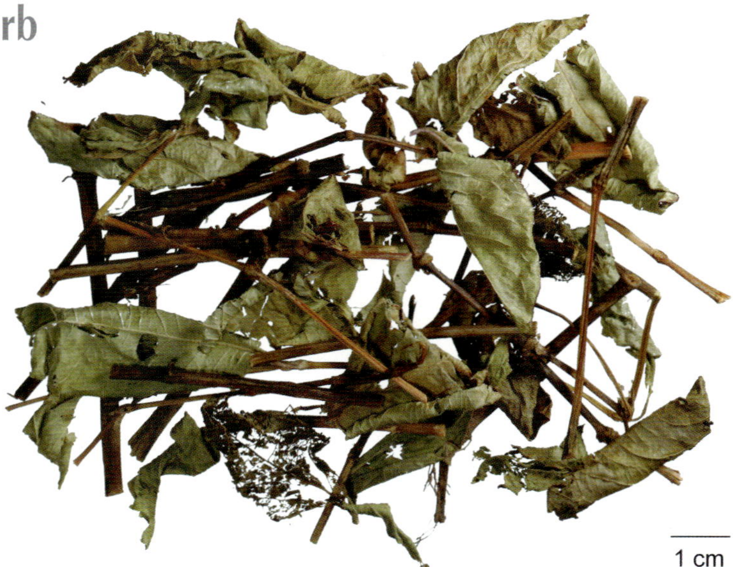

1 cm

Crude Drug

Source The whole herb of *Polygonum chinense* L. (Fam. Polygonaceae).

Distribution Mainly in Chinese provinces such as Fujian, Guangdong, Guangxi, Guizhou, Sichuan, Yunnan, Jiangxi and Zhejiang; also in Hong Kong.

Harvest & Processing Collect whole herbs between summer and autumn; use while fresh or dry under the sun.

Description Stem flattened and cylindrical, rameous (branched); 30-100 cm long; nodes slightly bulgy; nodes at lower part with fibrous roots. Outer surface pale green or dull purplish-brown, glabrous (without hairs), with fine ridges. Brittle, breaks easily; when broken, surface greyish-yellow, mostly hollow in the centre. Leaves alternate (borne singly at each node), mostly shrivelled and in fragments; when intact and smoothed out, blades ovate (egg-shaped in outline and attached at the broad end), oblong and orbicular (round), 5-10 cm long, 2-2.5 cm wide. Apex mucronate (with a short straight point), base truncate (squared as if cut off) or slightly rounded; entire (with continuous, even margin); upper surface dull green, underside lighter in colour, both sides nearly glabrous (without hairs); ocreae tubular, with oblique (with unequal sides) membranous apex. Odour: faint; taste: sour, slightly astringent.

Indications 1. Diarrhoea, hepatitis 2. Sore throat, diphtheria, whooping cough 3. Leukorrhagia 4. Otitis media, nebula, carbuncle, trauma 5. Vertigo, dizziness and tinnitus, hypertension

Chemical Composition Anthraquinones and flavonoids glycosides exist in the whole plant.

Herba Polygoni Perfoliati

Perfoliate Knotweed Herb

Gangbangui

杠板歸

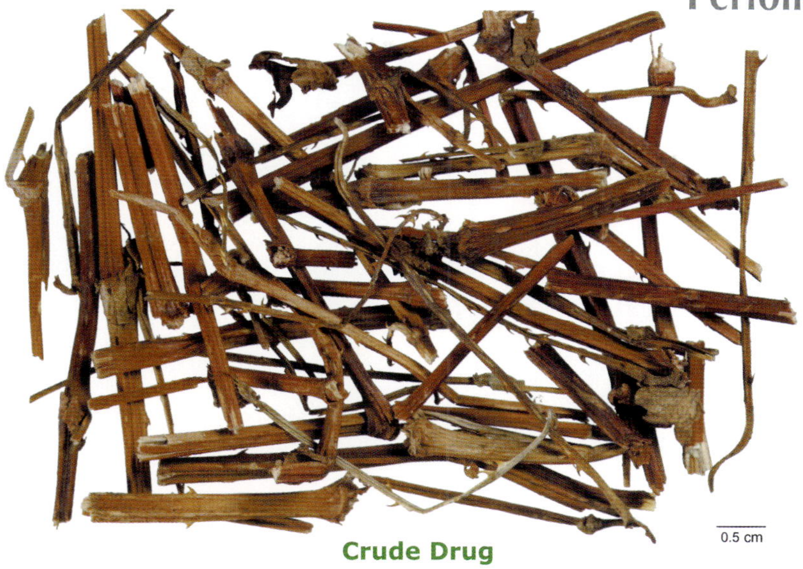

Crude Drug

Source The whole herb of *Polygonum perfoliatum* L. (Fam. Polygonaceae).

Distribution In Chinese provinces such as Jiangsu, Zhejiang, Fujian, Jiangxi, Guangdong, Guangxi and Sichuan; also in Hong Kong.

Harvest & Processing Cut off whole herbs between summer and autumn; use while fresh or dry by airing.

Description Stem slender, slightly quadrangular (four-angled); 1-5 mm in diameter; outer surface reddish-brown, brownish-yellow or yellowish-green, with barbs; nodes slightly bulgy, with annular (ring-like) scars left by ocreae; internodes 0.6-6 cm long; brittle, breaks easily; broken surface yellowish-white, with pith or hollow in the centre. Leaves alternate (borne singly at each node); blades mostly shrivelled or in fragments; when intact and smoothed out, almost the shape of equilateral triangles; pale brown or greyish-green; barbs sparsely growing along leaf margin, main veins on dorsal side and petioles. Short spikes acrogenous (growing from the apex) or growing at leaf axil; bracts orbicular (round); flowers small, mostly withered or fallen off. Odour: faint; taste: slightly sour.

Indications 1. Sores and boils, erysipelas, mumps, acute conjunctivitis, mastitis 2. Upper respiratory infection with fever and yellow sputum 3. Diarrhoea, jaundice, ascitis, oedema 4. Malaria

Chemical Composition Mainly contains flavonoid glycosides, anthraquinones and tannins.

Herba Portulacae

Purslane Herb
Machixian

馬齒莧

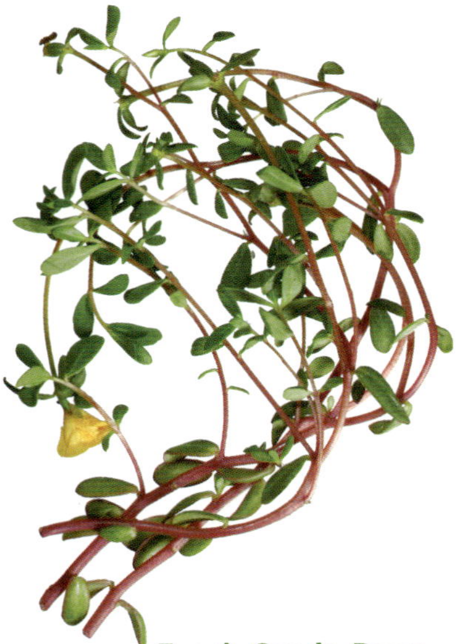

Frech Crude Drug

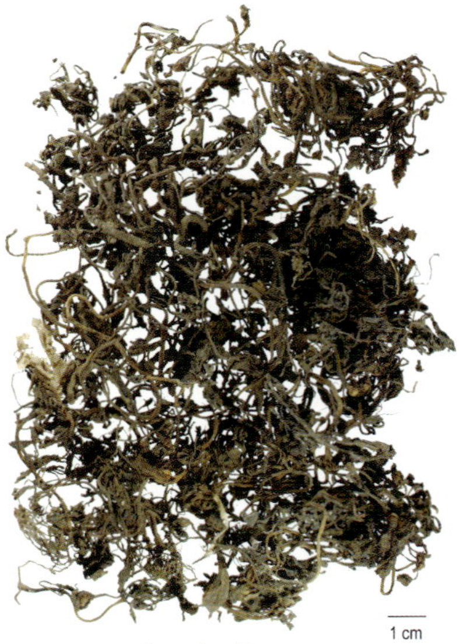

Crude Drug

Source
The whole herb of *Portulaca oleracea* L. (Fam. Portulacaceae).

Distribution
In all parts of China.

Harvest & Processing
Cut off whole herbs in August and September; wash away soil; remove foreign matter; blanch (or cook) in boiling water or steam, then take out and dry under the sun or by heat, alternatively use while fresh.

Description
Mostly shrivelled and curled into a mass. Stem cylindrical; 10-25 cm long, 1-3 mm in diameter; outer surface yellowish-brown to reddish-brown, marked with conspicuous twisting longitudinal grooves. Leaves crumble or fall off easily; when whole, blade obovate (egg-shaped in outline and attached at the narrower end), dull greenish-brown, 1-2.5 cm long, 0.5-1.5 cm wide. Apex blunt or slightly notched; entire (with continuous, even margin). Flowers rare, yellow, grown on herb tip. Capsules conical; about 5 mm long; dehiscent (splitting at maturity) with the top separating like a galeriform (cap-shaped) lid; containing numerous tiny black seeds. Odour: faint; taste: slightly sour, chewy.

Indications
1. Diarrhoea, dysentery, haemorrhoid 2. Eczema, dermatitis, carbuncle, herpes zoster, flat wart, vitiligo 3. Dysfunctional uterine bleeding, leukorrhagia

Chemical Composition
Mainly contains noradrenalin and large amounts of potassium salts (including potassium nitrate and potassium chloride).

Herba Potentillae Chinensis

Chinese Cinquefoil
Weilingcai

委陵菜

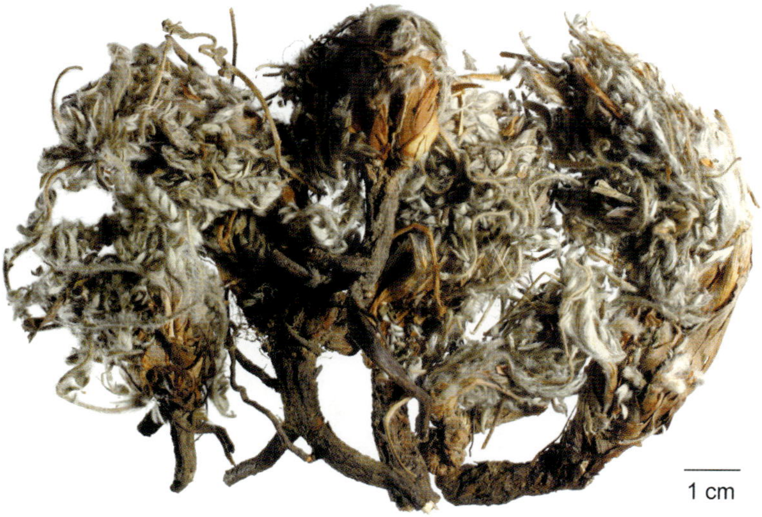

Crude Drug

Source The whole herb of *Potentilla chinensis* Ser. (Fam. Rosaceae).

Distribution Mainly in Chinese provinces such as Shandong, Liaoning, Jilin and Anhui.

Harvest & Processing Dig up whole herbs in spring or early summer before the plants put forth shoots; remove foreign matter; dry herbs under the sun.

Description Root conical or subconical, slightly curved, some rameous (branched); 5-17 cm long, 0.5-1 cm in diameter. Outer surface dull brown or dull purplish-red, marked with twisting longitudinal grooves; cork easily scales off; top part of root slightly bulgy, in some cases with 2-3 branches. Hard, breaks easily; broken surface shows radial rays and thin dull brown cortex, cortex often detached from xylem. Leaves basal, odd-pinnate (compound in a feather-like manner with an odd number of leaflets), petiolate (with a petiole); leaflets narrow and elliptical, margin pinnatipartite (parted in a feather-like manner); underside of leaflets and petiolules densely covered with greyish-white pubescence. Odour: faint; taste: astringent and slightly bitter.

Indications 1. Dysentery with bloody stools, chronic dysentery
2. Haemorrhoidal bleeding 3. Carbuncles and sores.

Chemical Composition Contains fumaric acid, gallic acid, protocatechnic acid and quercetin.

Note Customarily called '*Beizicao*'(North Gromwell Root) or '*Fanbaicao*' (Discoloured Cinpuefoil Herb) in Hong Kong.

Herba Potentillae Discoloris

Discolor Cinpuefoil Herb

Fanbaicao

翻白草

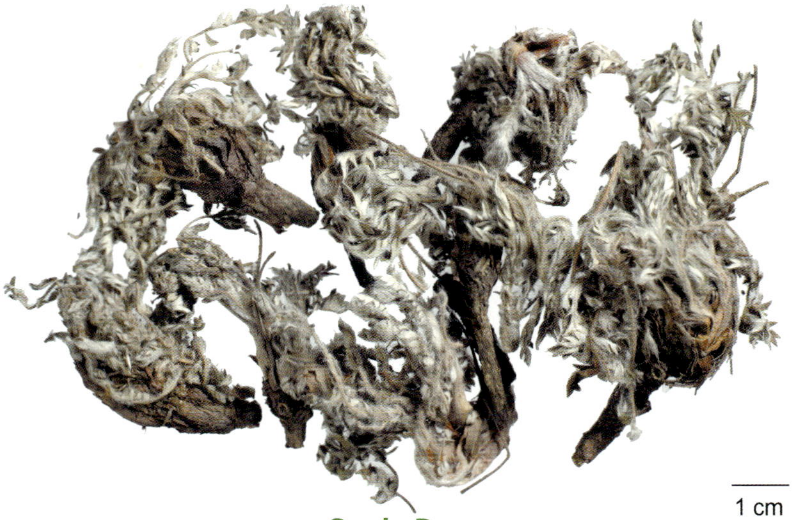

Crude Drug

Source The whole herb of *Potentilla discolour* Bge. (Fam. Rosaceae).

Distribution Mainly in Chinese provinces such as Hebei, Beijing and Anhui; also in most other regions of China.

Harvest & Processing Dig out whole herbs together with roots in summer and autumn; shake off soil; wash clean; dry under the sun.

Description Root tuber spindle-shaped or cylindrical, occasionally long and slender; marked with irregular twisting longitudinal grooves; 3-8 cm long Outer surface yellowish-brown or dull reddish-brown; cork relatively even. Hard and brittle; broken surface yellowish-white. Basal leaves caespitose (growing in tufts), odd-pinnate (compound in a feather-like manner with an odd number of leaflets), shrivelled and curled; leaflets 3-9, rectangular and orbicular (round), or narrow, oblong and elliptical terminal leaflet larger; leaflets dull green on upper surface, densely covered with while villi on underside; margin grossly serrate (with big saw-like teeth). Odour: faint; taste: sweet and slightly astringent.

Indications 1. Dysentery, diarrhoea, carbuncle 2. Menorrhagia, haemorrhoidal bleeding.

Chemical Composition Hydrolysable tannins, condensed tannins and flavonoids exist in the roots; the whole herb contains fumaric acid and gallic acid.

Herba Pyrolae

Pyrola Herb
Luxiancao

鹿銜草

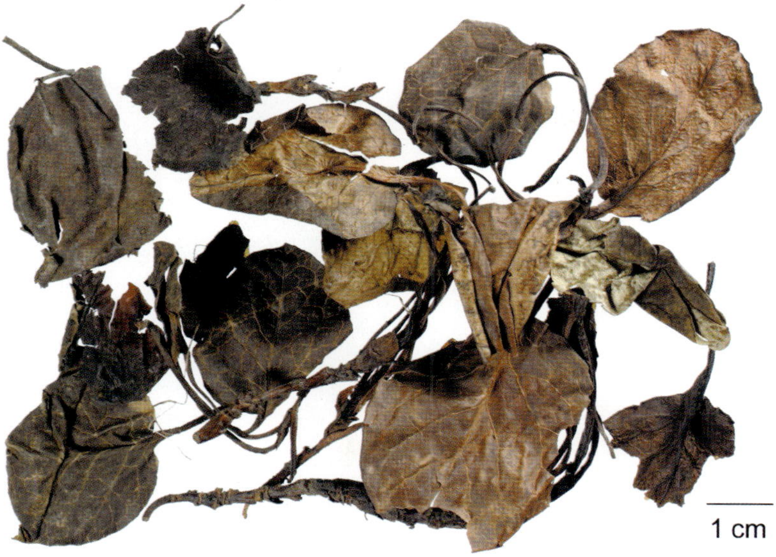

Crude Drug

Source The whole herb of *Pyrola decorata* H. Andr. (Fam. Pyrolaceae).

Distribution Mainly in Chinese provinces such as Henan, Gansu, Shaanxi, Zhejiang, Anhui, Jiangxi, Hubei, Hunan and Guangdong.

Harvest & Processing Harvest whole herbs anytime during the year, commonly in autumn; remove foreign matter; dry herbs under the sun until leaves soften and shrivel; smooth out leaves and heap herbs into piles to produce heat so that both sides of the leaves turn purplish-red or dull purplish-brown; dry again under the sun.

Description Brownish-green or close to light reddish-brown. Rhizome slender. Leaves alternate (borne singly at each node); 3-6 basal leaves; petioles 2-4 cm long, angulate (with ridges); blades coriaceous (leathery), quite thick, oblong and ovate (egg-shaped in outline and attached at the broad end), elliptical or oblong and elliptical; apex blunt but slightly pointed, mucronulate (with a very small, sharp tip); base broad and cuneate (wedge-shaped), decurrent (extending downwards) towards petiole; margin with sparse fine serrations. 5-8 flowers in a raceme; flowers broad and campanulate (bell-shaped); calyx 5-parted. Capsules dark brown, flattened and spherical.

Indications 1. Arthralgia with weakness of the loins and knees 2. Menorrhagia 3. Chronic cough caused by wasting diseases and pulmonary tuberculosis

Chemical Composition Mainly contains flavonoids such as kaempferol-3-O-glucoside.

Note According to *C.P.*, also used for medicinal purposes is the whole herb of *P. calliantha* H. Andr.

Herba Rabdosiae Serrae

Serrate Rabdosia Herb
Xihuangcao

溪黃草

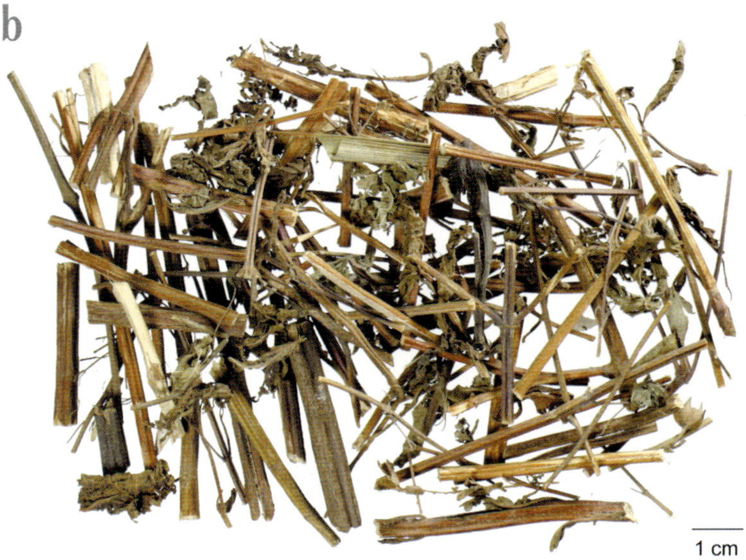

Crude Drug

Source The whole herb of *Rabdosia serra* (Maxim.) Hara (Fam. Labiatae).

Distribution Mainly in Chinese provinces such as Shanxi, Henan, Shaanxi, Gansu, Sichuan and Guizhou, and in northeastern and northern China.

Harvest & Processing Harvest above-ground parts in summer and autumn; remove foreign matter; dry under the sun.

Description Stems and branches quadrangular (four-angled), densely covered with retrorse (directed downwards or backwards) fine pubescence. Leaves opposite (borne in pairs at each node), often in fragments; intact leaves usually shrivelled; when smoothed out, leaves ovate (egg-shaped in outline and attached at the broad end), or ovate and lanceolate (lance-head shaped), with fine pubescence along veins on both sides. Cyme pedunculate (with a peduncle); panicle acrogenous (growing from the apex), formed by 5 to numerous florets. Bracts and bracteoles narrow and ovate to linear (long and narrow), densely covered with pubescence. Calyx campanulate (bell-shaped), about 1.5 mm long, outer surface with dense greyish-white pubescence and gland dots; calyx teeth triangular, of equal length with calyx tube. Corolla purple, about 5.5 mm long; corolla tube gibbous (swollen or enlarged on one side) near top of base; labrum with 4 even lobes, labium scaphoid (boat-shaped); pistil and style not protruding out of corolla.

Indications 1. Jaundice, acute hepatitis, cholangitis 2. Diarrhoea 3. Trauma 4. Toothache, gingivitis, aphthous ulcer of children.

Chemical Composition Mainly contains diterpene such as rabdoserrin A.

Herba Sarcandrae

Glabrous Sarcandra Herb
Zhongjiefeng
腫節風

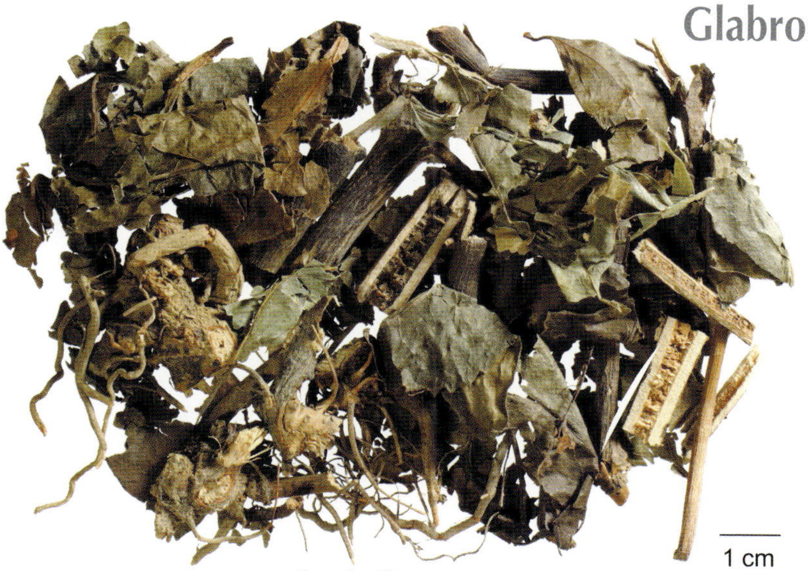

Crude Drug

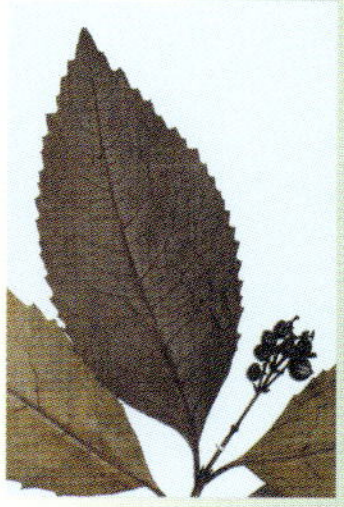

Glabrous Sarcandra Herb Magnified

Source The whole herb of *Sarcandra glabra* (Thunb.) Nakai (Fam. Chloranthaceae).

Distribution Mainly in Chinese provinces such as Jiangxi, Sichuan, Zhejiang and Guangxi; also in Hong Kong.

Harvest & Processing Harvest whole herbs in summer and autumn; remove foreign matter; dry under the sun.

Description Whole herb 50-120 cm long. Rhizome relatively thick, with dense long, strong and pliable rootlets. Stem cylindrical; nodes bulgy, ramose (with many branches); outer surface dull green to dull brown, marked with conspicuous fine longitudinal striae and scattered with longitudinal lenticels; brittle, breaks easily; when broken, surface with pith in the centre, or hollow in the centre. Leaves opposite (borne in pairs at each node), near coriaceous (leathery); blades ovate (egg-shaped) and lanceolate (lance-head shaped) to ovate and elliptical; outer surface green, dull greenish-brown to reddish-brown or brownish-red, smooth; margin grossly serrate(with big saw-like teeth), glands at tooth tips dull blackish-brown; petioles and base accrete (grow or join together) forming the shape of a sheath; spike acrogenous (growing from the apex), often rameous (branched). Odour: slightly fragrant; taste: slightly acrid.

Indications 1. Carbuncle, aphthous ulcer, gingivitis 2. Dysentery, filariasis 3. Trauma, stomachache, rheumatism, coronary heart diseases 4. Cough, dyspnoea 5. Cancer of lung, digestive system and leukemia

Chemical Composition Mainly contains istanbulin A and furmaric acid.

Herba Saururi

Chinese Lizardtail Rhizome or Herb

Sanbaicao

三白草

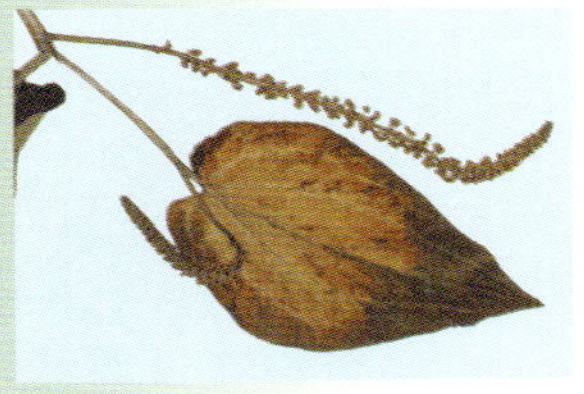

Chinese Lizardtail Rhizome or Herb Magnified

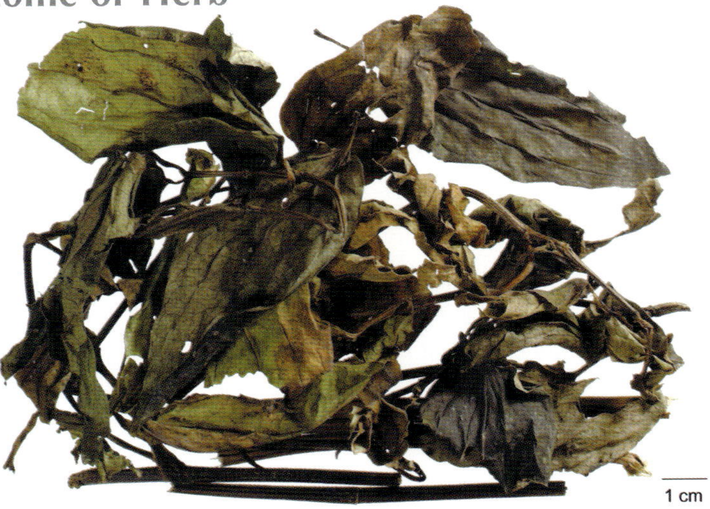

Crude Drug

Source The rhizome or whole herb of *Saururus chinensis* (Lour.) Baill. (Fam. Saururaceae).

Distribution Mainly in Chinese provinces such as Jiangsu, Zhejiang, Hunan and Guangdong; also in Hong Kong.

Harvest & Processing Collect rhizomes in autumn; collect whole herbs anytime during the year. Use while fresh or dry under the sun.

Description Rhizome cylindrical, with 4 longitudinal grooves, one of which relatively broad; when broken, surface yellow, fibrous, hollow in the centre. Leaves alternate (borne singly at each node), mostly shrivelled; when smoothed out, blades ovate (egg-shaped), or ovate and lanceolate (lance-head shaped); 4-15 cm long, 2-10 cm wide. Apex pointed, base cordate (heart-shaped); entire (with continuous, even margin); each leaf with 5 basal veins; petioles relatively long, with longitudinal wrinkles; Sometimes with dull brown racemes. Capsules subspherical. Odour: faint; taste: mild.

Indications 1. Dysuria, stranguria, urinary infection, nephritic oedema, morbid leukorrhoea 2. Boils, sores, eczema (external use).

Chemical Composition The whole plant contains essential oils with methyln-nonylketone as the main component.

Herba Saussureae Involucratae

Snow Lotus Herb
Tianshanxuelianhua

天山雪蓮花

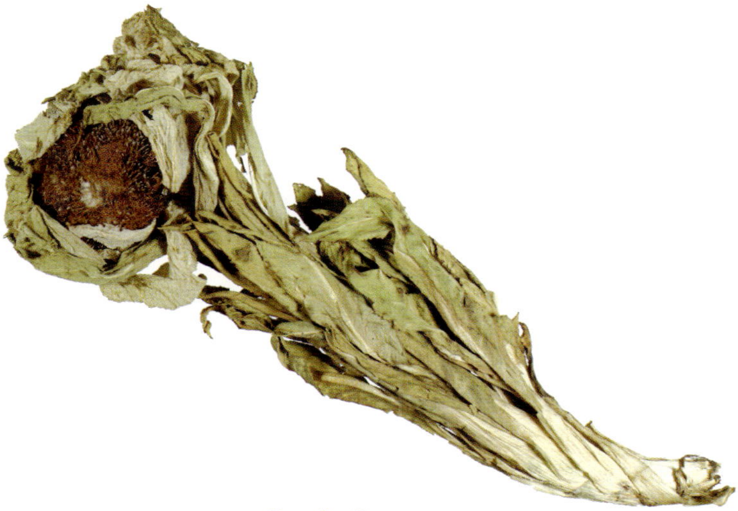

Crude Drug

Source The whole flower-bearing plant of *Saussurea involucrata* Kar. et Kir. (Fam. Compositae).

Distribution Mainly in Chinese provinces such as Qinghai and Gansu, and in Xinjiang.

Harvest & Processing Harvest whole plants in June and July during efflorescence; remove soil and sand; dry by airing.

Description Stem thick and strong, with a profusion of remnants of leaf base fibres. Leaves densely arranged; When whole and smoothed out, blade oblong and ovate (egg-shaped) or lanceolate (lance-head shaped); margin serrate (saw-like) and ciliate (with a marginal fringe of hairs; yellowish-green, more or less coriaceous (leathery). bracteal leaves oblong and ovate, or ovate; yellowish-white; membranous. 10-30 capitate inflorescences gathered closely into a spherical shape; phyllaries in 3-4 layers, outer layer mostly dull brown, outer surface covered densely with pubescence; inner layer brownish-yellow or yellowish-white, apex covered with pubescence. All flowers tubular in shape; corolla purplish-red; anthers purple; pistil with a 2-lobed stigma slightly longer than stamens. Achenes oblong and ovoid (egg-shaped), with longitudinal ribs, greyish-white; slightly bitter in taste.

Indications 1. Impotence, weakness of loin and knee 2. Rheumatism 3. Menstrual disorders, abdominal pain 4. Cough with copious watery whitish sputum

Chemical Composition Contains flavonoids, sesquiterpene lactones and sesquiterpene alkaloids.

Herba Saussureae Lanicepsis

Lanatehead Saussurea Herb
Xuelianhua

雪蓮花

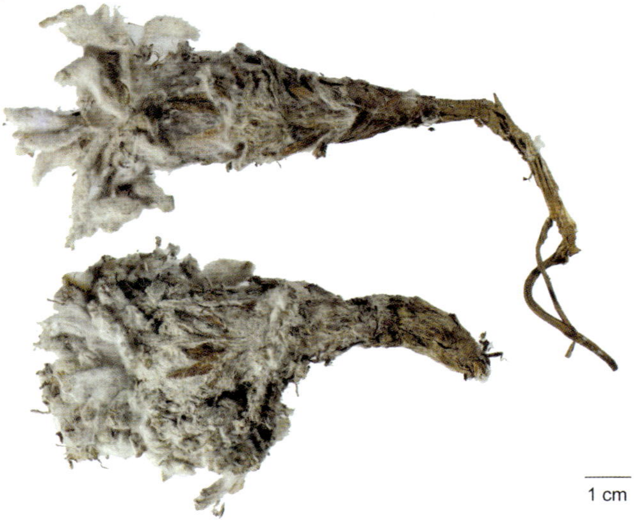

Crude Drug

Source The whole herb of *Saussurea laniceps* Hand.-Mazz. (Fam. Compositae).

Distribution Mainly in regions such as southwestern Sichuan province, eastern Tibet, and Yunnan province in China.

Harvest & Processing Harvest whole plants between June and July during efflorescence; remove soil; dry by airing.

Description Dry and shrivelled, resembling cotton balls; slightly obconical (inversely conical). Entire outer surface covered densely with white or pale yellow villi. Rhizome thick, reddish-brown, bark peels off easily. Leaves exceedingly dense, oblanceolate (inverse lance-head shaped) or spatulate (spoon-shaped); margin with undulate (wavy) shallow teeth. Capitate inflorescences numerous, sessile (without a supporting stalk), arranged at top part of stem in an ellipsoid (elliptical in long-section and circular in cross-section) and spicate (spike-like) manner; bracts linear (long and narrow) and lanceolate (lance-head shaped), densely covered with white tomenta. Involucre hemispherical; outer phyllaries linear and lanceolate, with dense growth of white tomenta; inner phyllaries lanceolate, covered with dull blackish-brown long hairs. Achenes pappi dull blackish-brown. Odour: faint; taste: mild.

Indications 1. Impotence, weakness and pain of the loins and knees 2. Menstrual disorders, morbid leukorrhoea 3. Arthralgia 4. Traumatic bleeding

Chemical Composition Scopoletin, umbelliferone and physcion exist in the whole plant.

Herba Schizonepetae

Fineleaf Schizonepeta Herb

Jingjie

荊芥

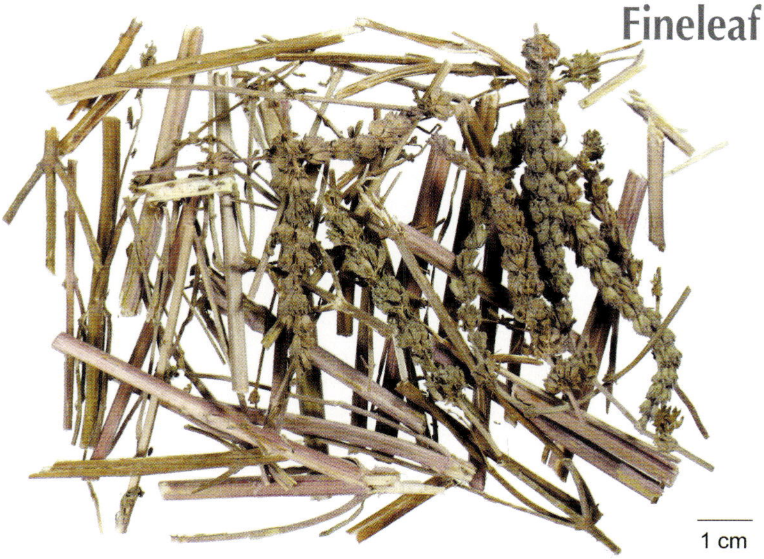

Crude Drug

Source The above-ground part of *Schizonepeta tenuifolia* (Benth.) Briq. (Fam. Labiatae).

Distribution Mainly in Chinese provinces such as Jiangsu, Zhejiang, Henan and Hebei.

Harvest & Processing Cut off above-ground parts in summer and autumn when flowers bloom to the tip and spikes turn green; remove foreign matter and dry under the sun to produce '*Jingjie*' (Fineleaf Schizonepeta Whole Herb). In northern China, spikes and stems are usually separated to produce '*Jingjie sui*' (Fineleaf Schizonepeta Spike) and '*Jingjie geng*' (Fineleaf Schizonepeta Stem).

Description Quadrangular (four-angled), upper part rameous (branched); 50-80 cm long, 2-4 mm in diameter. Outer surface pale yellowish-green or pale purplish-red, pubescent (covered with short, soft hairs); light in weight; brittle; broken surface off-white. Leaves opposite (borne in pairs at each node), mostly fallen off; blades parted into 3-5 pinnate (feather-shaped) divisions, each division slender. Spicate (arranged in spikes) verticillaster acrogenous (growing from the apex); 2-9 cm long, about 7 mm in diameter. Corolla mostly fallen off. Persistent calyx campanulate (bell-shaped); apex 5-toothed; pale brown or yellowish-green; pubescent. Nutlets brownish-black. Odour: aromatic; taste: slightly astringent, acrid-fresh.

Indications 1. Common cold, fever with anhidrosis 2. Headache 3. Sore throat 4. Scabies.

Chemical Composition Mainly contains essential oils with menthone as the main component.

Herba Scutellariae Barbatae

Barbated Skullcup Herb
Banzhilian

半枝蓮

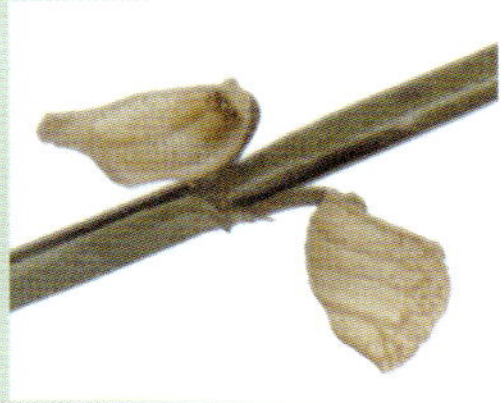

Barbated Skullcup Herb Magnified

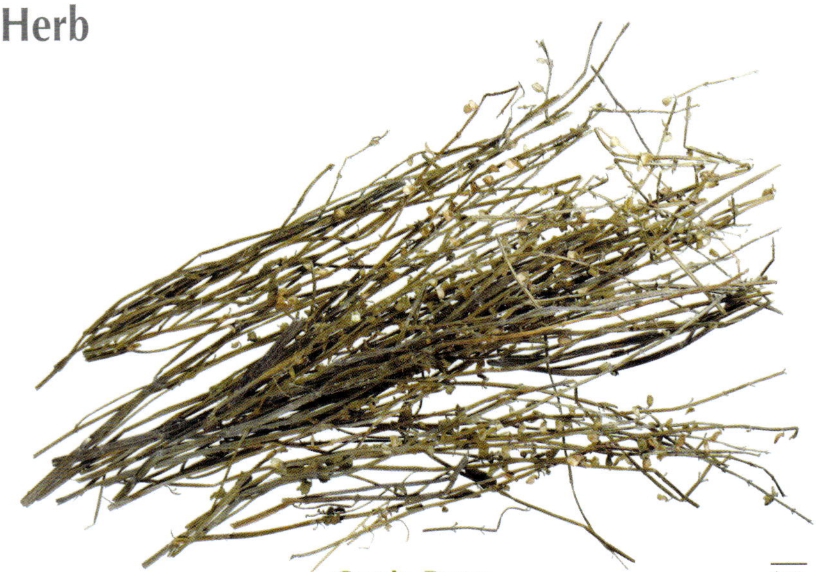

Crude Drug

Source The whole herb of *Scutellaria barbata* D. Don (Fam. Libiatae).

Distribution Mainly in Chinese provinces such as Hebei, Henan, Shanxi and Shaanxi; also in Hong Kong.

Harvest & Processing Collect whole herbs in summer and autumn when leaves flourish; remove foreign matter; wash clean; use while fresh or dry under the sun.

Description Whole herb 15-35 cm long; glabrous (without hairs) or sparsely hairy on floral axis. Roots slender. Stem caespitose (growing in tufts), relatively thin; quadrangular (four-angled); outer surface dull purple or brownish-green. Leaves opposite (borne in pairs at each node), with short petioles or nearly epetiolate (without a petiole); blades shrivelled; when intact and smoothed out, triangular and ovate (egg-shaped in outline and attached at the broad end), or lanceolate (lance-head shaped). Apex obtuse, base broad and cuneate (wedge-shaped); margin entire (continuous and even) or with a few inconspicuous crenations; upper surface dull green, underside greyish-green; brittle, break easily. Flowers solitary (occurring singly) at upper end of branches; corolla bilabiate (two-lipped), brownish-yellow or light bluish-purple, about 1.2 cm long, hairy. Nutlets flattened and spherical; light brown. Odour: faint; taste: slightly bitter.

Indications 1. General fatigue, abdominal pain and ascites 2. Cancer 3. Appendicitis, hepatitis 4. Gastrointestinal bleeding 5. Sores and carbuncles, pyodermas, snakebite, trauma (external use).

Chemical Composition Mainly contains flavonoid glycosides such as scutellarin.

Herba Selaginellae

Spikemoss
Juanbai

卷柏

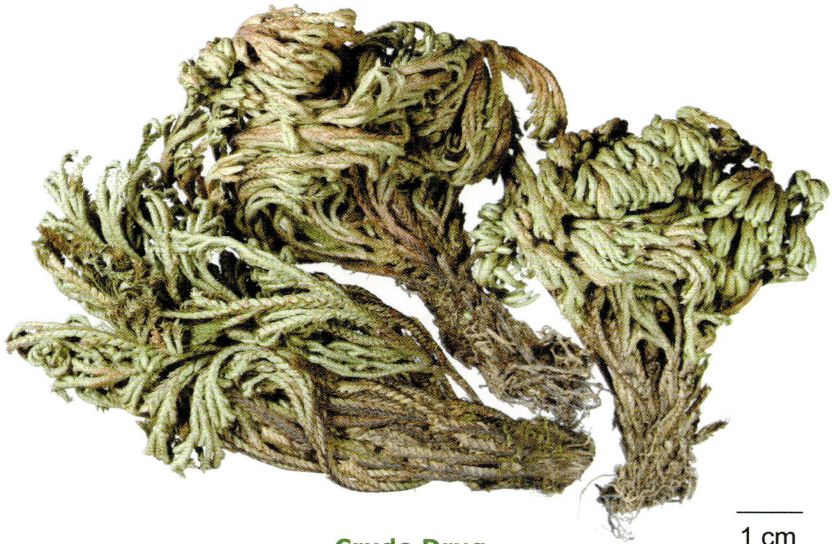

Crude Drug

Source The whole herb of *Selaginella tamariscina* (Beauv.) Spring (Fam. Selaginellaceae).

Distribution Mainly in Chinese provinces such as Hunan, Guangxi, Fujian, Sichuan, Shaanxi, Jiangxi and Zhejiang; also in Hong Kong.

Harvest & Processing Collect whole herbs anytime during the year; remove roots; wash clean; dry under the sun.

Description Curled into fist-like masses. Basal fibrous roots mostly cut off or cut short, leaving only remnants of root base. Branches caespitose (growing in tufts), flattened and with branchlets; green or brownish-yellow; curling inwards; densely covered with squamiform (scale-like) leaflets. Blades ovate (egg-shaped in outline and attached at the broad end), 1.5-2.5 mm long, about 1 mm wide; apex acute, with long light green to light brown aristae; margin membranous, unevenly serrulate (finely notched); central leaves arranged obliquely towards apex. Brittle, breaks easily. Odourless; taste: mild.

Indications 1. Amenorrhoea, dysmenorrhoea 2. Abdominal mass.

Chemical Composition Mainly contains sotetsuflavone, amentoflavone and hinokiflavone.

Note According to *C.P.*, also used for medicinal purposes is the whole herb of *S. pulvinata* (Hook. et Grev.) Maxim.

Herba Selaginellae Doederleinii

Doederlein's Spikemoss Herb

Shishangbai

石上柏

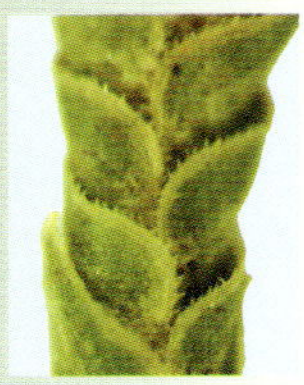

Doederlein's Spikemoss Herb Magnified

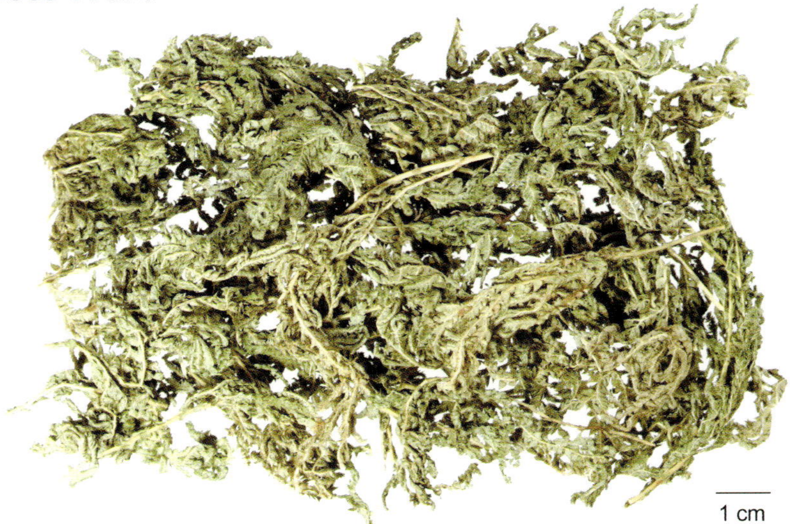

Crude Drug

Source The whole herb of *Selaginella doederleinii* Hieron (Fam. Selaginellaceae).

Distribution Mainly in Chinese provinces such as Anhui, Zhejiang, Jiangxi, Fujian, Taiwan, Hunan, Guangdong and Guangxi; also in Hong Kong.

Harvest & Processing Collect whole herbs anytime during the year; wash clean; use while fresh or dry under the sun.

Description Curled into a leafy mass. Main stem yellowish-green; branches often forked into prop roots. Leaves dimorphic (with two forms), pale green; lateral leaves and central leaves each in 2 rows; margin serrate (saw-like). Sporangiate spikes usually 2, acrogenous (growing from the apex) on shoot tips, quadrangular (four-angled); spores subspherical. Odour: fresh and fragrant; taste: slightly bitter.

Indications 1. Jaundice, hepatitis, cirrhosis, cholecystitis, diarrhoea, dysentery 2. Leukorrhagia 3. Cough, sore throat, silicosis 4. Bleeding 5. Certain kinds of cancer

Chemical Composition Mainly contains biflavonoids.

Herba Senecionis Scandentis

Climbing Groundsel Herb

Qianliguang

千里光

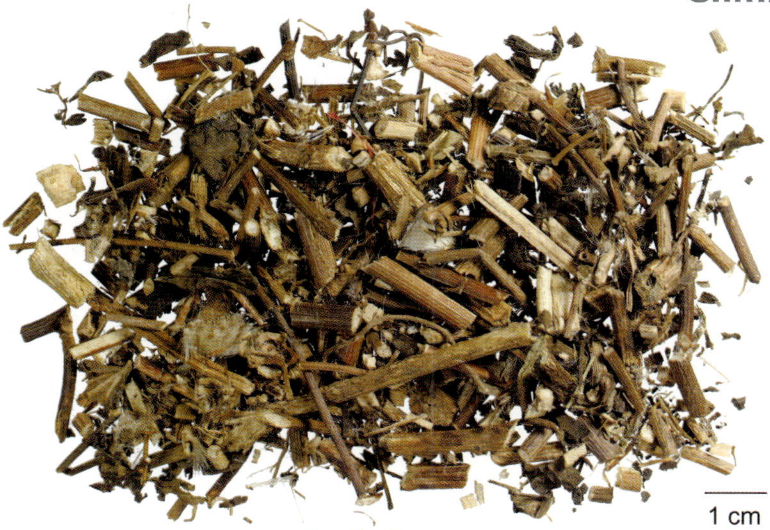

Crude Drug

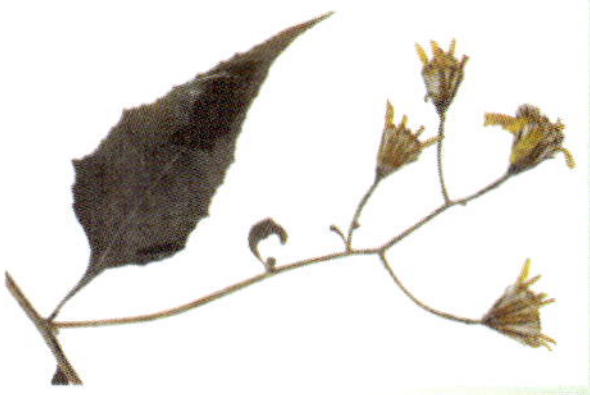

Climbing Groundsel Herb Magnified

Source The whole herb of *Senecio scandens* Buch.-Ham. (Fam. Compositae).

Distribution Mainly in Chinese provinces such as Guangxi and Yunnan; also in Hong Kong.

Harvest & Processing Harvest whole herbs in September and October; wash away soil; dry under the sun or use while fresh.

Description Whole herb 60-100 cm long, often cut into sections 3 cm long. Outer surface of stem reddish-brown or yellowish-brown; rough; marked with numerous twisting longitudinal grooves and yellowish-white fibre bundles. Brittle, breaks easily; when broken, surface reddish-brown, pith white. Leaves mostly curled, shrivelled and in fragments; when whole and smoothed out, blades in elliptical-triangular shape; margin irregular and serrate (saw-like). Achenes crowned in white pappi. Odour: slightly fragrant; taste: slightly bitter.

Indications 1. Sore throat, skin infection, erysipelas, appendicitis 2. Conjunctivitis, trachoma, keratitis, corneal ulcer 3. Diarrhoea, dysentery, leptospirosis 4. Eczema, weeping skin lesions.

Chemical Composition Mainly contains senecionine and favoranthin.

Herba Solani Nigri

Black Nightshade Herb
Longkui

龍葵

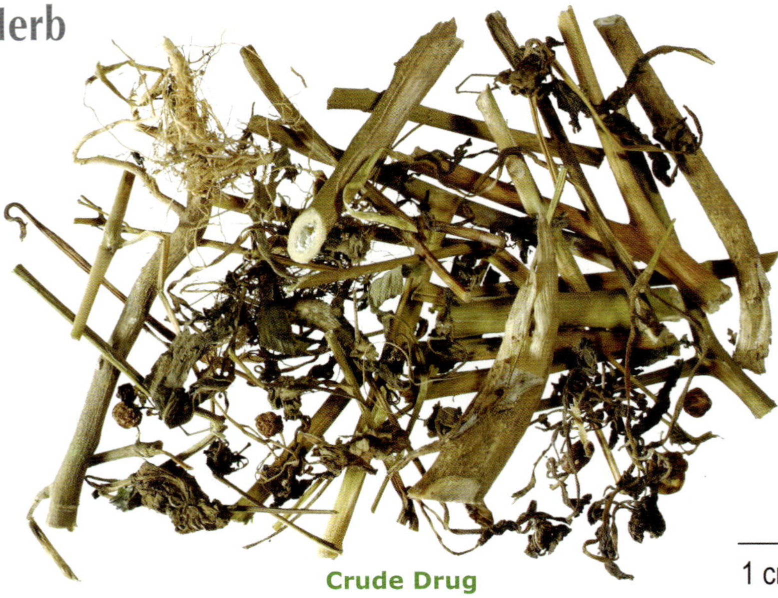

Crude Drug

1 cm

Source The whole herb of *Solanum nigrum* L. (Fam. Solanaceae).

Distribution In most regions of China, including Hong Kong.

Harvest & Processing Harvest whole herbs in summer and autumn; use while fresh or dry under the sun.

Description Stem cylindrical, ramose (with many branches); outer surface yellowish-green, marked with longitudinal wrinkles; hard and brittle; broken surface yellowish-white, hollowed. Leaves shrivelled or in fragments; when intact, blades ovate (egg-shaped) or elliptical. Apex acute or obtuse; margin entire (continuous and even), or with irregular undulate (wavy) teeth. Leaves dull green; both sides glabrous (without hairs) or sparsely pubescent (covered with short, soft hairs). Flowers and fruits rarely attached. Cyme scorpioid (shaped like a scorpion's tail), extra-axillary (outside of but close to the axil); with 4-6 florets; calyx reddish-brown; corolla brownish-yellow. Berries spherical, green and shrivelled. Seeds numerous, brown. Odour: faint; taste: mild.

Indications 1. Sores and boils, carbuncle, erysipelas 2. Trauma 3. Chronic bronchitis 4. Nephritic oedema

Chemical Composition Solasonine exists in the upper portion.

Herba Solidaginis

Common Goldenrod Herb

Yizhihuanghua

一枝黃花

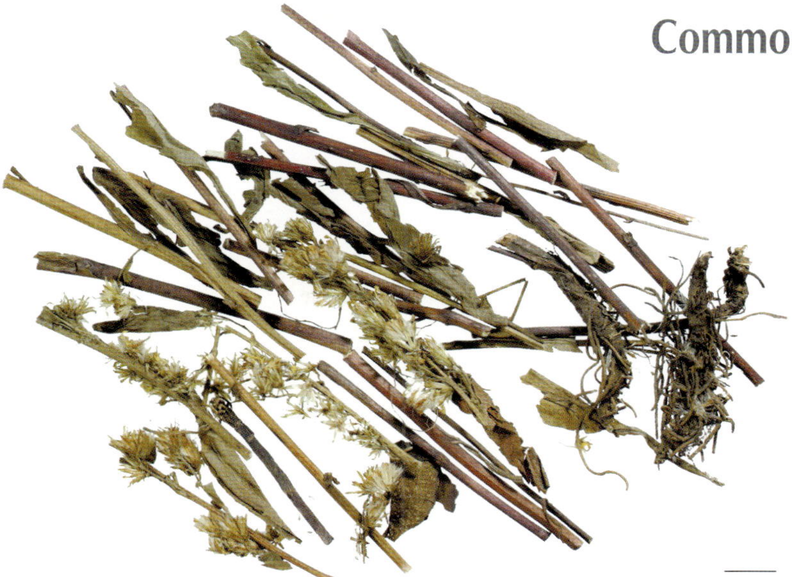

Crude Drug

1 cm

Source The whole herb of *Solidago decurens* Lour. (Fam. Compositae).

Distribution Mainly in regions south of the Yangtze River in China; also in Hong Kong.

Harvest & Processing Cut off whole herbs between summer and autumn; wash clean; use while fresh or dry under the sun.

Description Stem cylindrical; marked with longitudinal striae; smooth and glabrous (without hairs); stem apex sparsely hairy; hard and brittle, breaks easily; when broken, surface fibrous, with porous white pith in the centre. Leaf blades mostly in fragments and shrivelled; upper surface yellowish-green, underside pale green; when smoothed out, ovate (egg-shaped), or oblong and orbicular (round), or lanceolate (lance-head shaped), 4-10 cm long, 1.5-4 cm wide. Apex pointed, acuminate (tapering to a slender point) or obtuse, base constricted, forming aliform (wing-shaped) petioles; margin with sharp teeth; margin of upper part of leaves sparsely serrate (saw-like) and nearly entire (continuous and even), ciliate (with a marginal fringe of hairs). Capitate inflorescences growing densely at stem apex; bracts in 3 layers, membranous, persistent. Odour: fresh and fragrant; taste: bitter.

Indications 1. Influenza, headache, sore throat, cough with yellow sputum 2. Jaundice, diarrhoea, lower urinary tract infection 3. Carbuncles and sores 4. Venomous-snake bite.

Chemical Composition Mainly contains glycosides such as leiocarposide.

Herba Taraxaci

Dandelion

Pugongying

蒲公英

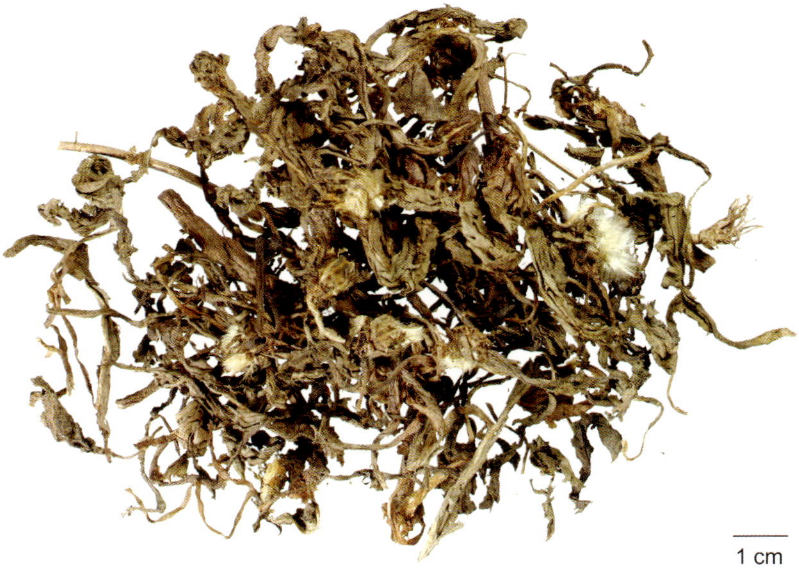

Crude Drug

Source The whole herb of *Taraxacum mongolicum* Hand.-Mazz. (Fam. Compositae).

Distribution Mainly in Chinese provinces such as Shanxi, Hebei and Shandong, and in northeastern China; also in most other regions of China, including Hong Kong.

Harvest & Processing Dig up whole herbs from spring to autumn when flowers start to bloom; remove foreign matter; wash clean; dry under the sun.

Description Shrivelled and curled leafy masses. Root conical, mostly curved; 3-7 cm long; outer surface reddish-brown, shrivelled; top part with reddish-brown or yellowish-white pubescence. Leaves basal, mostly shrivelled and in fragments; when intact, blades oblanceolate; dull greenish-brown or dull grey. Apex pointed or blunt; margin lobed or pinnatipartite; base attenuate, decurrent and stipitiform; main vein on underside prominent. Peduncle 1 to several, each with an acrogenous capitate inflorescence; phyllaries in many layers, with the inner one longer; corolla dull yellowish-brown or pale yellowish-white. Odour: faint; taste: slightly bitter.

Indications 1. Upper respiratory infection, acute tonsillitis, pharyngitis 2. Gastritism, cholecystitis 3. General fatigue 4. Abdominal pain 5. Pyodermas, snakebite (local application with juice of fresh plant)

Chemical Composition Mainly contains flavonoids such as *isoquercitrin (異槲皮甘)* and hyperin.

Note According to *C.P.*, also used for medicinal purposes is the whole herb of *T. sinicum* Kitag.

Herba Taxilli

Chinese Taxillus Twig
Sangjisheng
桑寄生

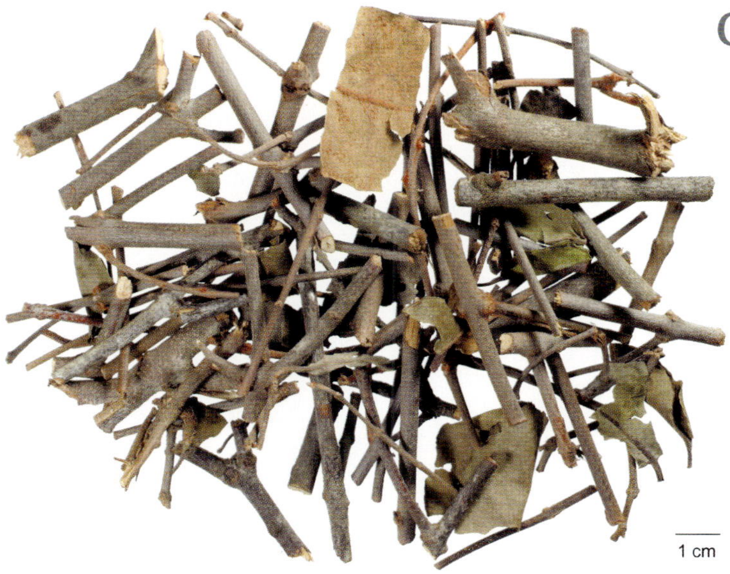

Crude Drug

Source The leaf-bearing twig of *Taxillus chinensis* (DC.) Danser (Fam. Loranthaceae).

Distribution Mainly in Chinese provinces such as Guangdong, Guangxi and Fujian; also in Hong Kong.

Harvest & Processing Harvest leaf-bearing twigs from winter to spring; remove thick stems; cut into sections and dry, or steam and dry.

Description Leaf-bearing twig cylindrical; 3-4 cm long, 0.2-1 cm in diameter. Outer surface dull reddish-brown or dull greyish-brown, marked with fine longitudinal striae and numerous small, protuberant brown lenticels; some young stems covered with reddish-brown pubescence. Hard. Broken surface uneven; cortex reddish-brown; xylem lighter in colour. Leaves mostly curled and with short petioles; when smoothed out, blade ovate (egg-shaped) or elliptical, 3-8 cm long, 2-5 cm wide; outer surface dull yellowish-brown; young leaves covered with fine pubescence. Apex obtuse, base orbicular (round) or broad cuneate (wedge-shaped); entire (with continuous, even margin); coriaceous (leathery). Odour: faint; taste: slightly astringent.

Indications 1. Rheumatism manifested as weakness of back and knees and weakness of extremities 2. Threatened abortion 3. Hypertension, angina pectoris, arrhythmia.

Chemical Composition Mainly contains flavonoids, such as quercetin and quercitrin.

Herba Verbenae

European Verbena Herb
Mabiancao

馬鞭草

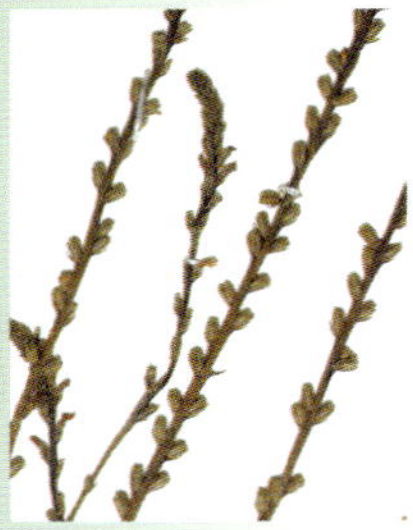

European Verbena Herb Magnified

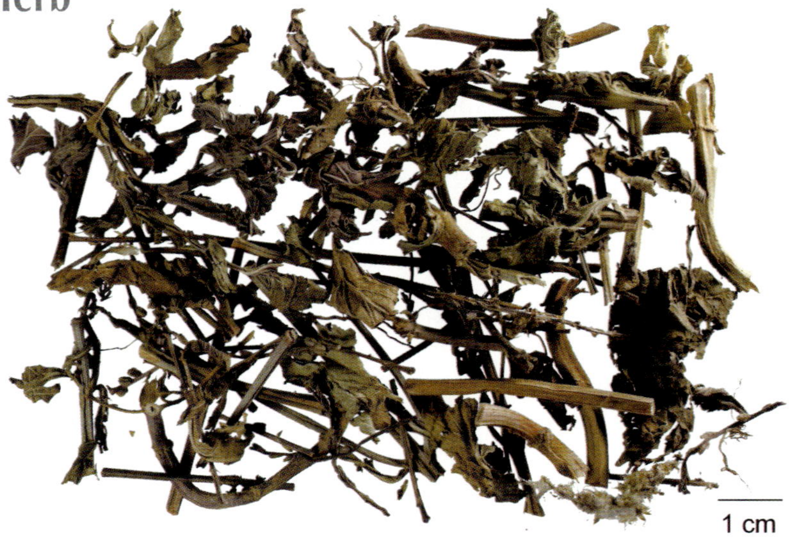

Crude Drug

Source The above-ground part of *Verbena officinalis* L. (Fam. Verbenaceae).

Distribution Mainly in Chinese provinces such as Hubei, Jiangsu, Guizhou and Guangxi; also in Hong Kong.

Harvest & Processing Cut off above-ground parts from July to October during efflorescence; remove foreign matter; dry under the sun.

Description Stem quadrangular (four-angled), ramose (with many branches), with longitudinal grooves on all sides; 0.5-1 m long; outer surface greyish-green or yellowish-green, rough, with sparse hairs. Hard and brittle, breaks easily; broken surface fibrous, with white pith in the centre, or hollowed Leaves opposite (borne in pairs at each node), greyish-green or dull greenish-brown, shrivelled, mostly in fragments; when intact and smoothed out, blades tripartite (parted into three divisions); margin serrate (saw-like). Spike slender, axillary (growing at axil) or acrogenous (growing from the apex); flowers small; flowers or fruits mostly fallen off, leaving only protuberant punctiform (dot-like) scars. Odourless; taste: bitter.

Indications 1. Diphtheria, sore throat, common cold, skin infection 2. Diarrhoea 3. Leucorrhalgia, menstrual disorders 4. Malaria, filariasis, hepatosplenomegaly, 5. Oedema, stranguria

Chemical Composition Mainly contains verbenalin and hastatoside.

Herba Visci

Coloured Mistletoe Herb

Hujisheng

槲寄生

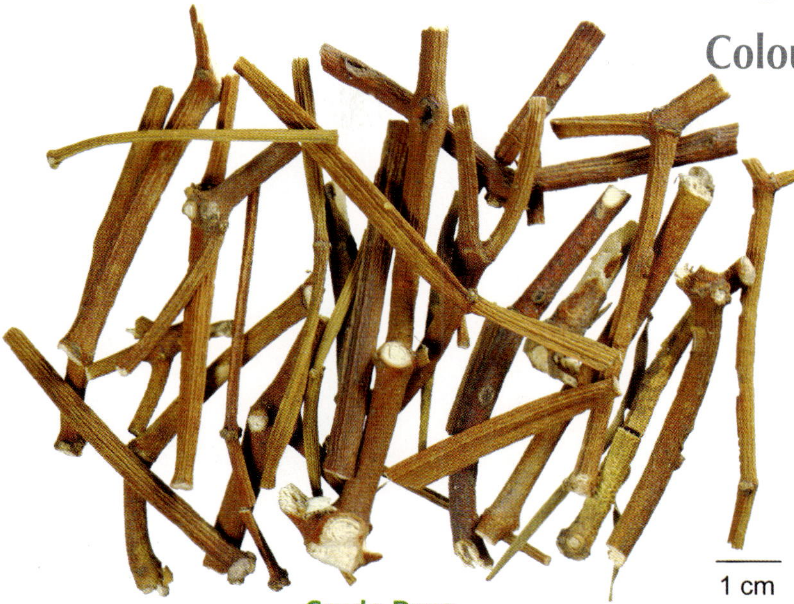

Crude Drug

Source The above-ground part of *Viscum coloratum* (Komar.) Nakai (Fam. Loranthaceae).

Distribution Mainly in northeastern and northern China, and in Chinese provinces such as Shaanxi, Gansu and Henan.

Harvest & Processing Cut off above-ground parts from winter to the following spring; remove thick stems; cut into sections; dry under the sun, or steam and dry.

Description Twigs cylindrical, 2-5 forked branches. Outer surface yellowish-green, golden-yellow or yellowish-brown, marked with longitudinal wrinkles; nodes bulgy, with branches or branch scars. Light in weight; brittle, breaks easily. When broken, surface uneven; cortex yellow; xylem lighter in colour, with radial rays; pith usually eccentric (not positioned directly on the central axis). Leaves opposite (borne in pairs at each node) on branch tips, fall off easily, epetiolate (without a petiole); blades oblong, elliptical and lanceolate (lance-head shaped). Apex obtuse, base cuneate (wedge-shaped); entire (with continuous, even margin); outer surface yellowish-green, marked with fine wrinkles; quinquenerved (with five main veins), with the middle 3 conspicuous; coriaceous (leathery). Berries spherical and shrivelled. Odourless; taste: slightly bitter, sticky when chewed.

Indications

1. Rheumatic arthralgia, pain and weakness of the loins and knees
2. Threatened abortion.

Chemical Composition Mainly contains flavonoids.

Herba Wedeliae

Chinese Wedelia Herb

Pengqiju

蟛蜞菊

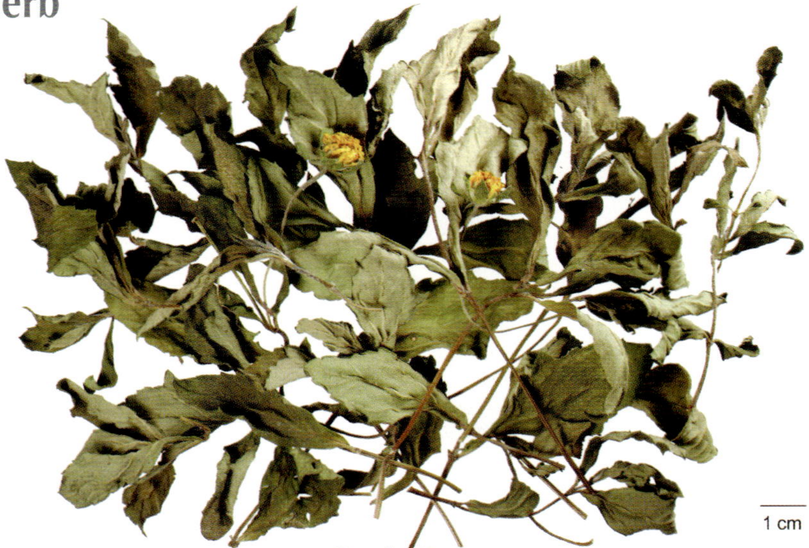

Crude Drug

Source The whole herb of *Wedelia chinensis* (Osb.) Merr. (Fam. Compositae).

Distribution Mainly in Chinese provinces such as Fujian, Guangdong, Hainan, Taiwan, Yunnan and Guangxi; also in Hong Kong.

Harvest & Processing Harvest whole herbs in spring and summer; use while fresh, or cut into sections and dry under the sun.

Description Stem cylindrical, curved; outer surface greyish-green or pale purple, marked with longitudinal wrinkles; nodes often with rootlets; young stem covered with pubescence. Leaves opposite (borne in pairs at each node), almost epetiolate (without a petiole), mostly shrivelled; when smoothed out, blade elliptical, or oblong, orbicular (round) and lanceolate (lance-head shaped). Apex mucronate (with a short straight point) or acuminate (tapering to a slender point); margin grossly-serrate (with big saw-like teeth) or undulate (wavy); upper surface dull greenish-brown, underside greyish-green, both sides covered with white pubescence. Capitate inflorescences usually solitary (occurring singly) at stem apex or leaf axil; peduncle and bracts covered with pubescence; bracts in 2 layers, greyish-green. Ligulate (strap-shaped) flowers and tubular flowers yellow. Odour: faint; taste: slightly astringent.

Indications 1. Respiratory tract infection, tonsillitis, mumps, diphtheria, pulmonary tuberculosis 2. Bleeding 3. Infectious hepatitis 4. Dysentery, haemorrhoid 5. Sores and boils

Chemical Composition Contains diterpenes and triterpenes.

Indigo Naturalis

Natural Indigo
Qingdai

青黛

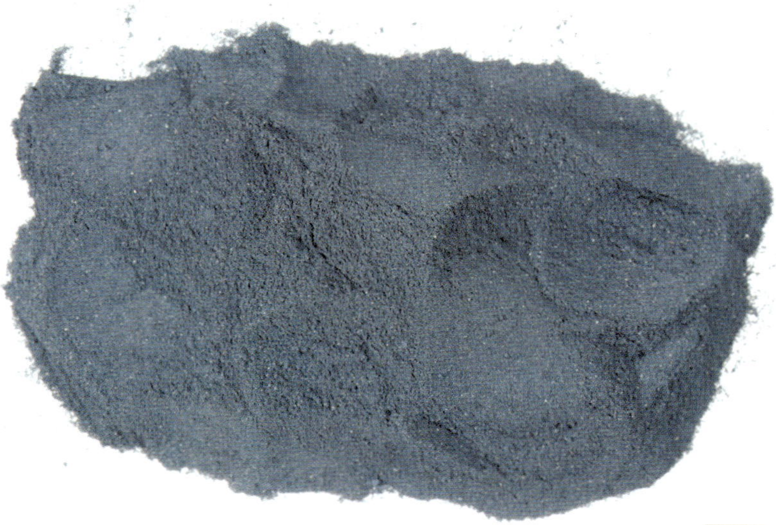

Crude Drug

Source The leaf or stem and leaf of *Baphicacanthus cusia* (Nees) Bremek. (Fam. Acanthaceae).

Distribution Mainly in Chinese provinces such as Fujian, Hebei, Jiangsu, Yunnan and Anhui.

Harvest & Processing Collect stems and leaves in summer and autumn; put in a big container or a wooden pail and soak in water for 2-3 days until the leaves have decayed and the stem bark peeled off; remove the waste; add 0.5 kg of lime into every 5 kg of stems and leaves and stir thoroughly; when the liquid changes from dark green to dark purplish-red, skim off the blue foam-like substance on the liquid surface; dry under the sun.

Description Dark blue powder, light in weight, flies into the air easily; or appears as irregular and poriferous (with numerous holes) lumps that turn into fine powder when rubbed with hands. Odour: slightly grassy; taste: mild.

Indications 1. Seasonal febrile diseases with thirst and eruptive exanthem, infantile epilepsy 2. Bleeding 3. Carbuncle, erysepilas, mumps, snake and insect bite 4. Sore throat, aphthous ulcer

Chemical Composition Mainly contains indirubin, indigo and isoindigo.

Note According to *C.P.*, also used for medicinal purposes is the powder or lumps prepared from the leaf or the stem and leaf of *Polygonum tinctorium* Ait. (Fam. Polygonaceae) and *Isatis indigotica* Fort. (Fam. Cruciferae).

Lignum Aquilariae Resinatum

Chinese Eaglewood
Chenxiang

沉香

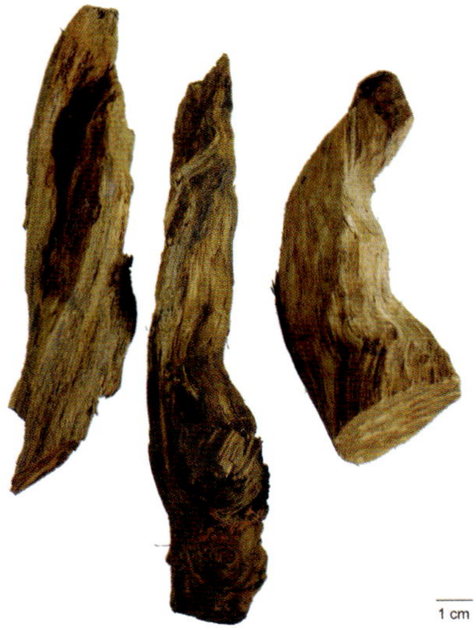

Crude Drug

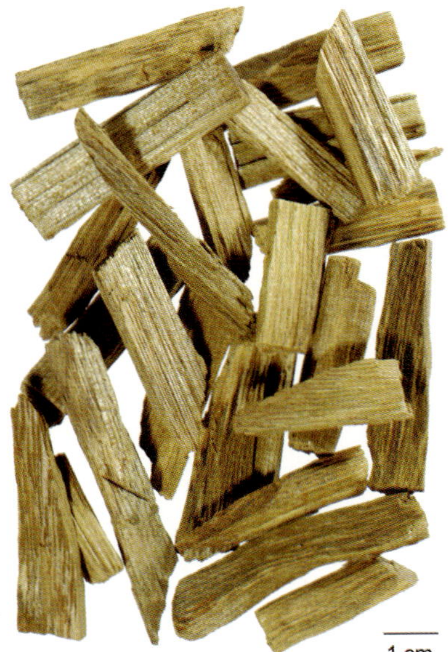

Decoction Pieces

Source

The heartwood, containing resin, of *Aquilaria sinensis* (Lour.) Gilg (Fam. Thymelaeaceae).

Distribution

Mainly in Chinese provinces such as Guangdong, Hainan, Guangxi, Fujian and Taiwan.

Harvest & Processing

Choose trees with trunks over 30 cm in diameter. At a point about 1.5-2 m from the ground, make several cuts on the trunks with a knife. The cuts should be separated from each other by a distance of about 30-50 cm, and about 3-4 cm deep to induce the secretion of resin. Several years later, collect heartwood.

Description

Irregular or placoid (plate-like) lumps, sometimes in small fragments. Outer surface uneven; marked with knife scars from processing; marked also with brownish-black, slightly lustrous patches containing resin and yellowish-white patches containing no resin. Texture loose; mostly do net sink in water. Fibres on broken surface spiniform (spine-shaped). Odour: with a distinctive fragrance; taste: slightly bitter. Produce dense smoke and a heavy aroma when burning, and ooze a black oily substance.

Indications

1. Distending pain in the chest and abdomen, vomiting and hiccup
2. Dysnoea

Chemical Composition

Mainly contains 2-(2-phenylethyl) chromones and sesquiterpenes such as baimuxinic acid.

Lignum Dalbergiae Odoriferae

Rosewood
Jiangxiang
降香

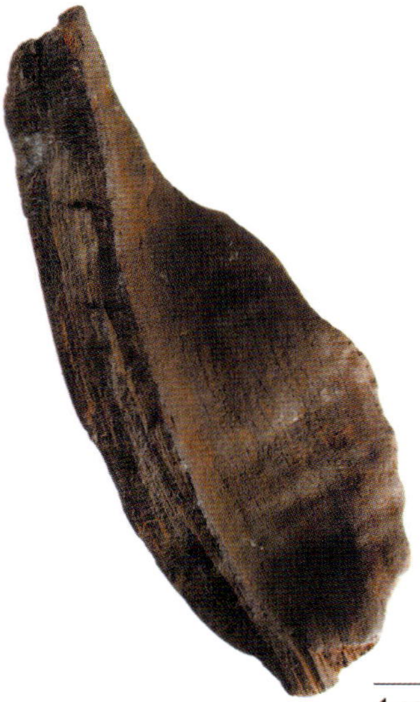

Crude Drug

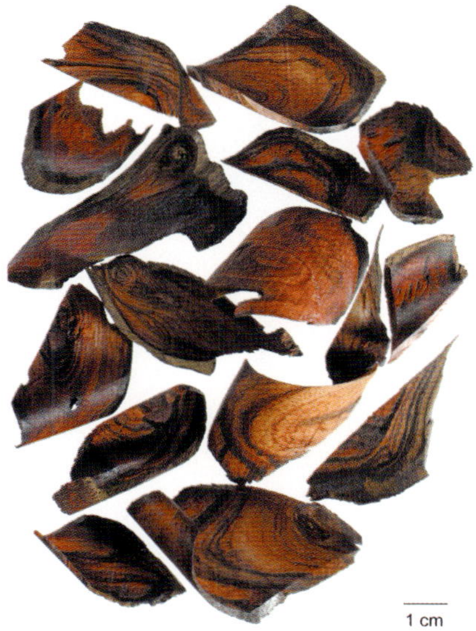

Decoction Pieces

Source The heartwood of the trunk and root of *Dalbergia odorifera* T. Chen (Fam. Leguminosae).

Distribution Mainly in Chinese provinces such as Guangdong, Hainan, Fujian, Guangxi and Yunnan.

Harvest & Processing Collect trunks and roots anytime during the year; remove cork and sapwood; dry in shaded areas.

Description Subcylindrical or irregular pieces; varying in size. Outer surface purplish-red to dull reddish-brown; cut surface with dense markings. Hard; highly oleaginous (oily); sink in water. Emit black smoke and oil when burned with fire, leaving behind white ashes. Odour: slightly fragrant; taste: slightly bitter.

Indications 1. Bleeding such as traumatic bleeding (external use), haemoptysis, and gastrointestinal bleeding 2. Chest Pain and abdominal pain.

Chemical Composition The heartwood of the roots mainly contains flavonoids such as formononetin, liquiritigenin and isoliquiritigenin.

Lignum Pini Nodi

Pine Nodular Branch
Yousongjie
油松節

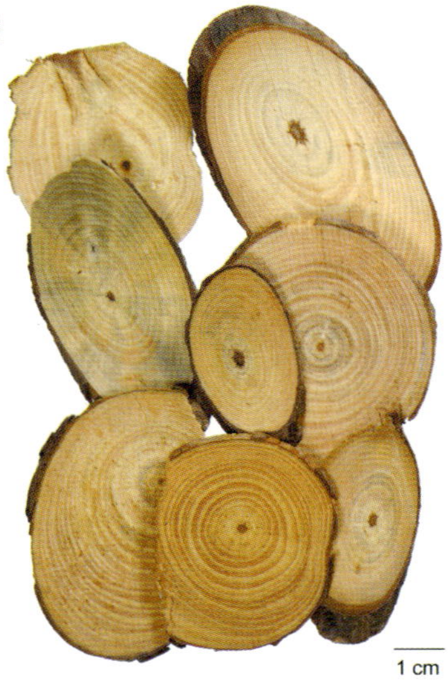

Decoction Pieces

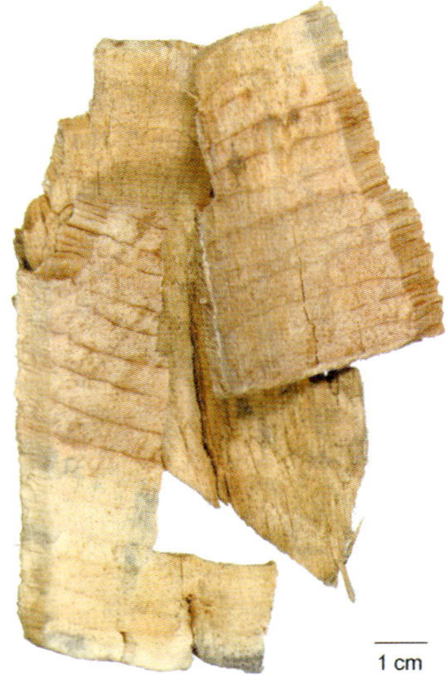

Decoction Pieces (length-wise cut slices)

Source The bulgy node on the stems and branches of *Pinus tabulaeformis* Carr. (Fam. Pinaceae) and of many other species of the same genus.

Distribution Mainly in Chinese provinces such as Liaoning, Hebei, Shandong, Henan, Shaanxi, Shanxi and Gansu.

Harvest & Processing Saw off bulgy nodes of trunks and branches, usually from lumbering or during factory processing; select and trim; dry under the sun or in shaded areas.

Description Disc-like sections, or irregular slices or pieces; varying in length and diameter. Outer surface brownish-yellow, greyish-brown or brownish-red; slightly rough; occasionally marked with brown to blackish-brown sebaceous (tallowy or fatty) maculae, or with cork remnants. Hard and heavy. When broken transversely, surface reveals pale brown xylem; heartwood in a darker shade, with concentric rings, occasionally scattered with poriform (pore-like) brown resin ducts, oleaginous (oily); pith small, pale yellowish-brown. When broken longitudinally, surface reveals unevenly distributed straight or oblique markings. Odour: with the distinctive fragrance of turpentine; taste: slightly bitter-acrid.

Indications 1. Arthralgia, ankylosis 2. Toothache (external use as gargle).

Chemical Composition Contains ursolic acid, isopimaric acid and essential oils.

Note Commonly sold are the node-bearing stems and branches of *Pinus tabulaeformis* Carr.

Lignum Sappan

Sappan Wood

Sumu

蘇木

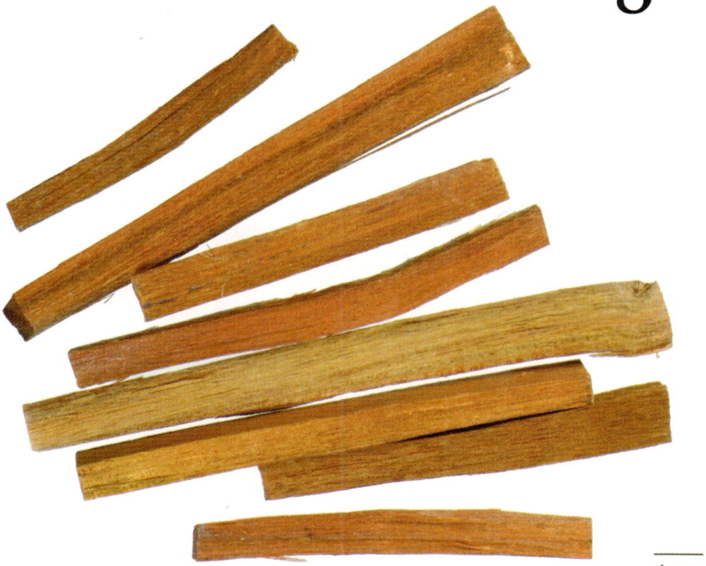

Decoction Pieces

Source The heartwood of *Caesalpinia sappan* L. (Fam. Leguminosae).

Distribution Mainly in Chinese provinces such as Taiwan, Guangdong, Guangxi and Guizhou.

Harvest & Processing Chop down trees anytime during the year, usually between May and July; remove cork and sapwood; take the yellowish-red or reddish-brown heartwood; dry heartwood under the sun; shave into thin strips or chop into small pieces for use.

Description Long and cylindrical or semi-cylindrical; in some cases with roots attached, forming a long, slightly curved, irregular rod-like piece or irregular verruciform (wart-shaped) piece; varying in length, 3-10 cm in diameter. Outer surface dull reddish-brown or yellowish-brown, with alternating red and yellow longitudinal striae; also marked with knife scars and small dented oil dots. Heavy in weight; hard, dense. When broken, surface strongly fibrous; when broken transversely, surface with conspicuous, suborbicular (almost round) concentric annulations (annual rings), sometimes with dull brown, brightly-dotted pith in the centre. Odour: slightly fragrant; taste: slightly sweet-astringent.

Indications 1. Amenorrhoea, dysmenorrhoea, lochiostasis 2. Pricking pain in the chest and abdomen 3. Trauma.

Chemical Composition Mainly contains essential oils with ocimene as the main component. Sappanin exists in the heartwood.

Medulla Junci

Common Rush
Dengxincao

燈心草

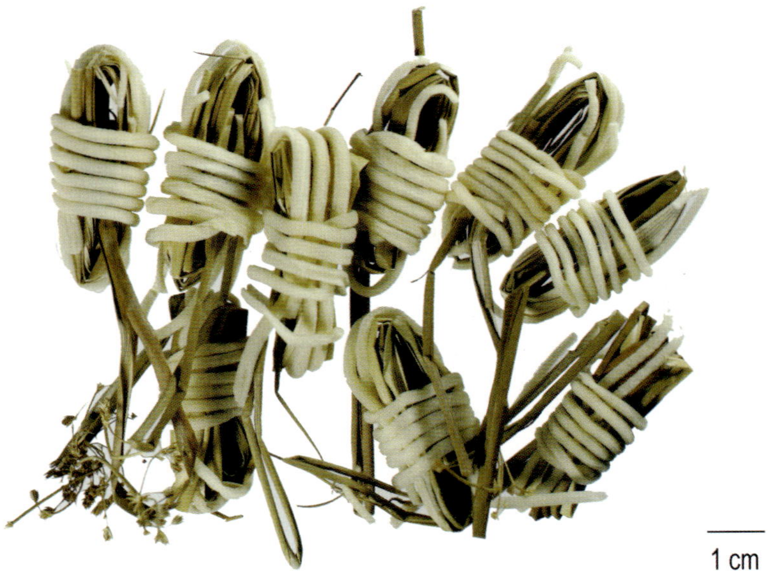

Crude Drug

Source The stem pith of *Juncus effuses* L. (Fam. Juncaceae).

Distribution Mainly in Chinese provinces such as Jiangsu, Sichuan, Fujian and Guizhou.

Harvest & Processing Cut off stems in summer and autumn; remove bark to get pith; dry pith under the sun; tie into bundles.

Description Slender and cylindrical; up to 90 cm long, 1-3 mm in diameter. Outer surface white or pale yellowish-white; marked with fine protuberant striae, and with pores in a spongilliform (spongy) pattern; slightly lustrous. Light in weight; soft and elastic, breaks easily when pulled; when broken, surface uneven and white. Odour: indistinct.

Indications Fidgetness and insomnia with oliguria and stranguria or with aphthous ulcer.

Chemical Composition Mainly contains effusol and juncunol.

Note In Hong Kong, commonly used is the stem pith, together with the rest of the whole herb, of *Juncus effusus* L.

Medulla Stachyuri

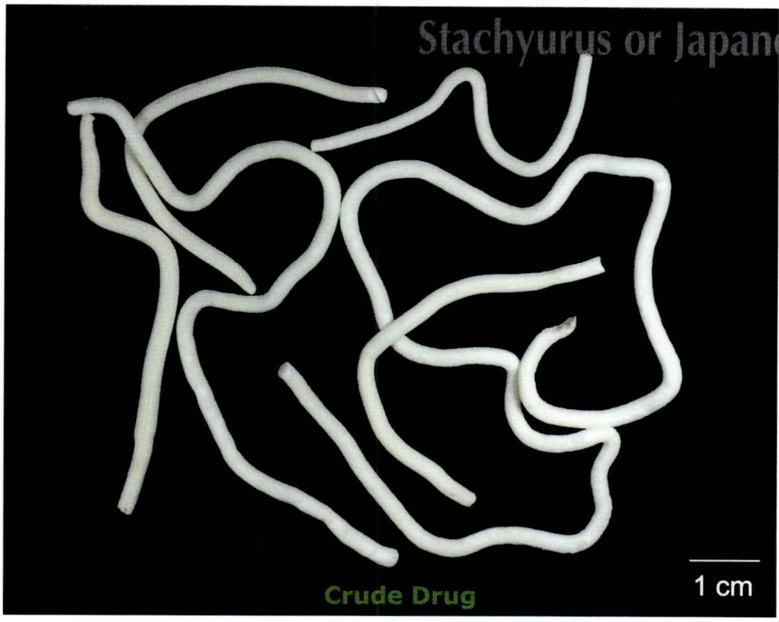

Crude Drug

Stachyurus or Japanese Helwingia Pith
Xiaotongcao
小通草

Source The stem pith of *Stachyurus himalaicus* Hook. f. et Thoms. (Fam. Stachyuraceae).

Distribution Mainly in Chinese provinces such as Shaanxi, Gansu, Jiangxi, Sichuan, Hubei, Guangxi and Yunnan.

Harvest & Processing Chop off young stems in autumn; trim off branches which are too fine or too thick; take out pith while fresh; straighten out with hands; dry under the sun.

Description Fine and cylindrical; varying in length, 0.4-1 cm in diameter. Outer surface white or yellowish, smooth with no markings. Light in weight; texture loose and soft, can be curled, flattens when kneaded; when broken, surface silver-white, lustrous, not hollow in the centre. Viscid and slippery on outer and broken surfaces after soaking in water. Odourless and tasteless.

Indications 1. Oliguria, urinary infection 2. Galactostasis, insufficient lactation.

Chemical Composition Contains polysaccharides and amino acids.

Note According to *C.P.*, also used for medicinal purposes is the stem pith of *S. chinensis* Franch. and *Helwingia japonica* (Thunb.) Dietr.

Medulla Tetrapanacis

Ricepaperplant Stem Pith
Tongcao

通草

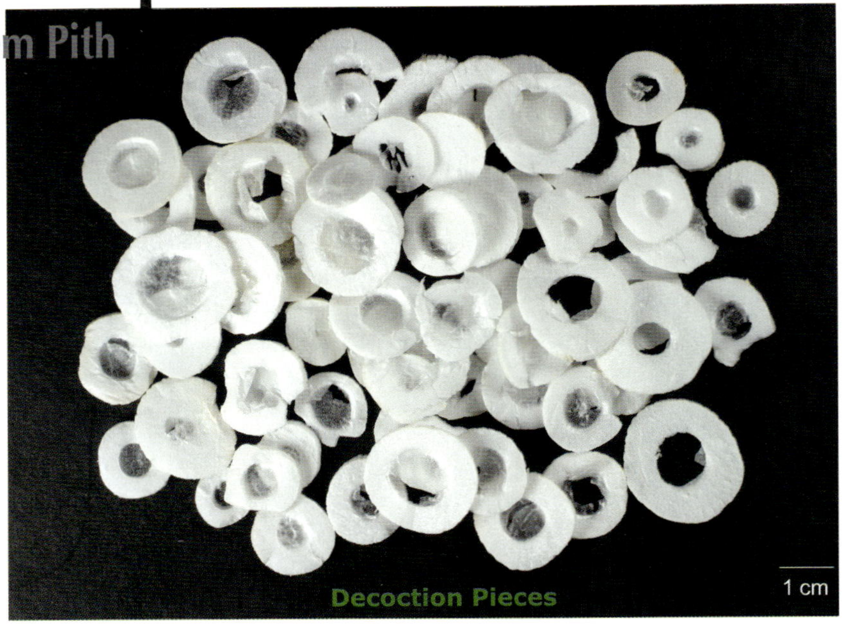

Decoction Pieces

Source The stem pith of *Tetrapanax papyriferus* (Hook.) K. Koch (Fam. Araliaceae).

Distribution Mainly in Chinese provinces such as Guizhou, Yunnan, Sichuan and Hubei.

Harvest & Processing Cut off stems 2-3 years old in autumn; cut into sections; poke out the pith with a small stick while fresh; straighten and dry under the sun.

Description Cylindrical; generally 20-40 cm long, 1-2.5 cm in diameter. Outer surface white or pale yellow; marked with shallow longitudinal grooves. Light in weight; texture loose and soft; slightly elastic, breaks easily. When broken, surface even, with silvery-white lustre; with a cavity or a translucent, orbicular (round) membrane in the centre; the cavity or membrane 0.3-1.5 cm in diameter. Longitudinal-section shows a scalariform (ladder-like) membrane. Odourless and tasteless.

Indications 1. Oedema, dysuria, urodynia 2. Agalactia, galactostasis.

Chemical Composition Contains amino acids, polysaccharides and fats.

Myrrha

Myrrh
Moyao
沒藥

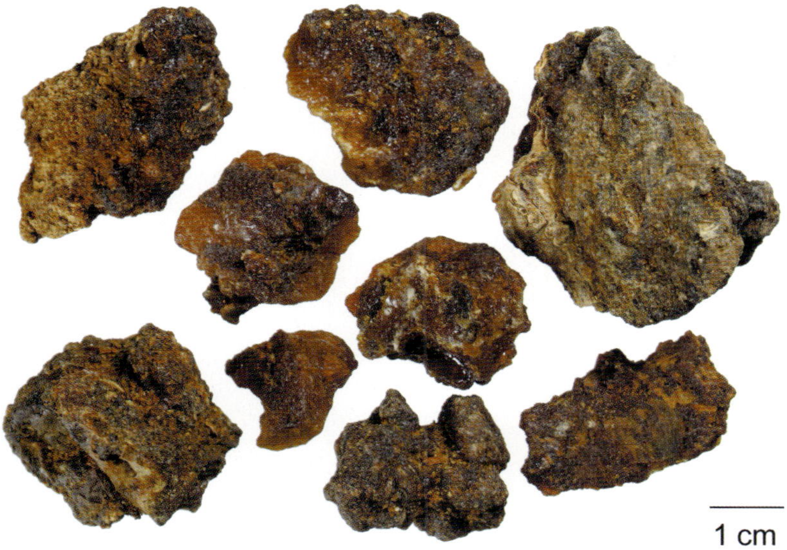

Crude Drug

Source The oleo-gum-resin secreted from the cortex of *Commiphora myrrha* Engler (*C. molmol* Engler) (Fam. Burseraceae) and other species of the same genus.

Distribution Mainly in places such as Somalia and Ethiopia in northeastern Africa, the southern Arabian Peninsula, and India.

Harvest & Processing Stab trees during November and February to let resin secrete from the wounds or cracks on the bark. Upon exposure to air, resin gradually turns from pale yellowish-white liquid into reddish-brown solids. Collect the solidified resin and remove foreign matter.

Description Irregular granules, or lumps of cohered granules; varying in size, generally about 2.5 cm in diameter, some up to 10 cm. Outer surface reddish-brown or yellowish-brown, uneven, covered with powder. Hard and brittle; broken surface granular, with brown oily lustre, and often with white maculae or striae; when sliced, surface translucent. Odour: fragrant and distinctive; taste: bitter and slightly acrid.

Indications 1.Angina pectoris, headache, chest and abdominal pain 2. Arthralgia, muscular spasm, numbness of limbs 3. Trauma 4. Amenorrhoea 5. Pyogenic skin infection

Chemical Composition Contains 25-35% resin with α,β-heerabomyrrholic acid as the main component.

Nux Prinsepiae

Hedge Prinsepia Nut
Ruiren

蕤仁

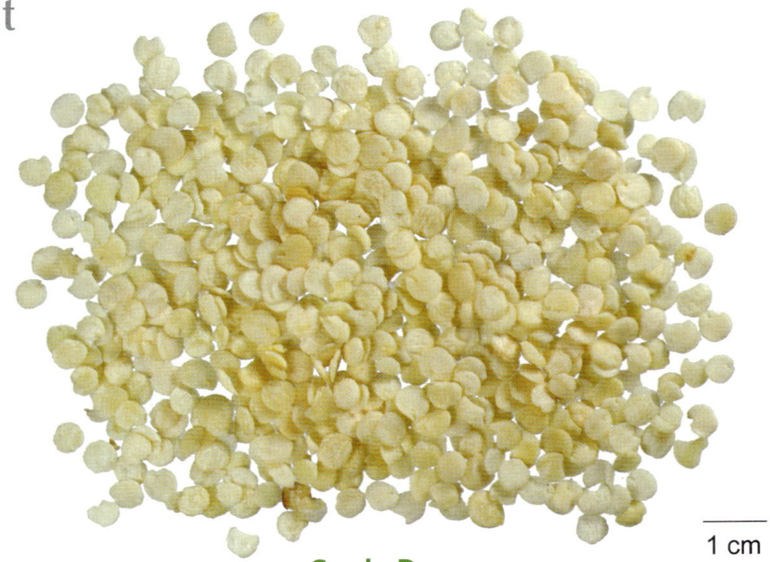

Crude Drug

Source The mature kernel of *Prinsepia uniflora* Batal. (Fam. Rosaceae).

Distribution Mainly in Chinese provinces such as Shanxi, Shaanxi, Gansu and Inner Mongolia.

Harvest & Processing Harvest mature fruits during summer and autumn; remove sarcocarp; wash clean; break pits to get kernels; dry under the sun. Commonly sold with testa removed.

Description Flattened and cordate (heart-shaped), or flattened and ovoid (egg-shaped), two sides slightly asymmetrical; 7-10 mm long, 6-8 mm wide, 3-5 mm thick. Outer surface light brown to dull brown; marked with dark reticulate (Netted) grooves and often with reddish-brown sarcocarp remnants. Hard. When cracked open, flat, suborbicular (almost round) or cordate seeds revealed. Seeds 6-7 mm long, about 5 mm wide, about 2 mm thick; testa reddish-brown, membranous; surface marked with 3-5 dark longitudinal venous (vein-like) striae on both sides; a short, pale-coloured hilum lies at the pointed end on the side; a chalaza lies at the round end between the two ends lies a dark raphe; cotyledons white, plump, oleaginous (oily). Odourless; taste: slightly bitter.

Indications 1. Conjunctivitis, blepharitis with impaired vision and photophobia.

Chemical Composition The seeds consist of proteins and fats.

Note According to *C.P.*, also used for medicinal purposes is the mature pit of *P. uniflora* Batal. *var.* serrata Rehd.

Olibanum

Frankincense
Ruxiang
乳香

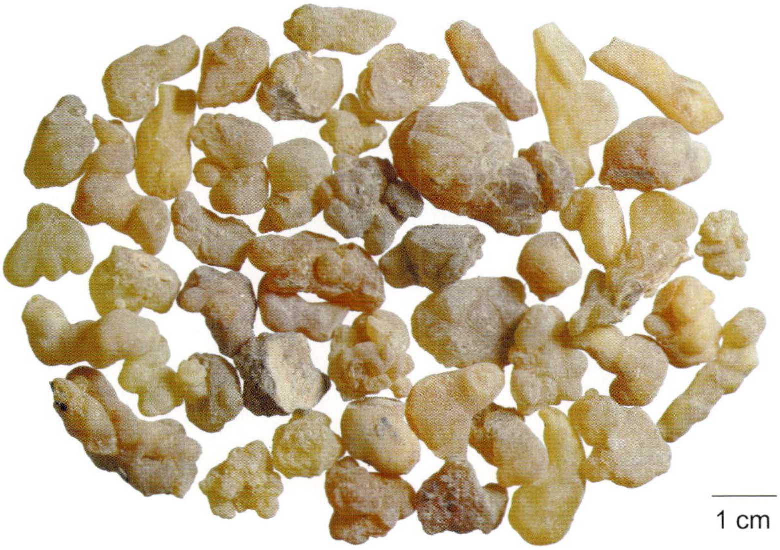

Crude Drug

Source The oleo-gum-resin secreted from the cut cortex of *Boswellia carterii* Birdwood (Fam. Burseraceae) and other species of the same genus.

Distribution Mainly in Somalia, Ethiopia and the southern Arabian Peninsula.

Harvest & Processing The cortex of frankincense trees has distinct (separate, not attached to like parts) resin ducts that usually produce resin in large quantities in spring. Cut a narrow groove on the bark from bottom up to let resin ooze and flow along the groove; harvest when resin solidifies into hard pieces a few days later. Put in airtight containers to avoid dust and store in shaded areas to avoid softening and colour change caused by heat.

Description Small mammilliform (nipple-shaped), lacrimiform (tear-shaped) or irregular pieces; 0.5-2 cm long, in some cases stuck together into a mass. Pale yellow, sometimes greenish or brownish-red; translucent; outer surface in some cases lustreless, often covered with a layer of off-white powder. Hard and brittle; broken surface waxy, lustreless, occasionally with glassy lustre. Odour: slightly fragrant; taste: slightly bitter, slightly hot. When chewed, first break into small fragments, then immediately soften to become gelatinous and sticky, turning saliva to milky-white.

Indications 1.Angina pectoris, headache, chest and abdominal pain 2. Arthralgia, muscular spasm, numbness of limbs 3. Trauma 4. Amenorrhoea 5. Pyogenic skin infection

Chemical Composition Mainly contains α, β-boswellic acid.

Omphalia

Thunder Ball

Leiwan

雷丸

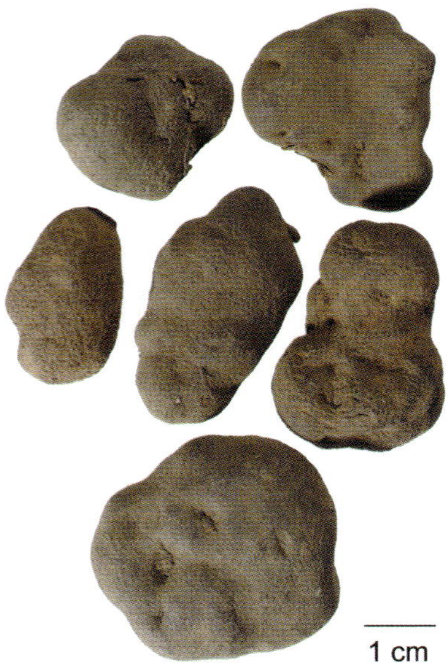

Crude Drug

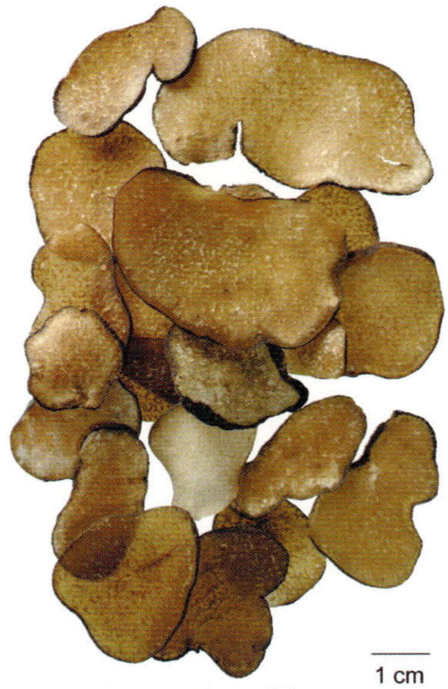

Decoction Pieces

Source The sclerotium of *Omphalia lapidescens* Schroet. (Fam. Tricholomataceae).

Distribution Mainly in Chinese provinces such as Sichuan, Yunnan, Guangxi and Shaanxi.

Harvest & Processing Dig out sclerotia in autumn; wash clean; dry under the sun.

Description Irregular or subspherical lumps; 1-3 cm in diameter. Outer surface dull greyish-brown or dull blackish-brown, marked with slightly raised reticulate (netted) wrinkles. Hard and solid, do not break easily; when broken, surface uneven, white or light greyish-yellow, granular or starchy, often marked with yellowish-brown marble-like markings formed by alternating translucent or opaque parts. Odourless; taste: slightly bitter. Slightly gritty and sticky when first chewed; eaves no residue even after prolonged chewing.

Indications Parasitosis such as taeniasis, oxyuriasis, ascariasis and ancylostomiasis.

Chemical Composition Mainly contains protease (S-4001) and polysaccharides.

Pericarpium Arecae

Areca Peel
Dafupi
大腹皮

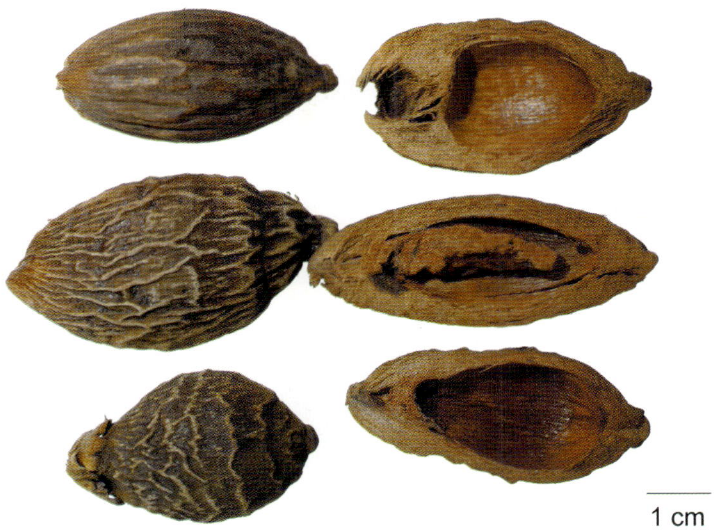

Crude Drug

Source The pericarp of *Areca catechu* L. (Fam. Palmae).

Distribution Mainly in Chinese provinces such as Hainan and Yunnan; also in provinces such as Fujian and Taiwan.

Harvest & Processing Collect immature fruits from winter to the following spring; boil and dry; cut length-wise into halves; peel off pericarp.

Description Pericarp cut length-wise into halves, each elliptical and gourd-ladle shaped; 5-7 cm long, about 3 cm wide. Exocarp surface greyish-yellow, marked with brown maculae and longitudinal cracks; endocarp dented, cordate (heart-shaped), yellowish-brown, smooth, hard; mesocarp fibrous. Whole pericarp loose in texture after being pounded; fibres pale yellow, resembling palm fibres. Light in weight; soft and pliable, easily torn along the length. Odour: faint; taste: slightly astringent.

Indications 1. Dyspepsia, constipation and dyschesia 2. Beriberi and oedema

Chemical Composition Mainly contains condensed tannins.

Petiolus Trachycarpi

Fortune Windmillpalm Petiole

Zonglü

棕櫚

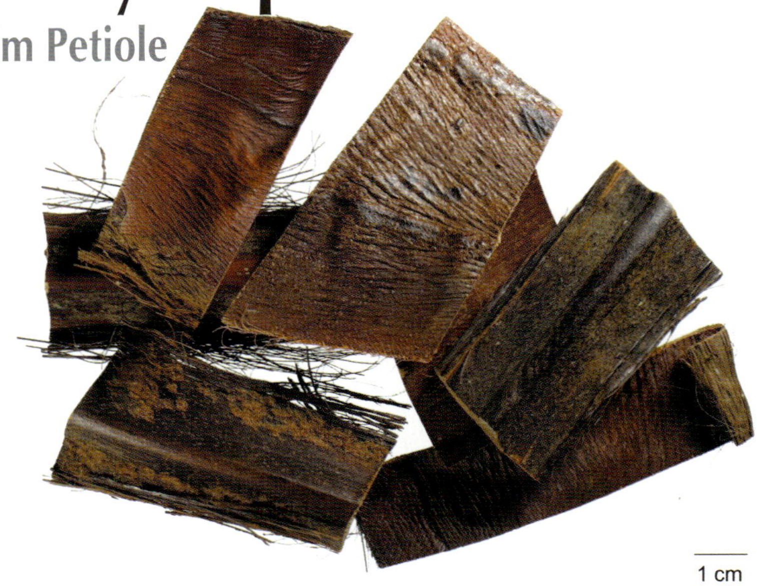

Crude Drug

Source The petiole of *Trachycarpus fortunei* (Hook. f.) H. Wendl. (Fam. Palmae).

Distribution Mainly in regions south of Yangtze River valley in China.

Harvest & Processing Harvest whole leaves, mostly in September and October; strip off basal petioles; shave off epidermal fibres; dry petioles under the sun.

Description Slate-like, reddish-brown; narrower and thicker at one end, broader and thinner at the other, varying in size. Dorsal side bulges at the centre in a triangular shape; Both sides smooth and covered with thick reddish-brown pubescence, in some cases pubescence has fallen off, revealing underlying longitudinal striae. Strong and pliable fibres exposed at removal of epidermis. Odourless; taste: mild.

Indications Bleeding such as haemoptysis, epistaxis, haematuria, haematochezia, dysfunctional uterine bleeding.

Chemical Composition Flavonoids such as glucoluteolin exist in the leaves.

Pollen Pini

Pine Pollen

Songhuafen

松花粉

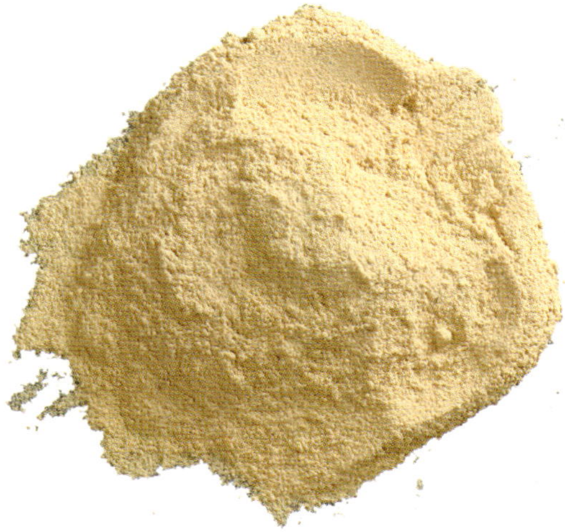

Crude Drug

1 cm

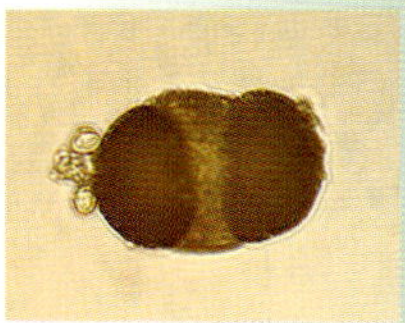

Pine Pollen Magnified

Source The pollen of *Pinus massoniana* Lamb. (Fam. Pinaceae).

Distribution Mainly in regions in Yangtze River valley in China; also in Hong Kong.

Harvest & Processing Collect male cones in April and May when flowers start to bloom; spread out in round, shallow bamboo baskets and dry under the sun; rub out pollen; remove foreign matter with fine sieves.

Description Bright yellow or pale yellow powder. Light in weight, flies into the air easily; smooth when twiddled with fingers. Odour: faint; taste: mild. Floats in water.
Pollen ellipsoid (elliptical in long-section and circular in cross-section) and smooth under a microscope, with a bulgy air-sac on either side; wall of air-sacs marked with conspicuous reticulate (netted) markings with triangular meshes.

Indications 1. Eczema, impetigo, erosion of the skin with exudation, diaper dermatitis 2. Traumatic bleeding.

Chemical Composition Mainly contains oils and fats.

Note According to *C.P.*, also used for medicinal purposes is the pollen of a few plants such as *P. tabulaeformis* Carr..

Pollen Typhae

Cattail Pollen
Puhuang

蒲黃

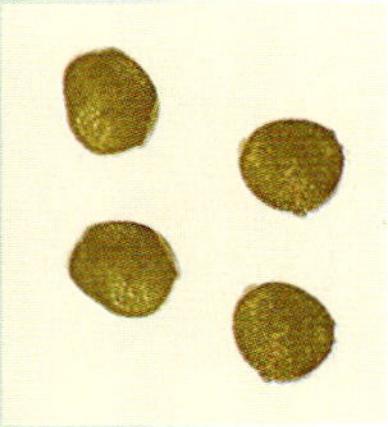

Cattail Pollen Magnified

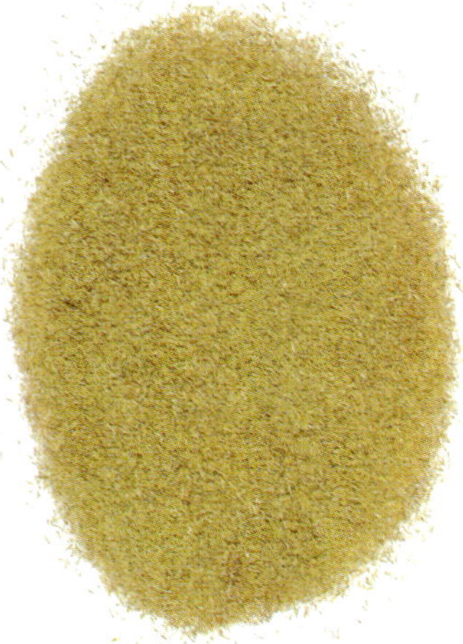

1 cm

Crude Drug (caopuhuang)

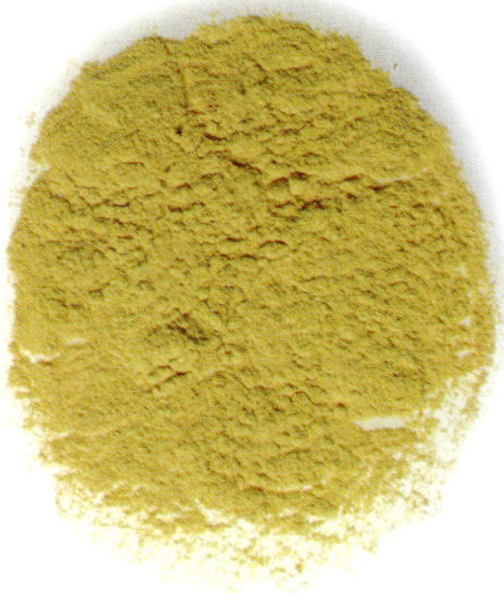

1 cm

Crude Drug (puhuang)

Source The pollen of *Typha angustifolia* L. (Fam. Typhaceae).

Distribution Mainly in Chinese provinces such as Jiangsu, Zhejiang, Shandong and Anhui.

Harvest & Processing Cut off male inflorescences at the tips of cattail spikes in June and July when flowers start to bloom; dry under the sun; pulverize; remove foreign matter to harvest pollen, customarily called '*Caopuhuang*' (Cattail Pollen with Flower); sieve further to collect pure pollen customarily called '*Puhuang*' (Cattail Pollen).

Description Powder bright yellow in colour, light in weight and loose in texture, flies in the air easily; smooth when twiddled with fingers, adheres to fingers; floats when placed in water. Odour: faint; taste: mild.

Indications 1. Dysmenorrhoea, abdominal pain during the puerperium, stomachache 2. Trauma 3. Bleeding 4. Aphthous ulcer 5. Dermatitis (external use).

Chemical Composition Mainly contains flavonoids such as typhaneoside.

Note According to *C.P.*, also used for medicinal purposes is the pollen of *T. orientalis* Presl.

Polyporus

Chuling
Zhuling

豬苓

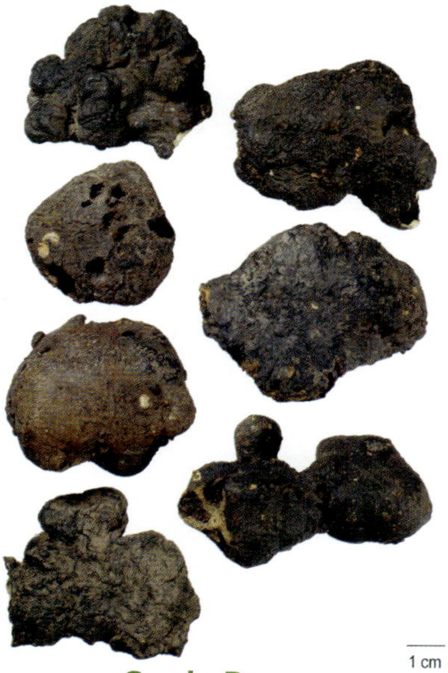

Crude Drug

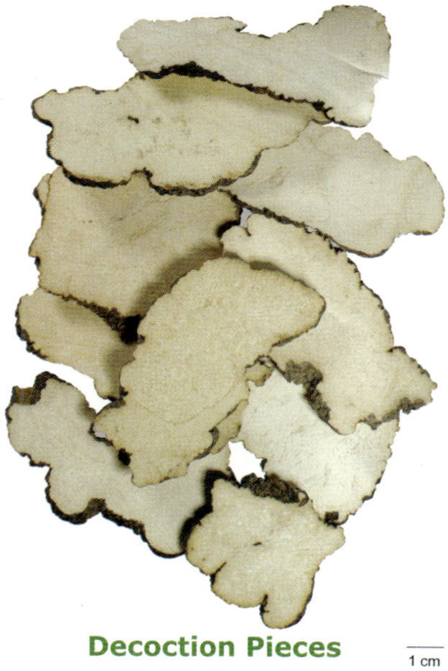

Decoction Pieces

Source

The sclerotium of *Polyporus umbellatus* (Pers.) Fries (Fam. Polyporaceae).

Distribution

Mainly in Chinese provinces such as Shaanxi, Yunnan, Henan and Shanxi. Mostly naturally grown, now successfully cultivated.

Harvest & Processing

Dig out sclerotia in spring and autumn; remove soil and sand; dry.

Description

Irregular pieces long, subspherical or flattened in shape, often rameous (branched); 5-25 cm long, 2-6 cm in diameter. Outer surface shrivelled or strumose (with cushion-like protuberances); greyish-black or brownish-black. Dense in texture but light in weight, floats in water. When broken, surface fine and smooth, relatively soft when pressed; off-white or yellowish-white, slightly granular. Odour: faint; taste: mild.

Indications

1. Odema, dysuria, stranguria, renal stone 2. Jaundice, chronic hepatitis 3. Leukorrhagia 4. Lung cancer, liver cancer, leukemia (IVI)

Chemical Composition

Contains polysaccharides and steroids such as polyporusterone A, B.

Poria

Indian Bread

Fuling

茯苓

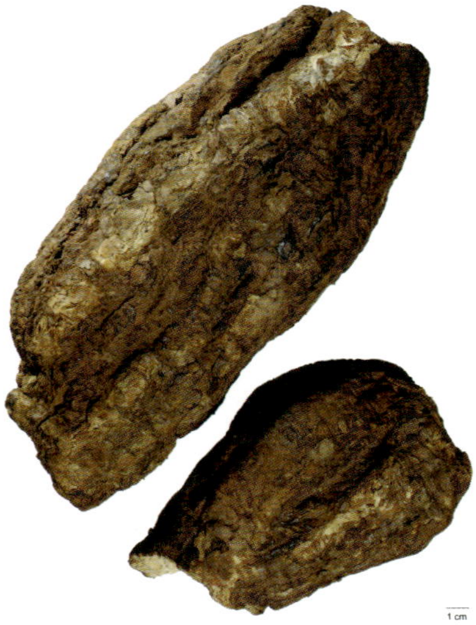

Crude Drug

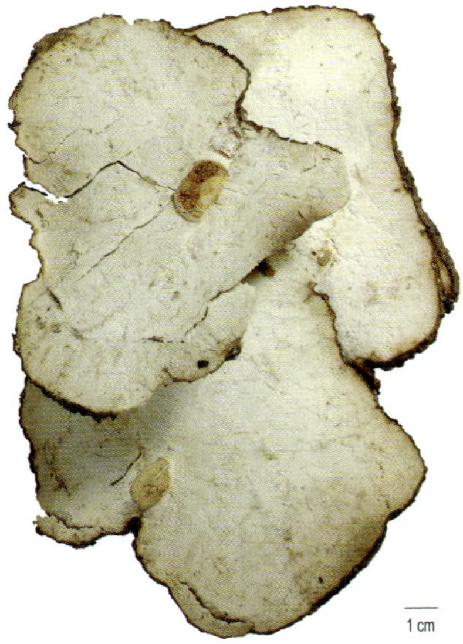

Decoction Pieces

Source The sclerotium of *Poria cocos* (Schw.) Wolf (Fam. Polyporaceae).

Distribution Mainly in Chinese provinces such as Yunnan, Hubei, Anhui and Guizhou. Cultivated or naturally grown.

Harvest & Processing Dig out wild Indian Bread mostly in pine forests from July to the following March, or collect cultivated Indian Bread between July and August in the second year after inoculation. Heap up fresh Indian Bread to let moisture evaporate; repeat a few times until wrinkles show on the outer surface and most moisture on the inside has been driven out; dry in shaded areas to produce '*Fuling ge*' (Intact Indian Bread).

Description *Fuling ge* (Intact Indian Bread): lumps subspherical, ellipsoid (elliptical in long-section and circular in cross-section) or irregular in shape; varying in size. Exoperidium thin and rough; reddish-brown to dull blackish-brown; marked with prominent, protuberant wrinkles. Heavy; hard and solid. Broken surface uneven; outer layer pale brown; inner part white and granular, very occasionally pale red.
Fuling kuai (Indian Bread in Pieces): pieces or slices cut from peeled Indian Bread; varying in size; sometimes with pine root remnants in the middle; white, pale red or pale brown.

Indications 1. Oedema, dysuria 2.Leukorrhagia 3. Cough 4. Diarrhoea, jaundice 5. Palpitaton, insomnia, dizziness, Chronic schizophrenia

Chemical Composition Contains triterpenes such as pachymic acid and eburicoic acid; also contains polysaccharides such as pachyman.

Pseudobulbus Cremastrae Seu Pleiones

Appendiculate Cremastra Pseudobulb

Shancigu

山慈菇

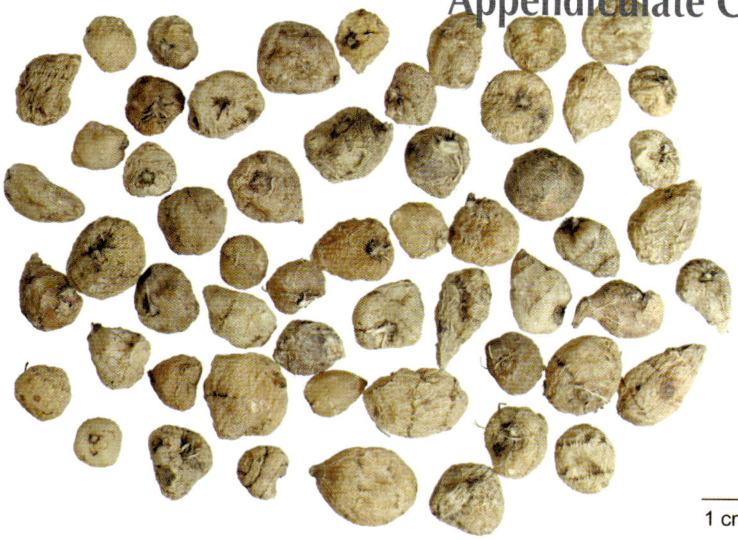

Crude Drug

Source The pseudobulb of *Cremastra appendiculata* (D. Don) Makino (Fam. Orchidaceae). Customarily called '*Mao Cigu*' (Hairy Appendiculate Cremastra Pseudobulb).

Distribution Mainly in chinese provinces such as Guizhou and Sichuan.

Harvest & Processing Collect pseudobulbs in summer and autumn; remove above-ground parts, soil and sand; group pseudobulbs according to size and cook thoroughly in boiling water; dry.

Description Flattened and spherical, or conical pieces irregular in shape; top end slightly protuberant, base with scars of fibrous roots; 1.5-3 cm long, bulgy part 1-2 cm in diameter. Outer surface yellowish-brown or reddish-brown, marked with longitudinal wrinkles or grooves; middle part with 2-3 slightly protuberant annular (ring-like) nodes; nodes with filiform (thread-like) fibres left by withered and rotted scale leaves. Hard, difficult to break; broken surface greyish-white or yellowish-white, slightly cuticular. Odour: faint; taste: mild, chewy.

Indications 1. Skin infection, scrofula and snakebite 2. Lymphosarcoma and cancer of breast, thyroid, skin, cervix, nasopharynx and oesophagus.

Chemical Composition Cremastosine I and II exist in the whole herb.

Note According to *C.P.*, also used for medicinal purposes is the pseudobulb of *Pleione bulbocodioides* (Franch.) Rolfe and *P. yunnanensis* Rolfe, both of which belong to the same family as *Cremastra appendiculata* (D. Don) Makino.

Radix Aconiti Brachypodi

Shortstalk Monkshood Root
Xueshangyizhihao

雪上一枝蒿

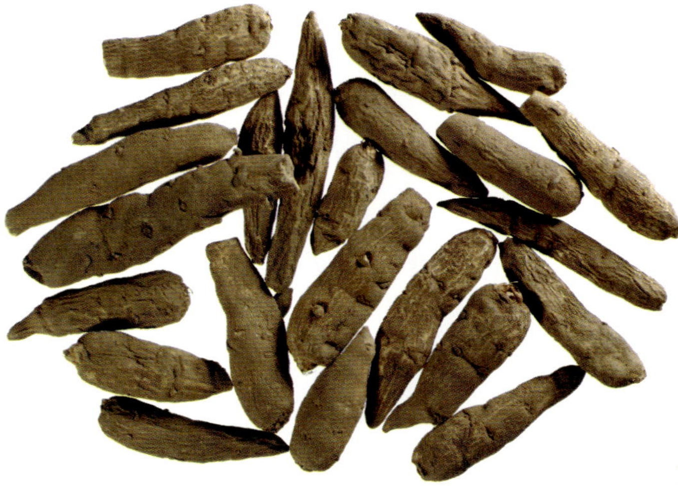

Crude Drug

1 cm

Source The root tuber of *Aconitum brachypodum* Diels. (Fam. Ranunculaceae).

Distribution Mainly in regions such as northwestern Yunnan province and western Sichuan province in China.

Harvest & Processing Dig up root tubers in late summer and early autumn; wash clean; dry under the sun; remove the surface.

Description Root tuber long and cylindrical, or conical; 2.5-7.5 cm long, 0.5-1.5 cm in diameter. Outer surface of lateral roots greyish-brown, smooth or marked with shallow wrinkles and scars of rootlets; hard and brittle, breaks easily; broken surface white, starchy, with a blackish-brown ring. Outer surface of axial root dark brown, marked with longitudinal wrinkles and remnants of lateral root base; broken surface uneven, with numerous clefts in the centre. Odour: faint; taste: tongue-numbing. Extremely toxic.

Indications 1. Rheumatism, trauma, acrodynia, toothache, sores, cancerous pain

Chemical Composition Mainly contains diterpene alkaloids.

Note Listed in Hong Kong as Category I (Toxic/Potent) Chinese Materia Medica.

Radix Aconiti Kusnezoffii

Kusnezoff Monkshood Root

Caowu

草烏

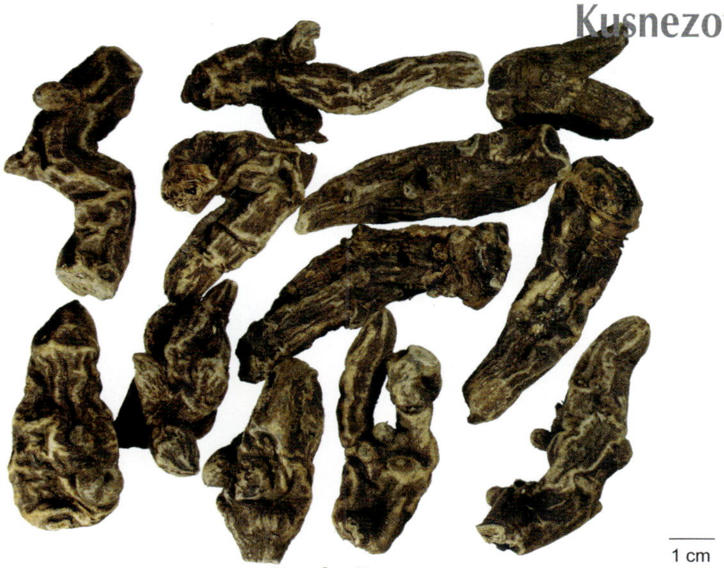

Crude Drug

Source The root tuber of *Aconitum kusnezoffii* Reichb. (Fam. Ranunculaceae).

Distribution Mainly in Chinese provinces such as Heilongjiang, Liaoning, Jilin and Hebei.

Harvest & Processing Dig out root tubers in autumn when leaves wither; remove rootlets, soil and sand; dry.

Description Irregular, long and conical, slightly curved; 2-7 cm long; 0.6-1.8 cm in diameter. Top end often with stem remnants and sparse remnants of adventitious root base; in some cases top end with a withered bud, one lateral side with an orbicular (round) or disc-like remnants of adventitious root base. Outer surface dull greyish-brown or dark reddish-brown, marked with longitudinal wrinkles, punctiform (dot-like) scars of rootlets and several strumiform (cushion-like) lateral roots. Hard; broken surface greyish-white or dull grey, with clefts; cambium ring polygonal and suborbicular (almost round); pith relatively large or hollow. Odourless; taste: pungent and tongue-numbing.

Indications 1. Rheumatic arthralgia 2. Sciatica 3. Hemiplegia, muscular spasm 4. Trauma 5. As local anaesthetic.

Chemical Composition Mainly contains alkaloids such as aconitine, mesaconitine and beiwutine.

Note Radix Aconiti Kusnezoffii is listed in Hong Kong as Category I (Toxic/Potent) Chinese Materia Medica, and the processed Radix Aconiti Kusnezoffii, Category II.

Radix Aconiti Lateralis Preparata

Prepared Common Monkshood Daughter Root

Fuzi

附子

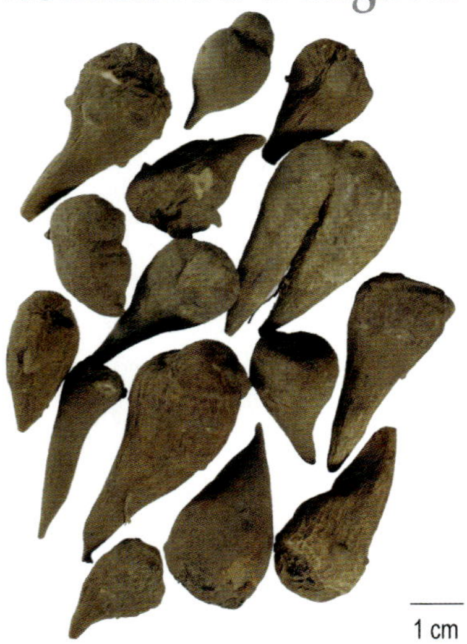

1 cm

Crude Drug

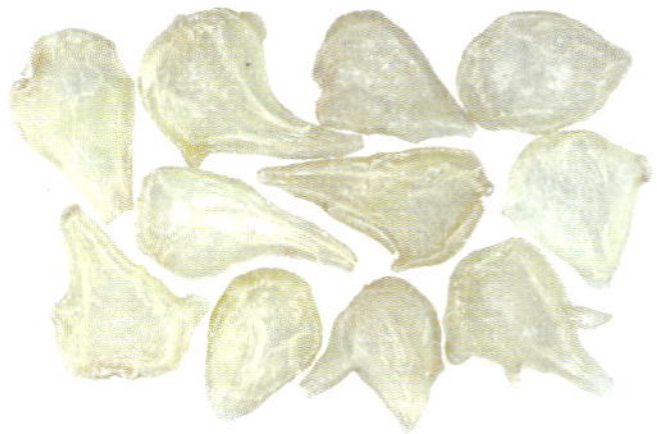

1 cm

Decoction Pieces (Baifupian)

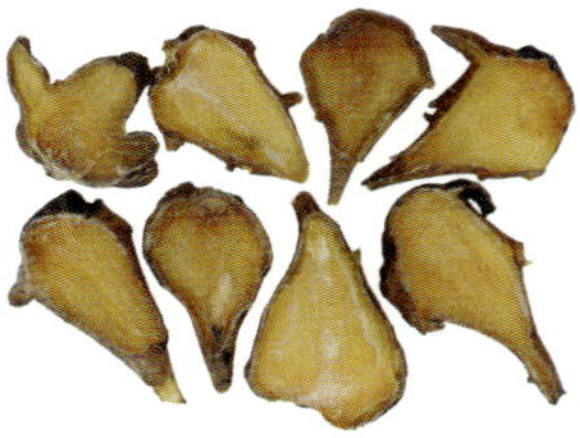

1 cm

Decoction Pieces (Heifupian)

Source The lateral root of *Aconitum carmichaeli* Debx. (Fam. Ranunculaceae).

Distribution Mainly in Chinese provinces such as Sichuan and Shaanxi.

Harvest & Processing Dig out whole plants from late June to early August; shake off soil and sand; take lateral roots (Common Monkshood Daughter Root) and remove fibrous roots. The lateral roots, commonly called '*Nifuzi*' (Earthy Common Monkshood Daughter Root), must be processed immediately. The directly dried '*Ni fuzi*' is called '*Sheng fuzi*' (Crude Common Monkshood Daughter Root).

Description Conical; 4-7 cm long, 3-5 cm in diameter. Outer surface greyish-black, covered with salt crystals; apex marked with dented bud scars; strumiform (cushion-like) branch roots or branch root scars on all sides. Heavy in weight. Cross-section dull greyish-brown, with a polygonal cambium ring; vessels inside cambium ring irregularly arranged. Odour: faint; taste: numbing, tongue-pricking.

Indications 1. Shock 2. Impotence, emission 3. Urinary frequency, oedema 4. Diarrhoea, constipation 5. Arthralgia, periarthritis of shoulder joint.

Chemical Composition Mainly contains alkaloids such as aconitine and mesaconitine.

Note Listed in Hong Kong as Category I (Toxic/Potent) Chinese Materia Medica, and the processed Radix Aconiti Lateralis Preparata, Category II.

Radix Adenophorae

Fourleaf Ladybell Root

Nanshashen

南沙參

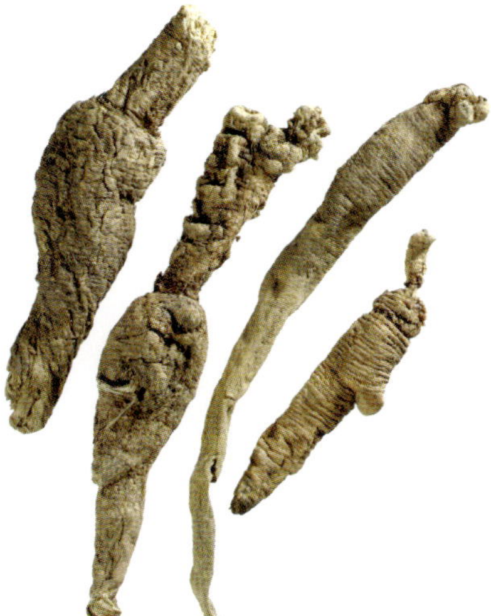

1 cm

Crude Drug

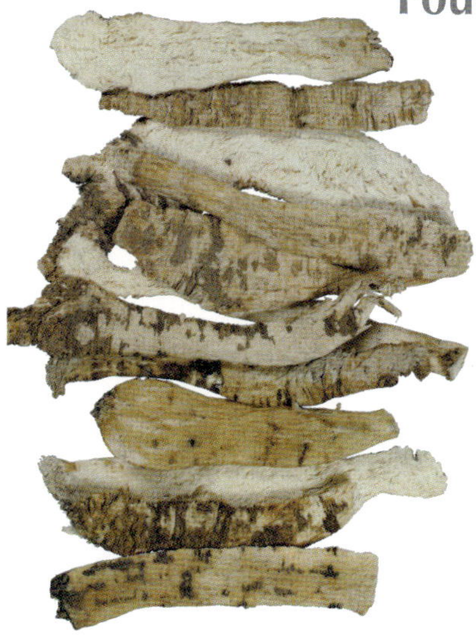

Decoction Pieces

1 cm

Source The root of *Adenophora tetraphylla* (Thunb.) Fisch. (Fam. Campanulaceae).

Distribution Mainly in Chinese provinces such as Anhui, Jiangsu, Zhejiang and Guizhou.

Harvest & Processing Dig out roots in spring and autumn; wash away soil; scrape away cork while fresh; wash clean; dry under the sun. Commonly used in Hong Kong in the form of length-wise cut slices.

Description Conical and slightly curved; 7-27 cm long, 0.8-3 cm in diameter. Top end with 1 or 2 rhizomes (rootstocks). After removal of cork, outer surface yellowish-white or pale brownish-yellow; dented parts often with cork remnants; upper part mostly with interrupted annulations of deep transverse striae, lower part with longitudinal striae and grooves. Light in weight; texture loose, breaks easily. When broken, surface uneven, marked with alternating yellow and white markings and numerous clefts. Odourless; taste: slightly sweet.

Indications 1. Rheumatic arthralgia 2. Sciatica 3. Hemiplegia, muscular spasm 4. Trauma 5. As a local anaesthetic.

Chemical Composition Mainly contains phenolic glycoside, such as shashenoside I, II, III.

Note According to *C.P.*, also used for medicinal purposes is the root of *A. stricta* Miq.

Radix Ampelopsis

Japanese Ampelopsis Root
Bailian

白蘞

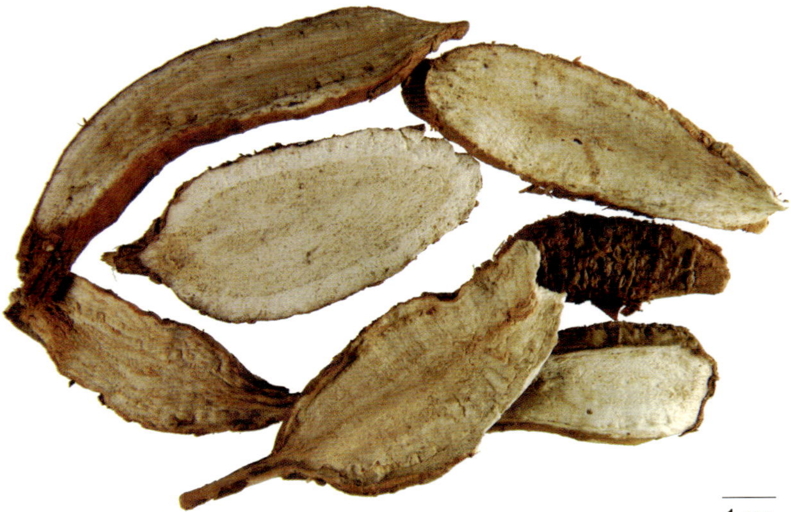

Crude Drug

Source The root tuber of *Ampelopsis japonica* (Thunb.) Makino (Fam. Vitaceae).

Distribution Mainly in Chinese provinces such as Henan, Hubei, Jiangxi and Anhui.

Harvest & Processing Collect root tubers in spring and autumn; remove stems and fine rootlets; wash root tubers clean; usually cut length-wise into two or four pieces or angled-cut into slices; dry under the sun.

Description Pieces cut length-wise are oblong and orbicular (round), or roughly spindle-shaped; 4-10 cm long, 1-2 cm in diameter. Outer surface reddish-brown or dull reddish-brown, marked with wrinkles, fine transverse striae and lalongate (transversely elongated) lenticels; bark flakes off easily; inner surface pale reddish-brown. When cut length-wise, surface marked with a protuberant ridge. When angled-cut, surface ovate (egg-shaped); 2.5-5 cm long, 2-3 cm wide. Cut surface powdery-white or light reddish-brown, marked with radial markings; margin relatively thick. Disperse dust when snapped. Odour: faint; taste: sweet.

Indications 1. Dermatitis, pyogenic skin infection, ulcerous disease of skin 2. Burns (external use).

Chemical Composition Mainly contains gallotannins.

Radix Angelicae Dahuricae

Dahurian Angelica Root
Baizhi

白芷

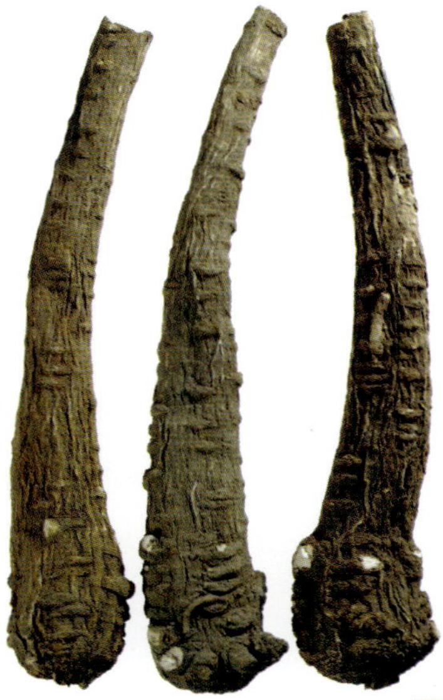

Crude Drug 1 cm

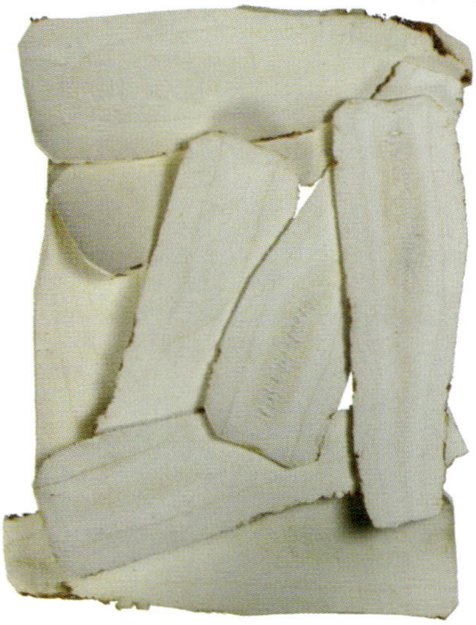

Decoction Pieces 1 cm

Source The root of *Angelica dahurica* (Fisch. ex Hoffm.) Benth. et Hook. f. *ex* Franch. et Sav. cv. Hangbaizhi (Fam. Umbelliferae).

Distribution Mainly in Chinese provinces such as Zhejiang and Sichuan.

Harvest & Processing Dig out roots between summer and autumn when leaves turn yellow; remove fibrous roots, soil and sand; dry under the sun or at low temperatures. Commonly used in Hong Kong in the form of length-wise cut slices.

Description Long and conical; 10-25 cm long, 1.5-2.5 cm in diameter. Outer surface greyish-brown or yellowish-brown; top part obtuse and quadrangular (four-angled), or suborbicular (almost round); surface marked with longitudinal wrinkles, branch root scars and lenticel-like, lalongate (transversely elongated) protuberances, sometimes arranged into 4 columns; top end marked with dented stem scars. Hard and solid; broken surface white or greyish-white, starchy; cambium ring brown, subquadrate (almost square) or suborbicular (almost round); cortex scattered with numerous brown oil dots. Odour: aromatic; taste: acrid, slightly bitter.

Indications 1. Common cold, sinusitis 2. Headache, toothache 3. Haemorrhoid complicated by anal fistula, haematochezia, 4. Burns, dermatitis and boils 5. Morbid leukorrhoea

Chemical Composition Mainly contains coumarins such as imperatorin and oxypeucedanin.

Note According to *C.P.*, also used for medicinal purposes is the root of *A. dahurica* (Fisch. *ex* Hoffm.) Benth. *et* Hook. f. *ex* Franch. *et* Sav. Qibaizhi.

Radix Angelicae Pubescentis

Doubleteeth Pubescent Angelica Root

Duhuo

獨活

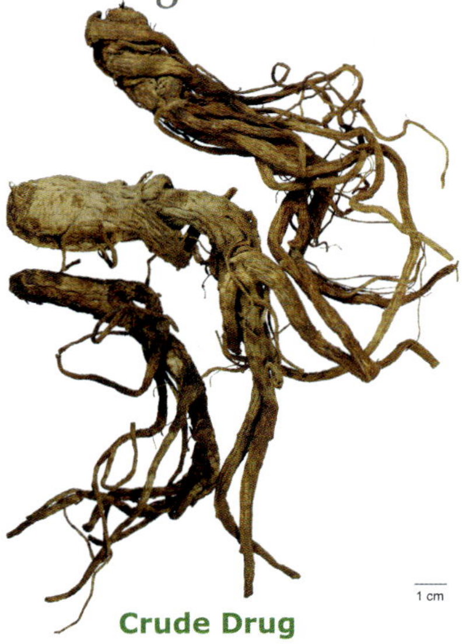

Crude Drug

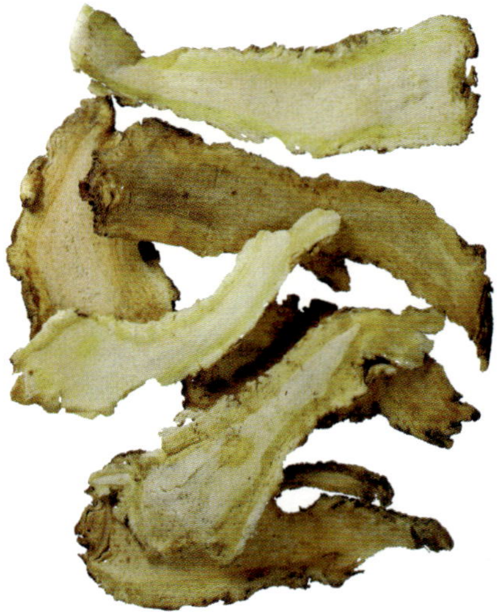

Decoction Pieces 1 cm

Source The root of *Angelica pubescens* Maxim. f. *biserrata* Shan et Yuan (Fam. Umbelliferae).

Distribution Mainly in Chinese provinces such as Hubei and Sichuan.

Harvest & Processing Dig out roots in early spring when shoots start to germinate, or in late autumn when leaves wither; remove stem remnants, fibrous roots and soil; dry by heat until half-dry; pile up for 2-3 days to soften; dry by heat again. Commonly used in Hong Kong in the form of length-wise cut slices.

Description Axial root thick and short, slightly cylindrical, with 2-3 branches or more at lower part; 10-30 cm long, 1.5-3 cm in diameter. Top part bulgy, marked with transverse wrinkles; top end dented or with stem and leaf scars. Outer surface dull greyish-brown or reddish-brown, marked with deep longitudinal wrinkles, protuberant lalongate (transversely elongated) lenticels and slightly protuberant rootlet scars. Relatively hard, softens when moistened. When broken, phloem greyish-white, scattered with numerous brown oil dots; cambium ring brown; xylem yellowish-brown. Odour: with a distinctive fragrance; taste: bitter-acrid, slightly tongue-numbing.

Indications 1. Arthralgia 2.Common cold, influenza with severe chill, low-grade fever and generalized pain 3. Toothache (external use).

Chemical Composition Mainly contains essential oils and coumarin.

Radix Angelicae Sinensis

Chinese Angelica
Danggui

當歸

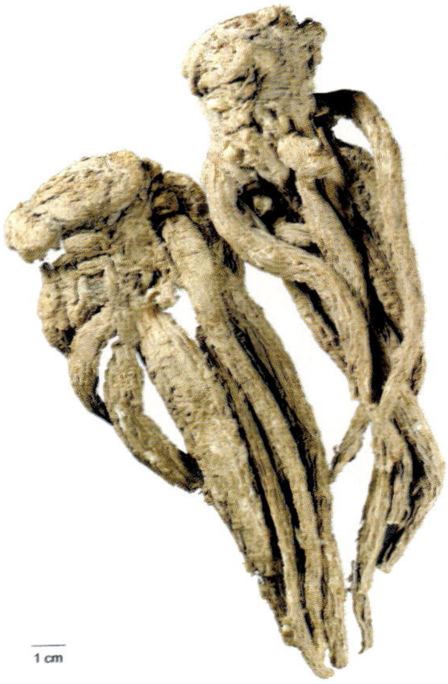

Crude Drug

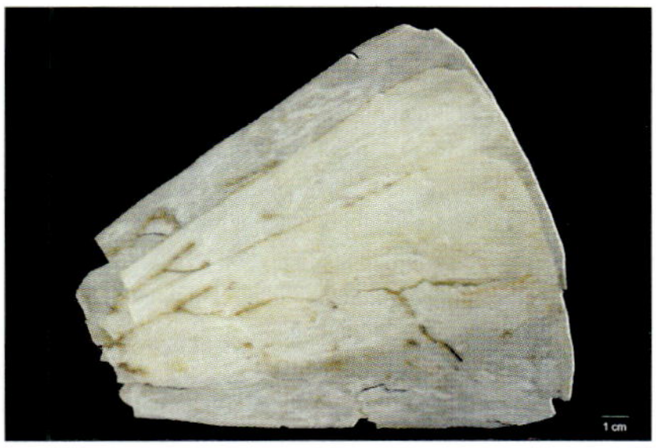

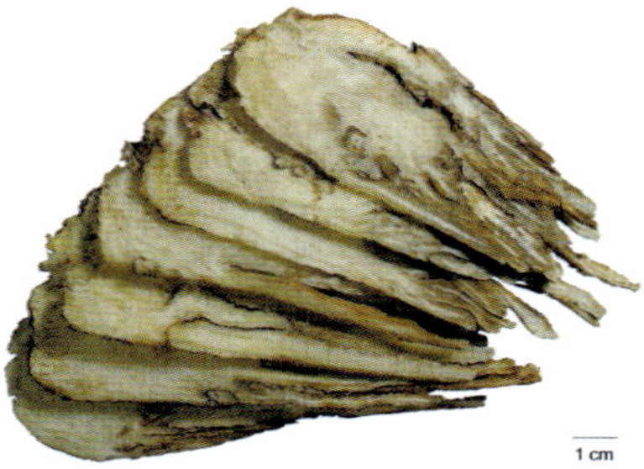

Decoction Pieces

Source The root of *Angelica sinensis* (Oliv.) Diels (Fam. Umbelliferae).

Distribution Mainly in Chinese provinces such as Gansu. Mostly cultivated.

Harvest & Processing Dig up roots after autumn, generally in the second year of cultivation; remove leaves, rootlets and soil; let stand to let the moisture inside evaporate briefly until the roots soften; tie into small bundles; dry slowly over low heat. Commonly used in Hong Kong in the form of length-wise cut slices of the top part or of the whole root.

Description Slightly cylindrical; upper part known as '*guitou*' (Angelica head), axial root known as '*guishen*' (Angelica body), branch roots known as '*gui wei*' (Angelica tails), whole root known as '*quangui*' ('whole Angelica'). Bark yellowish-brown to reddish-brown, marked with longitudinal wrinkles and lalongate (transversely elongated) lenticels; axial root thick and short, lower part with branch roots; branch roots thick at top part and tapering downwards, mostly twisted and marked with a few scars of rootlets. Soft and pliable; when broken, surface yellowish-white or pale yellowish-brown; cortex thick, marked with brown oil dots; cambium ring yellowish-brown; xylem lighter in colour, marked with radial markings; the core of broken surface of top part usually with pith and a cavity. Odour: heavily aromatic; taste: sweet, acrid and slightly bitter.

Indications 1. Anaemia 2. Menstrual disorders 3. Headache, abdominal pain, chest pain, coronary heart disease, rheumatism, trauma 4. Constipation 5. Carbuncles and sores

Chemical Composition Mainly contains essential oils with the ligustilide as the main component; also contains polyacetylene such as falcarindol.

Radix Ardisiae Crenatae

Coral Ardisia Root
Zhushagen

朱砂根

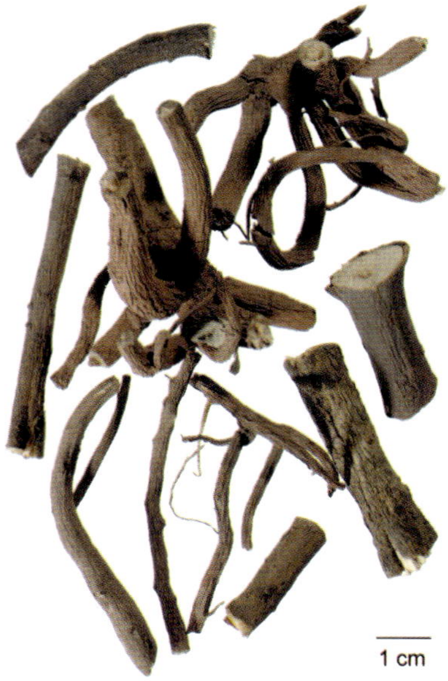

Crude Drug

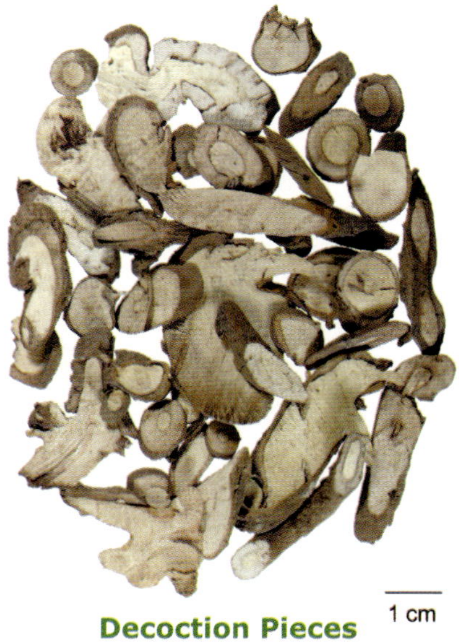

Decoction Pieces

Source The root of *Ardisia crenata* Sims (Fam. Myrsinaceae).

Distribution Mainly in Chinese provinces such as Guangxi, Guangdong, Jiangxi and Zhejiang; also in Hong Kong.

Harvest & Processing Dig up roots in autumn; cut into slices; dry under the sun or use while fresh.

Description Roots conglomerate (densely clustered) on slightly bulgy rhizome; cylindrical, slightly curving; 5-25 cm long, 2-10 cm in diameter. Outer surface dull greyish-brown or greyish-brown; with numerous longitudinal wrinkles and transverse or annular (ring-like) cracks; cortex and xylem separate easily. Hard and brittle, break easily. When broken, surface uneven; cortex thick, about half the size of broken surface, off-white or light purplish-red; xylem pale yellow. Odour: faint; taste: slightly bitter, acrid and tongue-pricking.

Indications 1. Sore throat 2. Rheumatism, trauma 3. Jaundice 4. Dysentery 5. Lymphangitis of lower limbs, mastitis, orchitis

Chemical Composition Mainly contains triterpene saponins such as ardicrenin.

Radix Ardisiae Gigantifoliae

Giganticleaf Ardisia Root

Zoumatai

走馬胎

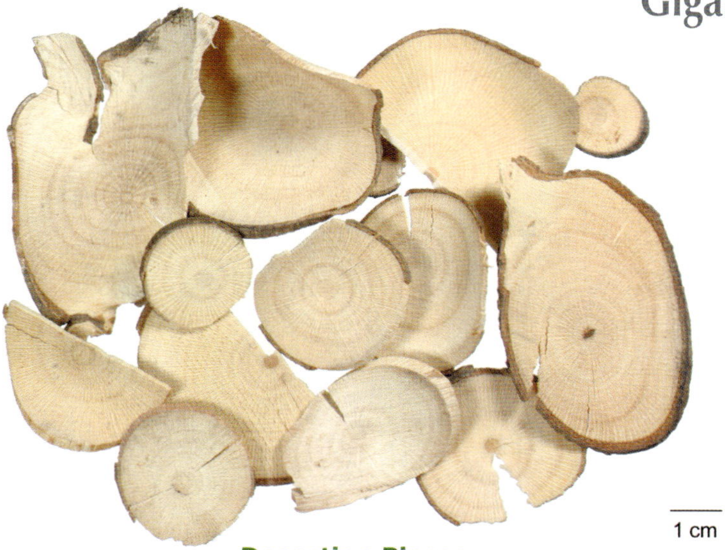

Decoction Pieces

Source The root and rhizome of *Ardisia gigantifolia* Stapf. (Fam. Myrsinaceae).

Distribution Mainly in Chinese provinces such as Guangdong and Guangxi; also in provinces such as Fujian, Jiangxi and Yunnan.

Harvest & Processing Collect roots and rhizomes in autumn; wash clean; use while fresh, or slice and dry under the sun.

Description Root irregular and cylindrical, slightly torose (cylindrical with alternate swellings and constrictions) and bulgy; varying in length, 1.5-4 cm in diameter. Outer surface dull greyish-brown or dull purplish; marked with longitudinal grooves; cortex falls off easily, about 2 mm thick. Hard, does not break easily. When broken, surface shows pale red cortex with purplish-red dots; xylem yellowish-white, with fine dense radial rays called '*juhua wen*' (chrysanthemum markings). Commercial products usually come in angled-cut slices about 2 mm thick. Odour: faint; taste: mild, slightly acrid.

Indications 1. Rheumatism 2. Postpartum lochiostasis, postpartum abdominal pain 3. Carbuncle, gangrene, cellulites, ulcerative skin lesion 4. Post traumatic swelling and pain

Chemical Composition Mainly contains 2-methyl-5-(Z-nonadec-14-engl)-vesorcinol and 5-(Z-nonadec-14-enyl)-resorcinol.

Radix Aristolochiae

Slender Dutchmanspipe Root
Qingmuxiang

青木香

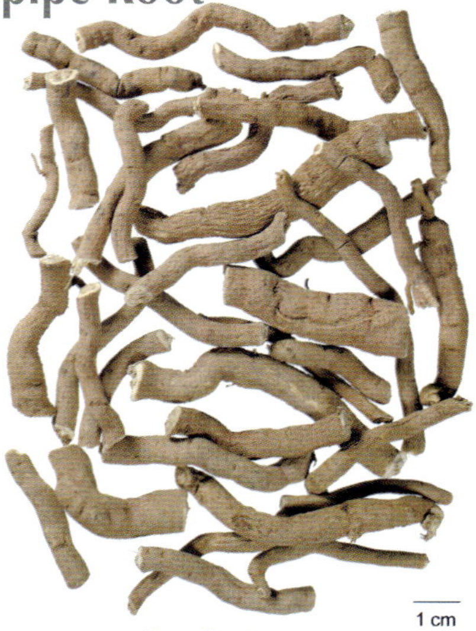

Crude Drug

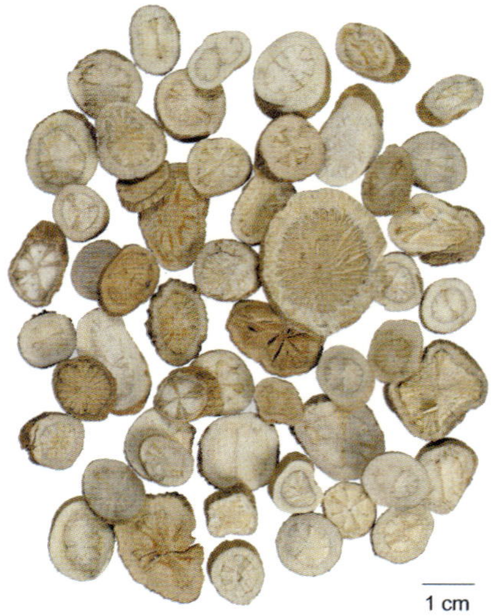

Decoction Pieces

Source The root of *Aristolochia debilis* Sieb. et Zucc. (Fam. Aristolochiaceae).

Distribution Mainly in Chinese provinces such as Jiangsu, Anhui, Zhejiang, Hunan and Sichuan.

Harvest & Processing Collect roots in spring and autumn; remove rootlets, soil and sand; dry under the sun.

Description Cylindrical, or slightly flattened and cylindrical, somewhat undulate (wavy); 3-15 cm long, 0.5-1.5 cm in diameter. Outer surface dull yellowish-brown or greyish-brown, marked with longitudinal wrinkles and scars of rootlets. Hard and brittle; when broken, surface shows faint cambium rings, pale yellow cortex, broad milky-white xylem rays, radial pale yellow xylem bundles and conspicuous vessel pores. Odour: fragrant and distinctive; taste: bitter.

Indications 1. Dizziness, headache and distending pain in the chest and abdomen 2. Carbuncles, boils 3. Snakebite, insect bite.

Chemical Composition Mainly contains alkaloids such as aristolochic acid A, B, C and tetrandrine.

Radix Aristolochiae Fangchi

Southern Fangchi Root

Guangfangji

廣防己

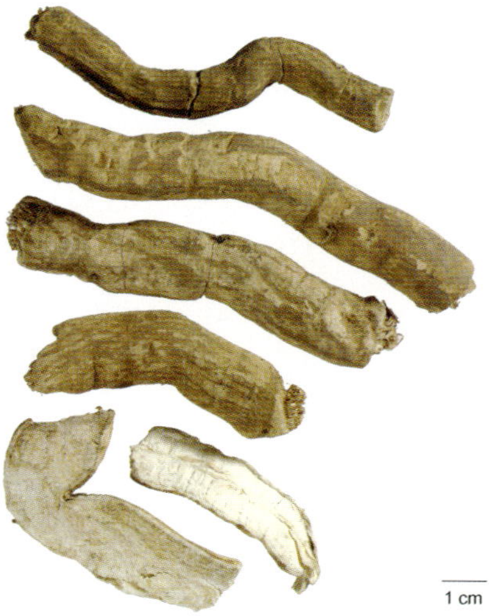

Crude Drug

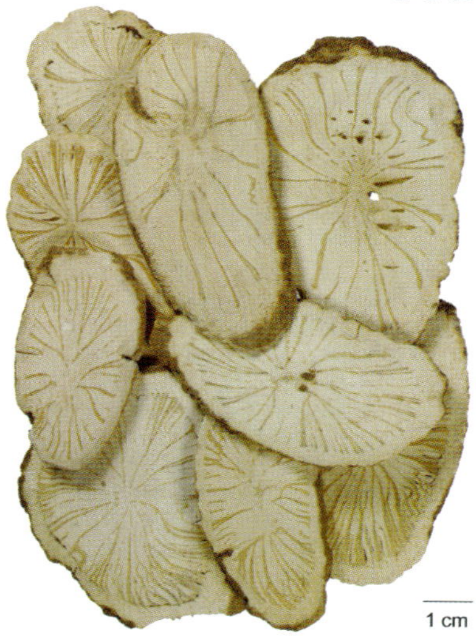

Decoction Pieces

Source The root of *Aristolochia fangchi* Y. C. Wu *ex* L. D. Chou et S. M. Hwang (Fam. Aristolochiaceae).

Distribution Mainly in Chinese provinces such as Guangdong and Guangxi.

Harvest & Processing Dig up roots in autumn and winter; wash clean; cut into sections; cut thick roots longitudinally into halves; dry under the sun.

Description Cylindrical or semi-cylindrical, slightly curved; 6-18 cm long, 1.5-4.5 cm in diameter. Outer surface greyish-brown, rough, marked with longitudinal grooves; roots with cork removed pale yellow and knife-scarred. Heavy, hard and solid, does not break easily; broken surface off-white, starchy, marked with radial, alternating greyish-brown and off-white striae. Customarily called '*chelun wen*'(wheel-spoke lines). Odourless; taste: bitter.

Indications 1. Arthralgia, acrodynia 2. Oedema, dysuria 3. Sores

Chemical Composition Mainly contains alkaloids such as aristolochic acid I and magnoflorine.

Radix Aristolochiae Heterophyllae

Yellowmouth Dutchmanspipe Root
Hanzhongfangji

漢中防己

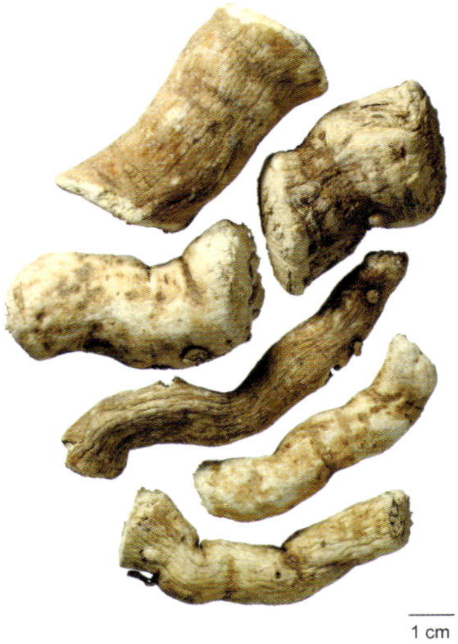

Crude Drug

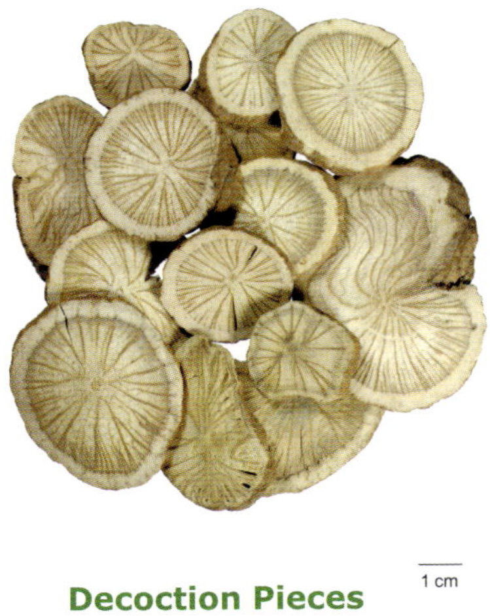

Decoction Pieces

Source
The root of *Aristolochia heterophylla* Hemsl. (Fam. Aristolochiaceae).

Distribution
Mainly in Chinese provinces such as Shaanxi, Hubei, Gansu and Sichuan.

Harvest & Processing
Collect roots in autumn; wash clean; cut into sections; cut thick ones length-wise into halves; dry under the sun.

Description
Cylindrical, slightly curved; 4-15 cm long, 1.5-3 cm in diameter; mostly pale yellowish-brown, with cork almost completely removed; cork remnants dull greyish-brown. Hard, does not break easily. Broken surface yellowish-white, starchy; cortex relatively thick; xylem with striae radiating from the centre, like wheel spokes, in a dichotomous (branched into two divisions) or tri-chotomous (branched into three divisions) manner. Odour: faint; taste: bitter-astringent.

Indications
1. Arthralgia, trauma, angina pectoris 2. Oedema, dysuria
3. Dyspnoeic cough, haemoptysis with copious expectoration
4. Hypertension 5. Lung cancer, squamous cell epithelioma.

Chemical Composition
Mainly contains aristolochic acid A and allantoin.

Radix Asparagi

Cochinchinese Asparagus Root
Tiandong
天冬

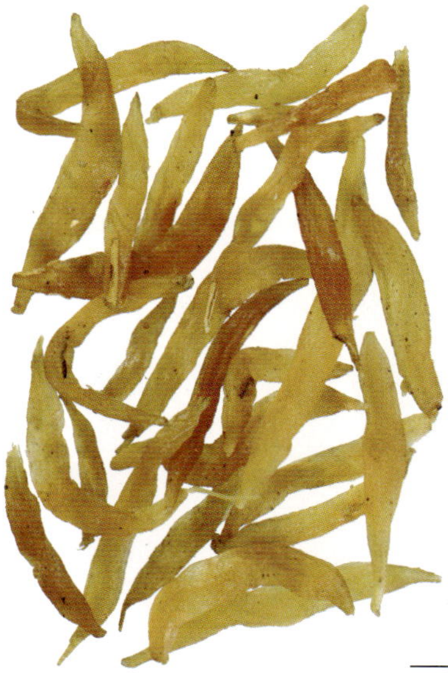

Crude Drug

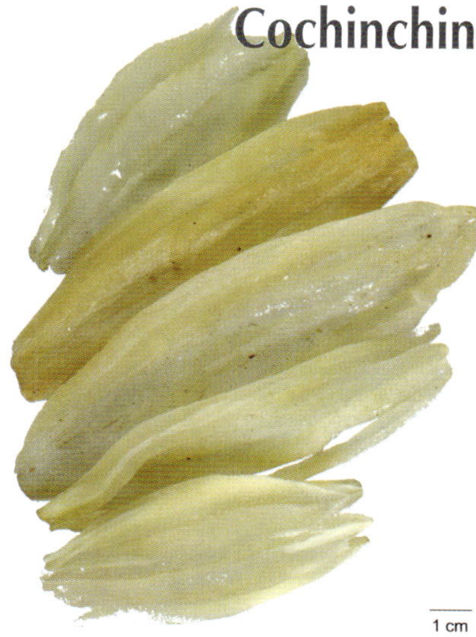

Decoction Pieces

Source The root tuber of *Asparagus cochinchinensis* (Lour.) Merr. (Fam. Liliaceae).

Distribution Mainly in Chinese provinces such as Guizhou, Sichuan and Guangxi; also in Hong Kong.

Harvest & Processing Collect root tubers in autumn and winter; wash away soil, remove top part and fibrous roots; cook or steam root tubers thoroughly; peel off cork while still hot; wash clean; dry under the sun. Commonly used in Hong Kong in the form of length-wise cut and compressed slices, with the woody core removed.

Description Oblong and spindle-shaped, slightly curved; 5-18 cm long, 0.5-2 cm in diameter. Outer surface yellowish-white to pale yellowish-brown; translucent; smooth or marked with longitudinal wrinkles of varying depths, and occasionally with remnants of greyish-brown cork. An opaque fine woody core visible when held against the light. Hard, or soft and smooth; sticky. When broken, surface cuticular, with a yellowish-white stele. Odour: faint; taste: sweet and slightly bitter.

Indications 1. Cough and sputum due to wasting disease 2. Chronic bronchitis 3. Thirst 4. Constipation 5. Pyogenic skin infection, snakebite (external use).

Chemical Composition Mainly contains steroidal saponins such as Asp-IV, Asp-V.

Radix Aucklandiae

Common Aucklandia Root
Muxiang

木香

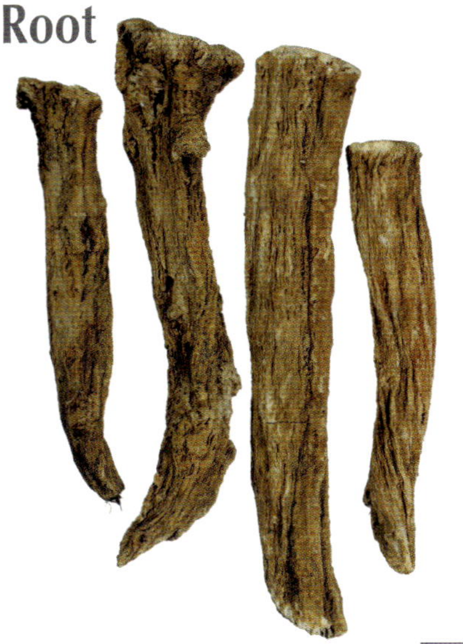

Crude Drug

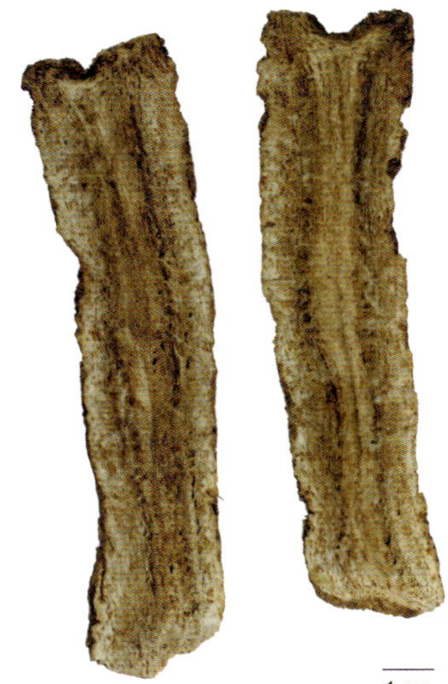

Decoction Pieces

Source The root of *Aucklandia lappa* Decne. (Fam. Compositae).

Distribution Mainly in Chinese provinces such as Yunnan (hence the name '*Yun muxiang*' [Yunnan Common Aucklandia Root]); also in provinces such as Sichuan and in Tibet.

Harvest & Processing Dig up roots of plants 2-3 years old in autumn and winter; remove leaves, rootlets and soil; cut roots into segments or slice length-wise into pieces; dry under the sun or by wind; remove cork. Commonly used in Hong Kong in the form of length-wise cut slices.

Description Cylindrical or semi-cylindrical; about 5-10 cm long, 0.5-5 cm in diameter. Outer surface yellowish-brown to dull greyish-brown; cork mostly removed; surface marked with conspicuous wrinkles, longitudinal grooves and scars of rootlets. Hard, solid and heavy; does not break easily. When broken, surface relatively even, dull greyish-brown to dull drown; cambium ring brown; with radial markings and scattered punctiform (dot-like) dull brownish oil cavities. Core of old roots often looks like withered wood. Odour: fragrant and distinctive; taste: slightly bitter.

Indications 1. Distending pain in the chest and epigastrium, tenesmus in dysentery 2. Diarrhoea, vomitting.

Chemical Composition Mainly contains dehydrocostus lactone and costunolide.

Radix Asparagi

Cochinchinese Asparagus Root
Tiandong
天冬

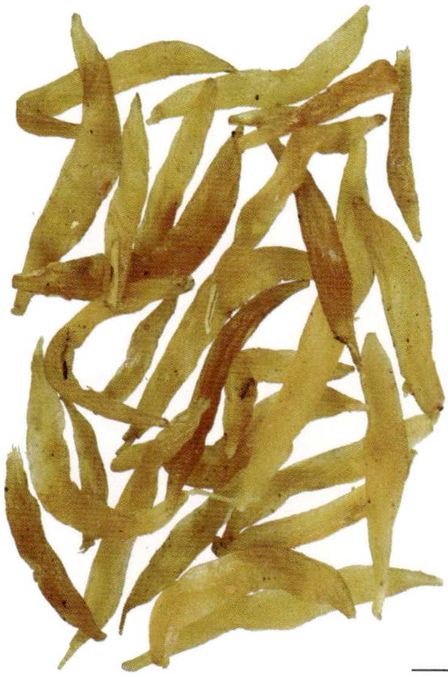

1 cm

Crude Drug

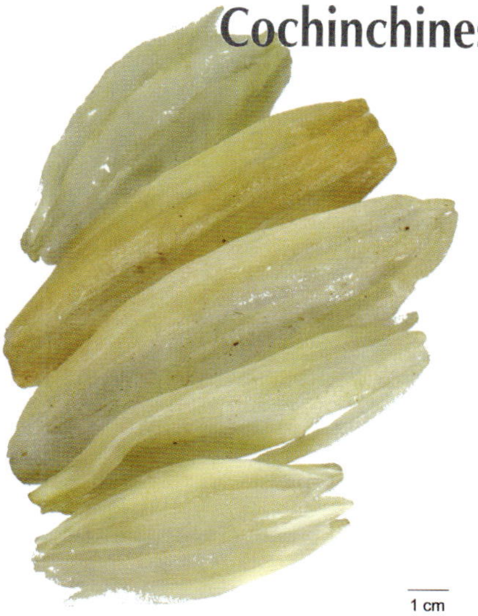

1 cm

Decoction Pieces

Source The root tuber of *Asparagus cochinchinensis* (Lour.) Merr. (Fam. Liliaceae).

Distribution Mainly in Chinese provinces such as Guizhou, Sichuan and Guangxi; also in Hong Kong.

Harvest & Processing Collect root tubers in autumn and winter; wash away soil, remove top part and fibrous roots; cook or steam root tubers thoroughly; peel off cork while still hot; wash clean; dry under the sun. Commonly used in Hong Kong in the form of length-wise cut and compressed slices, with the woody core removed.

Description Oblong and spindle-shaped, slightly curved; 5-18 cm long, 0.5-2 cm in diameter. Outer surface yellowish-white to pale yellowish-brown; translucent; smooth or marked with longitudinal wrinkles of varying depths, and occasionally with remnants of greyish-brown cork. An opaque fine woody core visible when held against the light. Hard, or soft and smooth; sticky. When broken, surface cuticular, with a yellowish-white stele. Odour: faint; taste: sweet and slightly bitter.

Indications 1. Cough and sputum due to wasting disease 2. Chronic bronchitis 3. Thirst 4. Constipation 5. Pyogenic skin infection, snakebite (external use).

Chemical Composition Mainly contains steroidal saponins such as Asp-IV, Asp-V.

Radix Asteris

Tatarian Aster Root
Ziyuan

紫菀

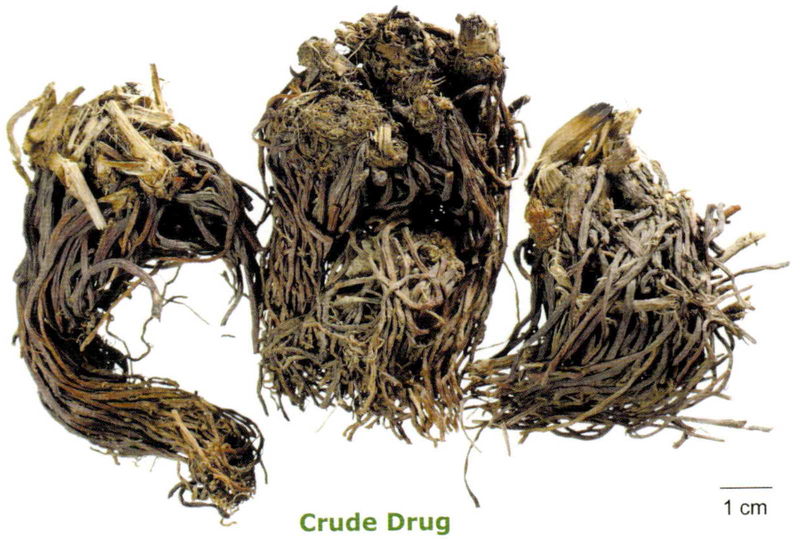

Crude Drug

Source The root and rhizome of *Aster tataricus* L. f. (Fam. Compositae).

Distribution Mainly in Chinese provinces such as Hebei, Anhui, Henan and Heilongjiang.

Harvest & Processing Dig out roots and rhizomes in spring and autumn; remove nodose (with nodes) rhizomes and soil; braid rootlets and dry rhizomes under the sun, or dry rhizomes under the sun without braiding.

Description Rhizome in irregular lumps; varying in size; top end with caudex and remnants of petiole base. Rootlets numerous, conglomerate (densely clustered) on rhizome; 3-15 cm long, 1-3 mm in diameter; usually braided. Outer surface purplish-red or greyish-red, marked with longitudinal wrinkles. Texture relatively soft and pliable; when broken, surface greyish-white, with purple rim. Odour: slightly fragrant; taste: sweet and slightly bitter.

Indications Various kinds of cough such as that caused by upper respiratory infection, non-productive cough with dyspnoea and chronic cough with bloody sputum

Chemical Composition Mainly contains triterpene saponins such as aster saponins A, B, C, D; Oilgopeptides such as asterin A, B.

Radix Astragali

Milkvetch Root

Huangqi

黃芪

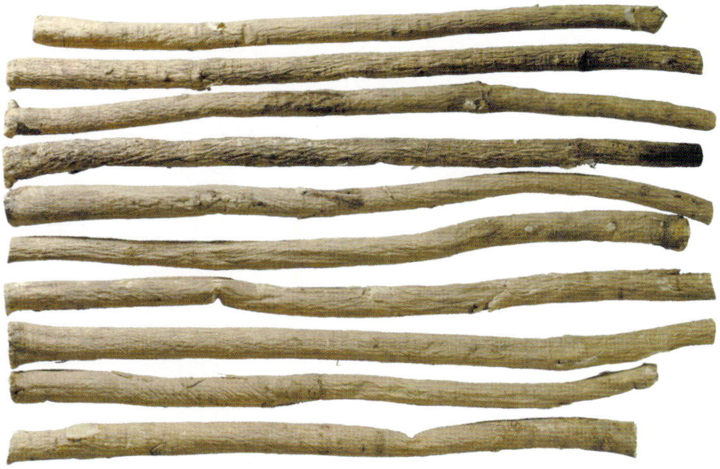

Crude Drug 5 cm

Source The root of *Astragalus membranaceus* (Fisch.) Bge. *var. mongholocus* (Bunge) Hsiao (Fam. Leguminosae).

Distribution Mainly in Chinese provinces such as Shanxi, Jilin and Hebei and in Inner Mongolia.

Harvest & Processing Dig out roots from September to November in autumn, or in spring before buds germinate; cut off rootstocks; shake off soil and sand; dry roots under the sun until half-dry; pile up for 1-2 days; dry under the sun again until completely dry; clip away lateral roots and fibrous roots; tie into small bundles. Commonly used in Hong Kong in the form of length-wise cut slices.

Description Cylindrical; thick at top and tapering downwards, seldom rameous (branched); 20-60 cm long, 1-3 cm in diameter. Outer surface pale yellowish-brown to dull dark brown; marked with conspicuous wrinkles and lalongate (transversely elongated) lenticels. Hard but slightly pliable; broken surface fibrous, starchy. Cross-section milky-white to pale yellow; xylem pale yellow, with fine and dense rays; phloem rays slightly curved; with clefts. Odour: distinctive and bean-like; taste: slightly sweet.

Indications 1. Perspiration caused by weakness or from no apparent cause 2. Chronic diarrhoea, rectal prolapse 3. General fatigue

Chemical Composition Mainly contains triterpene saponins such as astragaloside I, II, IV.

Note According to *C.P.*, also used for medicinal purposes is the root of *A. membranaceus* (Fisch.) Bge.

Radix Aucklandiae

Common Aucklandia Root
Muxiang

木香

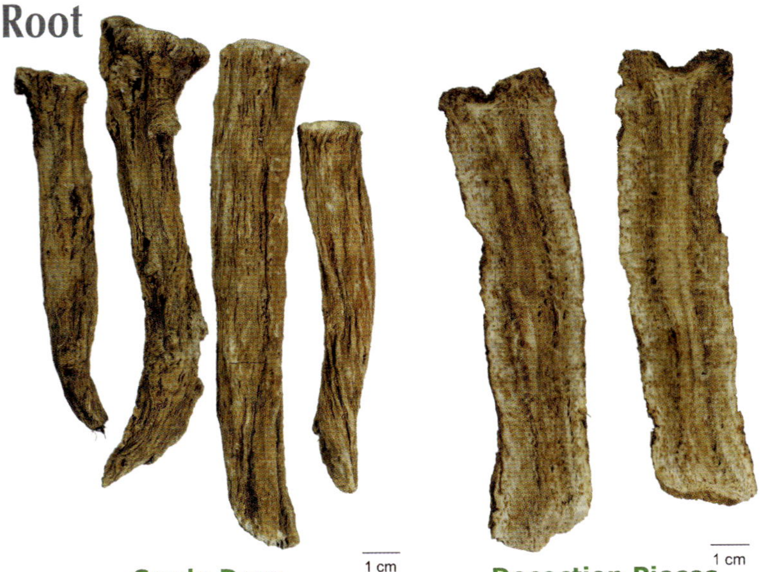

Crude Drug   Decoction Pieces

Source The root of *Aucklandia lappa* Decne. (Fam. Compositae).

Distribution Mainly in Chinese provinces such as Yunnan (hence the name '*Yun muxiang*' [Yunnan Common Aucklandia Root]); also in provinces such as Sichuan and in Tibet.

Harvest & Processing Dig up roots of plants 2-3 years old in autumn and winter; remove leaves, rootlets and soil; cut roots into segments or slice length-wise into pieces; dry under the sun or by wind; remove cork. Commonly used in Hong Kong in the form of length-wise cut slices.

Description Cylindrical or semi-cylindrical; about 5-10 cm long, 0.5-5 cm in diameter. Outer surface yellowish-brown to dull greyish-brown; cork mostly removed; surface marked with conspicuous wrinkles, longitudinal grooves and scars of rootlets. Hard, solid and heavy; does not break easily. When broken, surface relatively even, dull greyish-brown to dull drown; cambium ring brown; with radial markings and scattered punctiform (dot-like) dull brownish oil cavities. Core of old roots often looks like withered wood. Odour: fragrant and distinctive; taste: slightly bitter.

Indications 1. Distending pain in the chest and epigastrium, tenesmus in dysentery 2. Diarrhoea, vomitting.

Chemical Composition Mainly contains dehydrocostus lactone and costunolide.

Radix Bupleuri

Chinese Thorowax Root

Chaihu

柴胡

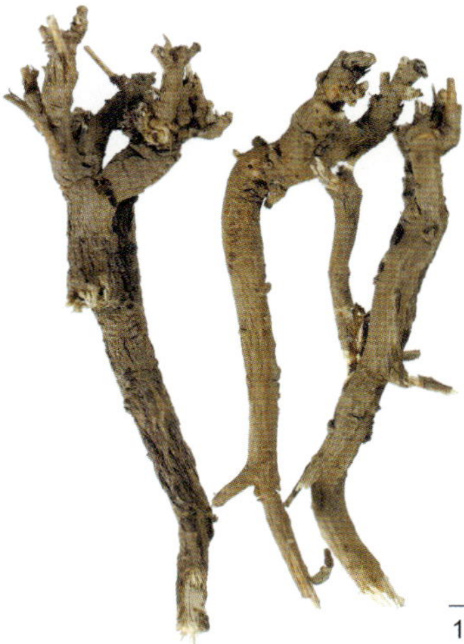

Crude Drug

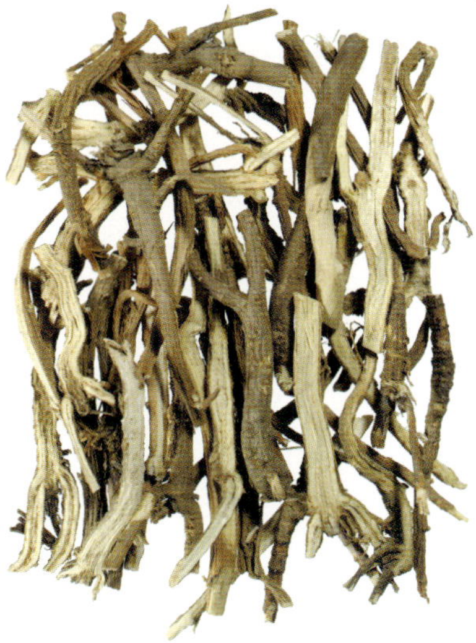

Decoction Pieces

1 cm

Source The root of *Bupleurum chinense* DC. (Fam. Umbelliferae). Customarily called "*Bei chaihu*"(North Chinese Thorowax Root).

Distribution Mainly in Chinese provinces such as Hebei, Liaoning, Jilin, Heilongjiang, Henan and Shaanxi.

Harvest & Processing Dig out roots in spring and autumn; remove leaves and soil; dry under the sun. Commonly used in Hong Kong in the form of length-wise cut slices.

Description Cylindrical, or long and conical; 6-15 cm long, 3-8 mm in diameter. Top part bulgy; top end with remnants of 3-15 caudexes or short fibrous leaf bases; lower part often rameous (branched). Outer surface dull blackish-brown or light brown, marked with longitudinal wrinkles, lateral root scars and lenticels. Hard and pliable, does not break easily. When broken, surface fibrous and lobate (lobe-like); cortex light brown; xylem yellowish-white. Odour: slightly fragrant; taste: slightly bitter.

Indications 1. Common cold 2. Fever 3. Cholecystitis 4. Menstrual disorders.

Chemical Composition Contains essential oils, and triterpene saponins such as saikosaponins a, d, s.

Note According to *C.P.*, also used for medicinal purposes is the root of *B. scorzonerifolium* Willd.

Radix Changii

Medicinal Changium Root
Mingdangshen

明黨參

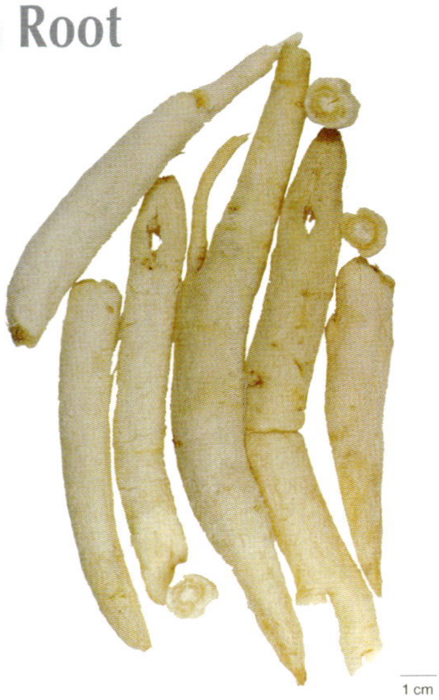

Crude Drug

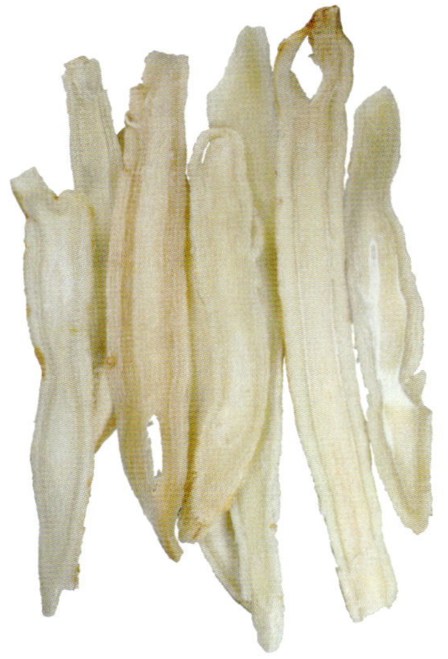

Decoction Pieces

Source The root of *Changium smyrnioides* Wolff (Fam. Umbelliferae).

Distribution Mainly in Chinese provinces such as Jiangsu, Zhejiang and Anhui.

Harvest & Processing Collect roots in April and May; remove fibrous roots; wash clean; boil thoroughly; scrape off cork; rinse; dry by airing. Commonly used in Hong Kong in the form of length-wise cut slices.

Description Slender and cylindrical, or long and spindle-shaped, or irregular long pieces; 6-20 cm long, 0.5-2 cm in diameter. Outer surface yellowish-white or pale brown; smooth or marked with longitudinal grooves and scars of fibrous roots; in some cases marked with reddish-brown maculae. Hard and brittle. Broken surface cuticular; cortex yellowish-white, peeled off easily; xylem off-white. Odour: faint; taste: mild.

Indications 1. Cough, dyspnoea, dryness of throat 2. Febrile diseases with regurgitation and vomiting 2. Skin infection

Chemical Composition Contains essential oils with methyl-6, 9-octadecadiynoate as the main component.

Radix Clematidis

Chinese Clematis Root
Weilingxian

威靈仙

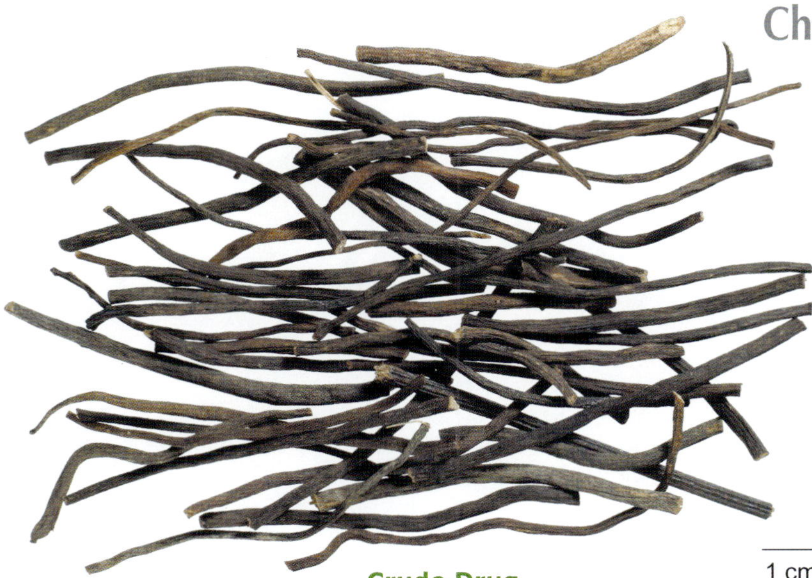

Crude Drug

1 cm

Source The root and rhizome of *Clematis chinensis* Osbeck (Fam. Ranunculaceae).

Distribution Mainly in Chinese provinces such as Jiangsu, Zhejiang, Jiangxi and Anhui; also in Hong Kong.

Harvest & Processing Dig out roots and rhizomes in autumn; remove soil and sand; dry under the sun.

Description Rhizome cylindrical; 1.5-10 cm long, 0.3-1.5 cm in diameter. Outer surface pale brownish-yellow; upper end with caudex remnants; lower part with numerous rootlets. Roots slender and cylindrical, slightly curved; 7-15 cm long, 1-3 mm in diameter. Outer surface dull blackish-brown, marked with fine longitudinal striae; cortex sometimes fallen off, exposing yellowish-white xylem. Rhizome relatively strong and pliable; broken surface fibrous. Roots hard and brittle, break easily; broken surface shows relatively broad cortex and pale yellow, slightly quadrate (square-shaped) xylem, often with clefts between cortex and xylem. Odour: faint; taste: mild.

Indications 1. Rheumatic arthritis 2. Acute tonsillitis, pharyngitis 3. Jaundice due to acute infectious hepatitis 4. Toothache.

Chemical Composition Contains protoanemonin and a variety of triterpene saponins.

Note According to *C.P.*, also used for medicinal purposes is the root and rhizome of *C. hexapetala* Pall. and *C. manshurica* Rupr.

Radix Chloranthi Serrati

Serrate Chloranthus Root

Jiji

及己

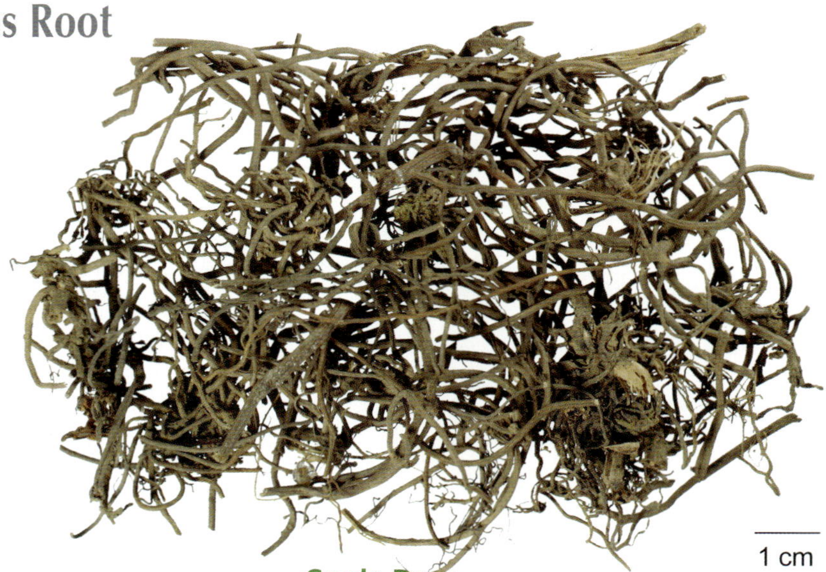

Crude Drug

Source The root of *Chloranthus serratus* (Thunb.) Roem. et Schult. (Fam. Chloranthaceae).

Distribution Mainly in Chinese provinces such as Anhui, Jiangsu, Zhejiang, Jiangxi, Fujian, Guangdong and Guangxi; also in Hong Kong.

Harvest & Processing Dig out roots in spring before efflorescence; remove shoots, soil and sand; dry under the sun.

Description Roots slender and cylindrical; about 10 cm long, 0.5-2 mm in diameter; outer surface earth-grey in colour, marked with scars of rootlets. Rhizome relatively short; about 3 mm in diameter; upper end with caudex remnants, lower part with numerous fine roots. Brittle. Broken surface relatively even; cortex greyish-yellow; xylem pale yellow. Odour: faint; taste: mild and bitter.

Indications 1. Trauma, fracture 2. Rheumatism 3. Amenorrhoea 4. Scabies and tinea, boils and sores, pruritus 5. Venomous-snake bite

Chemical Composition Contains neoacolamone.

Radix Cocculi Trilobi

Japanese Snailseed Root
Mufangji

木防己

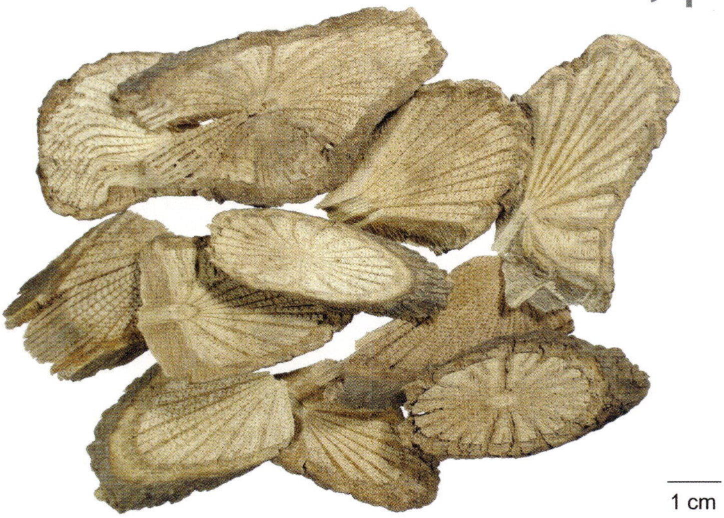

Decoction Pieces

Source The root of *Cocculus trilobus* (Thunb.) DC. (Fam. Menispermaceae).

Distribution Mainly in Shaanxi province and in southwestern, central and eastern regions of China; also in Hong Kong.

Harvest & Processing Dig out roots in spring and autumn, with the ones collected in autumn of better quality; remove stems, leaves and rootstocks; wash roots clean; dry under the sun.

Description Cylindrical or twisted, slightly torose (cylindrical with alternate swellings and constrictions); 10-20 cm long, 1-2.5 cm in diameter. Outer surface dull dark brown; marked with curved longitudinal grooves and sparse scars of branch roots. Hard; when broken, surface yellowish-white, marked with radial rays and pores. Odour: faint; taste: slightly bitter.

Indications 1. Arthralgia 2. Oedema, dysuria.

Chemical Composition Mainly contains alkaloids such as trilobine, magnoflorine.

Radix Codonopsis

Pilose Asiabell Root

Dangshen

黨參

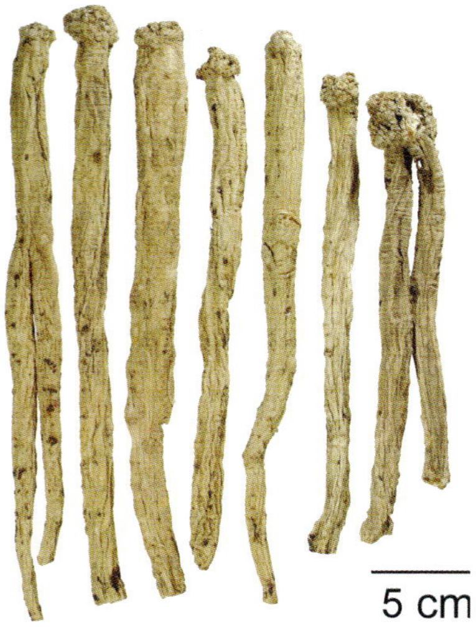

Crude Drug

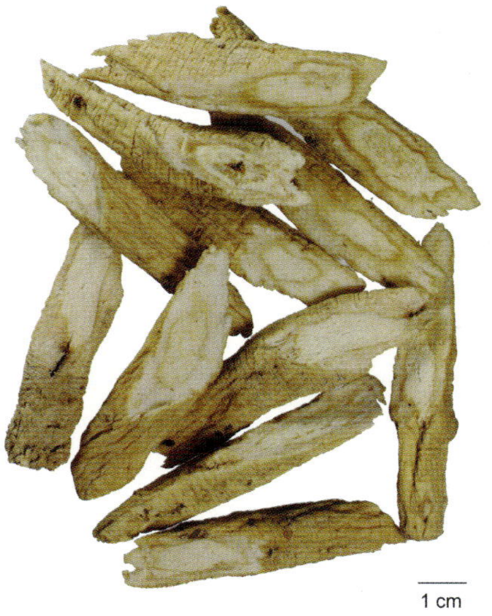

Decoction Pieces

Source The root of *Codonopsis pilosula* (Franch.) Nannf. (Fam. Campanulaceae).

Distribution Mainly in Chinese provinces such as Shanxi, Shaanxi, Gansu and Sichuan.

Harvest & Processing Dig out roots in autumn; remove above-ground parts and rootlets; wash away soil; dry until half-dry; rub 3-4 times; dry under the sun until nearly dry, then tie into bundles; dry under the sun again.

Description Long and cylindrical; outer surface yellowish-brown to greyish-brown. Top part of root with numerous verruciform (wart-shaped), protuberant stem scars and buds, with the top of each stem scar dented and punctiform (dot-like)-known as '*shizi panto*'. Dense transverse annulations below top part of root, gradually becoming sparse towards lower part; few or no transverse annulations on cultivated roots. Whole root marked with longitudinal wrinkles and scattered lalongate lenticels; scars of branch roots often with a gelatinous dull blackish-brown substance. Fairly hard, or fairly pliable. When broken, surface quite even, with clefts or radial markings; cortex pale yellowish-white to pale brown; xylem pale yellow, in the shape of a chrysanthemum. Odour: with a distinctive fragrance; taste: slightly sweet.

Indications 1. Anorexia, loose stool 2. Weakness, lassitude 3. Cough and dyspnoea, feeble voice 4. Dehydration 5. Rectal prolapse, uterine prolapse.

Chemical Composition Contains tangshenoside I, syringin, perlolyrine and atractylenolide.

Note According to *C.P.*, also used for medicinal purposes is the root of *C. pilosula* Nannf. var. *modesta* (Nannf.) L. T. Shen and *C. tangshen* Oliv.

Radix Crotonis Crassifolii

Thickleaf Croton Root
Jiguxiang

雞骨香

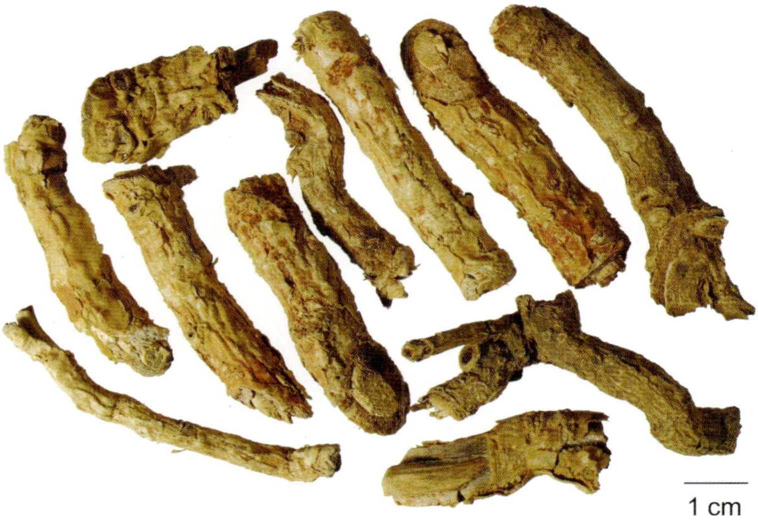

1 cm

Crude Drug

Source The root of *Croton crassifolius* Geisel. (Fam. Euphorbiaceae).

Distribution Mainly in southwestern China; also in Hong Kong.

Harvest & Processing Dig up roots anytime during the year; cut into slices; dry under the sun.

Description Slender and rod-like; 2-10 mm in diameter. Outer surface yellow or pale yellow, marked with longitudinal striae and protuberances; cork sometimes falls off. Brittle and breaks easily; broken surface uneven, fibrous. Cortex takes up about 1/3-1/4 of radius, pale yellow. Xylem yellow. Odour: slightly fragrant; taste: bitter-astringent.

Indications 1. All kind of pain such as distending pain of abdomen, pain due to rheumatism, hernia, pharyngitis, trauma

Chemical Composition Mainly contains sesquiterpenes such as cyperenoic acid.

Radix Curcumae

Turmeric Root Tuber

Yujin

鬱金

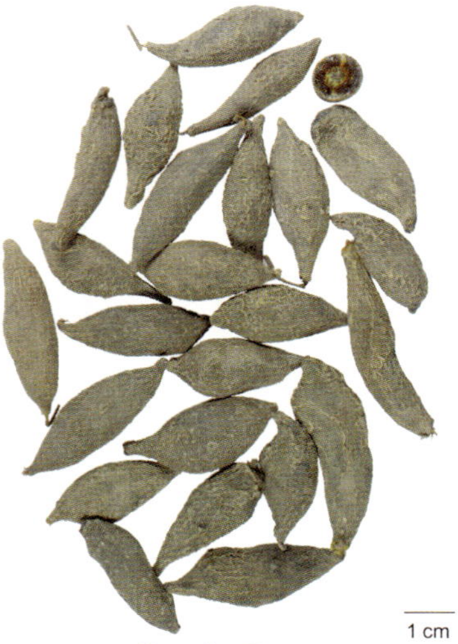

Crude Drug

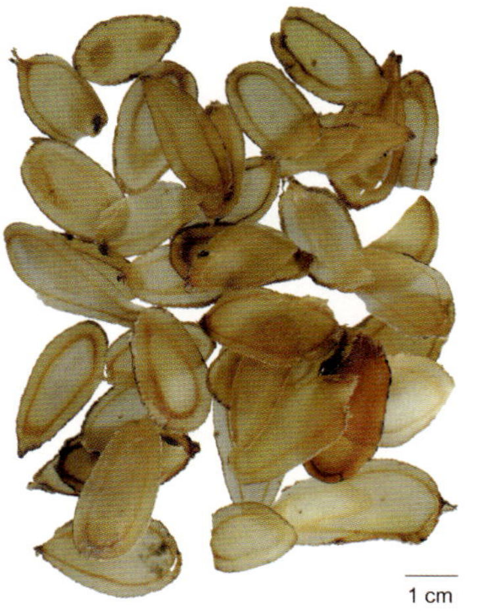

Decoction Pieces

Source The root tuber of *Curcuma wenyujin* Y. H. Chen et C. Ling (Fam. Zingiberaceae).

Distribution Mainly in Zhejiang province in China.

Harvest & Processing Dig out underground parts on dry sunny days in mid and late December of the year of plantation when leaves gradually wither; shake off soil; pick off root tubers; steam or cook for about 15 minutes; dry under the sun or by heat; remove fibrous roots.

Description Oblong and spherical, or ovoid (egg-shaped), slightly flattened, in some cases slightly curved, both ends acuminate (tapering to a slender point); 3.5-7 cm long, 1.2-2.5 cm in diameter. Outer surface dull greyish-brown or greyish-brown; marked with irregular longitudinal wrinkles, with the ridges of wrinkles lighter in colour. Hard. Broken surface greyish-brown or greyish-green, with waxy lustre; endodermis conspicuous. Odour: slightly fragrant; taste: slightly bitter.

Indications 1. Angina pectoris, trauma, bleeding 2. Menstrual disorders 3. Jaundice, hypochondriac mass 4. Apprenhension, epilepsy, psychosis, impairment of consciousness 5. Hyperlipidemia

Chemical Composition Mainly contains diarylheptanoids such as curcumin and demethoxycurcumin.

Note According to *C.P.*, also used for medicinal purposes is the root tuber of *C. longa* L., of *C. kwangsiensis* S. G. Lee *et* C. F. Liang and of *C. phaeocaulis* Val.

Radix Cyathulae

Medicinal Cyathula Root
Chuanniuxi
川牛膝

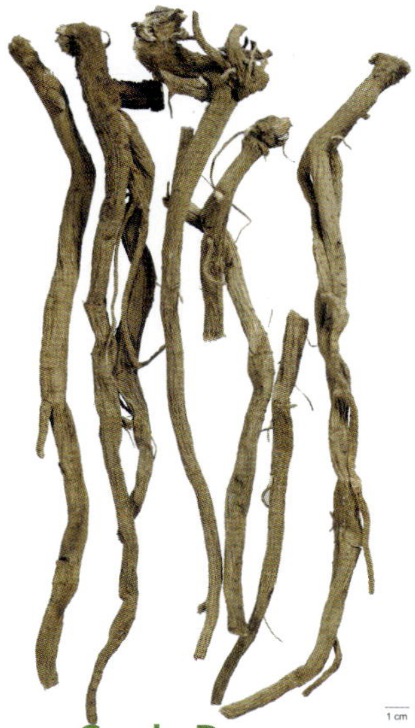

Crude Drug

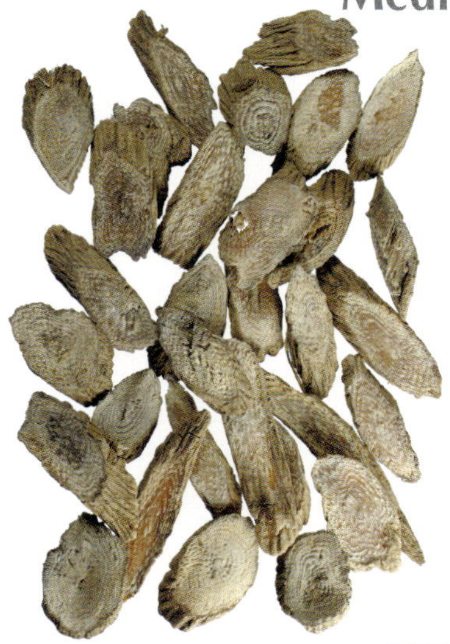

Decoction Pieces 1 cm

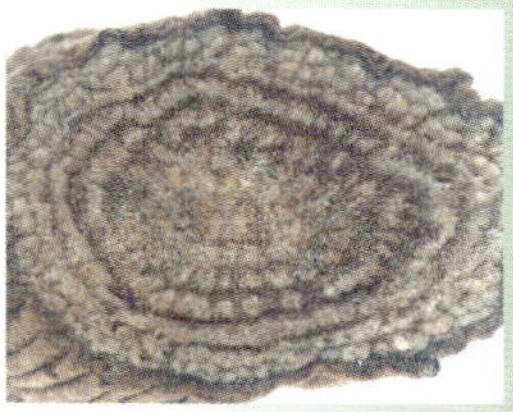

Medicinal Cyathula Root Magnified

Source The root of *Cyathula officinalis* Kuan (Fam. Amaranthaceae).

Distribution Mainly in Chinese provinces such as Sichuan, Yunnan and Guizhou. Naturally grown or cultivated.

Harvest & Processing Collect roots in autumn and winter; remove rootstocks, rootlets, soil and sand; dry roots by heat or under the sun until half-dry; heap up to drive out the moisture on the inside, then dry by heat or under the sun again.

Description Subcylindrical, slightly twisted, tapering towards the lower part or with a few branches; 30-60 cm long, 0.5-3 cm in diameter. Outer surface yellowish-brown or dull greyish-brown, marked with longitudinal wrinkles and scars of lateral roots; with many protuberant transverse lenticels; top end sometimes marked with remnants of rhizome and caudex. Strong and pliable, does not break easily; when broken, surface light yellow or brownish-yellow, with several concentric rings of punctiform (dot-like) vascular bundles. Odour: faint; taste: sweet.

Indications 1. Rheumatism 2. Haematuria 3. Amenorrhoea 4. Abdominal mass

Chemical Composition Mainly contains sterols such as cyasterone and amarasterone A.

Radix Cynanchi Atrati

Blackend Swallowwort Root and Rhizome

Baiwei

白薇

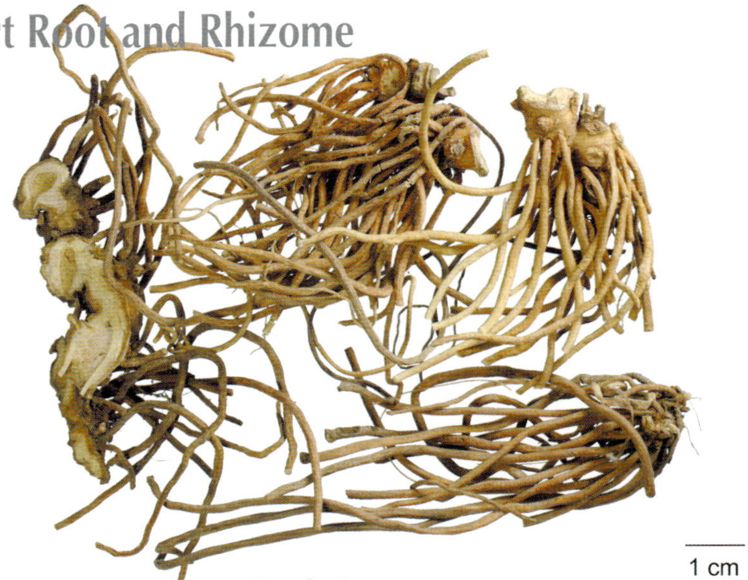

Crude Drug

Source The root and rhizome of *Cynanchum atratum* Bunge (Fam. Asclepiadaceae).

Distribution Mainly in Chinese provinces such as Shandong, Anhui, Liaoning and Hubei.

Harvest & Processing Collect roots and rhizomes in spring and autumn; wash clean and dry.

Description Slightly pony-tail in shape, mostly curved and curled. Rhizome thick and short, with nodes; upper part marked with round stem scars; lower part with numerous, conglomerate (densely clustered) fine long rootlets. Root 10-25 cm long, 1-2 mm in diameter; outer surface brownish-yellow; brittle, breaks easily; transverse section shows yellowish-white cortex and yellow or pale yellow xylem. Odour: faint; taste: slightly bitter.

Indications 1. Febrile diseases 2. Debility after delivery 3. Urinary tract infection 4. Sore throat, carbuncles and sores, Venomous-snake bite

Chemical Composition Mainly contains steroidal saponins such as cynatratoside A, B, C, D.

Note According to *C.P.*, also used for medicinal purposes is the root and rhizome of *C. versicolor Bge.*

Radix Cynanchi Paniculati

Paniculate Swallowwort Root

Xuchangqing

徐長卿

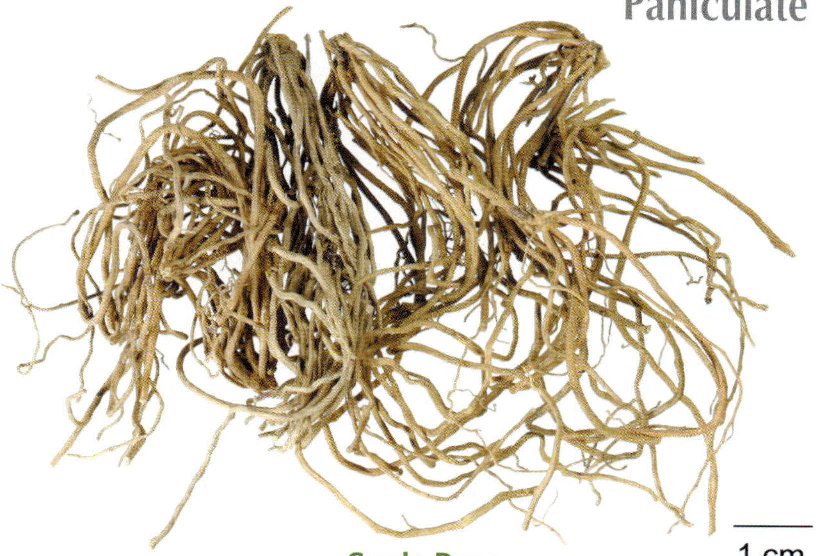

Crude Drug

Source The root and rhizome of *Cynanchum paniculatum* (Bunge) Kitag. (Fam. Asclepiadaceae).

Distribution In all parts of China, including Hong Kong.

Harvest & Processing Dig up roots and rhizomes in autumn; remove foreign matter; dry in shaded areas.

Description Rhizome irregular and cylindrical, with bulgy nodes; 0.5-3.5 cm long, 2-4 mm in diameter; top end with stem remnants; encircled by numerous slender roots. Root long and cylindrical, curved; 10-16 cm long, 1-1.5 mm in diameter; outer surface pale yellowish-white, pale brownish-yellow or brown, marked with very fine longitudinal wrinkles and fine, slender roots. Brittle, breaks easily. When broken, surface shows starchy and yellowish-white cortex; cambium ring pale yellow; xylem yellowish-brown and small. Odour: fragrant; taste: slightly acrid, numbs the tongue.

Indications 1. Arthralgia, lumbar strain, trauma, angina pectoris, biliary colic, abdominal pain, toothache (topical use) 2. Dermatitis, tinea, herpes zoster, psoriasis 3. Allergic rhinitis 4. Cough

Chemical Composition Contains neocynapanoside A.

Radix Dichroae

Antifeverile Dichroa Root
Changshan

常山

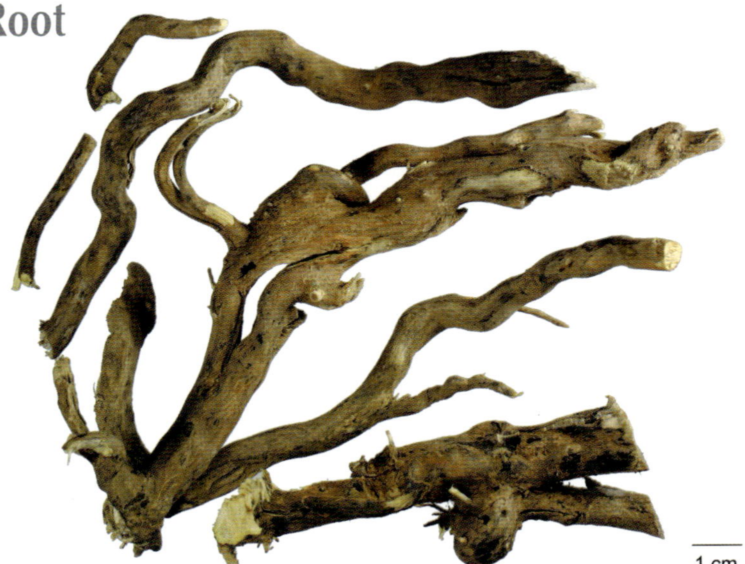

Crude Drug

Source The root of *Dichroa febrifuga* Lour. (Fam. Saxifragaceae).

Distribution Mainly in Chinese provinces such as Sichuan and Guizhou; also in Hong Kong.

Harvest & Processing Dig out roots in autumn; remove rootlets; wash clean; dry under the sun.

Description Cylindrical, often curved and twisted, in some cases rameous (branched); 9-15 cm long, 0.5-2 cm in diameter. Outer surface brownish-yellow, marked with fine longitudinal striae; bark peels off easily, exposing pale yellow xylem. Hard; does not break easily; a burst of powder when snapped; cross-section yellowish-white, with radial, off-white rays. Odourless; taste: bitter.

Indications 1. Malaria 2. Productive cough

Chemical Composition Mainly contains alkaloids such as dichroine and dichroidine.

Radix Dipsaci

Himalayan Teasel Root

Xuduan

續斷

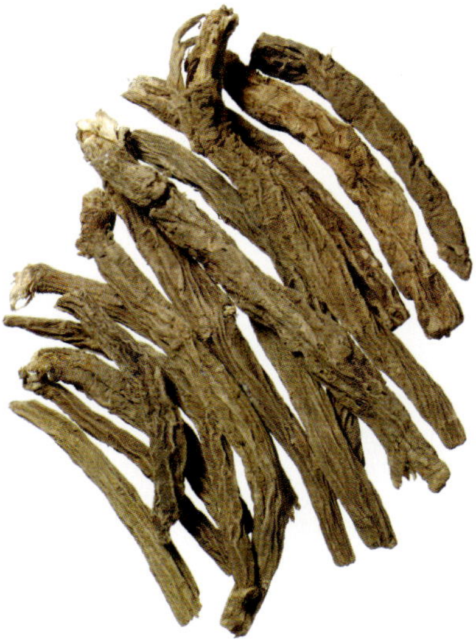

Crude Drug

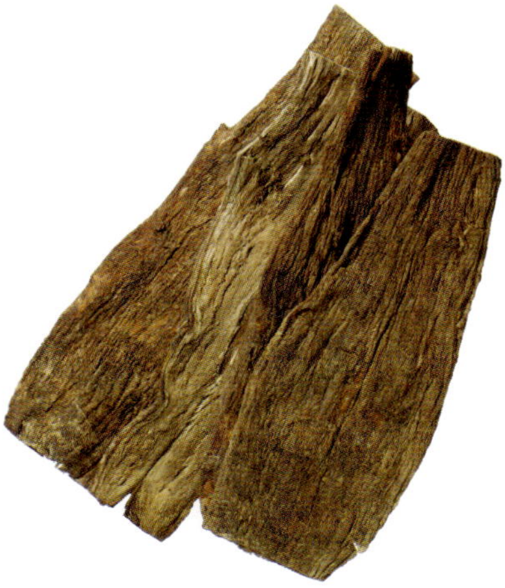

Decoction Pieces

Source

The root of *Dipsacus asperoides* C. Y. Cheng et T. M. Ai (Fam. Dipsacaceae).

Distribution

Mainly in Chinese provinces such as Hubei, Sichuan, Yunnan and Guizhou.

Harvest & Processing

Dig out roots in autumn; remove top parts and rootlets; dry over a small fire until half-dry; heap up to let moisture evaporate until the inside turns green; then dry by heat. Do not dry roots under the sun to aviod hardening. Commonly used in Hong Kong in the form of slices of the root cut length-wise and pounded flat.

Description

Long and cylindrical, slightly flattened and slightly curved; 5-15 cm long, 0.5-2 cm in diameter. Outer surface dull greyish-brown or reddish-brown; marked with conspicuous, twisted longitudinal wrinkles and grooves all over, and with lenticels and sparse scars of rootlets. Soft; dries and hardens on prolorged exposure to air; breaks easily. When broken, surface uneven; cortex dull brown at rim, blackish-green or brown at inner part; xylem dull yellowish-brown, with radial vessels. Odour: slightly fragrant; taste: bitter and slightly sweet, then astringent.

Indications

1.Backache, knee ache, rheumatism, trauma 2. Dysfunctional uterine bleeding, threatened abortion

Chemical Composition

Mainly contains iridoid glycosides such as sweroside and loganin.

Radix Echinopsis

Globethistle Root

Yuzhou Loulu

禹州漏蘆

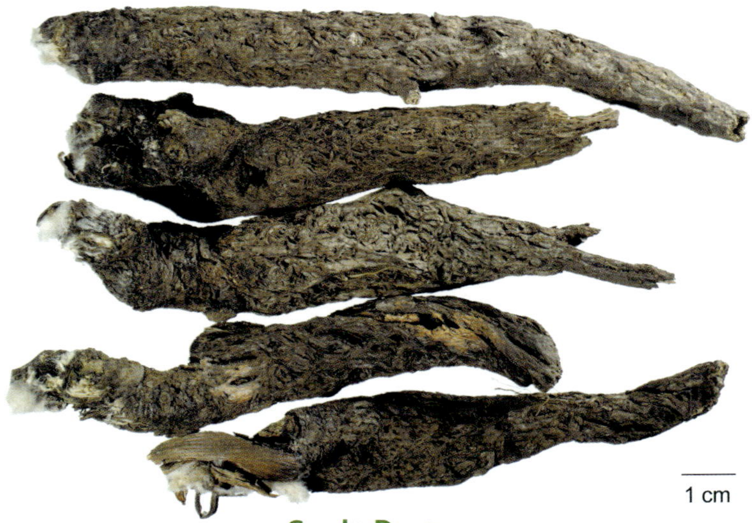

Crude Drug

Source The root of *Echinops latifolius* Tausch (Fam. Compositae).

Distribution Mainly in Chinese provinces such as Shandong and Henan, and in Inner Mongolia.

Harvest & Processing Dig up roots in spring and autumn; remove rootlets, soil and sand; use while fresh or dry under the sun.

Description Subcylindrical, slightly curved; varying in length, 0.5-1.5 cm in diameter. Outer surface earthy-yellow or greyish-brown, rough, marked with longitudinal wrinkles; apex with remnants of petiole vascular bundles, remnants hard, fibrous, brown and hair-like. Hard and brittle. Broken surface coarsely fibrous; cortex brown; xylem with alternating yellow and black striae arranged in the shape of chrysanthemum. Odour: faint; taste: slightly astringent.

Indications 1. Sores, carbuncles, pyogenic skin infection 2. Mastitis, galactostasis 3. Tuberculous of lymph node

Chemical Composition Mainly contains triterpenes such as taraxerol acetate and ursolic acid; also contains polyacetylenes such as echinoynethiophene.

Note According to *C.P.*, also used for medicinal purposes is the root of *E. grijisii* Hance.

Radix et Rhizoma Ephedrae

Ephedra Root
Mahuanggen
麻黃根

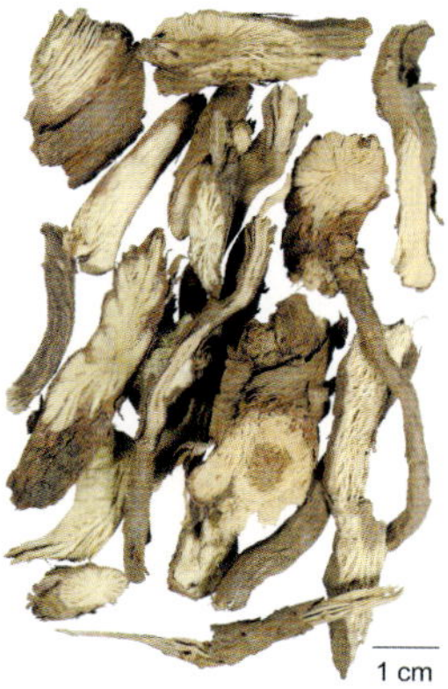

Decoction Pieces

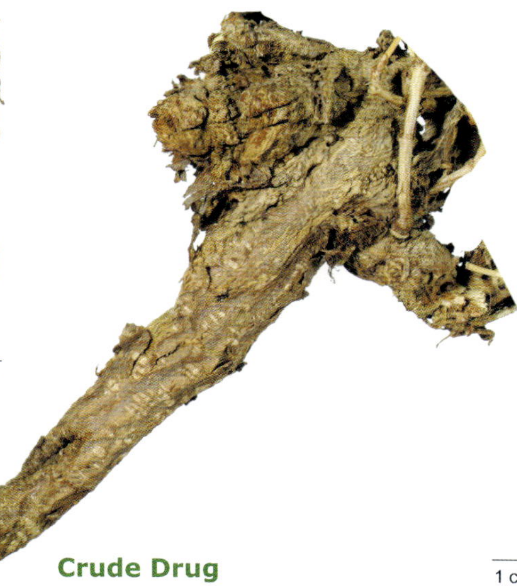

Crude Drug

Source The root or rhizome of *Ephedra sinica* Stapf (Fam. Ephedraceae).

Distribution Mainly in regions such as Xinjiang and Inner Mongolia in China.

Harvest & Processing Dig up roots or rhizomes after August; remove all rootlets, stems and shoots; dry rhizomes and roots under the sun.

Description Root mostly conical and cylindrical; rhizome relatively thin, cylindrical, slightly curved; 8-25 cm long, 0.5-1.5 cm in diameter. Outer surface of both root and rhizome reddish-brown or greyish-brown, marked with longitudinal wrinkles and scars of branch roots; bark rough, peels off easily. Upper part of root relatively thick; lower part relatively thin, often curved. Rhizome in even thickness, with bulgy nodes, internodes 0.7-2 cm long. Light in weight; hard and brittle, breaks easily. When broken, surface shows yellowish-white cortex and pale yellow or yellow xylem with radial rays; rhizome with pith at the centre. Odourless; taste: slightly bitter.

Indications Sweating such as spontaneous sweating, night sweating, postpartum sweating (external use)

Chemical Composition Mainly contains alkaloids such as ephedradine A, B, C, D.

Note According to *C.P.*, also used for medicinal purposes is the root or rhizome of *E. intermedia* Schrenk ex C. A. Mey.

Radix et Rhizoma Rhei

Rhubarb
Dahuang

大黃

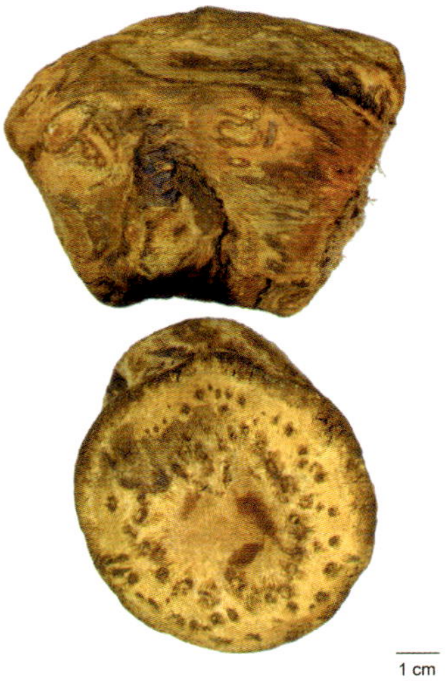

Crude Drug

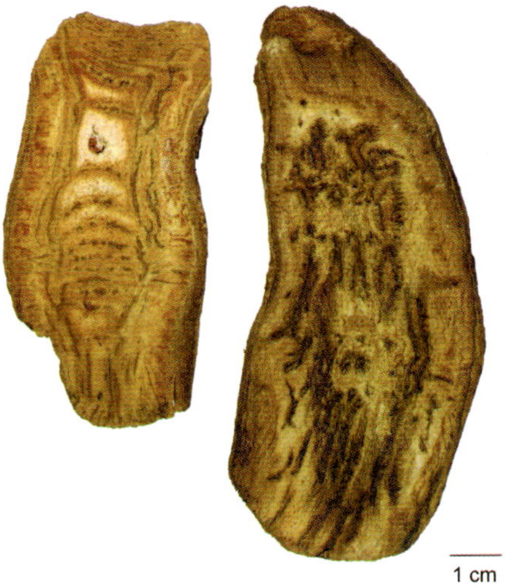

Decoction Pieces

Source The root and rhizome of *Rheum palmatum* L. (Fam. Polygonaceae).

Distribution Mainly in Chinese provinces such as Gansu, Qinghai and Sichuan, and in Tibet. Mostly cultivated.

Harvest & Processing Dig up roots and rhizomes in late autumn when leaves wither or in the following spring before germination; remove soil and rootlets; scrape off cork (do not use metal instruments); cut into slices or sections or process into egg shape or cylindrical shape; string pieces together and dry, or dry without stringing.

Description Subcylindrical, ovoid or hippocrepiform pieces, or irregular slices or sections. When cork is completely removed, outer surface yellowish-brown to reddish-brown; in some cases surface marked with off-white anomalous vascular bundles or with remnants of reddish-brown cork. Hard and solid. When broken, surface pale reddish-brown or yellowish-brown, granular. Pith in cross-section of rhizome relatively large; 'star-like' spots in cross-section, appearing in rings or scattered form. Cambium ring of root conspicuous; xylem well-developed, with radial rays and no star-like dots. Odour: fresh and fragrant; taste: bitter and slightly astringent; sticky when chewed, gritty, turns saliva yellow.

Indications 1. Constipation and intestinal obstruction, dysentery 2. Bleeding 3. Carbuncles and furuncles, burns and scalds 4. Amenorrhoea, postpartum abdominal pain 5. Jaundice

Chemical Composition Mainly contains anthraquinones such as emodin aloe-emodin; also contains condensed tannins.

Note According to *C.P.*, also used for medicinal purposes is the root and rhizome of *R. tanguticum* Maxim.ex Balf. and *R. officinale* Baill.

Radix et Rhizoma Sinopodophylli Hexandri

Chinese May-Apple Root and Rhizome

Guijiu

鬼臼

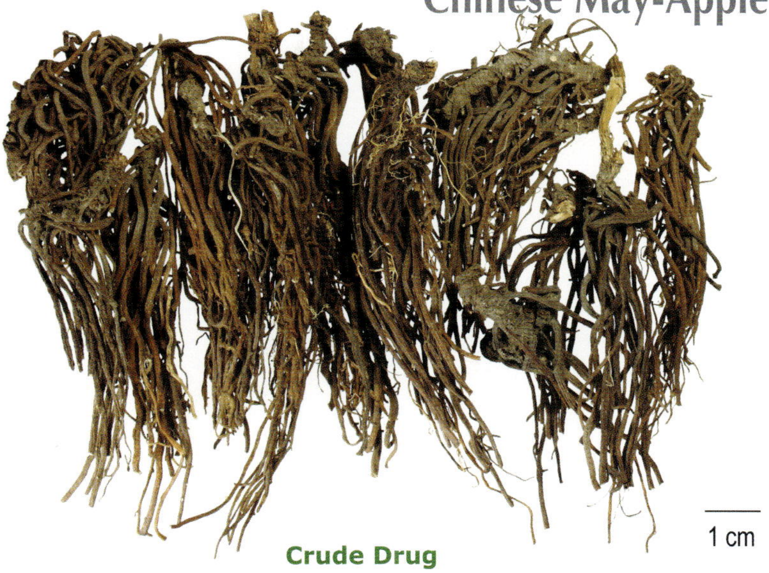

Crude Drug

Source The root and rhizome of *Sinopodophyllum hexandrum* (Royle) Ying (Fam. Berberidaceae).

Distribution Mainly in Chinese provinces such as Sichuan, Shaanxi and Gansu; also in provinces such as Qinghai, and in Tibet.

Harvest & Processing Dig up roots and rhizomes in spring and autumn; dry under the sun.

Description Rhizome in the form of irregular nodular pieces; each node subspherical, 0.8-1.2 cm in diameter; outer surface reddish-brown, with indistinct annulations and numerous rootlets and rootlet scars. Rootlets cylindrical; 1-3 mm in diameter; outer surface brownish-yellow, smooth, marked with fine longitudinal striae. Hard. Broken surface yellow, fibrous; when broken transversely, cortex on surface smooth; xylem bulgy, arranged in annular (ring-like) form; pith small, taking up about 1/4 of the diameter. Odour: faint; taste: bitter.

Indications 1. Rheumatism, trauma 2. Menstrual disorders, dysmenorrhoea 3. Abdominal pain 4. Cough

Chemical Composition Mainly contains lignans such as podophyllotoxin.

Note Also used for medicinal purposes is the root and rhizome of *Dysosma versipellis* (Hance M. Cheng ex Ying) and *D. pleiantha* (Hance) Woods, both of which belong to the same family as *Sinopodophyllum hexandrum* (Royle) Ying. The product processed from the three species are all listed in Hong Kong as Category I (Toxic/Potent) Chinese Materia Medica.

Radix et Rhizoma Thalictri

Meadowrue Root and Rhizome

Maweilian

馬尾連

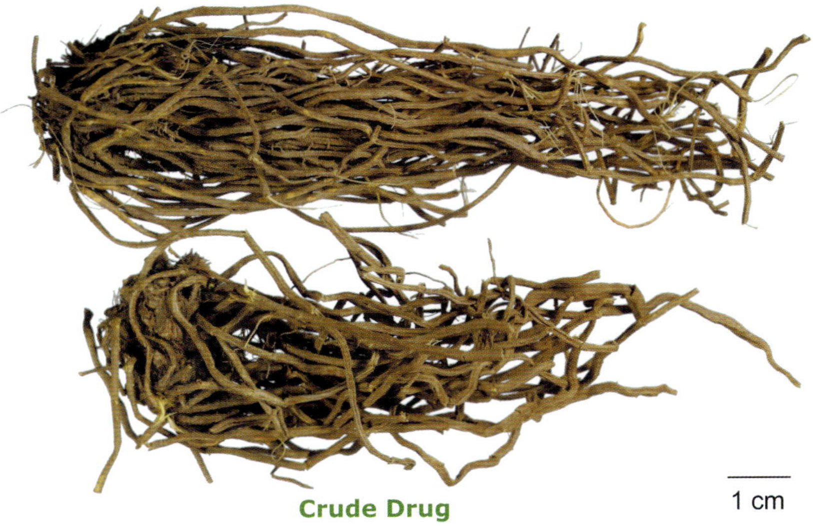

Crude Drug

Source The root and rhizome of *Thalictrum foliolosum* DC. (Fam. Ranunculaceae).

Distribution Mainly in Chinese provinces such as Sichuan and Yunnan, and in Tibet.

Harvest & Processing Dig out roots and rhizomes from September to the following February; cut away stem shoots; dry under the sun until half-dry; rub away cork; dry under the sun again.

Description Rhizome transverse, formed by several to over 10 confluent (running together or blending of one part into another) nodes; nodes with orbicular (round) hollow stem scars about 1 cm in diameter. Rootlets: several to over 10 in number, densely grown at underside of rhizome; 3 mm in diameter. Outer surface greyish-brown. Hard, breaks easily; broken surface shows orbicular golden-yellow woody core. Odour: faint; taste: slightly bitter.

Indications 1. Diarrhoea, dysentery, jaundice 2. Sores and boils 3. Red eyes, photophobia with lacrimation, conjunctivitis 4. Common cold with fever 5. Neoplasm

Chemical Composition Mainly contains a variety of alkaloids such as berberine, jatrorrhizine and palmatine.

Radix et Rhizoma Veratri Nigri

Falsehellebore Root and Rhizome

Lilu

藜蘆

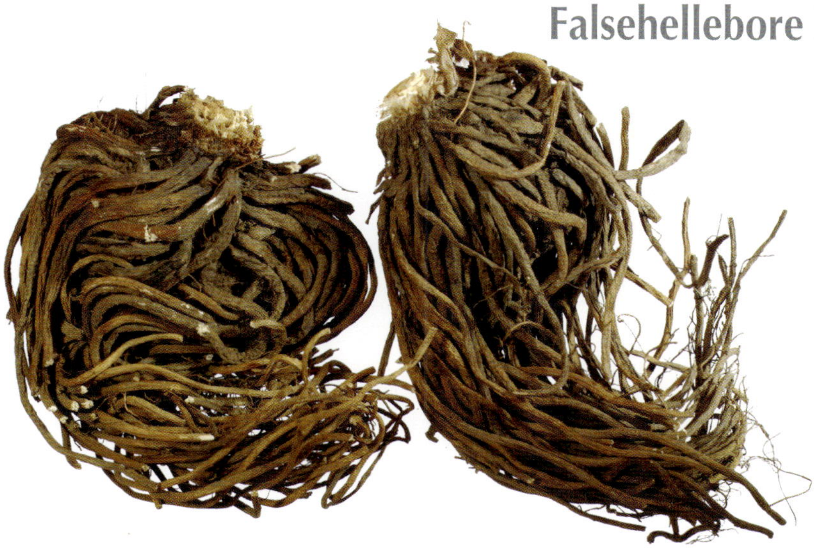

Crude Drug

Source The root or rhizome of *Veratrum nigrum* L. (Fam. Liliaceae).

Distribution Mainly in Chinese provinces such as Heilongjiang, Jilin, Liaoning, Hebei, Henan, Shandong, Shanxi, Jiangxi, Shaanxi, Gansu and Sichuan, and in Inner Mongolia and Xinjiang .

Harvest & Processing Dig up roots and rhizomes, usually in summer; remove above-ground leaves; wash clean; dry under the sun. Alternatively, dig up whole herbs; remove soil; dry under the sun.

Description Rhizome cylindrical; 2-4 cm long, 0.7-1.5 cm in diameter; outer surface brownish-yellow or earthy in colour; top part marked with remnants of leaf base and piliform (hair-like) fibre bundles, overgrown with rootlets on all sides. Root slender, slightly curved; 10-20 cm long, 1-4 mm in diameter; outer surface yellowish-white or dull greyish-brown, marked with relatively dense transverse wrinkles; lower part marked with numerous longitudinal wrinkles. Hard and brittle; broken surface off-white, with pale yellow stele in the centre; stele separates easily from cortex. Odour: faint; taste: extremely bitter, powder with a pronounced sternutatory (inducing sneezing) effect.

Indications 1. Cerebral vascular accident 2. Pharynigitis, laryngitis 3. Epilepsy.

Chemical Composition Mainly contains steroidal alkaloids.

Radix Eupatorii Chinensis

Chinese Eupatorium Root
Guangdongtuniuxi

廣東土牛膝

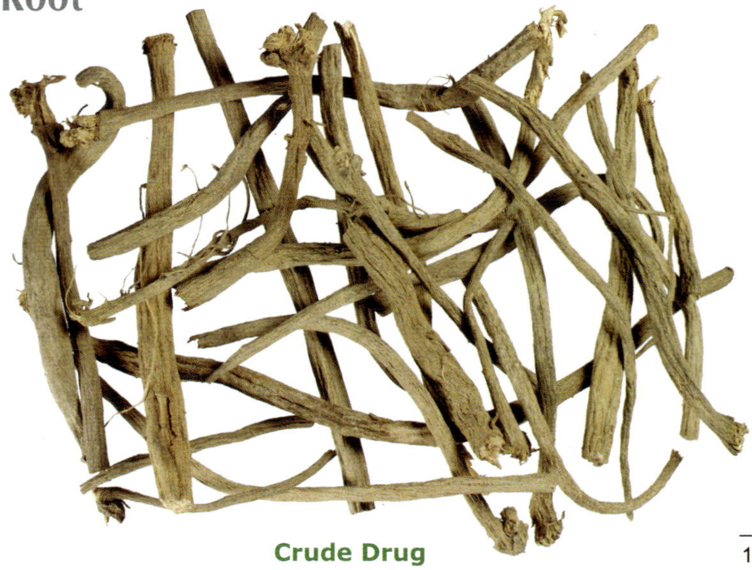

Crude Drug

1 cm

Source The root or whole herb of *Eupatorium chinense* L. (Fam. Compositae).

Distribution Mainly in Chinese provinces such as Guangdong and Guangxi; also in Hong Kong.

Harvest & Processing Dig up roots or whole herbs in autumn; remove soil; dry under the sun or use while fresh.

Description Root beard-like and cylindrical; 10-35 cm long, can reach 50 cm in length. Outer surface yellowish-brown. Hard and brittle, breaks easily; broken surface white. Stem and inflorescence pubescent (covered with short, soft hairs). Leaves simple (not separated into leaflets) and opposite (borne in pairs at each node); oblong and ovate (egg-shaped), or broad and ovate; crenate (with round-toothed edges); underside with pubescence and gland dots. Odour: slightly liquorice-like; taste: mild.

Indications 1. Pharyngitis, diphtheria 2. Haematemesis, haemoptysis 3. Dysentery with bloody stool 4. Trauma 5. Carbuncles and sores, burn and scald, venomous-snake bite

Chemical Composition Mainly contains essential oils and triterpenes.

Radix Euphorbiae Fischerianae

Langdu Root
Langdu
狼毒

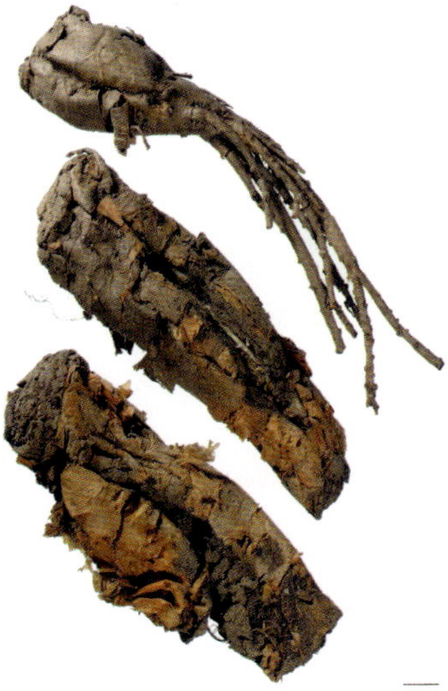

Crude Drug

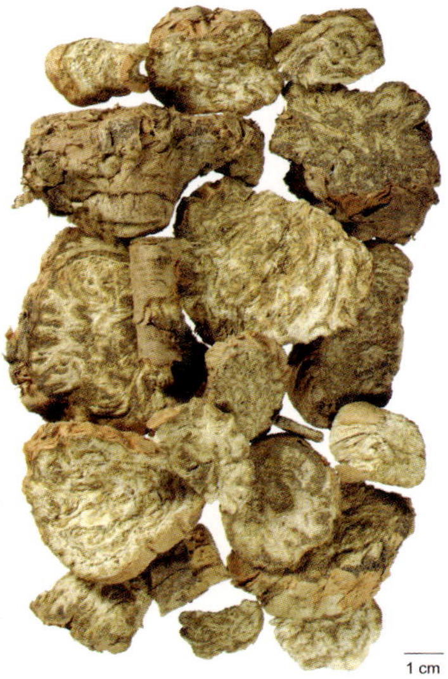

Decoction Pieces

Source ▶ The root of *Euphorbia fischeriana* Stend. (Fam. Euphorbiaceae).

Distribution ▶ Mainly in Chinese provinces such as Heilongjiang, Jilin, Liaoning, Hebei and Shanxi, and in Inner Mongolia.

Harvest & Processing ▶ Dig up roots in spring and autumn; remove leaves, soil and sand; cut into slices; dry under the sun.

Description ▶ Conical, or long and conical; cork greyish-brown, peels off easily, revealing brownish-yellow or brownish-red cortex. When cross-cut or cut at an angle, surface yellowish-white; marked with relatively conspicuous concentric annulations formed by anomalous vascular bundles. Light in weight; broken surface starchy. Odour: faint; taste: slightly bitter.

Indications ▶ 1. Psoriasis 2. Chronic bronchitis 3. Trichomonas vaginitis 4. Carbuncles, sores (external use).

Chemical Composition ▶ Mainly contains diterpenes such as langduin B and jolkinolide A, B.

Note ▶ Listed in Hong Kong as Category I (Toxic/Potent) Chinese Materia Medica is the unprocessed root of *E. fischeriana* Stend. and of *E. ebracteolata* Hayata and *Stellera chamaejasme* L. The processed Radix Euphorbiae Fischerianae is listed in Category II.

Radix Gentianae

Chinese Gentian
Longdan
龍膽

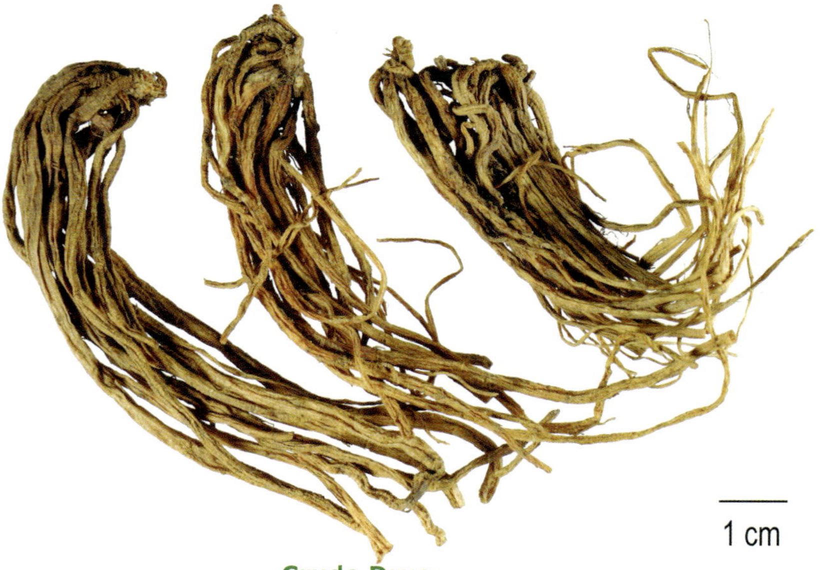

Crude Drug

Source The root and rhizome of *Gentiana scabra* Bunge (Fam. Gentianaceae).

Distribution Mainly in northeastern China.

Harvest & Processing Dig out roots and rhizomes in spring and autumn; remove remnants of above-ground stems; wash away soil; dry under the sun. The ones collected in autumn are of better quality.

Description Rhizome in the form of irregular pieces; outer surface dull greyish-brown or dark brown; top end marked with stem scars or remnants of caudexes; all sides and lower end with numerous slender roots. Roots cylindrical, slightly twisted; outer surface pale yellow or yellowish-brown; upper part usually with conspicuous transverse wrinkles; lower part thinner, marked with longitudinal wrinkles and scars of branch roots. Brittle, break easily. Broken surface slightly even; cortex yellowish-white or pale yellowish-brown; xylem paler in colour, with 5-8 xylem bundles arranged in an annular (ring-like) form, commonly known as "*jinmai dian*" (vein dots). Odour: faint; taste: quite bitter.

Indications 1. Jaundice, hypochondriac pain, bitter taste in the mouth 2. Leukorrhoea, vulvitis, eczema 3. Headache, flushed face, red eyes restlessness, hypertension 4. High fever with convulsion

Chemical Composition Mainly contains iridoid glycosides such as gentiopicroside and swertiamarin.

Note According to *C.P.*, also used for medicinal purposes is the root and rhizome of *G. triflora* Pall., of *G. manshurica* Kitag. and of *G. rigescens* Franch.

Radix Gentianae Macrophyllae

Largeleaf Gentian Root

Qinjiao

秦艽

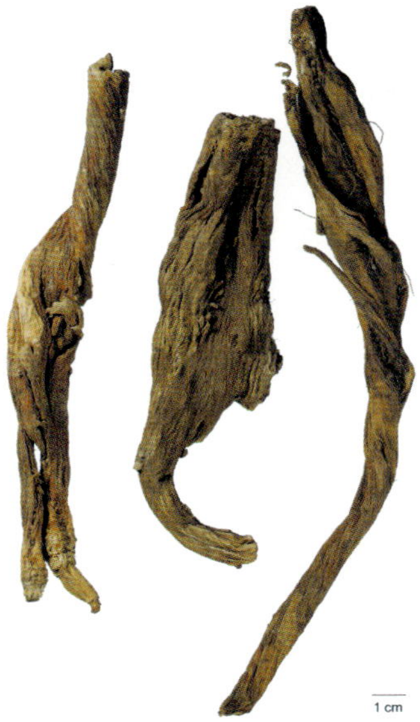

Crude Drug

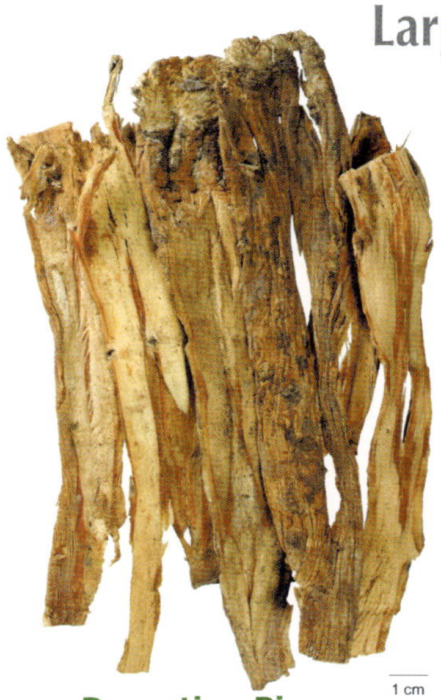

Decoction Pieces

Source The root of *Gentiana straminea* Maxim. (Fam. Gentianaceae).

Distribution Mainly in Chinese provinces such as Gansu, Shanxi and Shaanxi.

Harvest & Processing Dig out roots in spring and autumn; remove leaves and foreign matter dry under the sun. Commonly used in Hong Kong in the form of length-wise cut slices.

Description Subconical, mostly with several rootlets knotted and intertwined like a dough twist; 8-30 cm long, up to 7 cm in diameter. Outer surface reddish-brown; rough; marked with numerous twisted markings and mesh-like clefts. Texture loose, brittle, breaks easily; broken surface mostly looks withered.

Indications 1. Arthralgia, muscular spasm 2. Infantile malnutrition with fever, hectic fever 3. Jaundice, dysuria, dyschezia.

Chemical Composition Mainly contains iridoids such as swertiamarin.

Note According to *C.P.*, also used for medicinal purposes is the root of *G. macrophylla* Pall., of *G. crassicaulis* Duthie ex Burk., and of *G. dahurica* Fisch.

Radix Ginseng

Ginseng
Renshen

人參

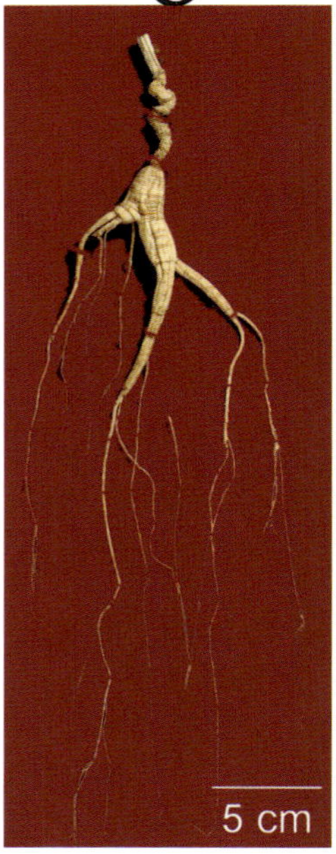

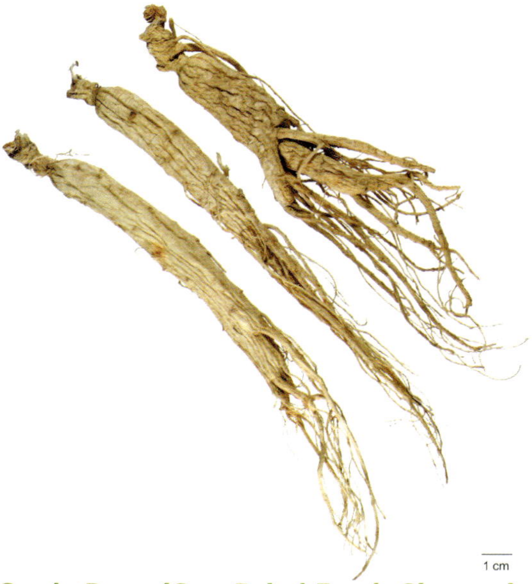

Crude Drug (Sun-Dried Fresh Ginseng)

Source The root of *Panax ginseng* C. A. Mey. (Fam. Araliaceae).

Distribution Mainly in Chinese provinces such as Jilin, Liaoning and Heilongjiang. Mostly cultivated.

Harvest & Processing Collect cultivated ginseng in autumn; wash clean; remove branch roots; dry ginseng under the sun or by heat to produce '*Shengshai shen*' (Sun-Dried Fresh Ginseng), or dry ginseng under the sun without removing branch roots to produce '*Quanxu Shengshai shen*' (Sun-Dried Whole Fresh Ginseng).

Description Axial root of Sun-Dried Fresh Ginseng spindle-shaped or cylindrical; outer surface greyish-yellow; upper part or entire root marked with sparse, shallow and interrupted thick transverse striae and conspicuous longitudinal wrinkles; lower part with 2-3 branch roots. Sun-Dried Whole Fresh Ginseng bears numerous fine long rootlets marked usually with indistinct small verruciform (wart-shaped) protuberances. Rhizome 1-4 cm long, 0.3-1.5 cm in diameter; mostly constricted and curved; with adventitious roots and sparse dented stem scars. Relatively hard. Transverse section pale yellowish-white, starchy; cambium ring brownish-yellow; cortex marked with punctiform (dot-like) yellowish-brown resin ducts and radial clefts. Odour: slightly fragrant and distinctive; taste: slightly bitter, gradually sweet.

Indications 1. General weakness, palpitations, forgetfulness. 2. Thirst and hyperhidrosis, anorexia 3. All kinds of chronic disease, post-haemorrhagic shock, collapse.

Chemical Composition Mainly contains triterpene saponins such as ginsenosides R_{b1}, R_{b2}, R_c, R_d, R_e, R_{g1}.

Radix Glehniae

Coastal Glehnia Root
Beishashen

北沙參

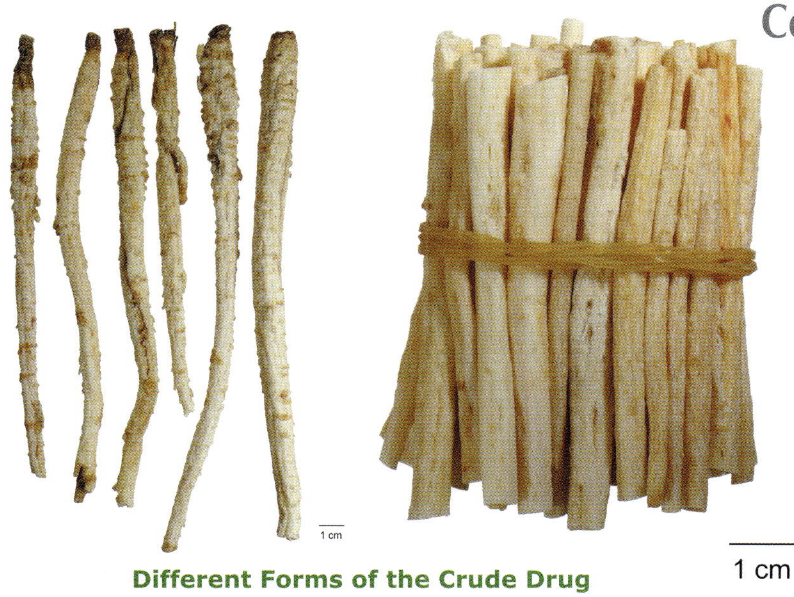

Different Forms of the Crude Drug

Source The root of *Glehnia littoralis* Fr. Schmidt ex Miq. (Fam. Umbelliferae).

Distribution Mainly in Chinese provinces such as Jiangsu and Shandong; also in Hong Kong.

Harvest & Processing Collect roots in summer and autumn; remove above-ground parts and rootlets; wash clean; dry briefly by airing; boil in boiling water; remove cork; dry roots under the sun or dry by heat, or dry directly under the sun after washing clean.

Description Slender and cylindrical; 15-45 cm long, 0.4-1.2 cm in diameter. Slender at the top, often marked with remnants of yellowish-brown rhizome base; thicker in the middle, getting slender again towards the end. Outer surface pale yellowish-white; relatively rough; with fine longitudinal wrinkles and grooves as well as punctiform (dot-like) brownish-yellow or white lenticels and scars of rootlets all over. Hard and brittle, breaks easily. Transverse section shows light yellowish-white cortex and yellow xylem; cortex and xylem separate easily, sometimes with clefts. Odour: distinctive; taste: slightly sweet.

Indications 1. Dry cough, chronic cough 2. Thirst in febrile diseases

Chemical Composition Mainly contains coumarins such as psoralen also contains essential oils.

Radix Glycyrrhizae

Liquorice Root
Gancao

甘草

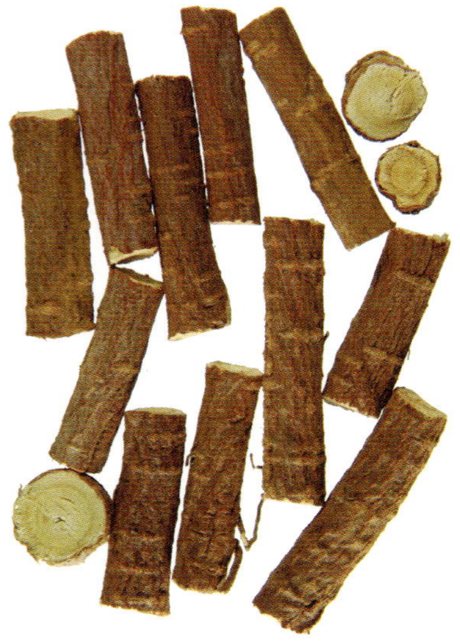

Crude Drug 1 cm

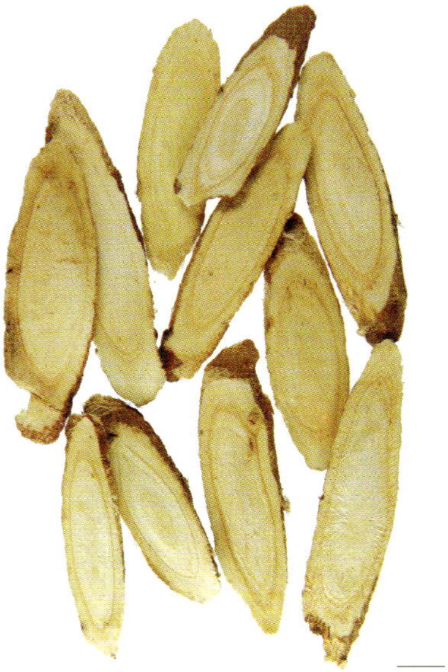

Decoction Pieces 1 cm

Source The root and rhizome of *Glycyrrhiza uralensis* Fisch. (Fam. Leguminosae).

Distribution Mainly in Chinese provinces such as Gansu, and in Xinjiang, Inner Mongolia and the western part of northeastern China.

Harvest & Processing Dig out roots and rhizomes in spring and autumn, with the ones collected in spring of better quality; cut away caudexes, young buds, branch roots and fibrous roots while fresh; cut roots and rhizomes into long sections; dry under the sun.

Description Root cylindrical; 25-100 cm long, 0.6-3 cm in diameter. Bark varies in tightness; reddish-brown or greyish-brown; marked with conspicuous longitudinal wrinkles, grooves and sparse rootlet scars; lenticels lalongate (transversely elongated). Hard and solid; heavy; when broken, surface slightly fibrous, yellowish-white, starchy, marked with a conspicuous cambium ring, radial markings and clefts. Rhizome cylindrical; outer surface with bud scars; cross-section with pith in the centre. Odour: faint; taste: sweet and distinctive.

Indications 1. Sore throat, cough 2. Gastric hyposecretion, gastroduodenal ulcer 3. Hysteria 4. Dermatitis and boils 5. Drug and food poisoning.

Chemical Composition Mainly contains triterpene saponins such as glycyrrhizin, also contains flavonoids such as liquiritin.

Note According to *C.P.*, also used for medicinal purposes is the root of *G. inflata* Bat. and of *G. glabra* L.

Radix Hedysari

Manyinflorescenced Sweetvech Root

Hongqi

紅芪

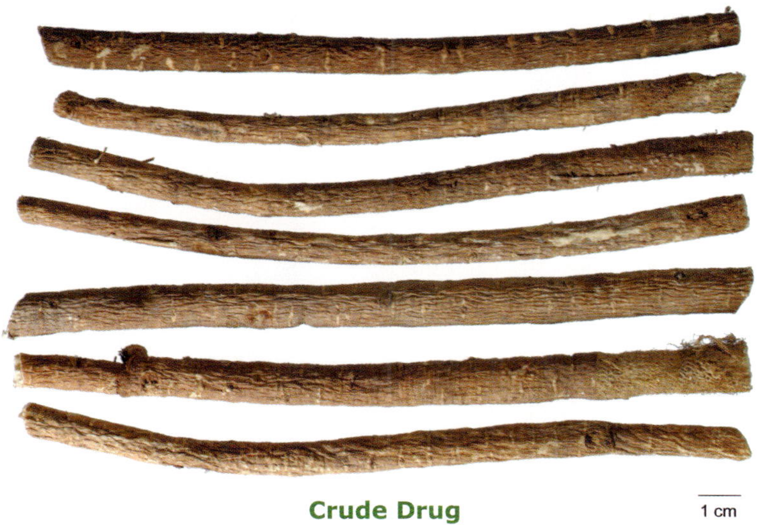

Crude Drug

Source The root of *Hedysarum polybotrys* Hand. -Mazz. (Fam. Leguminosae).

Distribution Mainly in Gansu province in China.

Harvest & Processing Dig up roots in autumn; wash clean; remove top part of roots and rootlets; dry the rest under the sun; bundle up.

Description Cylindrical, with few branches; 10-50 cm long, 0.8-2 cm in diameter. Outer surface dull reddish-brown, marked with longitudinal wrinkles and sparse scars of branch roots; lenticels lalongate (transversely elongated), slightly paler in colour, slightly protuberant. Cork peels off easily, exposing pale yellow cortex and fibres. Hard, difficult to break; broken surface fibrous, pale in colour, highly starchy. When broken transversely, surface reveals pale brown cortex, which takes up about 1/2-1/3 of the radius; cambium brown, arranged in rings; xylem dense. Odour: faint; taste: slightly sweet; bean-like when chewed.

Indications 1. Debility, anorexia and loose stools, anaemia, oedema, diabetes 2. Rectal prolapse 3. Bleeding 4. Spontaneous sweating 5. Abscess or boil difficult to burst

Chemical Composition Mainly contains isoflavonoids such as tormononetin.

Note According to *C.P.*, also used for medicinal purposes is a processed Radix Hedysari called '*Zhi hong qi*' (Prepared Manyinflorescenced Sweetvech Root).

Radix Helicteris

Narrowleaf Screwtree Root
Shanzhima

山芝麻

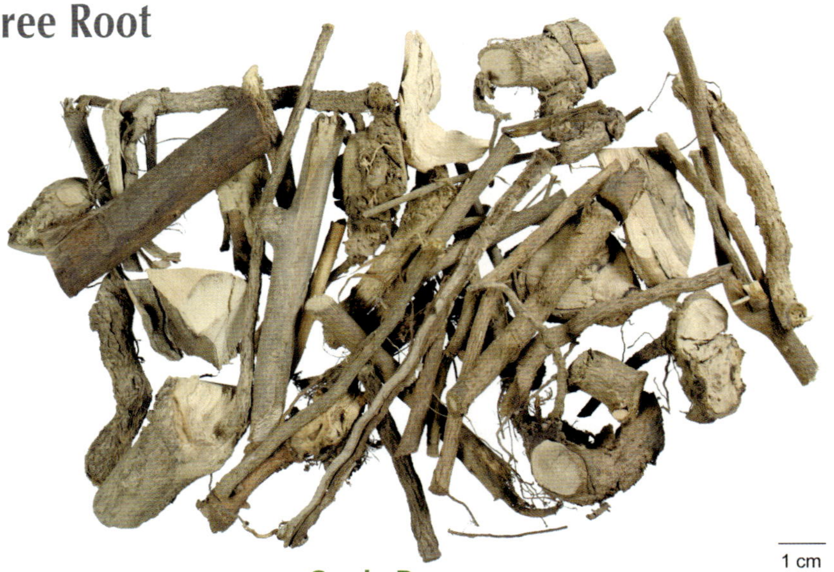

Crude Drug

Source The root of *Helicteres angustifolia* L. (Fam. Sterculiaceae).

Distribution Mainly in Chinese provinces such as Jiangxi, Fujian, Guangdong, Guangxi, Hunan, Taiwan, Yunnan and Guizhou; also in Hong Kong.

Harvest & Processing Collect roots anytime during the year; wash clean; cut into sections; dry under the sun.

Description Cylindrical, slightly twisted; top part often with nodular remnants of stems and branches; 15-25 cm long (commercial crude drugs usually cut into 2 cm-long pieces), 0.5-1.5 cm in diameter. Outer surface greyish-yellow to dull greyish-brown, occasionally with strong and pliable lateral roots or lateral root scars; cork rough, with cracks slanting longitudinally; cork of old roots scales off easily. Hard. When broken, cortex on surface dull brown or greyish-yellow, relatively thick, heavily fibrous, and peels off easily from xylem; xylem yellowish-white, with fine dense radial rays. Odour: slightly fragrant; taste: bitter and slightly astringent.

Indications 1. Febrile diseases 2. Upper respiratory infection, sore throat and cough with yellow sputum 3. Measles and mumps 4. Enteritis, dysentery, heamorrhoid 5. Carbuncles, scrofula

Chemical Composition Mainly contains triterpenes such as betulic acid and oleanolic acid.

Radix Ilicis Asprellae

Roughhaired Holly Root
Gangmeigen

崗梅根

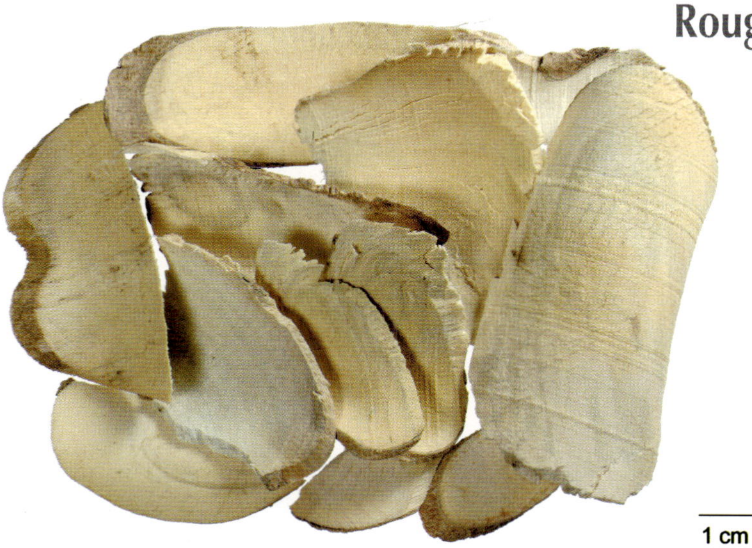

Decoction Pieces

Source The root of *Ilex asprella* (Hook. f. et Arn.) Champ. ex Benth. (Fam. Aquifoliaceae).

Distribution Mainly in Chinese provinces such as Guangdong, Guangxi, Fujian, Hunan and Jiangxi; also in Hong Kong.

Harvest & Processing Dig up roots in autumn; wash away soil; dry under the sun.

Description Somewhat cylindrical, slightly curved, rameous (branched); 30-50 cm long, 1.5-3 cm in diameter. Outer surface greyish-yellow to dull greyish-brown; marked with longitudinal wrinkles and scars of rootlets. Hard, does not break easily. Odour: faint; taste: bitter, then sweet. Commercially sold in the form of suborbicular (almost round) slices or sections; cortex relatively thin; xylem relatively broad, light yellow, marked with radial striae and numerous irregular annulations.

Indications 1. Common cold, cough, seasonal febrile diseases with thirst, headache and sore throat 2. Arthralgia 3. Angina pectoris

Chemical Composition Mainly contains lignans such as syringaresinol.

Radix Isatidis

Isatis Root
Banlangen
板藍根

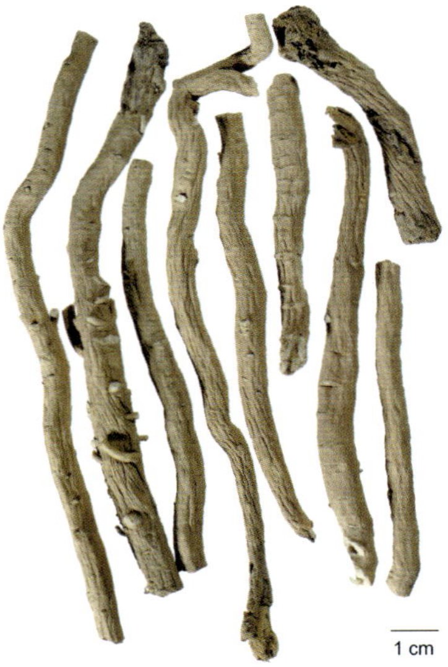

Crude Drug

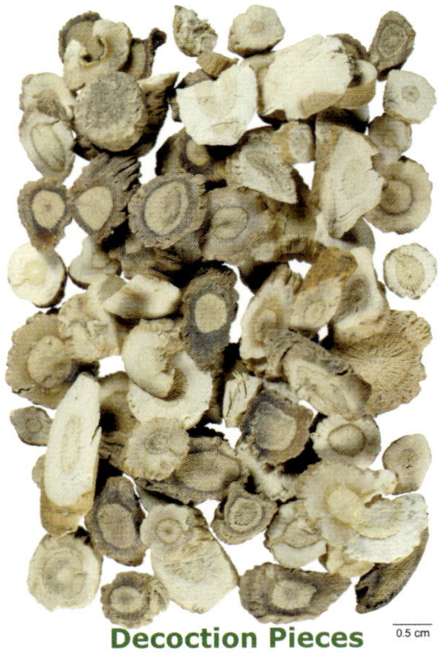

Decoction Pieces

Source The root of *Isatis indigotica* Fort. (Fam. Cruciferae).

Distribution Mainly in Chinese provinces such as Hebei and Jiangsu. Introduced to and cultivated in most regions of China.

Harvest & Processing Dig out roots in autumn; remove stemsand leaves; wash clean and dry under the sun; store in cool, dry places.

Description Cylindrical, slightly twisted; 10-20 cm long, 0.5-1 cm in diameter. Outer surface pale greyish-yellow or pale brownish-yellow, marked with longitudinal wrinkles, transverse lenticels and branch roots or branch root scars; top part slightly bulgy, with verticillate (arranged in whorls) dull green or dull brown remnants of petiole base, petiole scars and dense verruciform (wart-shaped) protuberances. Solid and slightly brittle. When broken, surface fairly even; bark yellowish-white, occupying about 1/2-3/4 of radius; xylem yellow.

Indications 1. Seasonal febrile diseases, pestilence 2. Mumps and other eruptive exanthem 3. Aphthous ulcer, sore throat.

Chemical Composition Mainly contains indigotin and indirubin.

Radix Kansui

Gansui Root

Gansui

甘遂

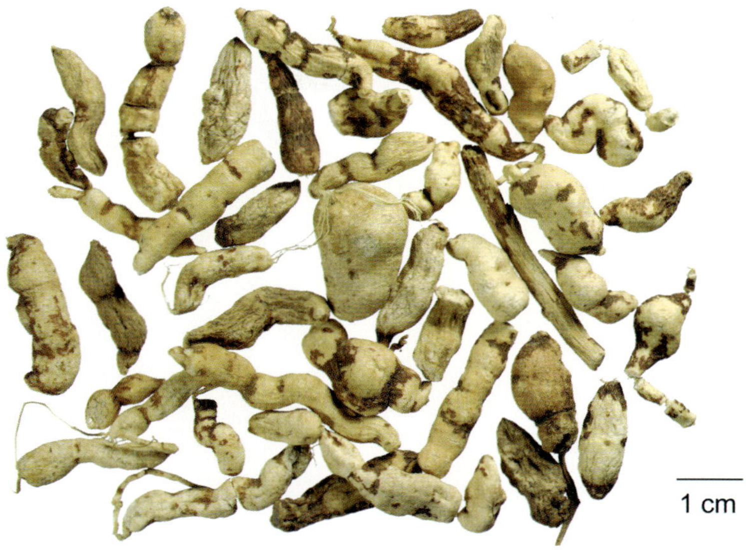

Crude Drug

Source The root tuber of *Euphorbia kansui* T. N. Liou ex T. P. Wang (Fam. Euphorbiaceae).

Distribution Mainly in Chinese provinces such as Shaanxi, Henan and Shanxi, and in Ningxia.

Harvest & Processing Dig out root tubers in spring before efflorescence or in autumn after shoots have withered; remove soil; wash clean; remove cork; dry under the sun.

Description Ellipsoid (elliptical in long-section and circular in cross-section), or long and cylindrical, or torose (cylindrical with alternate swellings and constrictions); 1-5 cm long, 0.5-2.5 cm in diameter. For the ones with cork removed, outer surface off-white or yellowish-white, with brown cork remnants at constrictions; for those with brownish-red cork intact, outer surface marked with conspicuous longitudinal grooves and a few lalongate (transversely elongated) lenticels. Brittle, breaks easily. Broken surface starchy; cortex off-white; xylem pale yellow, with radial markings. The long and cylindrical ones with strongly fibrous broken surface. Odour: faint; taste: slightly sweet, acrid, irritating.

Indications 1. Constipation, abdominal pain and distension, ileus 2. Bowel preparation before abdominal operation 3. Oedema, ascites, hydrothorax 4. Weeping skin infection, mumps (external use).

Chemical Composition Mainly contains euphornin, 2-euphorbol, tirucallol and kansuinine A, B.

Note Listed in Hong Kong as Category I (Toxic/Potent) Chinese Materia Medica, and the processed Radix Kansui, Category II.

Radix Knoxiae

Knoxia Root
Hongdaji
紅大戟

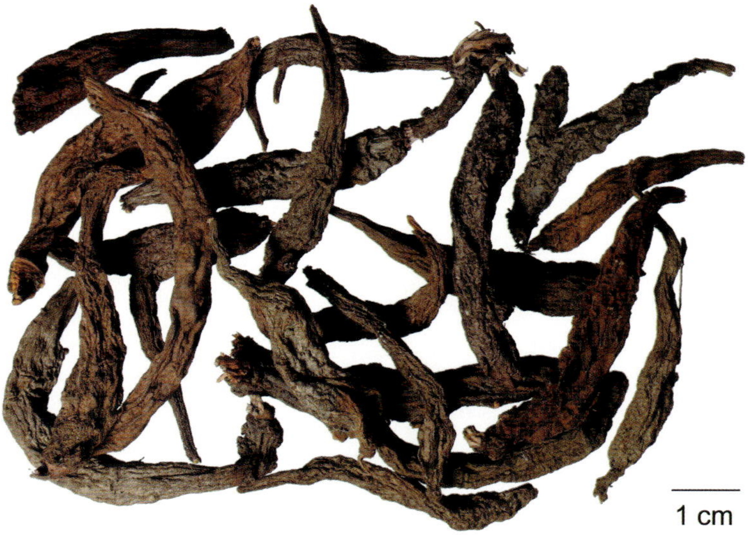

Crude Drug

Source The root tuber of *Knoxia valerianoides* Thorel et Pitard (Fam. Rubiaceae).

Distribution Mainly in Chinese provinces such as Fujian, Guangdong, Guangxi and Yunnan.

Harvest & Processing Dig up root tubers in autumn and winter; remove rootlets; wash clean; blanch in boiling water; dry.

Description Slightly spindle-shaped, or long and conical, usually without branches, slightly curved; 3-12 cm long, 0.6-1.2 cm in diameter. Outer surface brownish-red or greyish-brown, marked with twisted longitudinal wrinkles; top end with stem scars. Hard and solid, breaks easily. When broken, surface shows reddish-brown cortex and brownish-yellow xylem. Odourless; taste: sweet and slightly acrid. Sticky when moistened.

Indications 1. Hydrothorax, ascites 2. Carbuncles, sores, scrofula.

Chemical Composition Mainly contains anthraquinones such as damnacanthal and rubiadin.

Note Listed as slightly toxic in *C.P.*

Radix Linderae

Combined Spicebush Root

Wuyao

烏藥

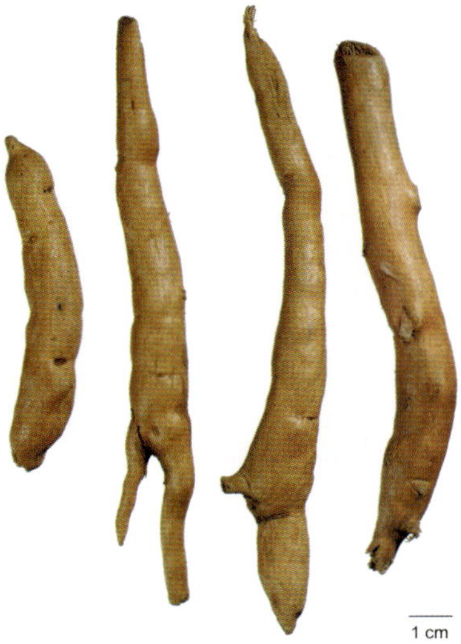

Crude Drug

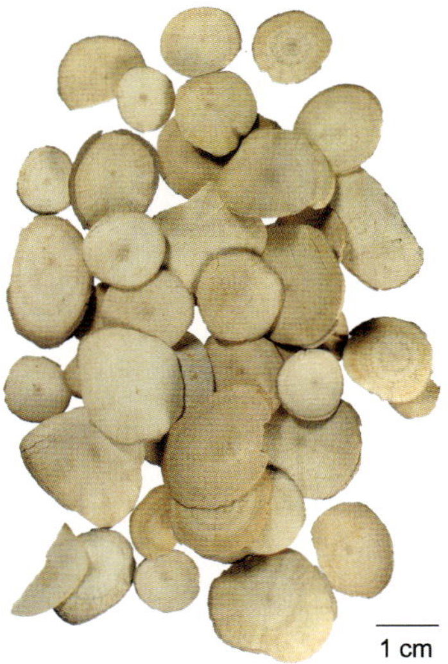

Decoction Pieces

Source The root tuber of *Lindera aggregate* (Sims) Kosterm. (Fam. Lauraceae).

Distribution Mainly in Chinese provinces such as Zhejiang, Anhui, Hunan, Guangdong and Guangxi.

Harvest & Processing Dig out root tubers anytime during the year; remove rootlets; wash clean; cut into slices while fresh and dry under the sun, or dry under the sun without slicing.

Description Mostly spindle-shaped; slightly curved. The ones with the middle part contracted and torose (cylindrical with alternate swellings and constrictions) are known as "*wuyao zhu*"(Combined Spicebush Root Pearls). 6-15 cm long, 1-3 cm in diameter; outer surface yellowish-brown or dull yellowish-brown; marked with longitudinal wrinkles and sparse rootlet scars. Hard; slices 0.2-2 mm thick; cut surface yellowish-white or pale yellowish-brown, with radial rays and annual rings, with the core darker in colour. Odour: fragrant; taste: slightly bitter, acrid, fresh.

Indications 1. Chest, gastric or abdominal pains 2. Dysmenorrhoea 3. Hernia pain 4. Rheumatic arthralgia with bone involvement, post traumatic pain

Chemical Composition Mainly contains sesquiterpenes such as linderol and linderane.

Radix Liriopes

Liriope Root Tuber
Shanmaidong

山麥冬

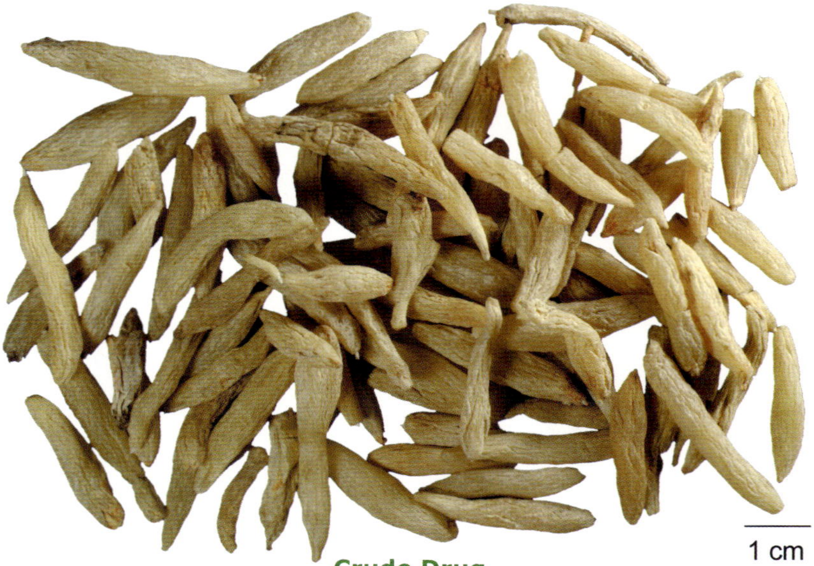

Crude Drug

Source The root tuber of *Liriope spicata* (Thunb.) Lour. *var. prolifera* Y. T. Ma (Fam. Liliaceae).

Distribution Mainly in Yangtze valley regions in Hubei province in China. Cultivated.

Harvest & Processing Cultivate liriopes between early and mid April and harvest in the following spring. Dig out root tubers; wash away sand and soil; dry under the sun or by heat; remove rootlets when dried; sieve away foreign matter.

Description Spindle-shaped, both ends slightly pointed; 1-3 cm long, 4-7 mm in diameter. Outer surface pale yellow to brownish-yellow; marked with irregular longitudinal wrinkles. Soft and pliable; hard and brittle when dried, breaks easily. Broken surface pale yellow to brownish-yellow, cuticular, with a small stele. Odour: faint; taste: sweet, sticky when chewed.

Indications 1. Dry coughs, thirst 2. Dysphoria, insomnia 3. Constipation.

Chemical Composition Mainly contains steroidal saponins.

Note According to *C.P.*, also used for medicinal purposes is the root tuber of *L. muscari* (Decne.) Baily.

Radix Lithospermi

Gromwell Root
Zicao
紫草

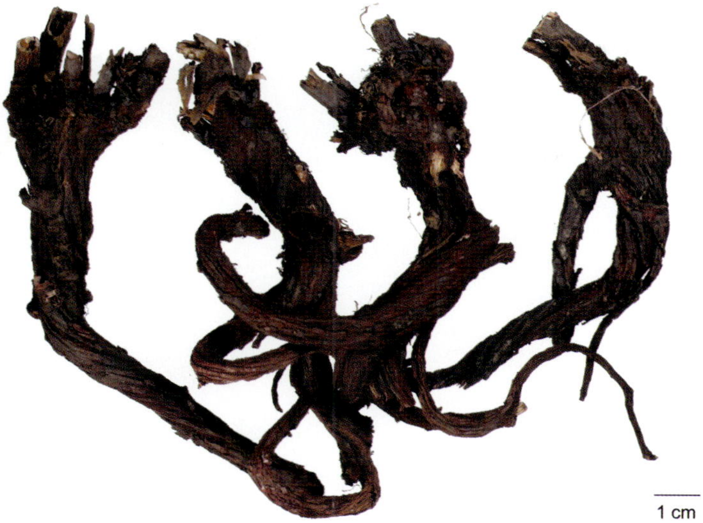

Crude Drug

Source The root of *Lithospermum erythrorhizon* Sieb. et Zucc. (Fam. Boraginaceae). Generally called '*Ying zicao*'(Hard Gromwell Root).

Distribution Mainly in Chinese provinces such as Heilongjiang, Liaoning, Jilin, Hebei, Henan, Shanxi, Shandong and Hunan.

Harvest & Processing Dig out roots in spring and autumn; remove soil; dry under the sun.

Description Conical or cylindrical, twisted, often rameous (branched); 7-15 cm long, 1-2 cm in diameter. Top part with caudex remnants. Outer surface purplish-red or purplish-black; rough; marked with longitudinal striae; cortex thin, falls off easily. Hard and brittle; when broken, surface uneven; cortex dark purple; xylem relatively large, greyish-yellow. Odour: distinctive; taste: sweet and slightly sour.

Indications 1. Measles and other eruptive exanthem, skin infection, eczema, burn 2. Constipation.

Chemical Composition Mainly contains naphthoquinones such as shikonin; also contains lithospermic acid.

Note According to *C.P.*, also used for medicinal purposes is the root of *Arnebia euchroma* (Royle) Johnst. and *A. guttata* Bunge, both of which belong to the same family as *L. erythrorhizon* Sieb. *et* Zucc.

Radix Morindae Officinalis

Morinda Root
Bajitian
巴戟天

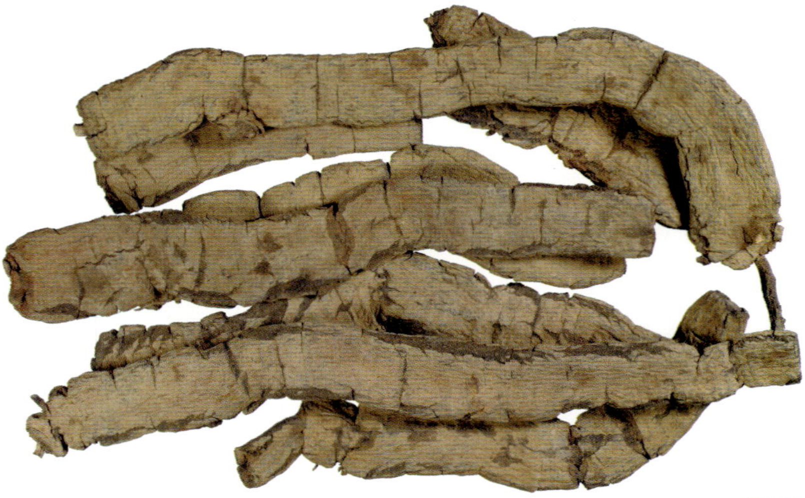

Crude Drug

Source The root of *Morinda officinalis* How (Fam. Rubiaceae).

Distribution Mainly in Chinese provinces such as Guangdong, Guangxi and Fujian.

Harvest & Processing Collect roots anytime during the year; clear away soil; remove fibrous roots; dry under the sun until nearly dry; pound gently to flatten; cut into segments 9-13 cm long; dry under the sun.

Description Flattened and cylindrical, slightly curved; varying in length, 0.5-2 cm in diameter. Outer surface greyish-yellow; rough; marked with longitudinal striae and transverse cracks; cortex occasionally with transverse cracks, exposing xylem the shape of stringed beads. Pliable. When broken, surface shows thick, purple or pale purple cortex; cortex separates easily from xylem; xylem hard, yellowish-brown or yellowish-white, 1-5 mm in diameter. Odourless; taste: sweet and slightly astringent.

Indications 1. Impotence, seminal emissions 2. Menstrual disorders 3. Pain in the lower abdomen, rheumatic arthralgia 4. Weakness of the extremities.

Chemical Composition Mainly contains anthraquinones such as rubiadin; also contains iridoid glycosides such as monotropein.

Radix Notoginseng

Sanchi

Sanqi

三七

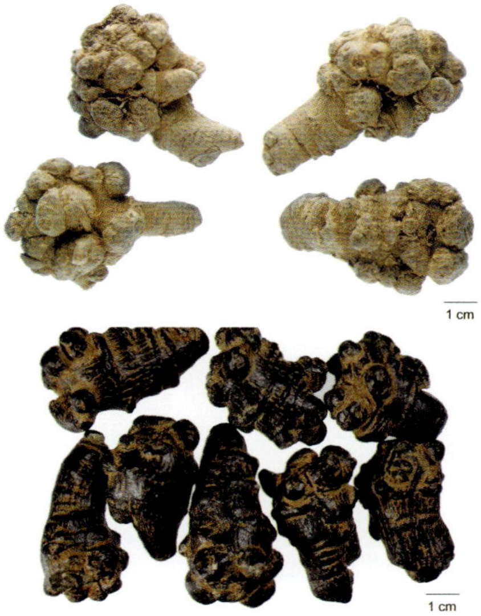

Crude Drug

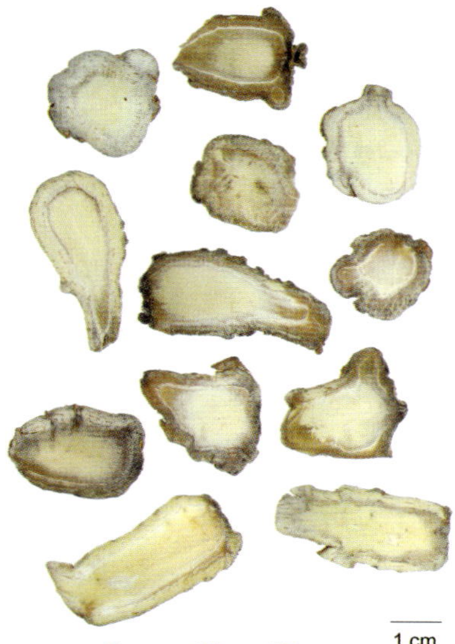

Decoction Pieces

Source The root of *Panax notoginseng* (Burk.) F. H. Chen (Fam. Araliaceae).

Distribution Mainly in Chinese provinces such as Guangxi and Yunnan. Mostly cultivated.

Harvest & Processing Collect roots in autumn before efflorescence, usually in the third or fourth year of cultivation; wash clean; separate axial roots, lateral roots from rhizomes; dry under sun until half-dry; knead repeatedly; remove cork. The *sanqi* commonly used in Hong Kong are roots which have been coloured with coal smoke and lustred with insect wax.

Description Axial root subconical or cylindrical. Outer surface dull greyish-brown or greyish-yellow, marked with interrupted longitudinal wrinkles, scars of branch roots and a few lenticels; apex marked with stem scars; with encircling strumiform (cushion-like) protuberances. Heavy; hard and solid; cortex and xylem often separate when crumbled. When broken, surface greyish-green, yellowish-green or greyish-white; cortex dotted with small brownish resin ducts; xylem slightly radial. Odour: light; taste: bitter, gradually sweet.

Indications 1. Various kinds of bleeding especially traumatic bleeding 2. Amenorrhoea, dysmenorrhoea 3. Coronary heart disease, angina pectoris, hyperlipidemia, chronic infectious hepatitis

Chemical Composition Mainly contains notoginsenosides and ginsenosides.

Radix Ophiopogonis

Dwarf Lilyturf Tuber
Maidong

麦冬

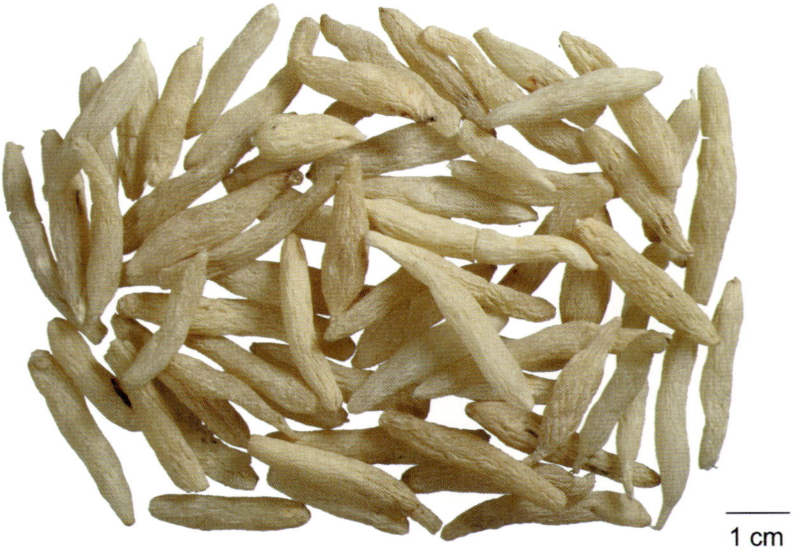

Crude Drug

Source The root tuber of *Ophiopogon japonicus* (Thunb.) Ker-Gawl. (Fam. Liliaceae).

Distribution Mainly in Chinese provinces such as Zhejiang and Sichuan; the ones from Zhejiang are known as '*Zhe maidong*'(Zhejiang Dwarf Lilyturf Tuber), and the ones from Sichuan, '*Chuan maidong*' (Sichuan Dwarf Lilyturf Tuber).

Harvest & Processing In Zhejiang, plants are collected from mid-April to late June in the third year of cultivation; in Sichuan, they are collected from early to mid April in the second year. Cut off root tubers; wash clean; dry repeatedly under scorching sun and pile up until nearly dry; remove fibrous roots; dry.

Description Spindle-shaped, both ends slightly pointed; 1.5-3 cm long, 3-6 mm in diameter in middle part. Outer surface yellowish-white or pale yellow; translucent; marked with fine, irregular and relatively deep longitudinal striae; one end often with small exposed stele. Pliable; when broken, surface yellowish-white, cuticular, translucent, with a small cylindrical stele in the centre. Odour: faint; taste: sweet and slightly bitter. Sticky when chewed.

Indications 1. Cough, pharyngitis, haemoptysis 2. Thirst 3. Anxiety

Chemical Composition Mainly contains steroidal saponins such as ophiopogonin A, B.

Radix Paeoniae Alba

White Peony Root
Baishao

白芍

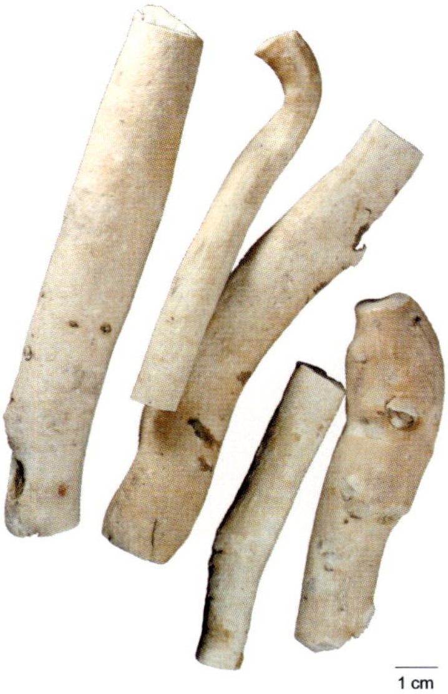

Crude Drug

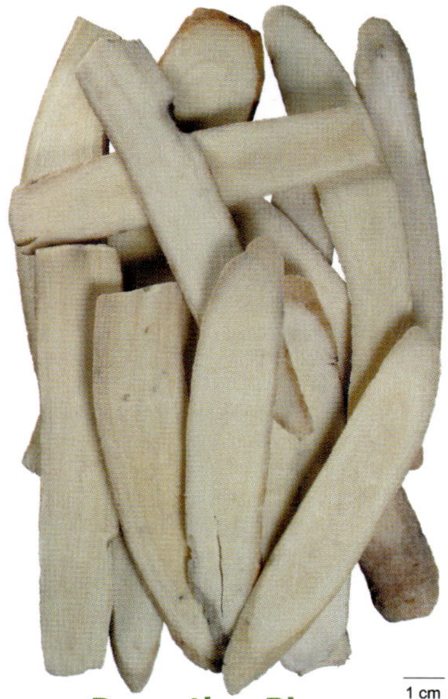

Decoction Pieces

Source The root of *Paeonia lactiflora* Pall. (Fam. Ranunculaceae).

Distribution Mainly in Chinese provinces such as Zhejiang, Anhui, Sichuan, Guizhou and Shandong.

Harvest & Processing Collect roots in summer and autumn; wash clean; remove the two ends and rootlets; peel cork after thoroughly boiled, or peel before boiling; dry roots under the sun.

Description Cylindrical, straight or slightly curved, two ends truncate (squared as if cut off); 5-18 cm long, 1-2.5 cm in diameter. Outer surface off-white or pale reddish-brown; smooth; marked with faint lalongate (transversely elongated) lenticels and longitudinal wrinkles, rootlet scars or remnants of reddish-brown cork. Hard and solid, does not break easily. Transverse section relatively smooth, off-white or slightly brownish-red, cuticular; cambium ring conspicuous; xylem marked with radial markings. Odour: faint; taste: slightly bitter, sour.

Indications 1. Menstrual disorders, dysfunctional uterine bleeding 2. Hypochondriac pain, abdominal pain and spasmodic pain of the limbs 3. Headache and dizziness 4. Sweating

Chemical Composition Mainly contains monoterpene glycosides such as paeonioflorin.

Radix Paeoniae Rubra

Red Peony Root
Chishao

赤芍

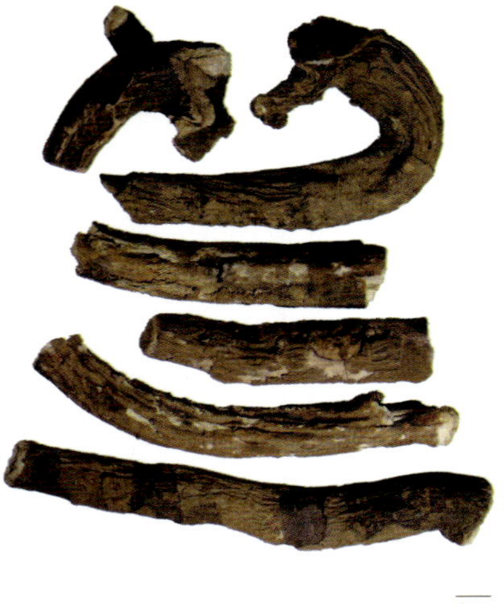

Crude Drug

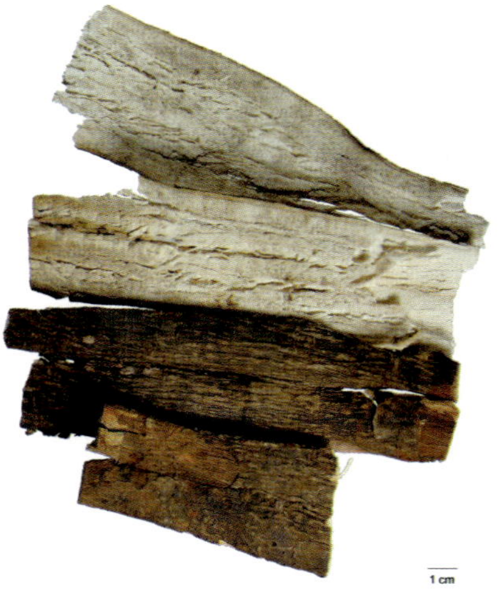

Decoction Pieces

Source The root of *Paeonia lactiflora* Pall. (Fam. Ranunculaceae).

Distribution Mainly in regions such as Inner Mongolia and in northeastern China; also in chinese provinces such as Hebei, Shaanxi, Shanxi and Gansu.

Harvest & Processing Collect roots in spring and autumn; remove rhizomes, rootlets, soil and sand; dry under the sun. Commonly used in Hong Kong in the form of length-wise cut and compressed slices.

Description Cylindrical and slightly curved; 5-40 cm long, 0.5-3cm in diameter. Outer surface reddish-brown; rough; marked with longitudinal grooves, wrinkles, scars of rootlets, and transverse protuberant lenticels; in some cases bark falls off easily. Hard and brittle, breaks easily. Transverse section pink-white or pink; cortex narrow; xylem with conspicuous radial markings; broken surface sometimes with clefts. Odour: slightly fragrant; taste: slightly bitter, sour-astringent.

Indications 1. Seasonal febrile diseases with eruptions 2. Bleeding 3. Menstrual disorders 4. Pain over chest, hypochondrium and abdomen, trauma 5. Skin infection, conjunctivitis.

Chemical Composition Mainly contains paeoniflorin and gallotannins.

Note According to *C.P.*, also used for medicinal purposes is the root of *P. veitchii* Lynch.

Radix Panacis Quinquefolii

American Ginseng
Xiyangshen
西洋參

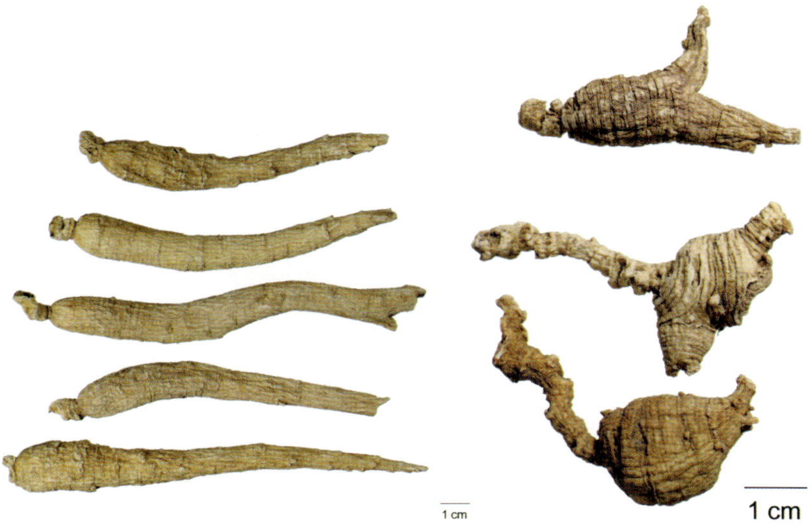

Different Forms of the Crude Drug

Source The root of *Panax quinquefolium* L. (Fam. Araliaceae).

Distribution Originated in Canada and the U.S.A; introduced and cultivated successfully in northeastern, northern and northwestern China.

Harvest & Processing Dig out roots in autumn; remove above-ground parts and soil; remove rootstocks, lateral roots and rootlets; wash roots clean; dry under the sun or at low temperatures.

Description Spindle-shaped, cylindrical or conical. Outer surface light yellowish-brown or yellowish-white; marked with transverse annulations and linear (long and narrow) lenticels, and with fine, dense, shallow longitudinal wrinkles and scars of rootlets. Lower middle part of axial root with one to several lateral roots, mostly broken. In some cases upper end with rhizome; annular (ring-like) nodes prominent; stem scar orbicular (round) or semi-orbicular, with adventitious roots remaining or already broken. Heavy; hard and solid, does not break easily. Transverse section even, light yellowish-white, slightly starchy; cortex with yellowish-brown punctiform (dot-like) resin ducts; cambium ring brownish-yellow; xylem arranged roughly in a radial pattern. Odour: faint but distinctive; taste: slightly bitter, gradually sweet.

Indications 1. Chronic cough, haemoptysis 2. Thirst, irritability and debility

Chemical Composition Mainly contains triterpene saponins such as ginsenosides Rb1, Rb2, Rc, Rd, Re.

Radix Patriniae Rupestris

Scabrous Patrinia Root

Mutouhui

墓頭回

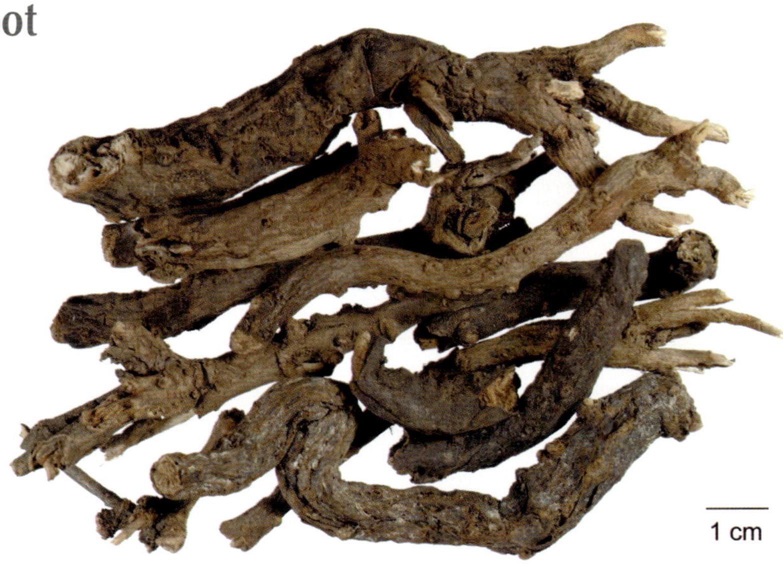

Crude Drug

Source The root of *Patrinia rupestris* (Pall.) Juss. *subsp*. scabra (Bunge) H. J. Wang (Fam. Valerianaceae).

Distribution Mainly in Chinese provinces such as Shanxi, Henan and Hebei.

Harvest & Processing Dig out roots in autumn; remove foreign matter; wash clean; dry under the sun.

Description Irregular and cylindrical, often curved; varying in length, 0.5-5 cm in diameter; top part thick and rameous (branched). Outer surface rough, reddish-brown, shrivelled, often strumose (with cushion-like protuberances); cork falls off easily, exposing brownish-yellow cortex. Broken surface fibrous, with radial clefts. Light in weight; texture loose. Odour: with a distinctive stink; taste: slightly bitter.

Indications 1. Appendicitis, dysentery, hepatitis 2. Conjunctivitis 3. Postpartum abdominal pain 4. Carbuncles, boils 5. Insomnia, neurasthenia.

Chemical Composition Mainly contains essential oils.

Radix Peucedani

Hogfennel Root
Qianhu
前胡

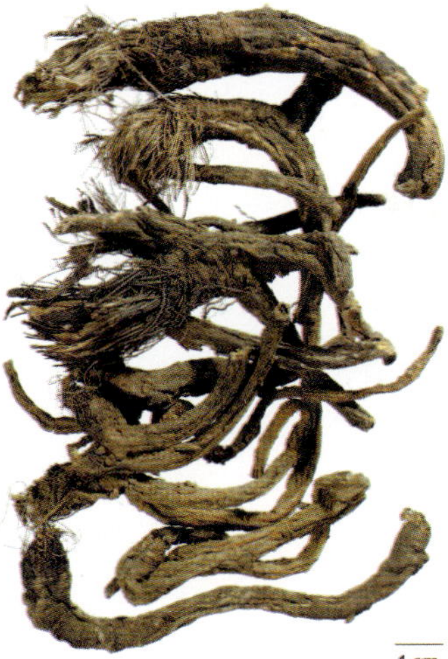

1 cm

Crude Drug
(Peucedanum praeruptorum)

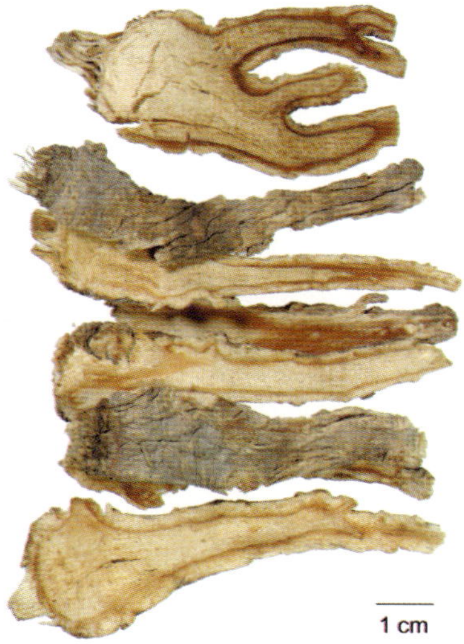

1 cm

Decoction Pieces
(Peucedanum praeruptorum)

Source The root of *Peucedanum praeruptorum* Dunn (Fam. Umbelliferae).

Distribution Mainly in Chinese provinces such as Zhejiang, Hunan and Sichuan.

Harvest & Processing Dig out axial roots in winter when plants have withered, or in early spring before plants put forth shoots; remove leaves, fibrous roots and soil; dry under the sun or by heat. Commonly used in Hong Kong in the form of length-wise cut slices.

Description Somewhat conical, cylindrical or spindle-shaped; slightly twisted; often rameous (branched) at lower part; branch roots mostly removed. Outer surface dull blackish-brown to greyish-yellow; centre of top part usually with stem scars and fibrous remnants of ocrea base. Relatively soft; dried ones hard, break easily. When broken, surface uneven, pale yellowish-white, with a brown cambium ring and radial markings; cortex takes up 3/5 of broken surface, pale yellow and scattered with numerous small brownish-yellow oil dots; xylem yellowish-brown. Odour: aromatic; taste: sweet, then slightly bitter-acrid.

Indications 1. Common cold, upper respiratory infection 2. Cough, copious expectoration.

Chemical Composition Mainly contains coumarins such as praeruptorin A, B.

Note According to *C.P.*, also used for medicinal purposes is the root of *P. decursivum* Maxim.

Radix Physochlainae

Funneled Physochlaina Root

Huashanshen

華山參

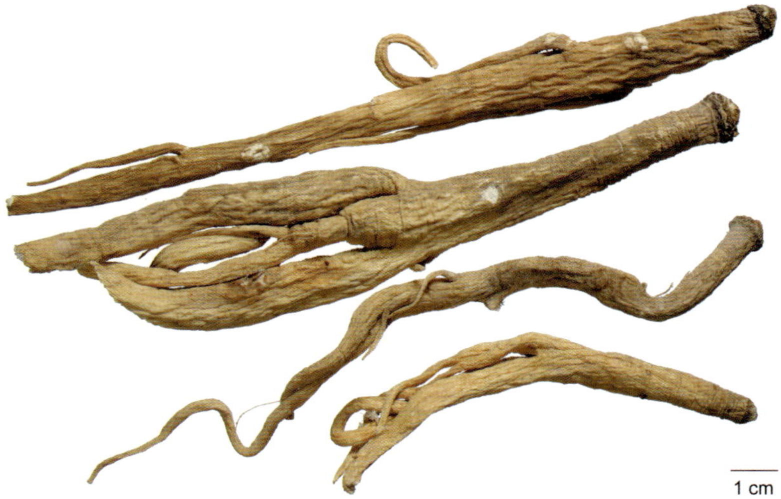

Crude Drug

Source The root of *Physochlaina infundibularis* Kuang (Fam. Solanaceae).

Distribution Mainly in regions such as Shaanxi province, western Henan province and southern Shanxi province in China.

Harvest & Processing Dig out roots in spring; remove rootlets; wash clean; dry under the sun.

Description Long and conical, or cylindrical, slightly curved, in some cases rameous (branched); 10-20 cm long, 1-2.5 cm in diameter. Top end often with 1 to several rhizome(s) marked with suborbicular (almost round) stem scars and verruciform (wart-shaped) protuberances. Lower part of axial root sometimes with 2-3 branches; outer surface reddish-brown or brown, marked with conspicuous wrinkles and lalongate (transversely elongated), yellowish-white lenticels; upper part marked with dense annulations. Relatively hard and brittle; broken surface uneven; cortex quite narrow, off-white; xylem wide, pale yellow, marked with fine dense radial markings. Odour: tobacco-like; taste: slightly bitter, a little tongue-numbing.

Indications 1. Cough and asthma with thin expectoration 2. Palpitation, insomnia

Chemical Composition Mainly contains alkaloids such as atropine and scopolamine.

Radix Phytolaccae

Pokeberry Root
Shanglu
商陸

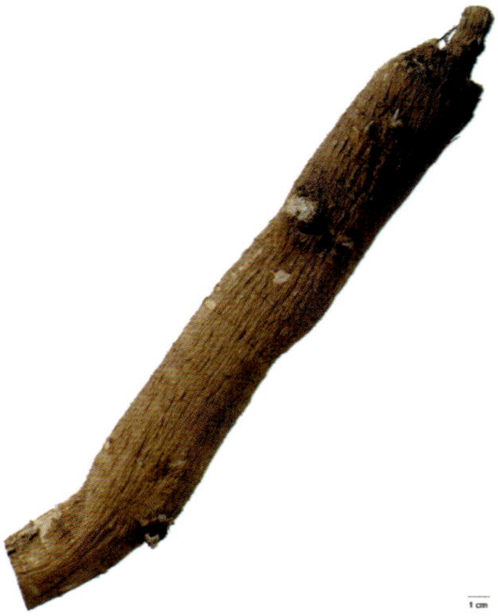

Crude Drug

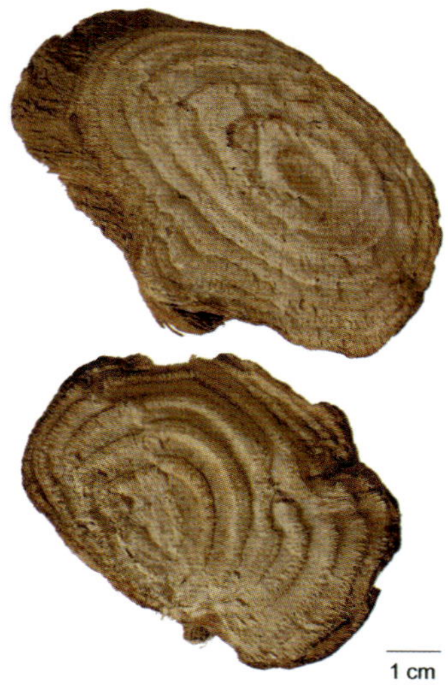

Decoction Pieces

Source The root of *Phytolacca acinosa* Roxb. (Fam. Phytolaccaceae).

Distribution Mainly in Chinese provinces such as Henan, Hubei and Anhui; also in Hong Kong.

Harvest & Processing Dig up roots from autumn to spring; remove fibrous roots, sand and soil; cut roots into pieces or slices; dry under the sun or dry in shaded areas.

Description Irregular cross-cut or length-wise cut pieces or slices; varying in thickness. Bark greyish-yellow or greyish-brown. Cross-cut slices curved and uneven, with shrivelled margin; 2-10 cm in diameter, 2-6 mm thick; cut surface light yellowish-brown or yellowish-white, xylem bulgy and marked with an anomalous structure of several protuberant concentric rings of anomalous vascular bundles–commonly called '*luopan wen*'(compass markings). Hard. Odour: faint; taste: sweet and mild, prolonged chewing numbs the tongue.

Indications 1. Oedema, ascites 2. Dysuria 3. Cervical erosion 4. Carbuncles and sores (external use).

Chemical Composition Mainly contains saponins such as phytolaccoside A, B, D, E.

Note According to *C.P.*, also used for medicinal purposes and listed as toxic is the root of *P. americana* L..

Radix Platycodonis

Platycodon Root
Jiegeng

桔梗

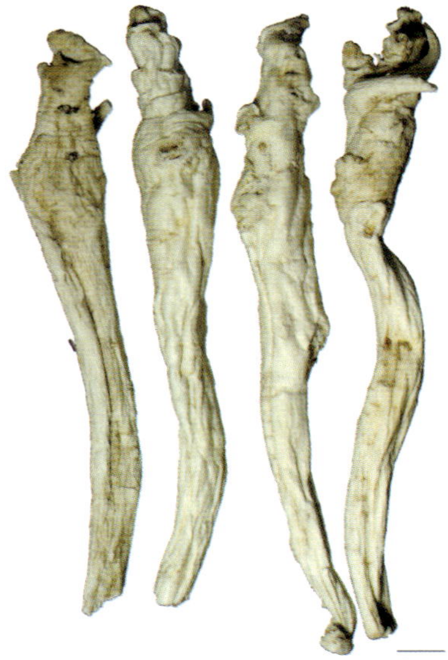

Crude Drug

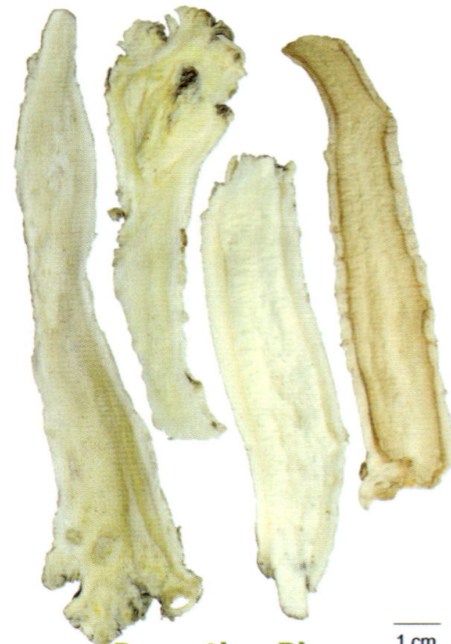

Decoction Pieces

Source The root of *Platycodon grandiflorum* (Jacq.) A. DC. (Fam. Campanulaceae).

Distribution Mainly in northeastern and northern China; also in Hong Kong.

Harvest & Processing Dig out roots in spring and autumn; remove soil and rootlets; scrape away cork while fresh or leave cork intact; dry under the sun. Commonly used in Hong Kong in the form of length-wise cut slices.

Description Cylindrical, or long and spindle-shaped, tapering towards the lower end; sometimes rameous (branched); slightly twisted. Outer surface white or pale yellowish-white; for roots with cork still attached, outer surface yellowish-brown to greyish-brown; marked with irregular, twisted longitudinal wrinkles, and with cicatrices and scars of rootlets resembling transverse lenticels; upper part with transverse striae. Top end with a relatively short rhizome; rhizome with several semilunar (half-moon shaped) stem scars. Brittle, breaks easily. When broken, surface uneven, with radial clefts; cortex off-white; cambium ring brown; xylem pale yellowish-white. Odourless; taste: slightly sweet, then bitter.

Indications 1. Colds, cough, bronchitis, copious expectoration 2. Sore throat.

Chemical Composition Mainly contains triterpene saponins such as platycodin A, C, D.

Radix Polygoni Multiflori

Fleeceflower Root

Heshouwu

何首烏

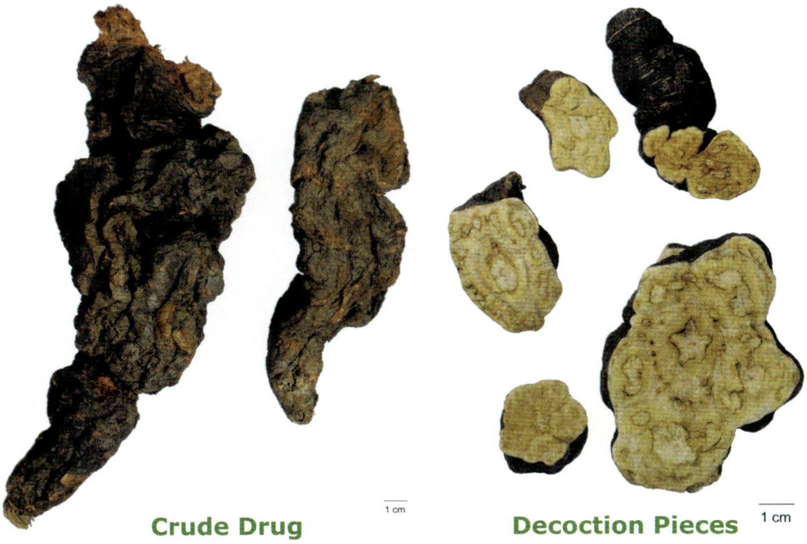

Crude Drug   Decoction Pieces

Source The root tuber of *Polygonum multiflorum* Thunb. (Fam. Polygonaceae).

Distribution Mainly in Chinese provinces such as Henan, Hubei, Guangxi and Guangdong; also in Hong Kong.

Harvest & Processing Collect root tubers in autumn and winter; slice off two ends; wash root tubers clean; dry under the sun. Cut large ones into slices about 2 cm thick; dry.

Description Lump-shaped or irregular spindle-shaped; 6-15 cm long, 4-12 cm in diameter. Outer surface reddish-brown or dull reddish-brown, uneven, marked with irregular, dense wrinkles and longitudinal grooves; lalongate (transversely elongated) lenticels, with a conspicuous root scar at either end. Hard, solid and heavy, does not break easily. Cut surface yellowish-brown or light reddish-brown, starchy; cortex marked with 4-11 rings of anomalous vascular bundles; xylem in the middle well-developed; sometimes with a woody core. Odour: faint; taste: slightly bitter, sweet-astringent.

Indications
1. Weakness, backache, knee pain, Premature greying of hair
2. Elevated serum cholesterol, coronary heart disease
3. Neurasthenia, insomnia, dizziness, sweating.

Chemical Composition Mainly contains emodin, rhein, chrysophanol, resveratrol and condensed tannins.

Note According to *C.P.*, also used for medicinal purposes is a processed Radix Polygoni Multiflori called '*Zhi heshouwu*' (Prepared Fleeceflower Root).

Radix Polygalae

Thinleaf Milkwort Root

Yuanzhi

遠志

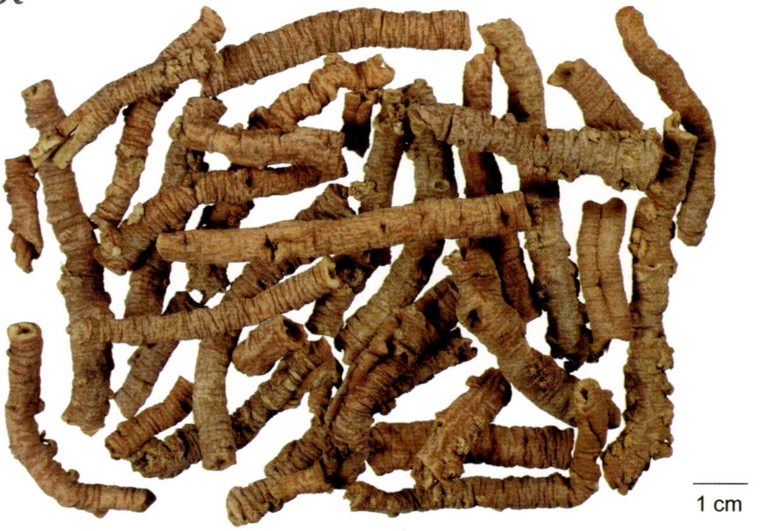

Decoction Pieces

Source The root of *Polygala tenuifolia* Willd. (Fam. Polygalaceae).

Distribution Mainly in Chinese provinces such as Shanxi, Shaanxi, Jilin and Henan.

Harvest & Processing Dig out roots in spring and autumn; remove stem remnants, rootlets and soil; dry under the sun. Alternatively, remove woody core (i.e. xylem) and dry under the sun to produce "*Yuanzhi rou*" (Thinleaf Milkwort Root Bark).

Description Cylindrical or double-tubular, with branch roots, slightly curved; 3-15 cm long, 3-8 mm in diameter. Outer surface greyish-yellow to greyish-brown; marked with relatively dense and deep transverse wrinkles and cracks; slightly nodular; occasionally with fine longitudinal striae and small verruciform (wart-shaped) scars of branch roots. Hard and brittle. When broken, surface shows brownish-yellow cortex and yellowish-white xylem; phloem detaches easily from xylem; for the ones with xylem removed, broken surface double-tubular. Odour: faint; taste: bitter and slightly acrid, throat-irritating when chewed.

Indications 1. Irritability, apprehension, palpitation, insomnia, excessive dreams 2. Convulsion, insanity 3. Productive cough with thick sputum 4. Skin infection, acute mastitis and breast nodules.

Chemical Composition Mainly contains triterpene saponins such as onjisaponins A, B, C, D; also contains xanthone.

Note According to *C.P.*, also used for medicinal purposes is the root of *P. sibirica* L.

Radix Pseudostellariae

Heterophylly Falsetarwort Root
Taizishen

太子參

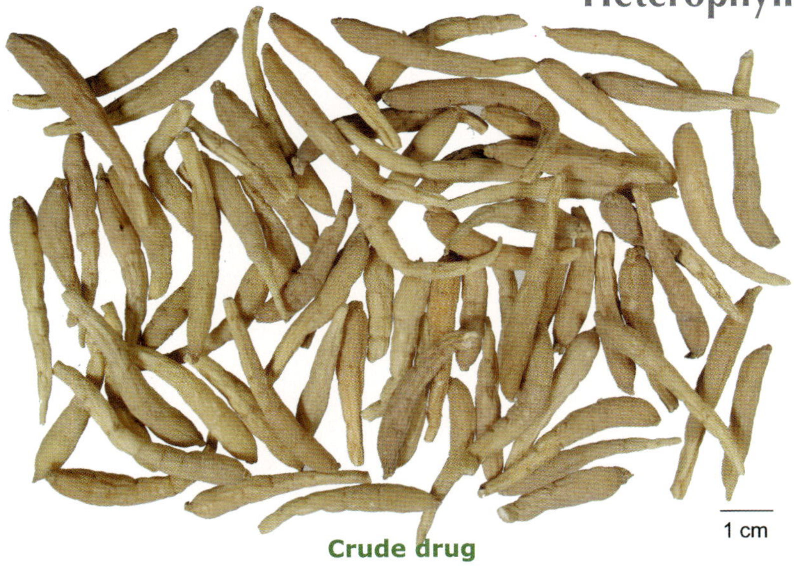

Crude drug

Source	The root tuber of *Pseudostellaria heterophylla* (Miq) Pax ex Pax et Hoffm. (Fam. Caryophyllaceae).
Distribution	Mainly in Chinese provinces such as Jiangsu, Shandong and Anhui.
Harvest & Processing	Dig up root tubers in summer when leaves wither; wash clean; remove rootlets; blanch root tubers in boiling water and dry under the sun, or dry directly under the sun.
Description	Slender and spindle-shaped or slender and rod-like, slightly curved; 2-10 cm long, 2-6 mm in diameter. Outer surface yellowish-white, relatively smooth, with light longitudinal wrinkles; dented parts of surface marked with scars of rootlets; top end with stem scars. Hard and brittle, breaks easily. When broken, surface smooth; either pale yellowish-white and cuticular, or off-white and starchy (if dried directly under the sun). Odour: faint; taste: slightly sweet.
Indications	1. Fatigue and anorexia 2. Debility after an attack of disease 3. Palpitation and thirst.
Chemical Composition	Contains heterophylin A, B.

Radix Pteroxygoni Giraldii

Girald Pteroxygonum Root
Hongyaozi

紅藥子

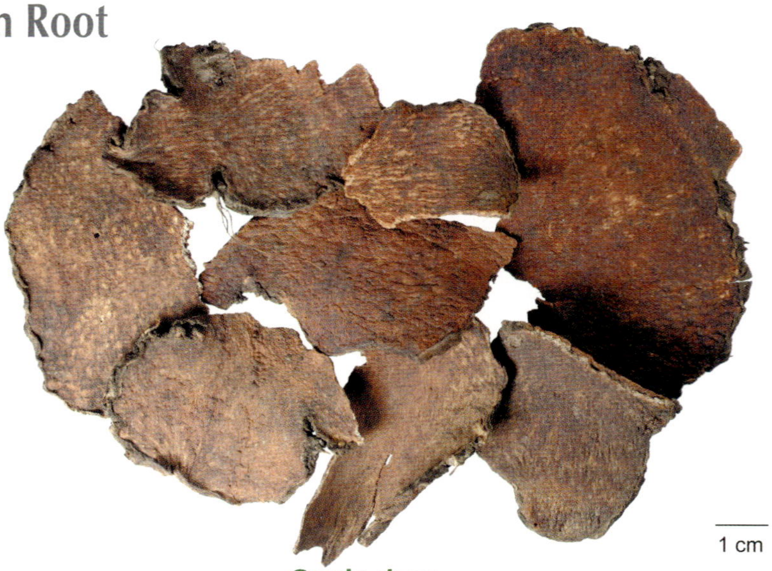

Crude drug

Source The root tuber of *Pteroxygonum giraldii* Damm. et Diels (Fam. Polygonaceae).

Distribution Mainly in Chinese provinces such as Shaanxi, Sichuan and Hebei.

Harvest & Processing Dig out root tubers in autumn; remove leaves and rootlets; wash away soil; slice root tubers; dry under the sun.

Description Lumps irregular in shape, or slightly cylindrical; 8-15 cm or above in length, 3-7 cm in diameter. Outer surface brownish-yellow; top part with numerous verruciform (wart-shaped) caudexes. Extremely hard, difficult to break. Cut surface dark yellow; xylem light yellow, annular (ring-like); some other light yellow anomalous vascular bundles scattered near pith. Odour: faint; taste: bitter.

Indications 1. Sore throat 2. Sores, furuncle, burn and scald 3. Gastrointestinal bleeding, epistaxis, dysfunctional uterine bleeding 4. Diarrhoea and dysentery 5. Rheumatism

Chemical Composition Contains trace amounts of anthraquinones and large amounts of tannins.

Radix Puerariae

Kudzuvine Root
Gegen
葛根

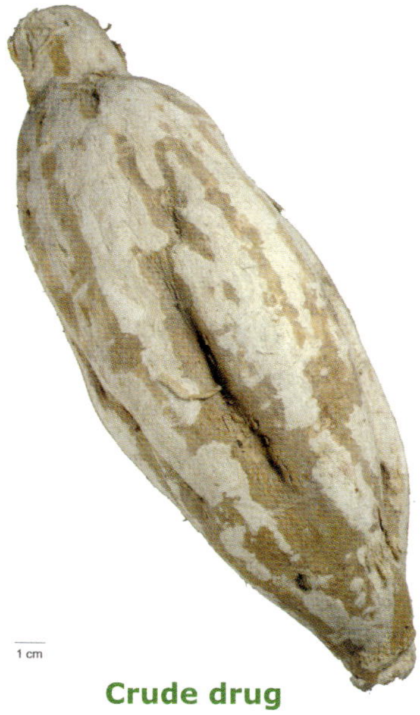

Crude drug

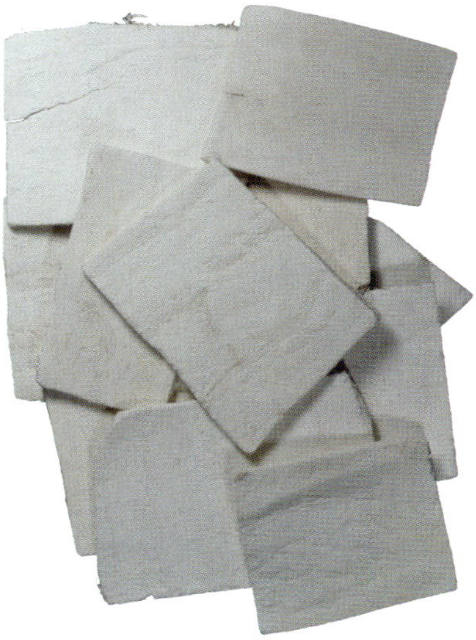

Decoction Pieces

1 cm

Source The root of *Pueraria thomsonii* Benth. (Fam. Leguminosae).

Distribution Mainly in Chinese provinces such as Hunan, Henan, Guangdong and Zhejiang; also in Hong Kong.

Harvest & Processing Dig out roots in spring and autumn; wash clean; remove cork; cut into slices; dry under the sun or dry by heat. Customarily used in Hong Kong in the form of angled-cut or length-wise cut slices.

Description Mostly rectangular; 5-35 cm long, 0.5-1 cm thick. Outer surface marked with longitudinal wrinkles; rough; sometimes with remnants of pale brown cork. Cut surface yellowish-white, with inconspicuous markings, heavily fibrous. Pliable. Odourless; taste: slightly sweet.

Indications 1. Common cold with fever 2. Thirst 3. Acute gastro-enteritis, diarrhoea 4. Palpitation.

Chemical Composition Contains daidzein and puerarin; also contains triterpene saponins.

Note According to *C.P.*, also used for medicinal purposes is the root of *P. lobata* (Willd.) Ohwi.

Radix Pulsatillae

Chinese Pulsatilla Root
Baitouweng

白頭翁

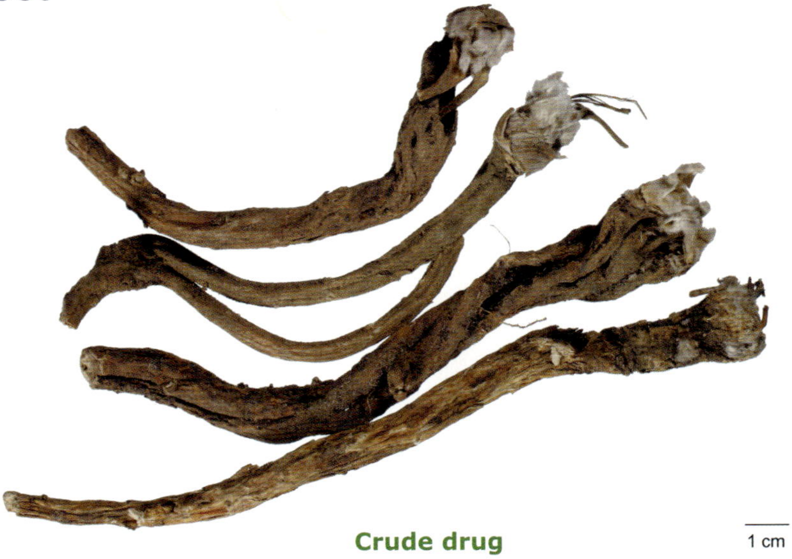

Crude drug

Source The root of *Pulsatilla chinensis*(Bunge) Regel (Fam. Ranunculaceae).

Distribution Mainly in northeastern, northern and eastern China.

Harvest & Processing Collect roots in spring and autumn; remove soil and sand; dry the roots.

Description Subcylindrical or conical, slightly twisted; 6-20 cm long, 0.5-2 cm in diameter. Outer surface yellowish-brown or reddish-brown; marked with irregular longitudinal wrinkles or grooves; cortex falls off easily, revealing pale yellow xylem; in some cases surface marked with reticulate (Netted) cracks or clefts; often withered into holes near top part. Top part slightly bulgy; with white villi; in some cases with remnants of sheath-like petiole base. Hard and brittle; transverse section shows yellowish-white or pale yellowish-brown cortex and pale yellow xylem. Odour: faint; taste: slightly bitter-astringent.

Indications 1. Amoebic dysentery, bacillary dysentery 2. Morbid leukorrhoea, vulval pruritus 3. Malaria 4. Epistaxis, haemorrhoidal bleeding

Chemical Composition Mainly contains pulchinenoside A, B, C, D and anemonin.

Radix Ranunculi Ternati

Catclaw Buttercup Root
Maozhaocao
貓爪草

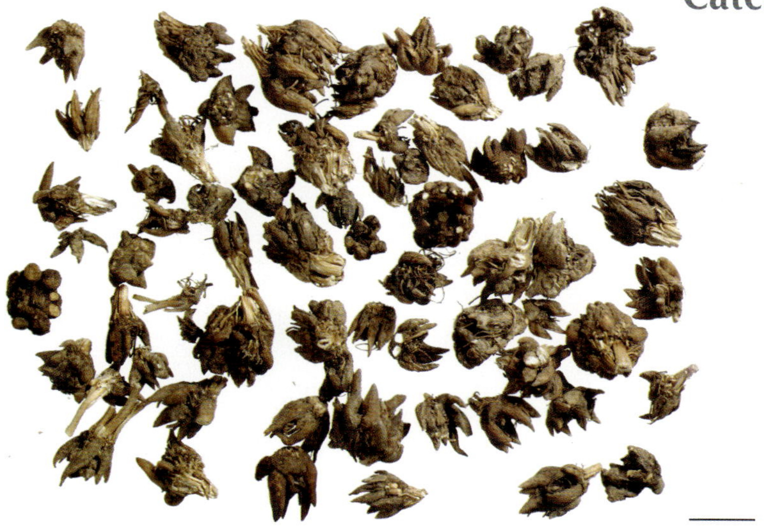

Crude drug

Source The root tuber of *Ranunculus ternatus* Thunb. (Fam. Ranunculaceae).

Distribution Mainly in regions around the middle and lower reaches of the Yangtze River in China.

Harvest & Processing Dig up root tubers in late autumn or early spring after 2-3 years of plantation; remove leaves and rootlets; wash away soil; dry under the sun.

Description Spindle-shaped, mostly 5-6 root tubers conglomerate (densely clustered), like a cat-claw; 3-10 mm long, 2-3 mm in diameter; apex with dull yellowish-brown stem remnants or stem scars. Outer surface dull yellowish-brown or greyish-yellow, colour darkens with time; marked with light longitudinal wrinkles, punctiform (dot-like) rootlet scars and remnants. Hard and solid; broken surface off-white or yellowish-white, hollow or solid, starchy. Odour: faint; taste: slightly sweet.

Indications 1. Scrofula without ulceration 2. Tuberculosis of lymph nodes.

Chemical Composition Contains ternatolide, γ keto δ valerolactone.

Radix Rehmanniae

Rehmannia Root
Dihuang

地黄

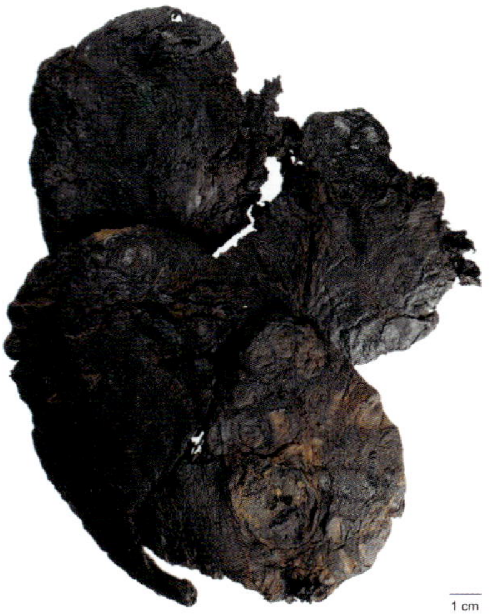

Crude Drug (Shengdihuang)

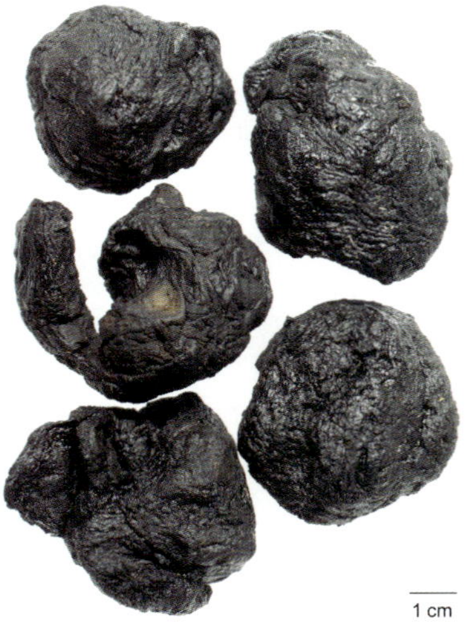

Crude Drug (Shudihuang)

Source The root tuber of *Rehmannia glutinosa* Libosch. (Fam. Scrophulariaceae).

Distribution Mainly in Chinese provinces such as Henan.

Harvest & Processing Dig out root tubers in autumn; remove rootstocks and rootlets; wash root tubers clean; use while fresh - commonly known as '*Xian dihuang*' (Fresh Rehmannia Root). Gently roast *Xian dihuang* until inside turns black and nearly dry; knead into lumps-commonly known as '*Sheng dihuang*' (Raw Rehmannia Root).

Description Mostly irregular pieces, or oblong and orbicular (round); middle part bulgy, narrower at two ends; 6-12 cm long, 3-6 cm in diameter. Some are small, long and rod-like, slightly flattened and gnarled. Outer surface greyish-black or greyish-brown; extremely wrinkled; lined with irregular transverse curves. Heavy; relatively soft and pliable, does not break easily. When broken, surface brownish-black or pitch-black, lustrous and sticky. Odourless; taste: slightly sweet.

Indications *Dried*: 1. Haemoptysis, epistaxis, menorrhagia 2. Menstrual disorders 3. Constipation
Processed: 1. Anaemia, Weakness 2. Nocturnal emission 3. Low-grade afternoon fever 4. Night sweating 5. Menorrhagia.

Chemical Composition Mainly contains iridoid glycosides such as catalpol and rehmannioside A, B, C, D.

Note According to *C.P.*, also commonly used is a processed Radix Rehmanniae called '*Shu dihuang*' (Prepared Rehmannia Root).

Radix Rhapontici

Uniflower Swisscentaury Root

Loulu

漏蘆

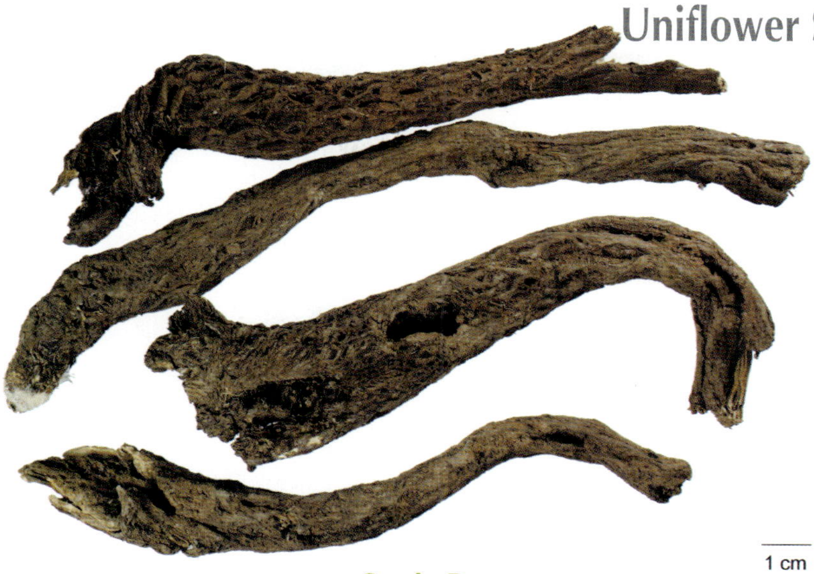

1 cm

Crude Drug

Source The root of *Rhaponticum uniflorum* (L.) DC. (Fam. Compositae).

Distribution Mainly in Chinese provinces such as Hebei, Liaoning and Shanxi.

Harvest & Processing Dig out roots in spring and autumn; remove rootlets, soil and sand; dry under the sun.

Description Conical or broken into slabs, mostly twisted; varying in length. Outer surface dull blackish-brown or dull brown, rough, marked with longitudinal grooves and rhombic, reticulate (netted) clefts; bark falls off easily; top part bulgy, with stem remnants and squamiform (scale-like) leaf bases, top end with greyish-white villi. Light in weight; brittle, breaks easily. When broken, surface uneven, often irregular and lamellate (composed of thin plates), greyish-yellow; core sometimes with stellate (star-shaped) clefts, often withered, greyish-black or brownish-black. Odour: distinctive; taste: slightly bitter.

Indications 1. Acute mastitis, galactostasis 2. Dermatitis 3. Haemorrhoid.

Chemical Composition Mainly contains triterpene saponins such as unifloroside, and sterols such as rhapontisterone.

Radix Rhodomyrti

Downy Rosemyrtle Root
Gangniangen

崗稔根

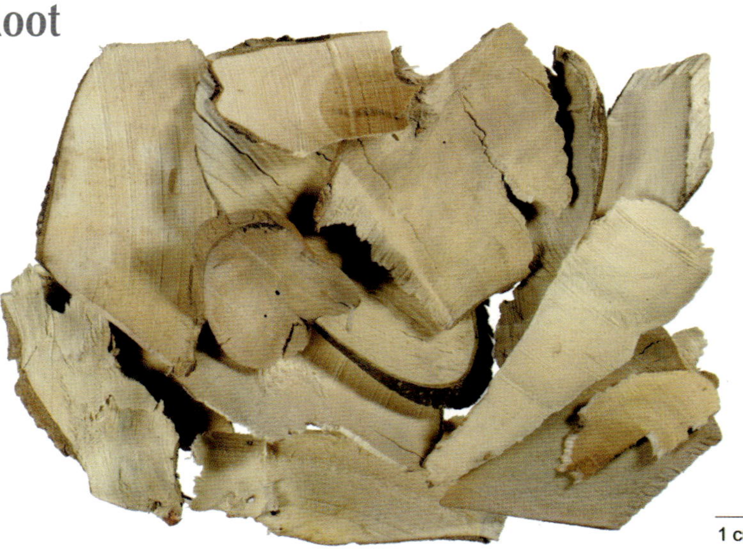

1 cm

Decoction Pieces

Source The root of *Rhodomyrtus tomentosa* (Ait.) Hassk. (Fam. Myrtaceae).

Distribution Mainly in Chinese provinces such as Guangdong, Guangxi, Fujian, Hunan and Jiangxi; also in Hong Kong.

Harvest & Processing Dig up roots in autumn; wash away soil; dry under the sun.

Description Somewhat cylindrical, slightly curved, rameous (branched). Outer surface greyish-yellow to dull greyish-brown; marked with longitudinal wrinkles and scars of rootlets. Hard, does not break easily. Odour: faint; taste: bitter-astringent, then sweet. Commercially sold in the form of suborbicular (almost round) slices or sections; cortex relatively thin, dull reddish-brown; xylem relatively broad, light brown, marked with dense radial striae and numerous annulations; central pith dented and punctiform (dot-like).

Indications 1. Jaundice, hypochondriac pain 2. Abdominal pain, vomiting, diarrhoea, dyspepsia 3. Lumbago, rheumatism, trauma, 4. Dysfunctional uterine bleeding 5. Anaemia, diabetes

Chemical Composition Mainly contains hydrolysable tannins such as pedunculagin and casuariin.

Radix Rubiae

India Madder Root

Qiancao

茜草

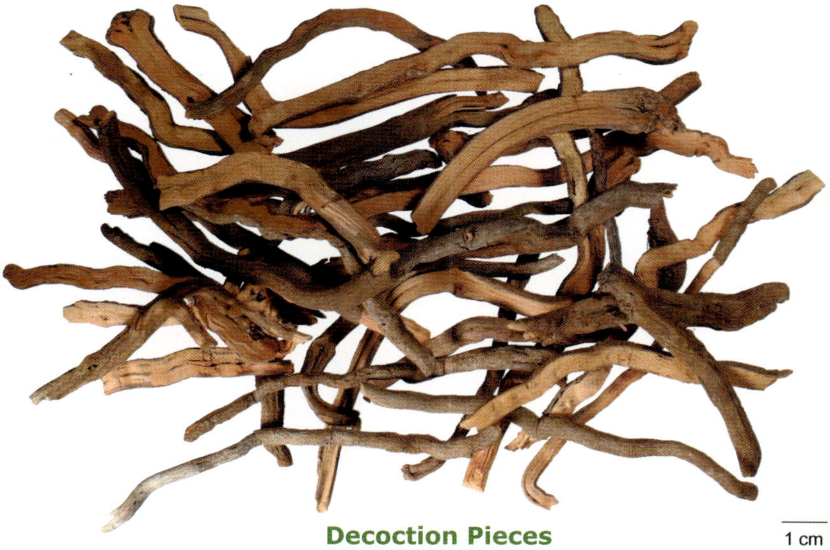

Decoction Pieces

Source The root of *Rubia cordifolia* L. (Fam. Rubiaceae).

Distribution Mainly in Chinese provinces such as Shaanxi, Shanxi and Henan; also in Hong Kong.

Harvest & Processing Dig out roots in autumn; those collected from mid-August to mid-September are of better quality. Remove shoots and soil; dry roots under the sun. Commonly used in Hong Kong in the form of length-wise cut slices.

Description Cylindrical, often curved or twisted; varying in thickness, 10-25 cm long, 0.2-1 cm in diameter. Outer surface reddish-brown or brown, marked with fine longitudinal wrinkles and sparse rootlet scars; cortex falls off easily, exposing yellowish-red xylem. Brittle, breaks easily. When broken, surface even; cortex narrow and purplish-red; xylem broad, light yellowish-red, with numerous vessel pores. Odour: faint; taste: slightly bitter.

Indications 1. Bleeding such as haemoptysis, epistaxis, dysfunctional uterine bleeding 2. Amenorrhoea 3. Arthralgia, post traumatic swelling and pain

Chemical Composition Mainly contains anthraquinones such as alizarin and xanthopurpurin.

Radix Salviae Miltiorrhizae

Danshen Root
Danshen

丹參

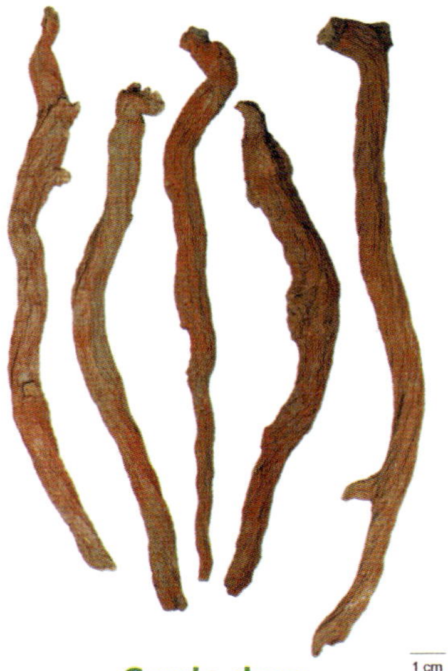

Crude drug

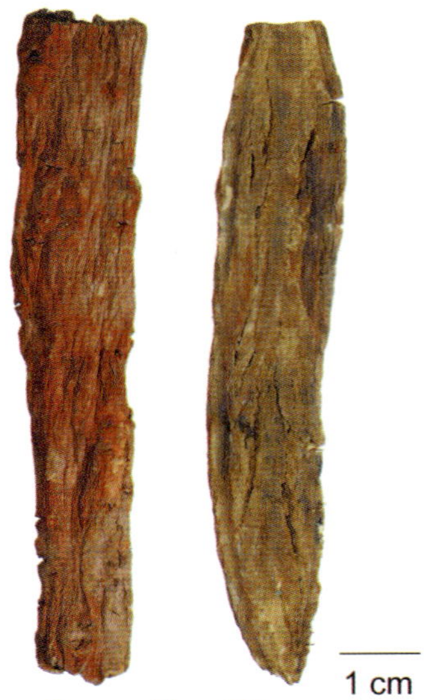

Decoction Pieces

Source The root and rhizome of *Salvia miltiorrhiza* bunge. (Fam. Labiatae).

Distribution Mainly in Chinese provinces such as Anhui, Jiangsu, Shandong and Sichuan. Cultivated or naturally grown.

Harvest & Processing Collect roots and rhizomes in spring and autumn; remove stems, leaves, sand, soil and rootlets; dry under the sun. Commonly used in Hong Kong in the form of length-wise cut slices.

Description Rhizome thick and short; top end sometimes with remnants of caudex; with a few long and cylindrical roots; slightly curved; some branches with fine rootlets; 10-20 cm long, 0.3-1 cm in diameter. Outer surface yellowish-red or dull red, rough, marked with longitudinal wrinkles; bark of old roots loose, mostly purplish-brown, and often scales off. Hard and brittle, breaks easily. When broken, surface with clefts, or fairly even and dense; cortex brownish-red; xylem greyish-yellow or dull purplish-brown, with radial yellowish-white vessels. Odour: faint; taste: slightly bitter-astringent.

Indications 1. Menstrual disorders, lochiorrhoea, lochiostasis 2. Abdominal pain, pricking pain in the chest, trauma, rheumatism 3. Irritability, palpitations and insomnia

Chemical Composition Mainly contains triterpenes such as tanshinone II_A , and polyphenolics such as salvianolic acid B.

Radix Sanguisorbae

Garden Burnet Root

Diyu

地榆

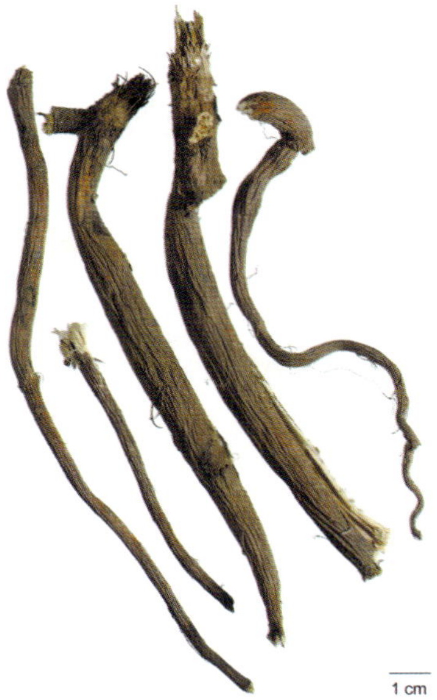

Crude drug

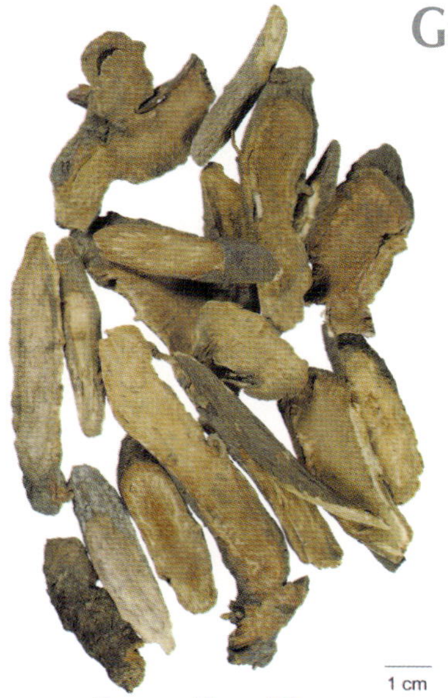

Decoction Pieces

Source The root of *Sanguisorba officinalis* L. (Fam. Rosaceae).

Distribution Mainly in Chinese provinces such as Shanxi and Shaanxi, and in Inner Mongolia and northeastern China.

Harvest & Processing Collect roots just before germination in spring or in autumn after plants have withered; remove rootlets; wash roots clean and then dry; or cut into slices while fresh and then dry.

Description Cylindrical or irregular spindle-shaped, slightly curved; 5-25 cm long, 0.5-2 cm in diameter. Outer surface dull greyish-brown, reddish-brown or dull purple; rough; with longitudinal wrinkles, transverse cracks and scars of branch roots. Hard and brittle. Transverse section relatively smooth, pink or pale yellow; xylem relatively light in colour, with radial markings. Odour: faint; taste: bitter and astringent. Slices irregular and orbicular (round), or elliptical; 2-5 mm thick; cut surface purplish-red or reddish-brown.

Indications 1. Haemoptysis, haematuria, bleeding haemorrhoids 2. Diarrhoea, chronic gastro-enteritis 3. Burns (external use).

Chemical Composition Contains tannins and a variety of triterpene saponins such as sanguisoubin.

Note According to *C.P.*, also used for medicinal purposes, and commonly known as '*Mian Diyu*' (Fibrous Garden Burnet Root), is the root of *S. officinalis* L. *var. longifolia* (Bert.) Yüet Li.

Radix Saposhnikoviae

Divaricate Saposhnikovia Root

Fangfeng

防風

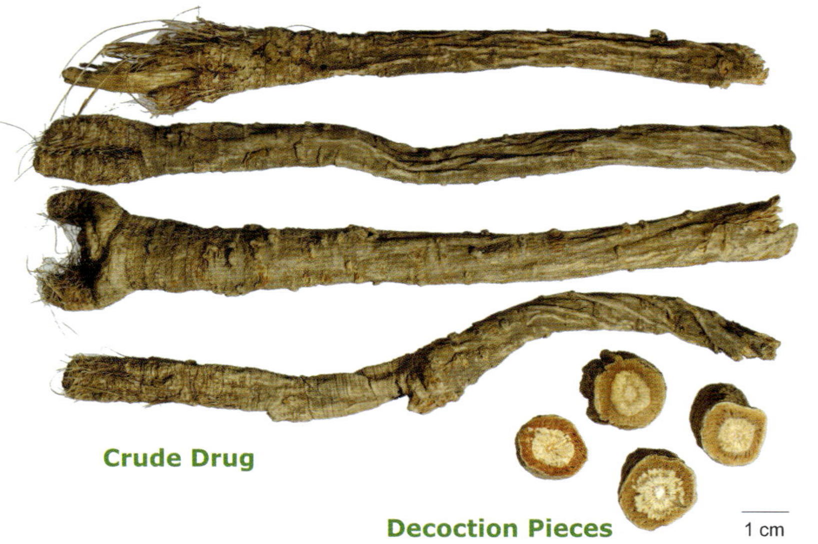

Crude Drug

Decoction Pieces

1 cm

Source
The root of *Saposhnikovia divaricata* (Turcz.) Schischk. (Fam. Umbelliferae).

Distribution
Mainly in eastern Inner Mongolia and northeastern China; customarily called "*Guan fangfeng*"(Gate Divaricate Saposhnikovia Root). Mostly cultivated nowadays.

Harvest & Processing
Dig out roots in spring and autumn; remove caudexes, fibrous roots, soil and sand; dry under the sun until nearly dry; tie up in small bundles; dry under the sun again.

Description
Long and cylindrical, tapering at lower part, in some cases slightly curved; 15-30 cm long, 0.5-2 cm in diameter. Top part with dense, conspicuous annulations; annulations mostly with reddish-brown, piliform (hair-like) remnants of leaf base. Outer surface greyish-brown, rough; marked with longitudinal wrinkles, numerous lalongate (transversely elongated) lenticels and protuberant, punctiform (dot-like) rootlet scars. Light in weight; loose in texture, breaks easily. Broken surface uneven; cortex light brown, with clefts, scattered with yellowish-brown oil dots; xylem light yellow; core in the shape of chrysanthemum. Odour: distinctive; taste: slightly sweet.

Indications
1. Common cold, headache, dizziness 2. Migraine, rheumatic arthritis.

Chemical Composition
Mainly contains coumarins, polyacetylene and essential oils.

Radix Scrophulariae

Figwort Root
Xuanshen

玄參

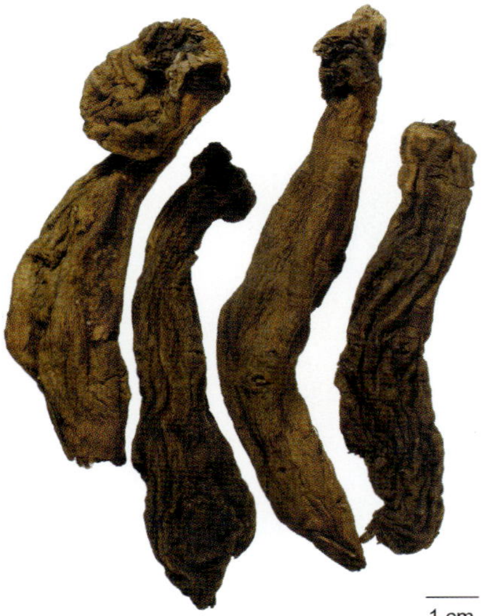

1 cm

Crude Drug

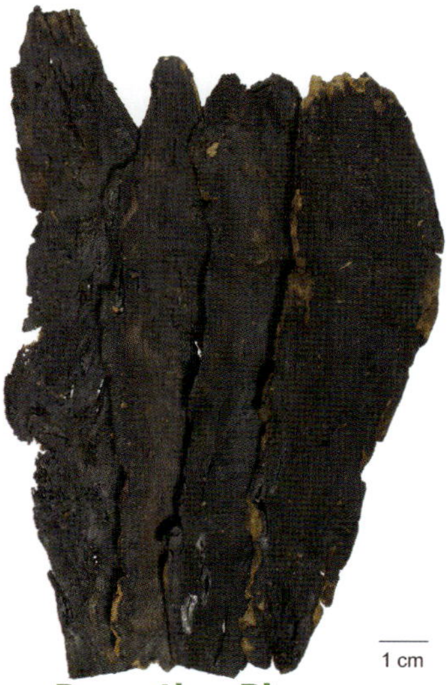

1 cm

Decoction Pieces

Source The root of *Scrophularia ningpoensis* Hemsl. (Fam. Scrophulariaceae).

Distribution Mainly in Chinese provinces such as Zhejiang, Hubei, Jiangsu and Jiangxi.

Harvest & Processing Collect roots in winter; remove rootstocks, rootlets, root buds, soil and sand; dry roots until half-dry; heap up to let moisture evaporate until the inside turns black; dry again under the sun or by heat. Commonly used in Hong Kong in the form of length-wise cut slices.

Description Conical, thicker in the middle or thick at the upper part and slender at the lower; 6-20 cm long, 1-3 cm in diameter. Outer surface greyish-yellow or reddish-brown, marked with conspicuous longitudinal grooves and transverse lenticels. Hard, does not break easily. Transverse section relatively smooth, pitch-black and slightly lustrous. Odour: caramel-like; taste: sweet and slightly bitter. If immersed in water, water will turn ink-black.

Indications 1. Polydipsia due to febrile diseases 2. Constipation. 3. Rashes, dermatitis, boils and scrofula 4. Gingivitis, tonsillitis, pharyngitis, acute lymphadenitis

Chemical Composition Mainly contains iridoid glycosides such as harpagide and harpagoside.

Radix Scutellariae

Baical Skullcap Root
Huangqin

黄芩

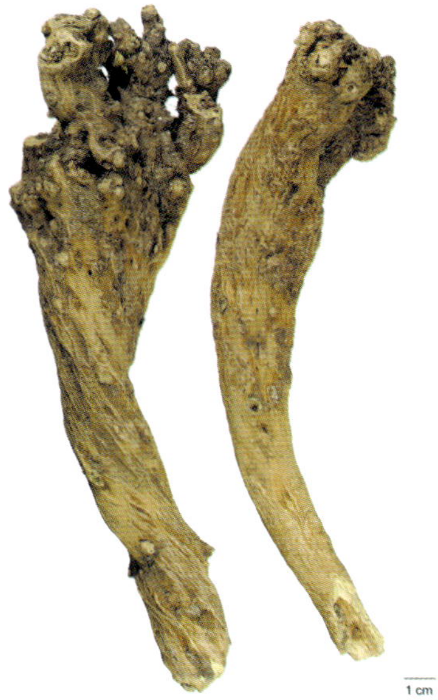

Crude drug

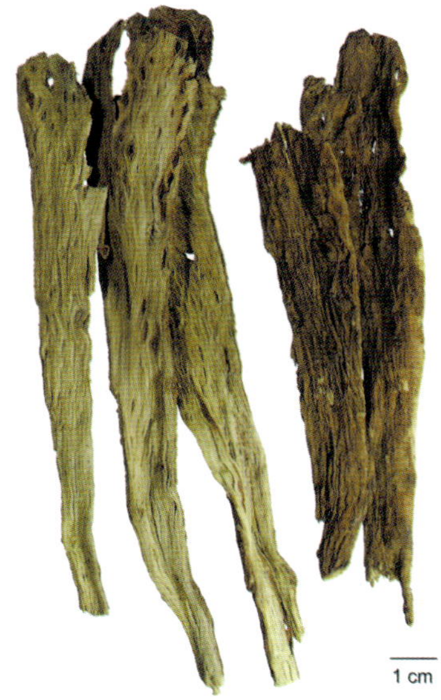

Decoction Pieces

Source: The root of *Scutellaria baicalensis* Georgi (Fam. Labiatae).

Distribution: Mainly in Chinese provinces such as Hebei, Shanxiand Liaoning, and in Inner Mongolia.

Harvest & Processing: Dig out roots in spring and autumn; remove soil and sand; dry roots under the sun until half-dry, then remove cork; dry under the sun again. Commonly used in Hong Kong in the form of length-wise cut slices.

Description: Conical and twisted; 8-25 cm long, 1-3 cm in diameter. Outer surface brownish-yellow or dark yellow, marked with sparse verruciform (wart-shaped) rootlet scars; top end with stem scars or caudex remnants; upper part relatively rough, with twisted longitudinal wrinkles or irregular, reticulate (netted) striae; lower part marked with fine longitudinal striae and fine wrinkles. Hard and brittle, breaks easily; when broken, surface yellow, with a reddish-brown core. Old roots with a dull brown or brownish-black and withered or hollow core are called '*Kuqin*'(Withered Baical Skullcap Root). New roots are called '*Ziqin*'(Young Baical Skullcap Root) or '*Tiaoqin*'(Slender Baical Skullcap Root). Odour: faint; taste: bitter.

Indications: 1. Jaundice, enteritis, peptic ulcer 2. Sore throat, cough with yellow sputum, hyperpyrexia with polydipsia 3. Haemoptysis, epistaxis 4. Carbuncles and sores 5. Threatened abortion

Chemical Composition: Mainly contains flavonoids such as baicalein and baicalin.

Radix Semiaquilegiae

Muskroot-like Semiaquilegia Root
Tiankuizi

天葵子

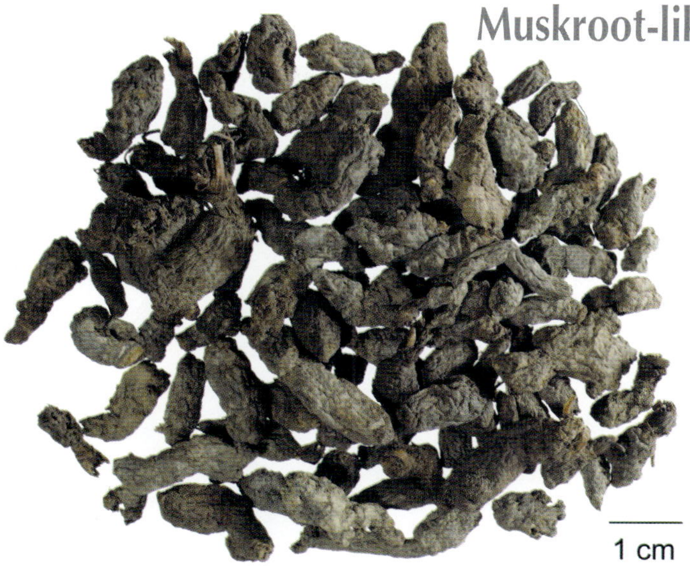

1 cm

Crude drug

Source The root tuber of *Semiaquilegia adoxoides* (DC.) Makino (Fam. Ranunculaceae).

Distribution Mainly in Chinese provinces such as Hunan, Hubei, Jiangsu, Guizhou and Anhui.

Harvest & Processing Dig up root tubers in May before plants completely wither; remove from larger ones all remnants of leaves; dry the larger ones under the sun; remove rootlets and soil.

Description Irregular, short and cylindrical, spindle-shaped or lump-shaped; slightly curved; very occasionally with 2-3 short branches; 1-3 cm long, 0.5-1 cm in diameter. Outer surface dull brown to greyish-black, marked with irregular wrinkles and rootlets or scars of rootlets; top end often marked with remnants of caudex and leaf base and covered with several layers of sheath-like dull yellowish-brown scales; usually bulgy in the middle. Relatively soft, breaks easily. When broken, surface shows off-white cortex; xylem yellowish-brown or yellowish-white, with markings roughly in a radial pattern. Odour: faint; taste: sweet, slightly bitter and acrid.

Indications 1. Carbuncle, sores, boils and scrofula 2. Mastitis 3. Venomous-snake bite.

Chemical Composition Contains alkaloids.

Radix seu Caulis Acanthopanacis Senticosi

Manyprickle Acanthopanax
Ciwujia

刺五加

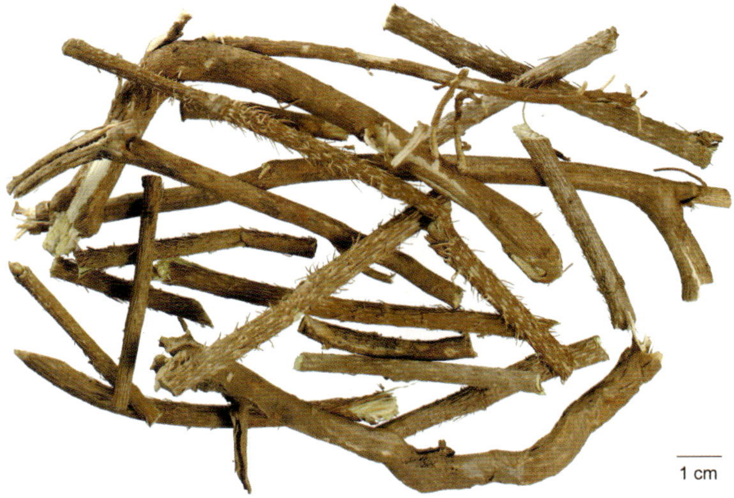

Crude Drug

Source The root, and rhizome or stem of *Acanthopanax senticosus* (Rupr. et Maxim.) Harms (Fam. Araliaceae).

Distribution Mainly in Chinese provinces such as Heilongjiang, Jilin, Liaoning, Hebei and Shaanxi.

Harvest & Processing Dig out roots, and rhizomes or stems in spring and autumn; remove soil; cut into sections and dry under the sun.

Description Root cylindrical and mostly twisting; 0.3-1.5 cm in diameter. Outer surface dull greyish-brown or dull blackish-brown, marked with conspicuous wrinkles; bark relatively thin, surface greyish-yellow where bark has fallen off. Hard; broken surface yellowish-white and fibrous. Odour: with a distinctive fragrance; taste: slightly acrid, a little bitter, astringent.

Stem cylindrical; varying in length. Old branches dull greyish-brown, marked with longitudinal cracks, inermous (without thorns or spines); young branches dull yellowish-brown, densely echinulate (with very small prickles or spines). Hard, does not break easily. When broken, cortex thin and yellowish-white; xylem broad and light yellow; pith in the centre. Odour: faint; taste: slightly acrid.

Indications 1. Chronic rheumatism with weakness of extremities, infantile paralysis 2. Insomnia, excessive dreams, palpitation 3. Loose stool, anorexia 4. Leukopenia 5. Coronary heart disease

Chemical Composition Eleutheroside A, B, C, D, E exist in the roots. The stems mainly contain eleutheroside B_1.

Radix seu Rhizoma Nardostachyos

Nardostachys Root and Rhizome

Gansong

甘松

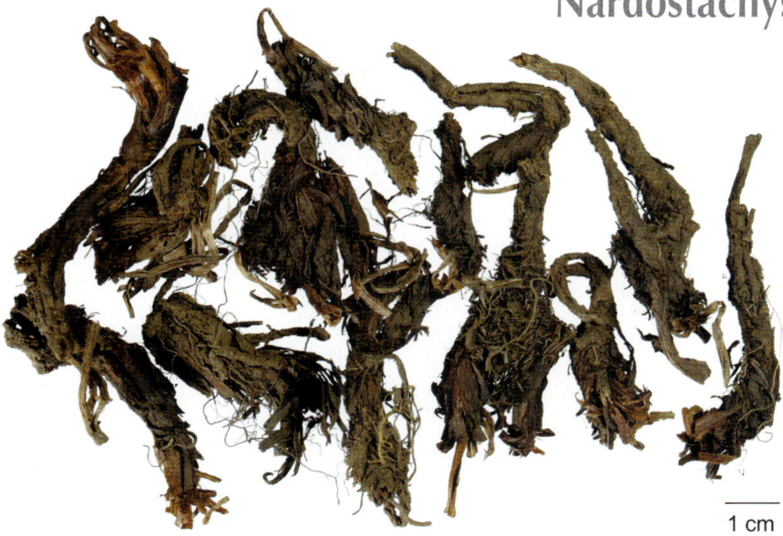

1 cm

Crude Drug

Source The root and rhizome of *Nardostachys chinensis* Batal. (Fam. Valerianaceae).

Distribution Mainly in Sichuan province in China; also in provinces such as Qinghai and Gansu.

Harvest & Processing Collect roots and rhizomes in spring and autumn, preferably in autumn; clear away soil and sand; do not wash with water to avoid losing the fragrance; remove remnants of stems and rootlets; dry roots and rhizomes under the sun or in shaded areas.

Description Slightly conical, curving gently most of the time, thick on top and tapering downwards; 5-18 cm long. Rhizome short; top part with base remnants of above-ground stems and multi-layers of fibrous, or membranous and lamellar (like thin plates) remnants of withered leaf base, with the outer layers brownish-black and the inner layers brown or yellow. Root singular or branched; 6-16 cm long, 0.3-1 cm in diameter; outer surface shrivelled, reddish-brown, with rootlets and fibrous roots. Texture loose and brittle; breaks easily. Transverse section rough; cortex dark brown, often lobate (divided into lobes); xylem yellowish-white. Odour: distinctive; taste: bitter, acrid and refreshing.

Indications 1. Stomachache, vomit, anorexia. 2. Toothache 3. Foot oedema (external use).

Chemical Composition Mainly contains sesquiterpenes, such as nardostachone and nardosinone.

Note According to *C.P.*, also used for medicinal purposes is the root and rhizome of *N. jatamansi* DC.

Radix Sophorae Flavescentis

Lightyellow Sophora Root
Kushen

苦參

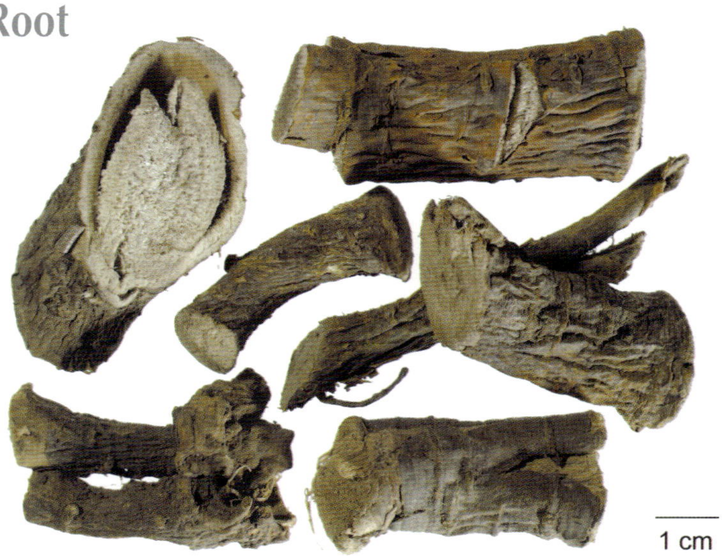

Crude drug

Source The root of *Sophora flavescens* Ait. (Fam. Leguminosae).

Distribution Mainly in Chinese provinces such as Shanxi, Henan and Hebei.

Harvest & Processing Dig out roots in spring and autumn; cut away top parts; remove rootlets and soil; dry under the sun, or cut into slices while fresh and dry under the sun.

Description Long and cylindrical; lower part often rameous (branched); 10-30 cm long, 1-2 cm in diameter. Outer surface greyish-brown or brownish-yellow, marked with conspicuous longitudinal wrinkles and lalongate (transversely elongated) lenticels; bark often cracked and rolling outwards, exposing smooth, yellow xylem. Hard, difficult to break. Broken surface fibrous and yellowish-white; cortex and xylem conspicuously distinct from each other; with radial markings and clefts; sometimes with concentric annulations. Odour: faint; taste: extremely bitter.

Indications 1. Diarrhoea 2. Abdominal pain 3. Trichomonas vaginitis, pruritus vulvae, burns (external use).

Chemical Composition Mainly contains alkaloids such as matrine, and flavonoids such as kuraridin.

Radix Sophorae Tonkinensis

Vietnamese Sophora Root and Rhizome

Shandougen

山豆根

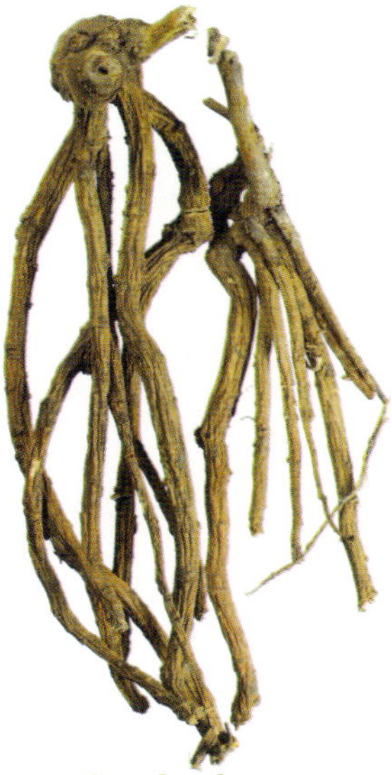

1 cm

Crude drug

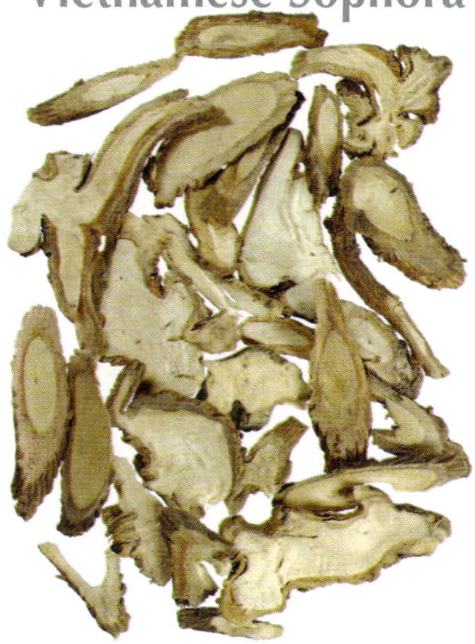

1 cm

Decoction Pieces

Source The root and rhizome of *Sophora tonkinensis* Gagnep. (Fam. Leguminosae).

Distribution Mainly in Chinese provinces such as Guangxi, Guizhou, Yunnan and Guangdong.

Harvest & Processing Collect roots and rhizomes in autumn; remove foreign matter; wash clean; dry under the sun.

Description Rhizome nodular, irregular in shape, lalongate (transversely elongated); top end often with remnants of stem base or stem scars; several roots growing beneath the remnants. Root long and cylindrical, occasionally rameous (branched), slightly curved; varying in length, 0.7-1.5 cm in diameter; outer surface brown or blackish-brown, marked with irregular longitudinal wrinkles and protuberant lalongate (transversely elongated) lenticels. Hard, difficult to break. Broken surface fairly even; cortex pale yellowish-brown; xylem pale yellow. Odour: bean-like; taste: extremely bitter.

Indications 1. Sore throat 2. Laryngocarcinoma, early stage of lung cancer.

Chemical Composition Mainly contains alkaloids such as matrine and oxymatrine; also contains flavonoids such as maackiain and sophoranone.

Note Listed in Hong Kong as Category I (Toxic/Potent) Chinese Materia Medica.

Radix Stellariae

Starwort Root
Yinchaihu

銀柴胡

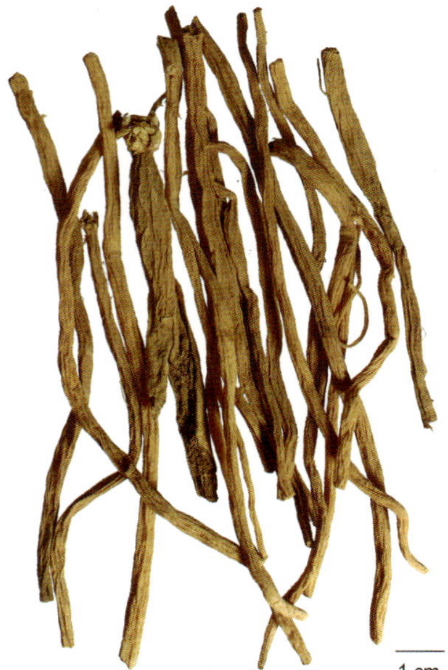

Crude drug 1 cm

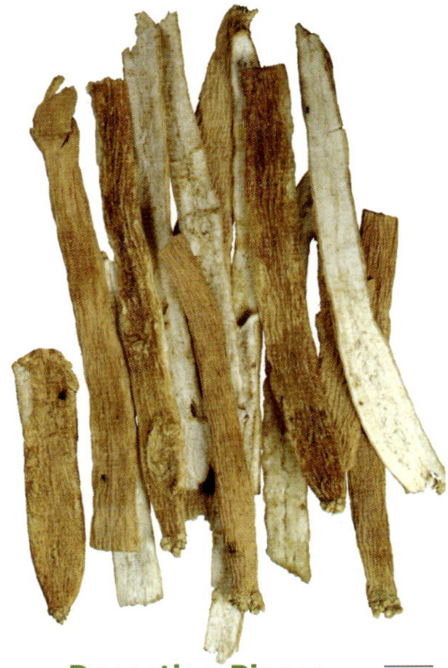

Decoction Pieces 1 cm

Source The root of *Stellaria dichotoma* L. *var. lanceolata* Bunge (Fam. Caryophyllaceae).

Distribution Mainly in Chinese provinces such as Gansu and Shanxi, and in Ningxia and Inner Mongolia.

Harvest & Processing Dig up roots in spring and summer at germination, or after autumn when leaves wilt. For cultivated plants, dig up roots in mid-September of the third year of planting or in mid-April of the fourth year. Remove stem remnants and rootlets as well as soil and sand; dry roots under the sun.

Description Subcylindrical, occasionally rameous (branched); 15-40 cm long, 1-2.5 cm in diameter. Outer surface light brownish-yellow to light brown; marked with twisting longitudinal wrinkles and scars of branch roots; mostly marked with minute poriform (pore-like) or disciform (disc-like) indentations customarily called '*shayan*'(sand pits). Top part of root slightly bulgy, with numerous, dense verruciform (wart-shaped) protuberances of buds or stem base remnants, customarily called '*zhenzhu pan*'(tray of pearls). Hard and brittle, breaks easily. Broken surface uneven, rather loose, with clefts; cortex very thin; xylem with alternating yellow and white radial markings. Odour: faint; taste: sweet.

Indications 1. Hectic fever 2. Infant malnutrition with fever.

Chemical Composition Contains stellaria cyclopeptide I.

Radix Stemonae

Stemona Root

Baibu

百部

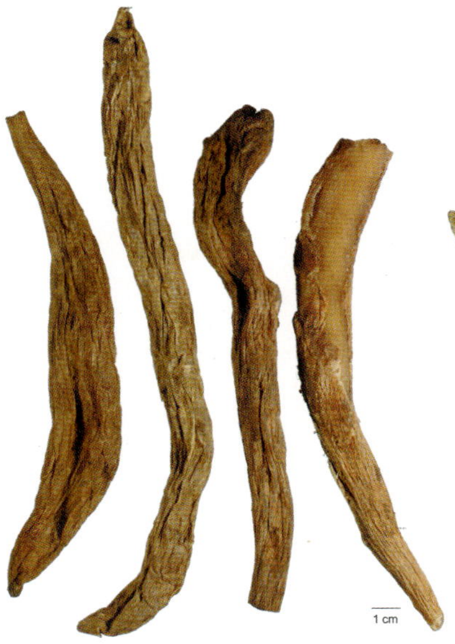

Crude drug

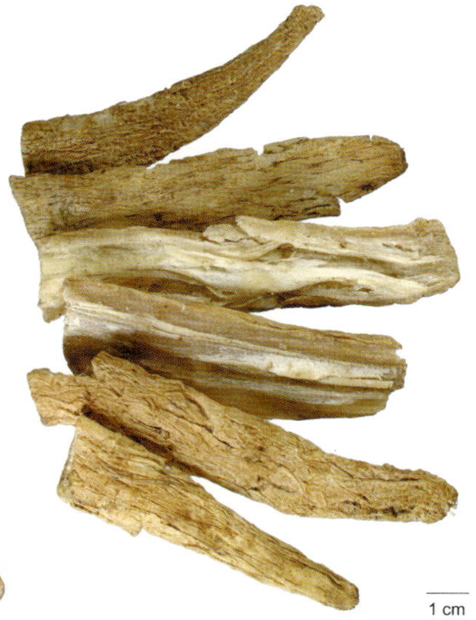

Decoction Pieces

Source The root tuber of *Stemona sessilifolia* (Miq.) Miq. (Fam. Stemonaceae).

Distribution Mainly in Chinese provinces such as Anhui, Jiangsu, Zhejiang and Hubei; also in Hong Kong.

Harvest & Processing Collect root tubers in spring and autumn; remove fibrous roots; steam or boil root tubers thoroughly in hot water; dry under the sun.

Description Spindle-shaped, long and relatively narrow at the top end, shrivelled and curved; 5-12 cm long, 0.5-1 cm in diameter. Outer surface yellowish-white or pale brownish-yellow; marked with irregular, deep longitudinal grooves and occasional transverse wrinkles. Brittle. When broken, surface even, cuticular, pale yellowish-brown or yellowish-white, cortex relatively broad; stele flat and shrunken. Odour: faint; taste: sweet and bitter.

Indications
1. Cough, cough due to pulmonary tuberculosis, whooping cough
2. Threadworm infestation.

Chemical Composition Mainly contains alkaloids such as stemonine and stemonidine.

Note According to *C.P.*, also used for medicinal purposes is the root tuber of *S. japonica* (B1.) Miq. and *S. tuberosa* Lour.

Radix Stephaniae Tetrandrae

Fourstamen Stephania Root

Fangji

防己

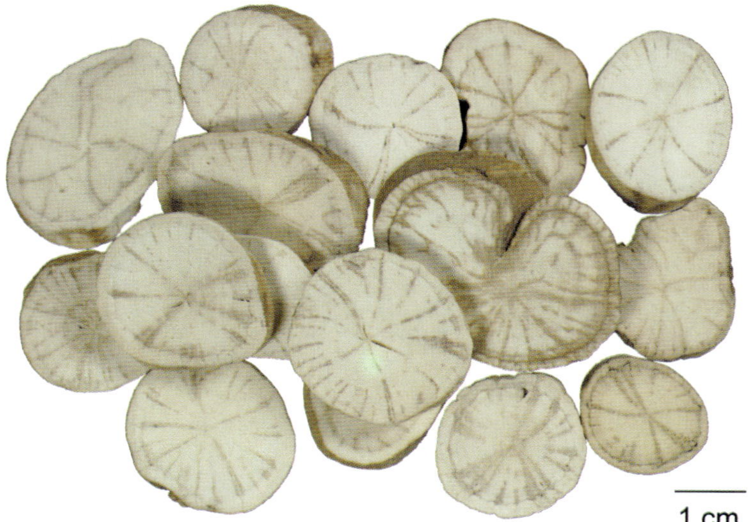

Decoction Pieces

Source The root of *Stephania tetrandra* S. Moore (Fam. Menispermaceae).

Distribution Mainly in Chinese provinces such as Zhejiang, Anhui, Hubei and Hunan; also in Hong Kong.

Harvest & Processing Dig out roots in autumn; wash clean; remove cork; put under the sun until half-dried; cut into sections, with the bigger ones cut again longitudinally; dry.

Description Root section somewhat cylindrical, semi-cylindrical or lamellar (like a thin plate), bent; 5-10 cm long, 1-5 cm in diameter. Outer surface pale greyish-yellow; curved part often with deep, transverse grooves, and node-like protuberances in between the grooves. Hard and solid; heavy in weight. Broken surface even, greyish-white, starchy; with the xylem taking up most of the surface, and sparse radial markings commonly known as "*chelun wen*"(wheel-spoke lines). Odour: faint; taste: bitter.

Indications 1. Oedema and dysuria, oliguria 2. Arthralgia 3. Scabies, tinea, carbuncle 4. Hypertension.

Chemical Composition Mainly contains alkaloids such as tetrandrine and berbamine.

Radix Tinosporae

Tinospora Root
Jinguolan

金果欖

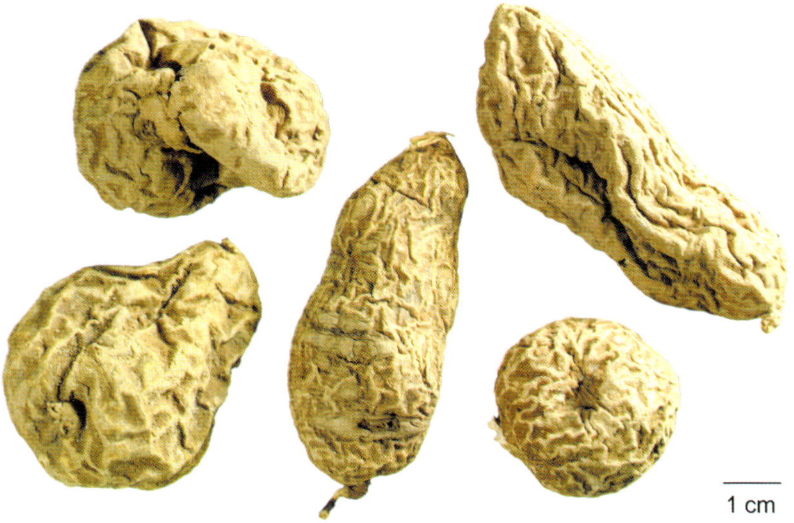

Crude drug

Source The root tuber of *Tinospora sagittata* (Oliv.) Gagnep. (Fam. Menispermaceae).

Distribution In Chinese provinces such as Guangxi, Hunan, Hubei, Sichuan and Guizhou; also in Hong Kong.

Harvest & Processing Dig out root tubers between September and November; remove stems and rootlets; wash clean and slice; dry by heat or under the sun.

Description Irregular, long and spindle-shaped, or irregular lumps in shape; varying in size, 5-10 cm long, 3-6 cm in diameter. Outer surface yellowish-brown or pale brown; shrivelled and uneven; marked with deep irregular wrinkles. Both ends often with remnants of rootlet base. Hard; when broken, surface yellowish-white and starchy. Odourless; taste: bitter.

Indications 1. Sore throat 2. Carbuncles, boils 3. Diarrhoea, dysentery 4. Epigastric pain.

Chemical Composition Mainly contains alkaloids such as palmatine and jatrorrhizine.

Note According to *C.P.*, also used for medicinal purposes is the root tuber of *T. capillipes* Gagnep.

Radix Trichosanthis

Snakegourd Root
Tianhuafen

天花粉

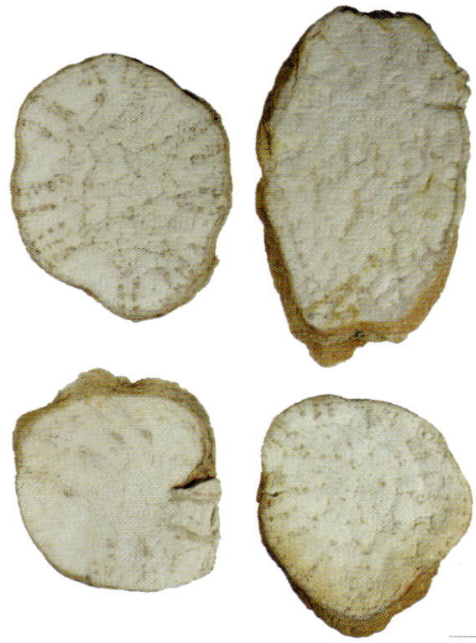

Crude drug

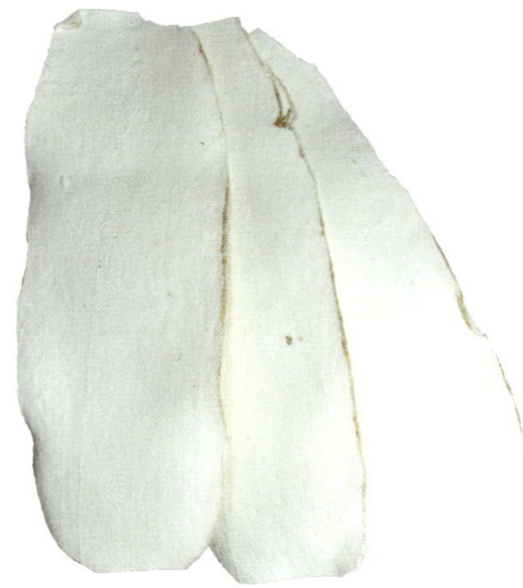

Decoction Pieces

Source The root of *Trichosanthes kirilowii* Maxim. (Fam. Cucurbitaceae).

Distribution Mainly in Chinese provinces such as Henan, Shandong, Jiangsu and Anhui.

Harvest & Processing Collect roots in autumn and winter; wash away soil; scrape off cork; cut roots into segments; dry under the sun or by heat. Commonly used in Hong Kong in the form of length-wise cut slices.

Description Irregular and cylindrical, spindle-shaped or blade-shaped; 8-16 cm long, 1.5-5.5 cm in diameter. Outer surface yellowish-white or pale brownish-yellow; marked with longitudinal wrinkles, rootlet scars and slightly dented lalongate (transversely elongated) lenticels, and occasionally with remnants of yellowish-brown cork. Hard and solid. When broken, surface white or pale yellow, highly starchy; when cross-cut, surface marked with yellow pores of vessels arranged roughly in a radial pattern; when cut length-wise, surface marked with yellow striae of xylem vessels. Odourless; taste: slightly bitter.

Indications 1. Thirst in febrile disease, diabetes 2. Dry cough 3. Mastitis and sores

Chemical Composition Mainly contains trichosanthin.

Note According to *C.P.*, also used for medicinal purposes is the root of *T. rosthornii* Harms.

Radix Tripterygii

Common Threewingnut Root

Leigongteng

雷公藤

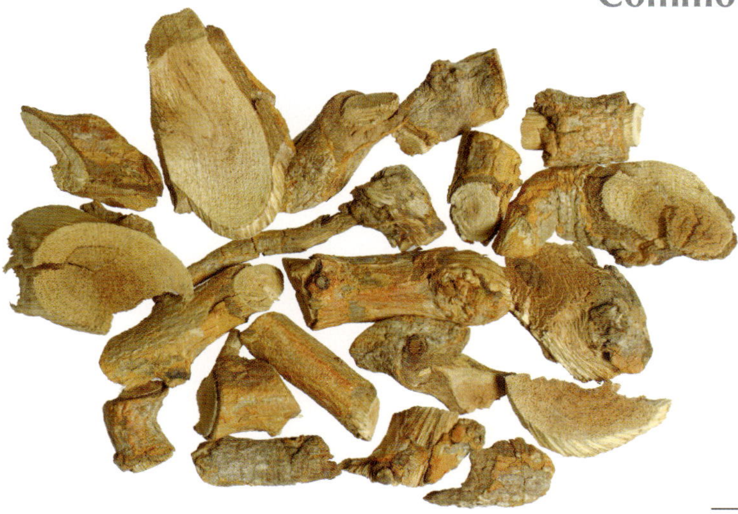

1 cm

Decoction Pieces

Source The root of *Tripterygium wilfordii* Hook. f. (Fam. Celastraceae).

Distribution Mainly in Chinese provinces such as Fujian, Zhejiang, Anhui and Hunan.

Harvest & Processing Dig up roots in autumn; remove soil; dry under the sun, or remove cork and then dry under the sun. Usually cut and sold in sections or slices of various lengths.

Description Cylindrical, twisted, often with remnants of stem base. Outer surface earthy to yellowish-brown in colour, rough, marked with dense longitudinal grooves and annular (ring-like) or semi-annular clefts; cork often peels off, exposing orange-yellow cortex; cortex falls off easily, exposing yellowish-white xylem. Hard; when snapped, powder flies in the air; broken surface fibrous. When broken transversely, surface shows laminiform (consisting of layers) orange-yellow cork layer; phloem reddish-brown; xylem yellowish-white, marked with dense, needle-eye like pits and relatively conspicuous radial rays. Odour: faint but distinctive; taste: bitter and slightly acrid.

Indications 1. Rheumatism, rheumatoid arthritis, sciatica 2. Auto-immue diseases such as lupus erythematosus, glomerular nephritis, nephrotic syndrome 3. Vasculitis, eczema, dermatitis, psoriasis

Chemical Composition Mainly contains alkaloids such as wilfordine and wilforine; also contains sesquiterpene such as tritptolide.

Radix Vladimiriae

Common Vladimiria Root
Chuanmuxiang

川木香

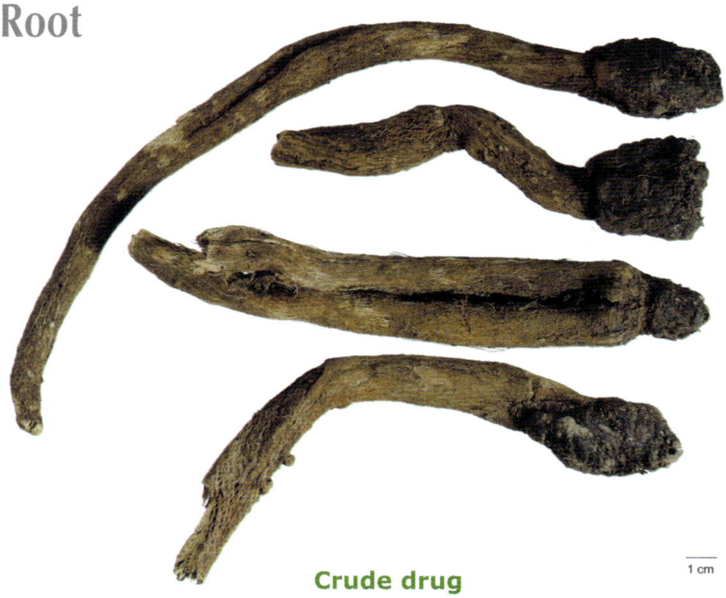

Crude drug

Source The root of *Vladimiria souliei* (Franch.) Ling (Fam. Compositae).

Distribution Mainly in Chinese provinces such as Sichuan, and in Tibet.

Harvest & Processing Collect roots in autumn; remove rootlets and foreign matter; dry roots. Customarily used in Hong Kong in the form of length-wise cut slices.

Description Cylindrical (commonly known as '*Tiegan muxiang*' [Iron-rod Common Vladimiria Root]) or semi-cylindrical with longitudinal grooves (commonly known as '*Caozi muxiang*' [Trough Common Vladimiria Root]), slightly curved; 10-30 cm long, 1-3 cm in diameter. Outer surface dull yellowish-brown or reddish-brown, marked with longitudinal wrinkles. Where bark has fallen off, fine loofah-shaped markings are visible. Top part of root occasionally marked with black viscous gummy substance. Relatively light in weight; hard and brittle, breaks easily. When broken, surface yellowish-white or yellow, with sparse deep yellowish oil dots and clefts; xylem broad, with radial rays; in some cases core withered. Odour: slightly fragrant; taste: bitter, sticky when chewed.

Indications 1. Abdominal distension, anorexia 2. Abdominal pain 3. Dysentery.

Chemical Composition Mainly contains sesquiterpenes such as mokkolactone.

Note According to *C.P.*, also used for medicinal purposes is the root of *V. souliei* (Franch.) Ling *var. cinerea* Ling.

Radix Wikstroemiae

Indian Stringbush Root
Liaogewang

了哥王

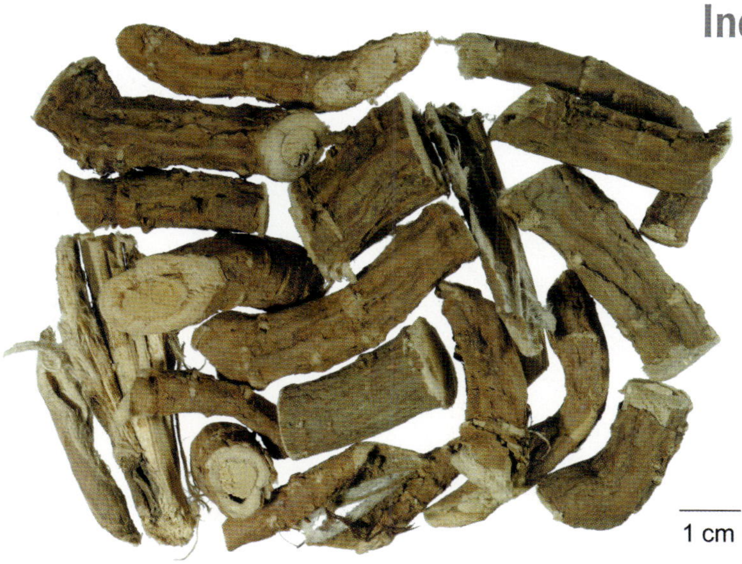

Crude drug

Source The root and stem of *Wikstroemia indica* (L.) C. A. Mey. (Fam. Thymelaeaceae).

Distribution Mainly in Chinese provinces such as Guangdong, Guangxi, Jiangxi, Fujian, Hunan and Guizhou; also in Hong Kong.

Harvest & Processing Collect roots and stems in summer; dry in shaded areas or use while fresh.

Description Root cylindrical, with branch roots; 0.5-3 cm in diameter. Outer surface yellowish-brown to greyish-brown; marked with irregular, heavy longitudinal wrinkles, transverse lenticels and slightly protuberant scars of branch roots. Strong and pliable. When broken, surface shows off-white cortex 1.5-4 mm thick and easily detached from xylem; xylem pale yellow, with radial striae. Odour: faint; taste: slightly bitter; prolonged chewing causes a burning, unpleasant seasation.

Indications 1. Carbuncles and sores, scrofula 2. Arthralgia 3. Trauma 4. Snake and insect bite.

Chemical Composition Stem and stem bark mainly contain diterpenes and coumarins.

Radix Zanthoxyli

Shinyleaf Pricklyash Root

Liangmianzhen

兩面針

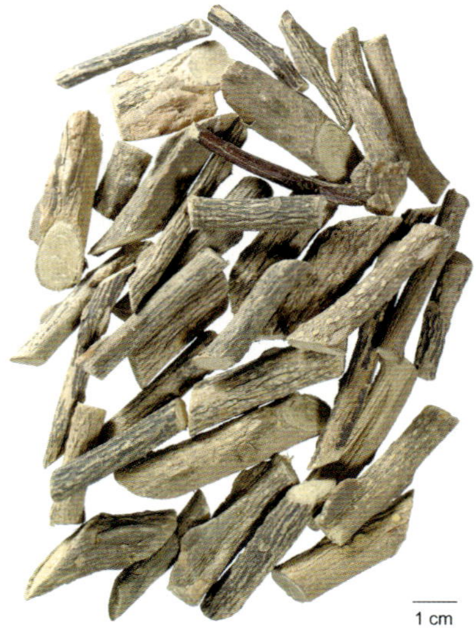

Crude drug

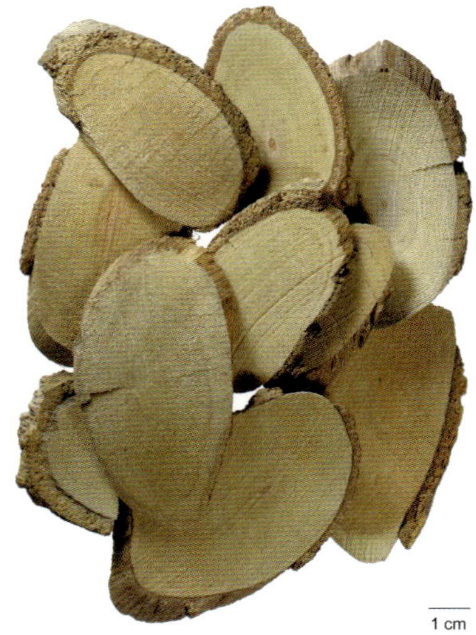

Decoction Pieces

Source The root of *Zanthoxylum nitidum* (Roxb.) DC. (Fam. Rutaceae).

Distribution Mainly in Chinese provinces such as Fujian, Hunan, Guangxi, Guangdong, Yunnan and Taiwan; also in Hong Kong.

Harvest & Processing Harvest roots anytime during the year; wash clean; cut into slices; dry under the sun or use while fresh. Commonly sold in the form of irregular slices or sections 1-4 mm thick. Hard.

Description Cylindrical and slightly curved; 0.7-5 cm or above in diameter. Outer surface dark brownish-yellow to light brown, marked with heavy longitudinal wrinkles, occasionally with transverse clefts; lenticels protuberant, suborbicular (almost round), bright yellow or dull yellowish-brown. When broken transversely, surface shows thin cork; cortex light brown, with slightly lustrous dark yellow maculae; xylem greyish-yellow, with concentric annulations and dense pores. Hard. Odour: slightly fragrant; taste: pungent, tongue-numbing and bitter.

Indications 1. Trauma, rheumatic arthralgia, stomachache, toothache 2. Venomous-snake bite 3. Burn and scalds.

Chemical Composition Mainly contains alkaloids such as nitidine and chelerythrine.

Note Listed as slightly toxic in *C.P.*

Radix Zanthoxyli Avicennae

Avicennia Pricklyash Root

Yingbubo

鹰不泊

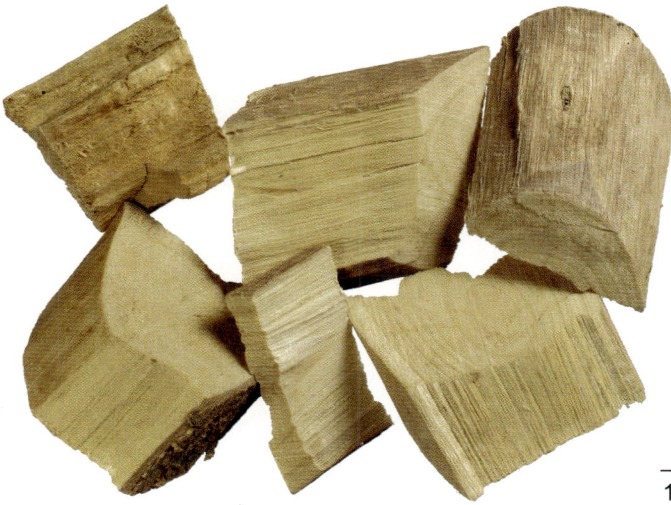

1 cm

Crude drug

Source The root of *Zanthoxylum avicennae* (Lam.) DC. (Fam. Rutaceae).

Distribution Mainly in Chinese provinces such as Guangdong, Guangxi, Fujian and Jiangxi; also in Hong Kong.

Harvest & Processing Dig up roots anytime during the year; wash clean; cut into slices; dry under the sun.

Description Cylindrical; varying in length, 0.8-3 cm or above in diameter. Outer surface yellowish-brown; marked with numerous deep longitudinal grooves. Hard, does not break easily. When broken, surface bright yellow; annulations visible on thicker roots; outer side of cortex brownish-black, inner side light brown; xylem dull yellow. Taste: slightly bitter, tongue-numbing.

Indications 1. Rheumatism, trauma, lumbago 2. Abdominal pain, jaundice, chronic hepatitis 3. Oedema 3. Leukorrhagia 4. Common cold, cough, whooping cough 5. Appendicitis

Chemical Composition Mainly contains alkaloids such as nitidine and magnoflorine.

Ramulus Cinnamomi

Cassia Twig
Guizhi

桂枝

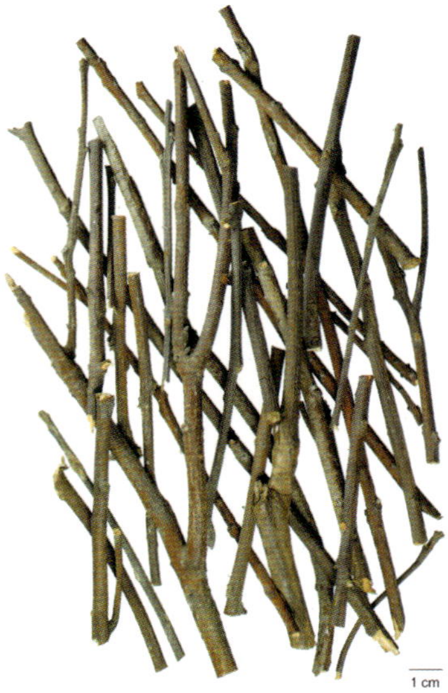

Crude drug

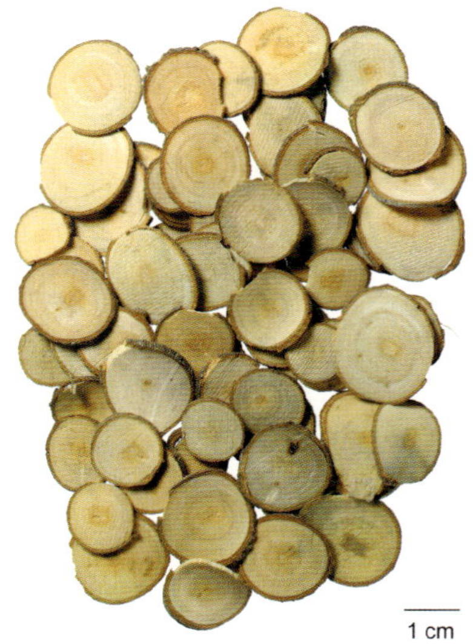

Decoction Pieces

Source The twig of *Cinnamomum cassia* Presl (Fam. Lauraceae).

Distribution Mainly in Chinese provinces such as Guangxi, Guangdong and Fujian; also in Yunnan province and Hong Kong.

Harvest & Processing Clip off twigs two years after field planting; remove foliage; dry twigs under the sun. Alternatively, collect branches clipped off or coppice shoots hacked off during trimming; dry under the sun.

Description Long and cylindrical, ramose (with many branches); 30-70 cm long, 0.3-1 cm in diameter at the thick end. Outer surface brownish-red or reddish-brown, marked with fine wrinkles and small verruciform (wart-shaped) scars of leaves, branches and buds; lenticels punctiform (dot-like) or elliptical-punctiform. Hard and brittle, breaks easily. When broken, surface shows reddish-brown cortex; xylem yellowish-white to light yellowish-brown; pith somewhat quadrate (square-shaped). Odour: with a distinctive fragrance; taste: sweet and slightly acrid, cortex with a stronger taste.

Indications 1. Common cold, cough, dizziness 2. Palpitation, precordial pain 3. Arthralgia 4. Amenorrrhoea, dysmenorrhoea 5. Dysuria, oedema

Chemical Composition Mainly contains essential oils with cinnamaldehyde as the main component.

Ramulus Uncariae cum Uncis

Gambir Plant

Gouteng

鉤藤

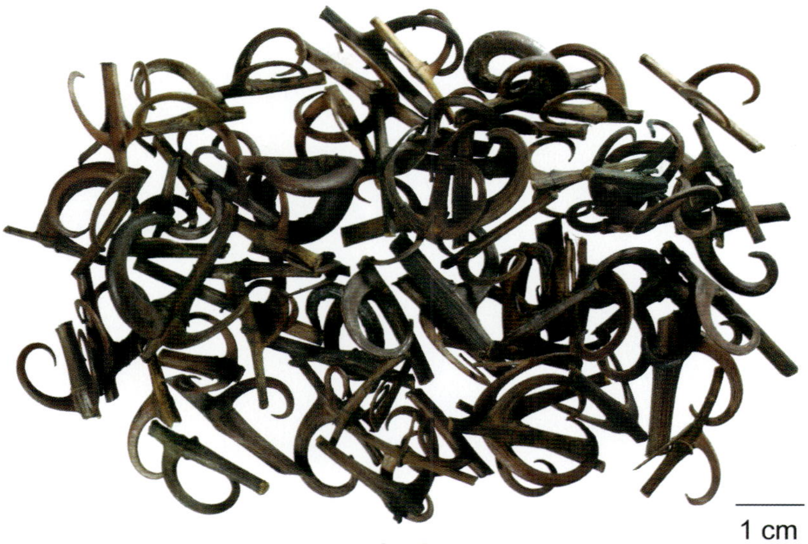

1 cm

Crude drug

Source The hook-bearing twig of *Uncaria rhynchophylla* (Miq.) Jacks. (Fam. Rubiaceae).

Distribution Mainly in Chinese provinces such as Guangxi, Guangdong, Hubei and Hunan.

Harvest & Processing Collect hook-bearing twigs in autumn and winter; cut into short sections; dry under the sun, or steam and dry under the sun.

Description Short sections of hook-bearing twigs. Twigs cylindrical or somewhat quadrangular (four-angled); outer surface reddish-brown to purplish-red, marked with fine longitudinal striae, smooth and glabrous (without hairs). Most branch nodes with a pair of hooks, hooks opposite (borne in pairs at each node) and curving downwards; occasionally only one side of node with a hook, the other side with a protuberant scar. Hooks slightly flat or slightly orbicular (round); apex narrow and pointed; base slightly orbicular, flat and broad. Light in weight; strong and pliable. When broken, cortex fibrous; pith yellowish-white, loose like sponge, or shrivelled into a cavity. Odourless; taste: mild.

Indications 1. Infantile convulsions, hyperpyrexia, frequent night crying of infants 2. Headache due to common cold, neural headache 3. Dizziness and blurred vision due to hypertension.

Chemical Composition Mainly contains alkaloids such as rhynchophylline.

Note According to *C.P.*, also used for medicinal purposes is the hook-bearing twig of *U. macrophylla* Wall., of *U. hirsuta* Havil., of *U. sinensis* (Oliv.) Havil. and of *U. sessilifructus* Roxb.

Receptaculum Nelumbinis

Lotus Receptacle
Lianfang

蓮房

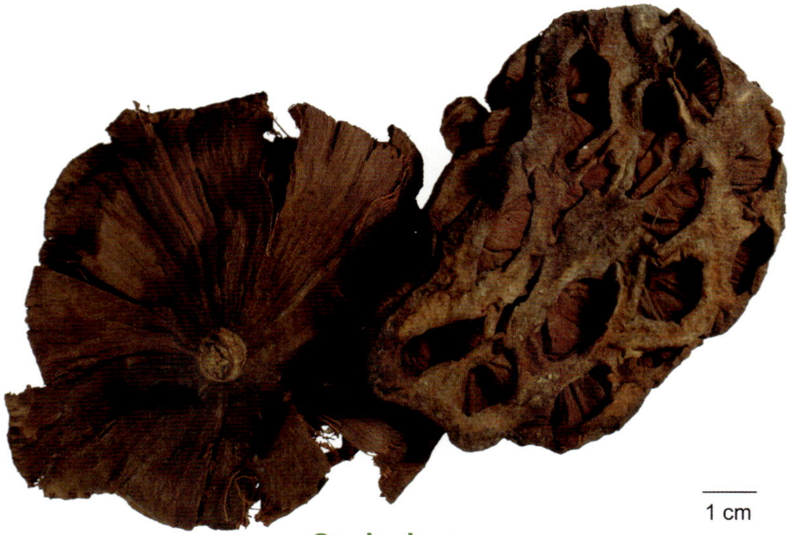

Crude drug

Source The receptacle of *Nelumbo nucifera* Gaertn. (Fam. Nymphaeaceae).

Distribution In most regions of China, including Hong Kong.

Harvest & Processing Cut off lotus seedpods in autumn when fruits are ripe; remove seeds and pedicels; dry under the sun.

Description Obconical (inversely conical) or funnelform, with numerous cracks; 5-8 cm in diameter, 4-6 cm thick. Outer surface greyish-brown; marked with fine longitudinal striae and wrinkles, or cracked and fibrous at some parts. Horizontal surface orbicular (round) and even, with numerous small orbicular holes left after removal of seeds; base with remnants of pedicel base or pedicel scars. Light in weight; texture soft. When cut open length-wise, numerous clefts revealed, giving it a sponge-like appearence. Odour: faint; taste: slightly astringent.

Indications Bleeding such as menorrhagia, dysfunctional uterine bleeding, haematuria, haemorrhoidal bleeding, and excessive postpartum bleeding.

Chemical Composition Mainly contains hyperoside.

Resina Ferulae

Chinese Asafetida
Awei

阿魏

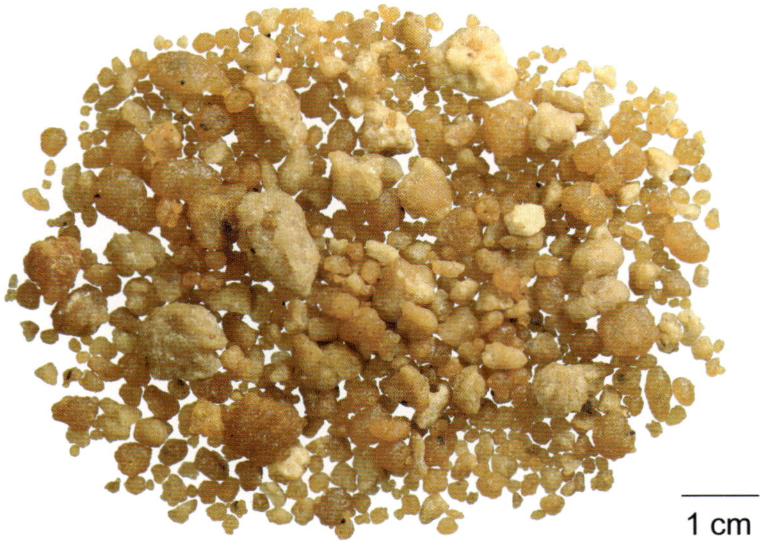

Crude drug

Source The resin of *Ferula sinkiangensis* K. M. Shen (Fam. Umbelliferae).

Distribution Mainly in Ili in the Xinjiang region of China.

Harvest & Processing In late spring and early summer, i.e. from full efflorescence to early fruit period, slant-cut downwards from the upper part of the stem to induce resin secretion; make a new cut each time when resin stops oozing; repeat 3-5 times; put the resin collected into containers and dry in well-ventilated and cool places.

Description Irregular or lacrimiform (tear-shaped) hard lumps, in some cases lipoid (fat-like), occasionally semi-fluid. In varying shades of colour, greyish-white, waxy yellow or light brownish-yellow. Hard lumps hard as white wax; light in weight; broken surface slightly porous and clefted; freshly cut surface relatively light in colour, colour darkens with time. Lipoid pieces viscid; greyish-white, colour darkens after long storage. When water is added, resin turns to white emulsion when ground. Odour: with a heavy and lasting garlic-like stink; taste: slightly bitter, pungent as garlic, fairly tongue-irritating and gives a burning sensation.

Indications 1. Dyspepsia 2. Abdominal mass 3. Abdominal pain due to parasitosis.

Chemical Composition Mainly contains essential oils and coumarins.

Note According to *C.P.*, also used for medicinal purposes is the resin of *F. fukanensis* K. M. Shen.

Resina Garciniae Morellae

Gamboge Tree Rasin

Tenghuang

藤黃

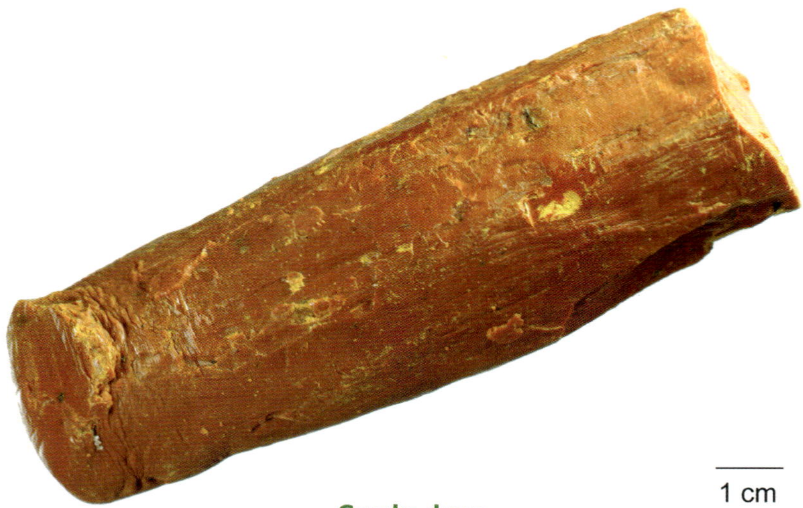

Crude drug

Source The gum resin of *Garcinia morella* Desr. (Fam. Guttiferae).

Distribution Originated in countries like India, Thailand, Vietnam, Cambodia and Malaysia. Cultivated in Guangdong and Guangxi provinces in China.

Harvest & Processing Before efflorescence make a spiroid (spiral-like) cut at about 3 m from the ground on the cortex of the trunks; insert a bamboo container into the wound to collect the emerging resin; steam dry over heat; scrape off resin with a knife.

Description Fistular (hollow and cylindrical) or irregular lumps; 3-5 cm in diameter; reddish-yellow or orange-brown. Outer surface covered with yellowish-green powder and marked with longitudinal striae. Brittle, break easily. Broken surface smooth, conchiform (shell-like) or hollow, with dull yellowish-brown and waxy lustre. When water is added, gum resin turns into yellow emulsion when ground; burn when thrown into fire. Odour: faint; taste: pungent.

Indications 1. Carbuncle, Pyodermas 2. Ulcerative gingivitis, dental caries (external use)

Chemical Composition Mainly contains xanthone such as gambogic acid.

Note Resina Garciniase Morellae listed in Hong Kong as Category I (Toxic/Potent) Chinese Materia Medica and the processed Resina Garciniae Morellae, Category II.

Resina Liquidambaris

Beautiful Sweetgum Resin
Fengxiangzhi
楓香脂

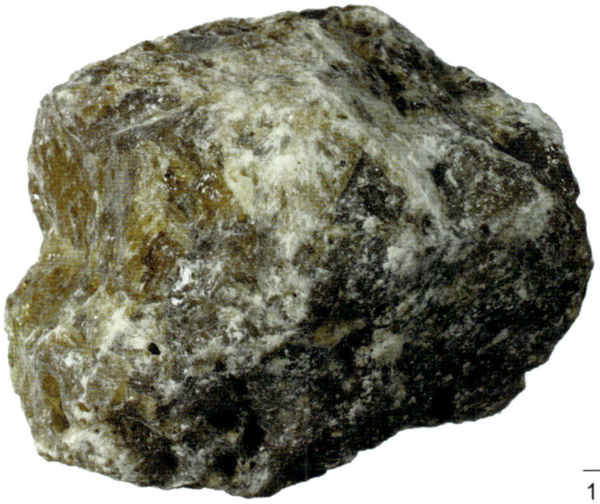

1 cm

Crude drug

Source The resin of *Liquidambar formosana* Hance (Fam. Hamamelidaceae).

Distribution Mainly in Chinese provinces such as Zhejiang, Jiangxi, Fujian and Yunnan; also in Hong Kong.

Harvest & Processing In summer, bore holes around the tree trunk at 15-20 cm from the root and with sufficient space between the holes. Repeat the process up the tree trunk at the same vertical intervals. Collect resin from November to the following March; dry under the sun or dry naturally.

Description Irregular lumps, or subspherical granules; varying in size, mostly 0.5-1 cm in diameter, occasionally up to 3 cm. Outer surface pale yellow to yellowish-brown, translucent or opaque. Brittle; breaks easily; broken surface marked with glassy lustre. Odour: fresh and fragrant, fragrance stronger when burning; taste: mild.

Indications 1. Trauma, swelling and pain of carbuncle and boil 2. Bleeding such as haemoptysis, epistaxis and traumatic haemorrhage.

Chemical Composition Mainly contains essential oils.

Rhizoma Acori Tatarinowii

Grassleaf Sweetflag Rhizome
Shichangpu

石菖蒲

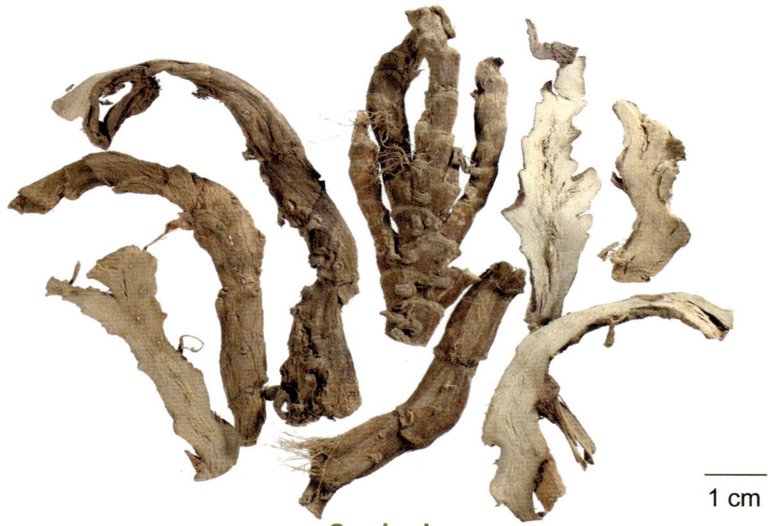

Crude drug

Source The rhizome of *Acorus tatarinowii* Schott. (Fam. Araceae).

Distribution Mainly in Chinese provinces such as Sichuan, Zhejiang, Jiangxi and Jiangsu; also in Hong Kong.

Harvest & Processing Collect rhizomes in autumn and winter; remove leaves and fibrous roots; wash away soil; dry rhizomes under the sun.

Description Flattened and cylindrical, mostly curved, often branched; 3-20 cm long, 0.3-1 cm in diameter. Outer surface reddish-brown or greyish-brown; rough; marked with annular (ring-like) nodes of various density, length of internodes varies between 2-8 mm; marked with fine longitudinal striae; one side marked with remnants of fibrous roots or punctiform (dot-like) root scars; leaf scars triangular, arranged in an alternate pattern; with remnants of hairy and squamiform (scale-like) leaf base. Hard. Transverse section fibrous, off-white or reddish; endodermis ring conspicuous; broken surface with numerous punctiform (dot-like) vascular bundles and brown oil dots. Odour: aromatic; taste: bitter and slightly acrid.

Indications 1. Chronic gastritis, feeling of oppression in the chest 2. Delirium, deafness, tinnitus 3. Rheumatic arthritis, lumbago.

Chemical Composition Mainly contains essential oils with α, β, γ -asarone and elemicin as the main components.

Rhizoma Acori Tatarinowii

Rhizoma Alismatis

Oriental Waterplantain Rhizome

Zexie

澤瀉

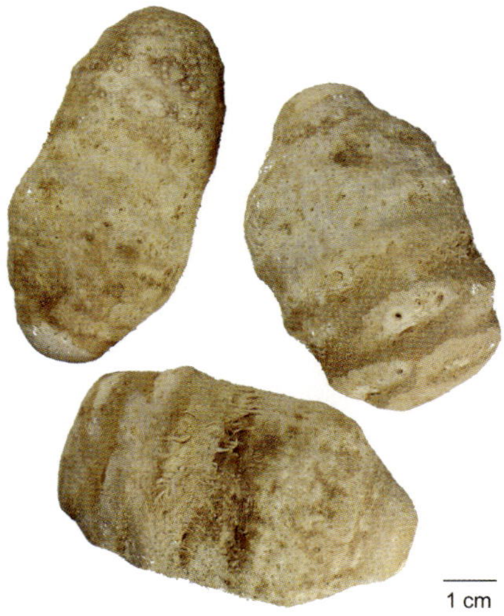

Crude drug

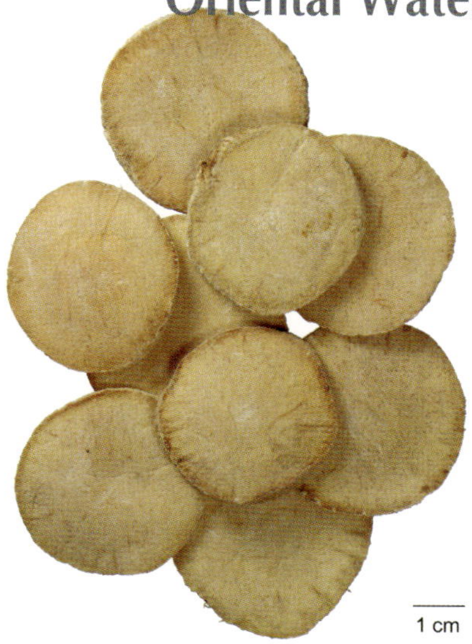

Decoction Pieces

Source The tuber of *Alisma orientale* (Sam.) Juzepcz (Fam. Alismataceae).

Distribution Mainly in Chinese proviuces such as Fujian, Sichuan and Jiangxi.

Harvest & Processing Dig out tubers in winter; remove leaves and fibrous roots, and shave off cork; wash tubers clean; dry by heat. Alternatively, put tubers in a bamboo basket to remove fibrous roots and cork; dry under the sun.

Description Subspherical, ellipsoid (elliptical in long-section and circular in cross-section) or obovoid (inverse egg-shaped); 2-7 cm long, 2-6 cm in diameter; outer surface yellowish-white or pale yellowish-brown. For tubers with cork remnants, outer surface pale brown and marked with irregular, shallow transverse annulations and numerous small, protuberant scars of fibrous roots; both annulations and scars especially dense at the bottom. Hard and solid; when broken, surface yellowish-white, starchy, poriferous (with numerous pores). Odour: faint; taste: slightly bitter.

Indications 1. Nephritic oedema, pyelitis, dysuria 2. Enteritis, diarrhoea.

Chemical Composition Mainly contains triterpenes such as alisol A, B, C.

Rhizoma Alpiniae officinarum

Lesser Galangal Rhizome
Gaoliangjiang

高良薑

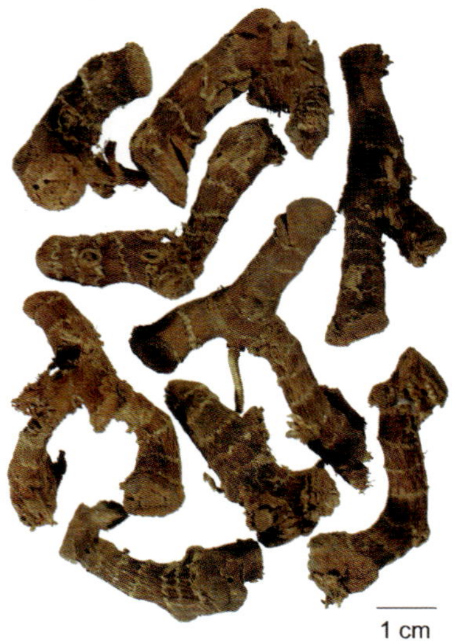

Crude drug

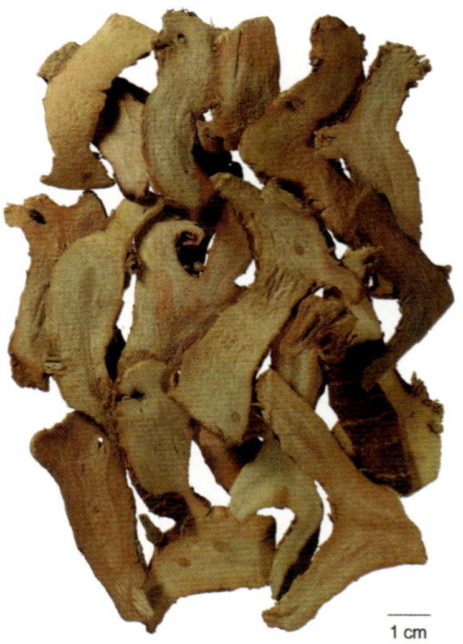

Decoction Pieces

Source The rhizome of *Alpinia officinarum* Hance (Fam. Zingiberaceae).

Distribution Mainly in Chinese provinces such as Guangdong and Guangxi.

Harvest & Processing Dig out rhizomes in late summer and early autumn; remove fibrous roots and scale remnants; wash clean; cut into sections; dry under the sun.

Description Cylindrical, mostly curved, rameous (branched); 5-9 cm long, 1-1.5 cm in diameter. Outer surface brownish-red to dull brown, marked with dense longitudinal wrinkles and greyish-brown undulate (wavy) annular (ring-like) nodes; internodes 0.2-1 cm long; one side with orbicular (round) root scars. Pliable but strong, does not break easily. When broken, surface greyish-brown to reddish-brown, fibrous; stele takes up about 1/3 of the diameter. Odour: fragrant; taste: pungent.

Indications 1. Epigastric pain, vomiting, dyspepsia 2. Gastric and duodenal ulcer, chronic gastritis 3. Acute gastroenteritis.

Chemical Composition Mainly contains flavonoids such as galangin; also contains essential oils with eugenol as the main component.

Rhizoma Anemarrhenae

Common Anemarrhena Rhizome

Zhimu

知母

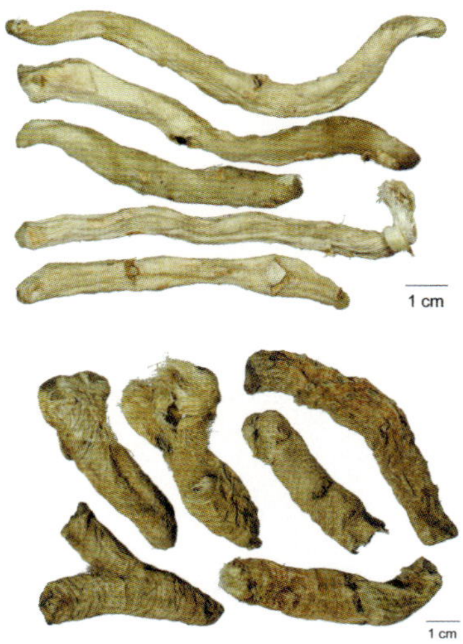

Crude drug

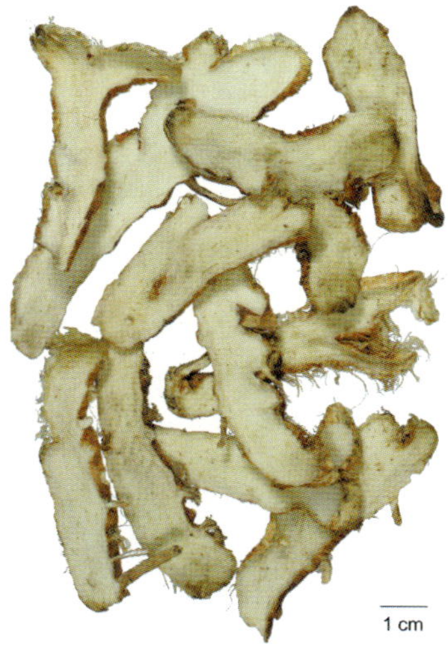

Decoction Pieces

Source
The rhizome of *Anemarrhena asphodeloides* Bunge (Fam. Liliaceae).

Distribution
Mainly in Chinese provinces such as Hebei, Shanxi and Shaanxi, and in Inner Mongolia.

Harvest & Processing
Collect rhizomes in spring and autumn; remove base remnants and fibrous roots; dry rhizomes under the sun to produce '*Mao zhimu*'(Hairy Common Anemarrhena Rhizome). Alternatively, peel off cork while fresh; dry rhizomes under the sun to produce '*Guang zhimu*'(Glabrous Common Anemarrhena Rhizome).

Description
Mao zhimu: Rod-like, slightly curved and flat, occasionally with branches. Top end with light yellow leaf scars and stem scars; upper surface with a dented groove, and annular (ring-like) nodes arranged closely; dense yellowish-brown remnants of leaf base on nodes; underside bulgy and slightly shrivelled, marked with dented or protuberant punctiform (dot-like) root scars. Hard, breaks easily; when broken, surface yellowish-white. Taste: slightly sweet, slightly bitter; sticky when chewed. Commonly used in Hong Kong in the form of length-wise cut slices.
Guang zhimu: Outer surface white; with twisted grooves; sometimes with leaf scars and root scars.

Indications
1. Hyperpyrexia, hectic fever 2. Polydipsia 3. Cough with thick yellow sputum and difficult expectoration 4. Constipation

Chemical Composition
Mainly contains timosaponins A-I, A-II, A-III, A-IV, B-I, B-II and anemaran A, B, C, D.

Rhizoma Anemones Raddeanae

Radde Anemone Rhizome
Liangtoujian

兩頭尖

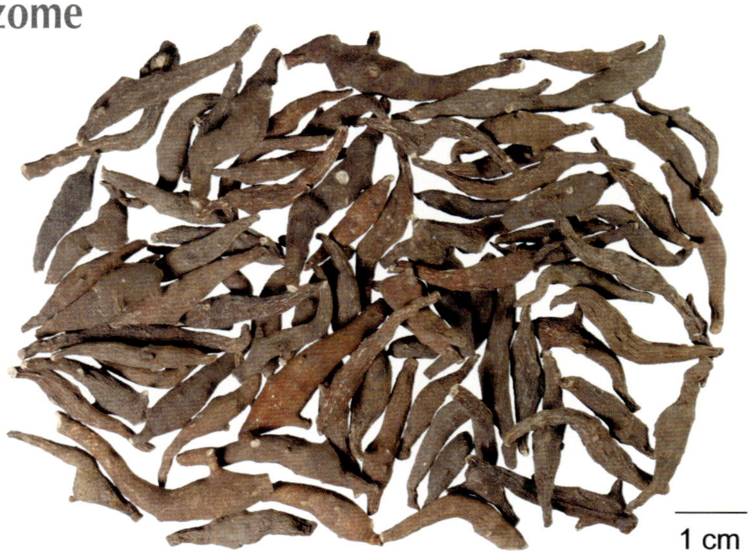

Crude drug

Source The rhizome of *Anemone raddeana* Regel (Fam. Ranunculaceae).

Distribution Mainly in Chinese provinces such as Shandong, Liaoning, Jilin and Heilongjiang.

Harvest & Processing Dig up rhizomes in summer; remove stem remnants and rootlets; dry rhizomes under the sun.

Description Oblong and spindle-shaped, both ends fine and pointed, slightly curved, relatively bulgy near one end; 1-3 cm long, 2-7 mm in diameter. Outer surface reddish-brown or brownish-black, marked with fine longitudinal wrinkles; bulgy part marked with 1-3 fin-like, protuberant scars of branch roots; outer surface occasionally with 3-5 indistinct annular (ring-like) nodes. Hard and brittle, breaks easily; when broken, surface fairly smooth, off-white or dull greyish-brown, cuticular. Odour: faint; taste: mild, then slightly bitter and hot-numbing.

Indications 1. Rheumatoid arthritis with muscular contracture 2. Carbuncles with ulceration.

Chemical Composition Mainly contains diosgenin and raddeanin Ro, A, B, C, D.

Note Listed as toxic in *C.P.*

Rhizoma Anemonis Altaicae

Irkutsk Anemone Rhizome

Jiujiechangpu

九節菖蒲

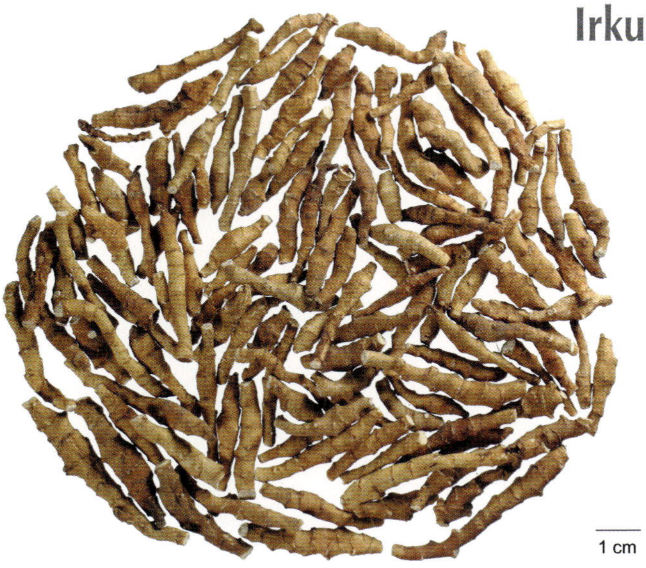

Crude drug

Source The rhizome of *Anemone altaica* Fisch. ex C.A. Mey. (Fam. Ranunculaceae).

Distribution Mainly in Shaanxi province in China.

Harvest & Processing Harvest rhizomes from crops planted for five years or more in May or June before leaves wilt; remove soil and sand; dry under the sun, then rub to remove rootlets; sieve out foreign matter.

Description Oblong and spindle-shaped, slightly curved; 1-4 cm long, 3-5 mm in diameter. Outer surface brownish-yellow to dull brown; marked with numerous semi-annular protuberant nodes and scale-leaf scars arranged in a slanted, alternate manner; each node marked with 1-3 protuberant root scars. Hard and brittle, breaks easily; when broken, surface smooth, white, starchy, marked with vascular bundles in the form of 6-12 pale yellow dots arranged in a ring. Odour: faint; taste: slightly sour.

Indications 1. Fever with impairment of consciousness, epilepsy, neurosis 2. Deafness and tinnitus 3. Anorexia, distending pain in the chest and the abdomen 4. Carbuncles, sores (external use).

Chemical Composition Contains essential oils with cedrol as the main component.

Rhizoma Anemonis Altaicae

Rhizoma Arisaematis

Jackinthepulpit Tuber
Tiannanxing

天南星

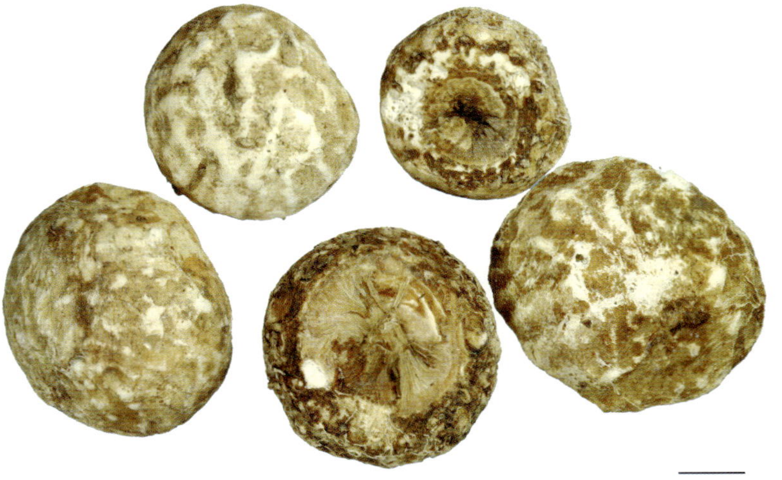

Crude Drug

1 cm

Source The tuber of *Arisaema erubescens* (Wall.) Schott (Fam. Araceae).

Distribution Mainly in Chinese provinces such as Henan, Hebei, Shandong, Anhui and Jiangsu.

Harvest & Processing Dig out tubers in autumn and winter when leaves wither; remove fibrous roots and cork; dry the tubers.

Description Flattened and spherical; 1-2 cm thick, 1.5-6.5 cm in diameter. Outer surface off-white or pale brown; relatively smooth; top end with dented stem scars, whole tuber encircled with punctiform (dot-like) root scars; periphery occasionally with small, flattened and spherical lateral buds. Hard, does not break easily; broken surface uneven, white and starchy. Odour: slightly acrid; taste: hot-numbing.

Indications 1. Productive cough with feeling of oppression in the chest 2. Dizziness, cerebral vascular accident, hemiplegia, facial palsy, numbness of extremities. 3. Skin infection, scrofula, snakebite.

Chemical Composition Contains paeonol and aurantiamide acetate.

Note According to *C.P.*, also used for medicinal purposes are the tuber of *A. heterophyllum* Bl. and *A. amurense* Maxim., and the processed Rhizoma Arisaematis called '*Dannanxing*'(Bile Arisaema). The unprocessed tuber of *A. erubescens* (Wall.) Schott and the two species mentioned above is listed in Hong Kong as Category I (Toxic/Potent) Chinese Materia Medica, and the processed product *Dannanxing*, Category II.

Rhizoma Atractylodis

Atractylodes Rhizome
Cangzhu
蒼朮

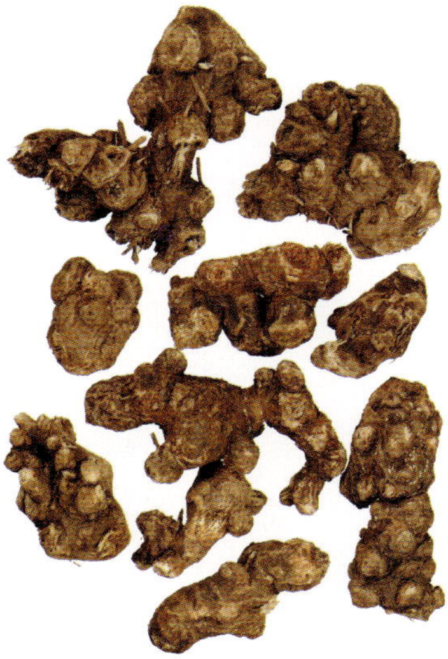

1 cm

Crude Drug

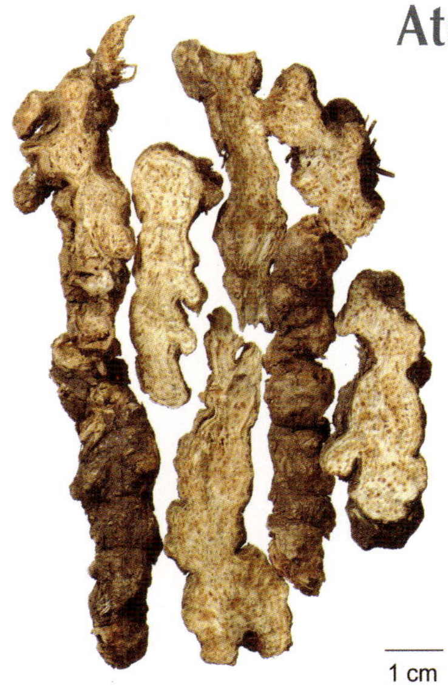

1 cm

Decoction Pieces

Source The rhizome of *Atractylodes lancea* (Thunb.) DC. (Fam. Compositae).

Distribution Mainly in Chinese provinces such as Hubei, Jiangsu and Henan.

Harvest & Processing Dig out rhizomes in spring and autumn; remove soil and sand; dry under the sun; remove rootlets.

Description Irregular and nodular, or slightly torose (cylindrical with alternate swellings and constrictions); sometimes curved; usually without branches. Outer surface yellowish-brown to greyish-brown, marked with fine longitudinal grooves, wrinkles and sparse remnants of rootlets; nodes often with constrictions of shallow, transverse grooves; internodes with orbicular (round) stem scars, one end often with caudex remnants, occasionally with stem scars. Hard and solid; breaks easily. When broken, surface slightly uneven, off-white or yellowish-white, scattered with numerous orange-yellow or brownish-red oil cavities; acerose (needle-shaped) white crystals formed after exposure for a relatively long time. Odour: with a heavy aroma; taste: slightly sweet, bitter and acrid.

Indications 1. Oedema 2. Vomiting, diarrhoea, anorexia, abdominal distension 3. Night blindness, blurring of vision 4. Rheumatism 5. Eczema, weeping skin lesions.

Chemical Composition Mainly contains essential oils with sesqutiterpene as the main component.

Note According to *C.P.*, also used for medicinal purposes is the rhizome of *A. chinensis* (DC.) Koidz.

Rhizoma Atractylodis Macrocephalae

Largehead Atractylodes Rhizome
Baizhu

白术

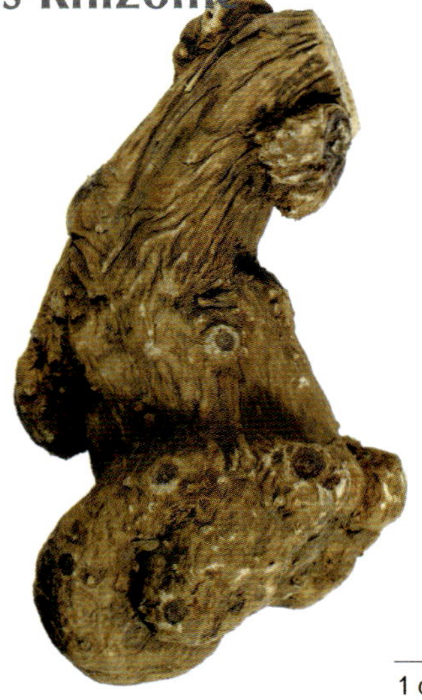

Crude drug

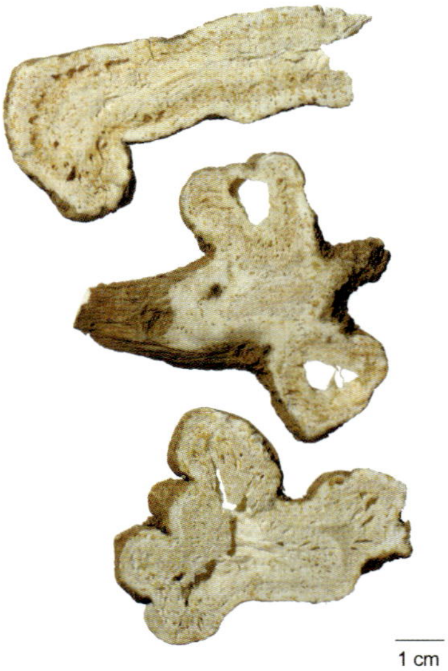

Decoction Pieces

Source The rhizome of *Atractylodes macrocephala* Koidz. (Fam. Compositae).

Distribution Mainly in Chinese provinces such as Zhejiang, Anhui, Hubei and Hunan. Mostly cultivated.

Harvest & Processing Collect rhizomes 2-3 years old in late October; remove stems, leaves and rootlets; dry rhizomes by heat to produce '*Hongzhu*' (Fire-Dried Largehead Atractylodes Rhizome), or dry under the sun to produce '*Shengshai zhu*' (Sun-Dried Largehead Atractylodes Rhizome).

Description Plump pieces irregular in shape; 3-13 cm long, 1.5-7 cm in diameter. Outer surface greyish-yellow or greyish-brown; marked with irregular strumiform (cushion-like) protuberances, interrupted longitudinal wrinkles and grooves, and scars of rootlets; top end marked with caudex remnants and bud scars. Hard, does not break easily. When broken, surface uneven; transverse section of *Shengshaizhu* pale yellowish-white to pale brown, with chrysanthemum markings and scattered brownish-yellow oil dots; transverse section of *Hongzhu* cuticular, deeper in colour and with clefts. Odour: fresh and fragrant; taste: sweet and slightly acrid; slightly sticky when chewed.

Indications 1. Anorexia, abdominal distension, chronic diarrhoea, weakness 2. Oedema, oliguria 3. Spontaneous sweating 4. Threatened abortion and morning sickness 5. Arthralgia

Chemical Composition Mainly contains essential oils with atractylon as the main component.

Rhizoma Atractylodis

Rhizoma Belamcandae

Blackberrylily Rhizome
Shegan
射干

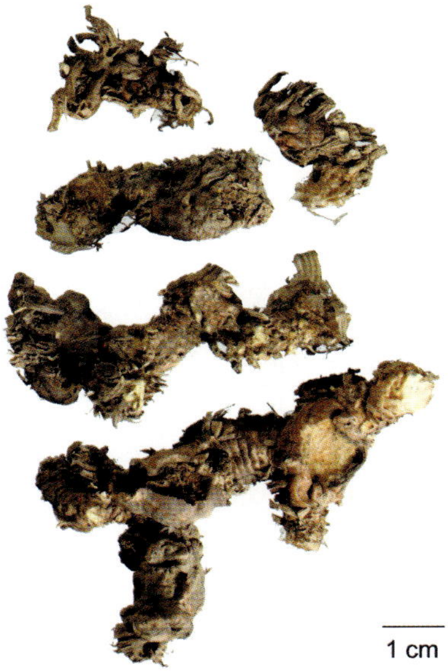

Crude drug

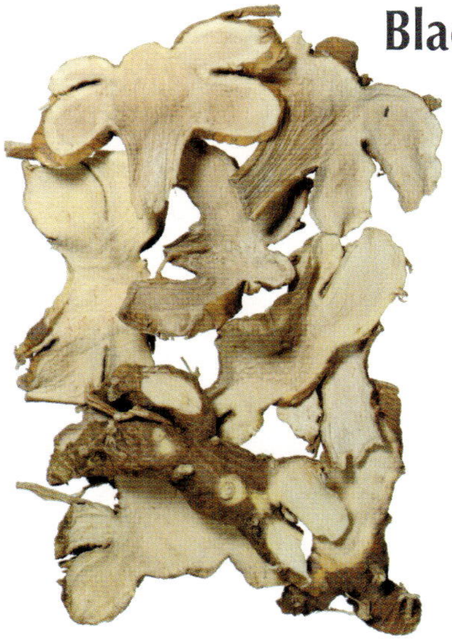

Decoction Pieces

1 cm

Source The rhizome of *Belamcanda chinensis* (L.) DC. (Fam. Iridaceae).

Distribution Mainly in Chinese provinces such as Henan, Hubei and Jiangsu; also in Hong Kong.

Harvest & Processing Dig out rhizomes in early spring or late autumn; remove leaves; dry under the sun until half-dry; scorch away fibrous roots; dry under the sun again. Commonly used in Hong Kong in the form of length-wise cut slices.

Description Irregular and nodular; 3-10 cm long, 1-2 cm in diameter. Outer surface dull yellowish-brown, reddish-brown or dull blackish-brown; shrivelled; marked with relatively dense annulations. Upper part with several disciform (disc-like) dented stem scars, occasionally with remnants of caudex; lower part with rootlet remnants and root scars. Hard; when broken, surface yellow and granular. Odour: faint; taste: bitter and slightly acrid.

Indications
1. Expectoration, retropharyngeal abscess and sore throat
2. Tracheitis, parotitis, tonsillitis.

Chemical Composition Mainly contains isoflavonoids such as irigenin and tectorigenin.

Rhizoma Bistortae

Bistort Rhizome
Quanshen

拳參

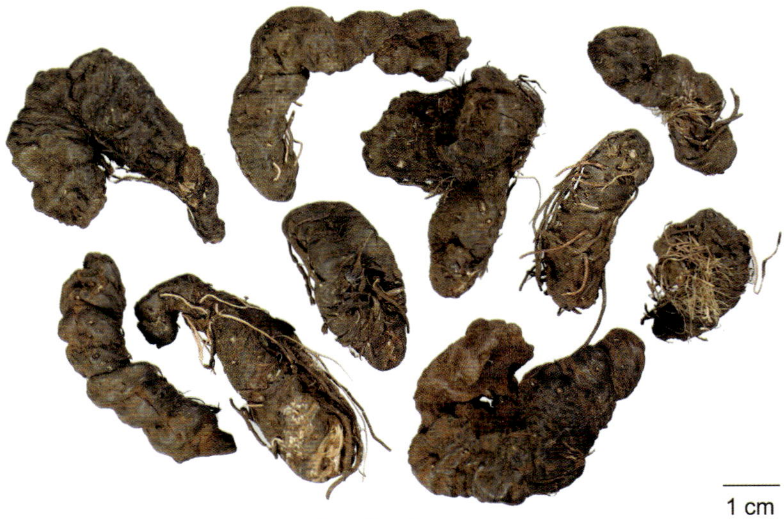

Crude drug

Rhizoma Bistortae

Source The rhizome of *Polygonum bistorta* L. (Fam. Polygonaceae).

Distribution Mainly in Chinese provinces such as Shandong, Jiangsu and Hubei, and in northern and northwestern China.

Harvest & Processing Dig up rhizomes in spring when plants germinate, or in autumn when leaves are about to wilt; remove soil and sand; dry rhizomes under the sun; remove rootlets.

Description Flattened and rod-like, or flattened, cylindrical and curved, slightly narrower at both ends, or tapering towards one end; in some cases curled up; 6-13 cm long, 1-2.5 cm wide. Outer surface dull purplish-brown or purplish-black, rough; one side protuberant, the other fairly flat and occasionally slightly grooved; whole rhizome marked with dense annulations and remnants of rootlets or root scars. Hard. When broken, surface light brownish-red; vascular bundles yellowish-white, punctiform (dot-like), arranged in a ring. Odourless; taste: bitter and astringent.

Indications 1. Diarrhoea, enteritis 2. Bleeding haemorrhoid 3. Dermititis 4. Stomatitis, gingivitis (external use).

Chemical Composition Mainly contains gallic acid, hydrolysable tannins, condensed tannins and anthraquinones.

Rhizoma Bletillae

Common Bletilla Tuber

Baiji

白及

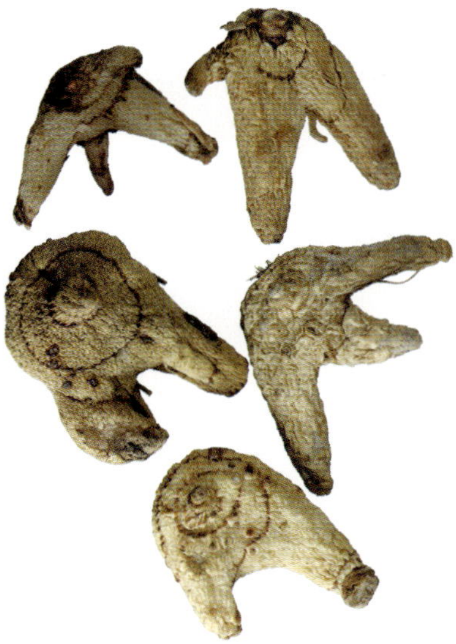

Crude drug 1 cm

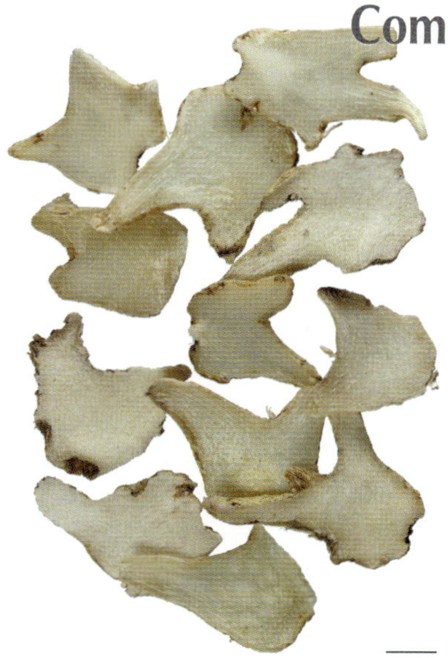

Decoction Pieces 1 cm

Source The tuber of *Bletilla striata* (Thunb.) Reichb. f. (Fam. Orchidaceae).

Distribution Mainly in Chinese provinces such as Guizhou, Sichuan, Yunnan, Hubei and Jiangxi; also in Hong Hong.

Harvest & Processing Collect tubers in summer and autumn; remove fibrous roots; wash clean; process immediately to prevent tubers from turning black; boil or steam thoroughly; dry under the sun until half-dry; remove cork; dry under the sun again.

Description Irregular, flattened and round or rhombic; usually with 2-3 claw-like branches; 1.5-5 cm long, 0.5-1.5 cm thick. Upper part marked with protuberant stem scars; lower part carries marks of being joined to another tuber. Outer surface greyish-white or yellowish-white, with several concentric rings encircling the stem scar; nodes marked with remnants of punctiform (dot-like) brown scars of fibrous roots. Hard; does not break easily. When broken, surface off-white, translucent, cuticular, scattered with punctiform vascular bundles. Odourless; taste: bitter, sticky when chewed.

Indications Various kinds of bleedings such as haemoptysis due to pulmonary tuberculosis and bronchiectasis, gastrointestional bleeding, epistaxis and traumatic bleeding etc.

Chemical Composition Mainly contains bibenzyl and dihydrophenanthrene.

Rhizoma Bolbostemmatis

Paniculate Bolbostemma
Tubeimu

土貝母

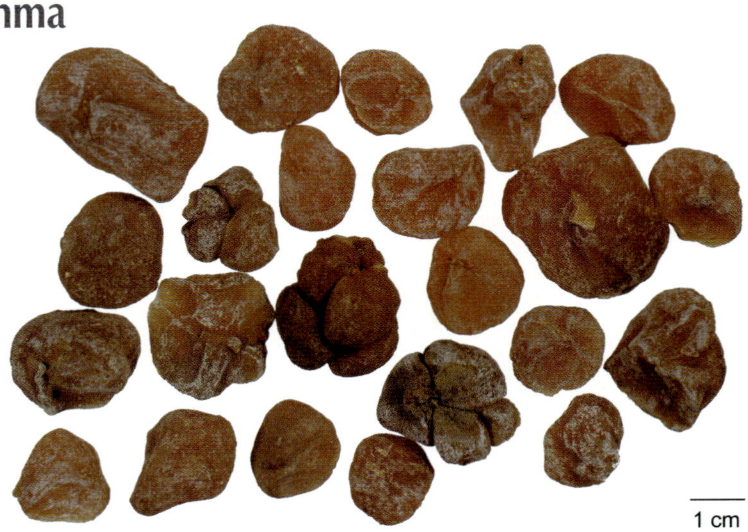

Crude Drug

Source The subterranean fleshy bulb of *Bolbostemma paniculatum* (Maxim.) Franquet (Fam. Cucurbitaceae).

Distribution Mainly in Chinese provinces such as Henan, Shanxi, Shaanxi and Hebei.

Harvest & Processing Collect bulbs in autumn; peel off succulent white scale leaves; wash clean; boil thoroughly; dry under the sun.

Description Irregular pieces; often broad in the middle; 0.5-1.5 cm long, 0.7-2-3 cm wide. Outer surface dull brown or light reddish-brown; translucent when thoroughly boiled; uneven and furrowed. Ventral side usually marked with a longitudinal groove; base marked with light-coloured scars and base remnants of bulb axis; dorsal side usually bulgy or polygonal. Hard, do not break easily. When crushed, surface cuticular, relatively smooth. Odour: with a slight burnt smell; taste: slightly sweet and then slightly bitter-acrid. Slightly sticky.

Indications 1. Breast abscess, breast cancer 2. Scrofula, lumps, boils and sores 3. Snake and insect bites

Chemical Composition Mainly contains tubeimosides.

Rhizoma Chuanxiong

Szechwan Lovage Rhizome
Chuanxiong
川芎

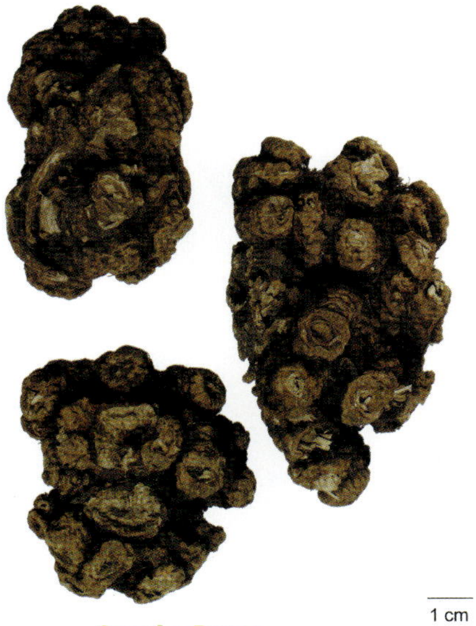

Crude Drug

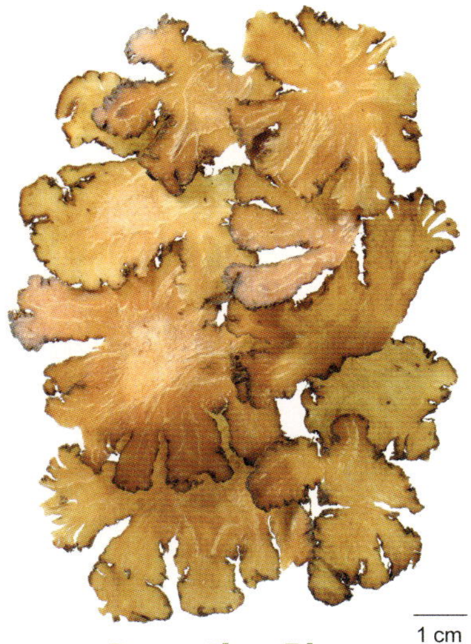

Decoction Pieces

Source The rhizome of *Ligusticum chuanxiong* Hort. (Fam. Umbelliferae).

Distribution Mainly in Chinese provinces such as Sichuan, Hubei, Shaanxi and Jiangxi. Cultivated.

Harvest & Processing Collect rhizomes in summer when bulgy nodes on stems become prominent and slightly purplish in colour; remove stems, leaves and soil; air to dry until half-dry and then dry by heat; remove rootlets.

Description Irregular and nodular, fist-shape a pieces; 2-7 cm in diameter. Outer surface dull yellowish-brown, rough and wrinkled, with numerous protuberant annular (ring-like) nodes; top end with dented suborbicular (almost round) stem scars; lateral side of lower part and annular nodes with numerous small strumiform (cushion-like) root scars. Hard and solid, do not break easily. When broken, surface yellowish-white or greyish-yellow, with an undulate (wavy) cambium ring and criss-crossing striae, scattered with punctiform (dot-like) yellowish-brown oil cavities. With a distinctive and strong fragrance; taste: bitter, acrid, slightly tongue-numbing and then slightly sweet.

Indications 1. Menstrual disorders 2. Dizziness, headache, chest pain 3. Aversion to cold 4. Abdominal pain with mass formation, post traumatic swelling and pain 5. Rheumatic arthralgia

Chemical Composition Mainly contains alkaloids such as chuanxiongzine also contains essential oils.

Rhizoma Cibotii

Cibot Rhizome

Gouji

狗脊

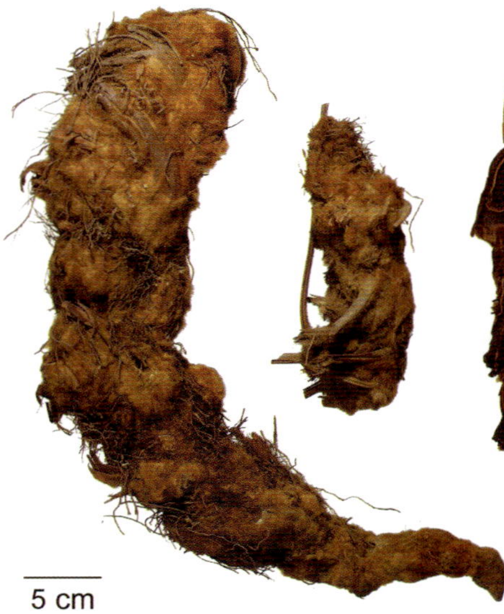

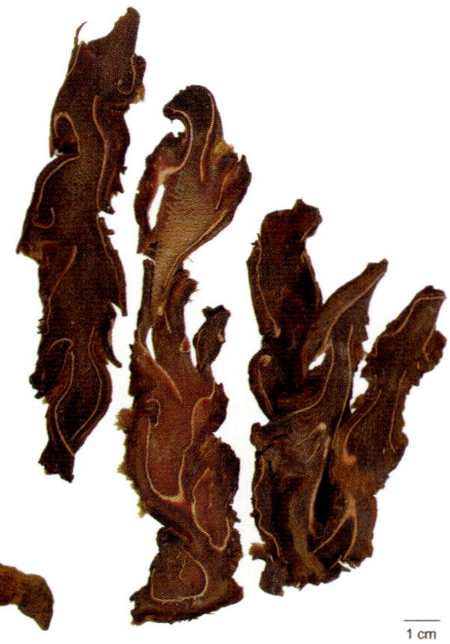

Crude drug　　　　Decoction Pieces

Source The rhizome of *Cibotium barometz* (L.) J. Sm. (Fam. *Dicksoniaceae*).

Distribution Mainly in Chinese provinces such as Fujian and Sichuan; also in Hong Kong.

Harvest & Processing Dig out rhizomes in autumn and winter; remove sand and soil; dry. Alternatively, shave off hard roots, petioles and golden-yellow pubescence, then slice into thick pieces and dry under the sun to produce '*Sheng Goujipian*' (Raw Cibot Rhizome Slice); or steam, dry under the sun until nearly dry, slice into thick pieces and then dry to produce '*Shu Goujipian*' (Steamed Cibot Rhizome Slice).

Description Irregular, long and rod-like; 10-60 cm long, 2-20 cm in diameter. Outer surface dark brown, covered with golden-yellow pubescence; upper part with several reddish-brown remnants of petiole base, lower part with black rootlets. Hard, difficult to break. Odourless; taste: mild and slightly astringent. When sliced, irregular in shape, long and strip-like; with uneven edges; occasionally with remaining golden-yellow pubescence. Outer surface dark brown; cut surface light brown, relatively smooth, with a protuberant brownish-yellow xylem annulation or stria. Hard and brittle, breaks easily; starchy.

Indications 1. Chronic rheumatism, backache, weakness and stiffness of lower limbs 2. Urinary frequency, enuresis, leukorrhagia.

Chemical Composition Mainly contains pterosin R, onitin and onitin-2'-0- β -D-glucoside.

Rhizoma Cimicifugae

Largetrifoliolious Bugbane Rhizome

Shengma

升麻

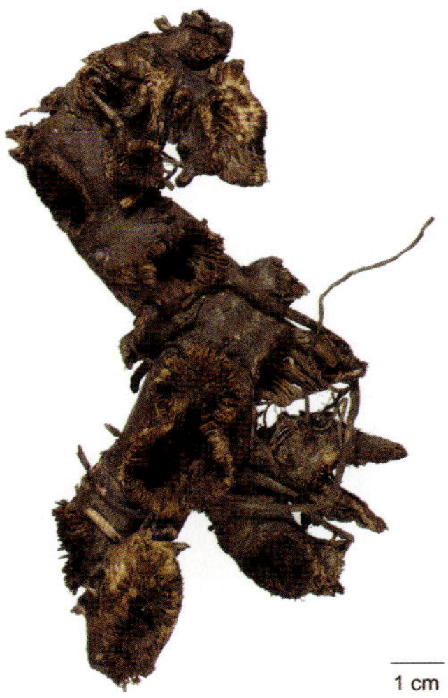

Crude drug

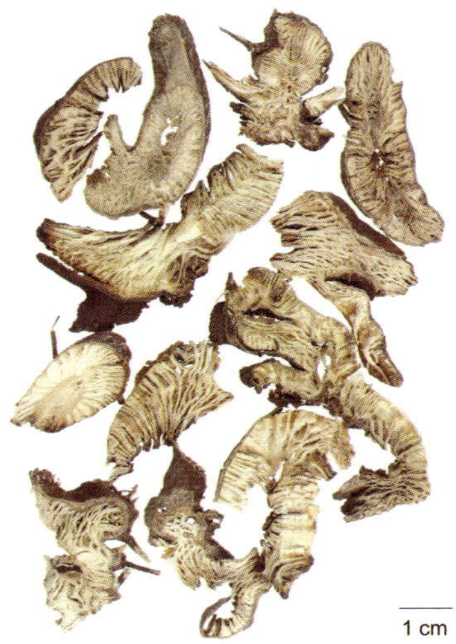

Decoction Pieces

Source The rhizome of *Cimicifuga heracleifolia* Kom. (Fam. Ranunculaceae).

Distribution Mainly in Chinese provinces such as Liaoning, Jilin, Heilongjiang, Hebei, Shanxi and Shaanxi.

Harvest & Processing Collect rhizomes in autumn; remove soil and sand; dry under the sun until rootlets are dry, then burn or remove rootlets; dry under the sun again.

Description Long and irregular pieces, nodular, with many rootlets ; 10-20 cm long, 2-4 cm in diameter. Outer surface dull blackish-brown or reddish-brown; rough and uneven; marked with hard remnants of fine rootlets. Upper part marked with several orbicular (round) hollow scars of caudex; inner surface of hollows marked with reticulate (netted) grooves. Lower part uneven, with scars of rootlets. Light in weight; hard, do not break easily. When broken, surface uneven, with clefts; fibrous; yellowish-green or pale yellowish-white. Odour: faint; taste: slightly bitter and astringent.

Indications

1. Toothache, headache, sore throat and aphthous ulcers
2. Chronic diarrhoea and rectal prolapse, uterine prolapse
3. Measles and eruptive exanthem

Chemical Composition Mainly contains triterpene saponins such as cimicifugoside.

Note According to *C.P.*, also used for medicinal purposes is the rhizome of *C. dahurica* (Turcz.) Maxim. and *C. foetida* L.

Rhizoma Coptidis

Golden Thread
Huanglian

黃連

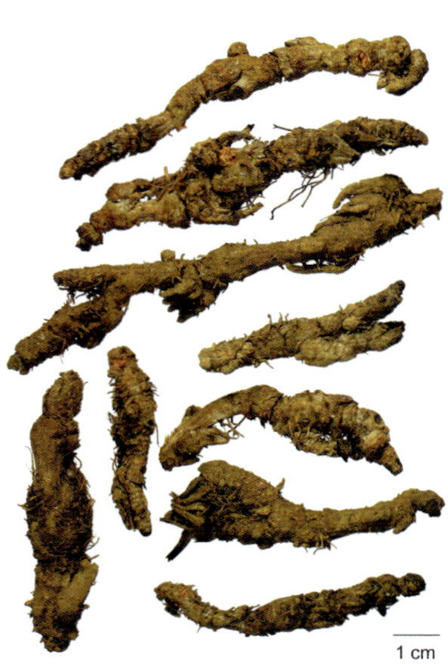

Crude drug

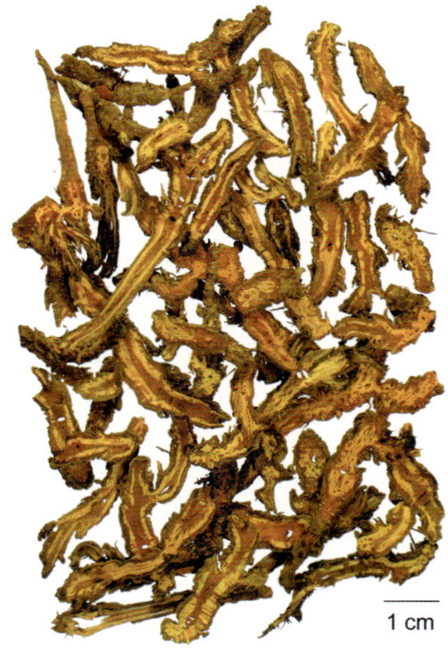

Decoction Pieces

Source The rhizome of *Coptis chinensis* Franch. (Fam. Ranunculaceae). Customarily called "*Weilian*"(Bitter Golden Thread).

Distribution Mainly in Sichuan province in China; also in provinces such as Hubei, Shaanxi and Gansu. Mostly cultivated.

Harvest & Processing Dig out rhizomes in autumn; remove rootlets and foreign matter; dry.

Description With many fine rootlets clustered into a bundle; often curved, resembling a chicken claw. Single rhizome 3-6 cm long, 3-8 mm in diameter. Outer surface greyish-yellow or dull yellowish-brown, rough, with irregular, nodular protuberances, rootlets and remnants of rootlet base; in some cases internode surface smooth like haulm. Upper part mostly with remnants of dull brown scale leaves; top end often with remnants of stems or petioles. Hard; when broken, surface uneven; cortex orange-red or dull brown; xylem bright yellow or orange-yellow, arranged in a radial form; pith sometimes hollow. Odour: faint; taste: extremely bitter.

Indications 1. Aphthous ulcer, bacillary dysentery, gastroenteritis 2. Fever and irritation, insomnia 3. Haemoptysis, epistaxis 4. Eczema, carbuncles and sores, 5. Conjunctivitis

Chemical Composition Mainly contains alkaloids such as berberine and coptisine.

Note According to *C.P.*, also used for medicinal purposes is the rhizome *of C. deltoidea* C. Y. Cheng et Hsiao and *C. teeta* Wall.

Rhizoma Corydalis

Yanhusuo Tuber

Yanhusuo

延胡索

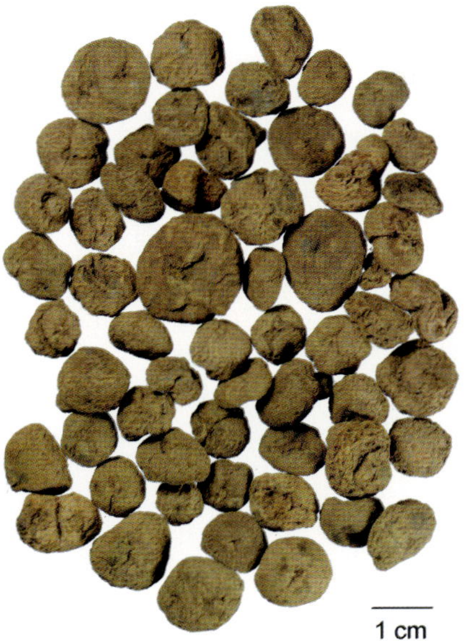

Crude drug

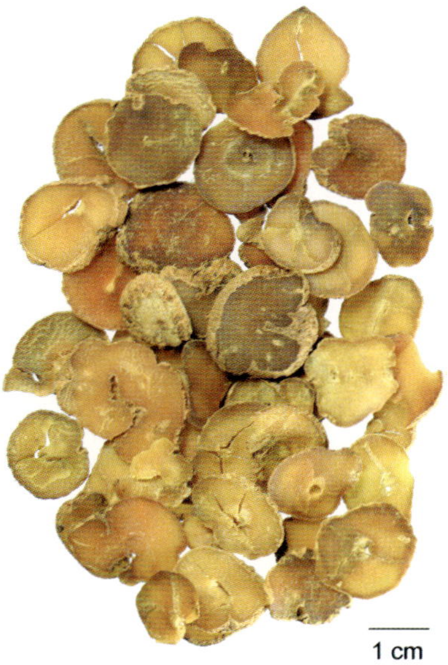

Decoction Pieces

Source The tuber of *Corydalis yanhusuo* W. T. Wang (Fam. Papaveraceae).

Distribution Mainly in Chinese provinces such as Zhejiang, Hubei, Hunan and Jiangsu.

Harvest & Processing Dig out tubers in early summer (May-July) when leaves wither; remove fine roots; wash clean; boil thoroughly; dry under the sun.

Description Somewhat flattened and spherical; 0.5-1.5 cm in diameter. Outer surface yellow or dull yellowish-brown, with irregular reticulate (netted) wrinkles. Top end with slightly dented stem scars; base often with verruciform (wart-shaped) protuberances, or a slight dent like a navel. Hard and brittle; broken surface yellow, cuticular, with waxy lustre. Odour: faint; taste: bitter.

Indications 1. Headache, abdominal pain 2. Dysmenorrhoea 3. Dysfunctional uterine bleeding

Chemical Composition Mainly contains alkaloids such as corydaline and tetrahydropalmatine.

Rhizoma Curculiginis

Common Curculigo Rhizome
Xianmao

仙茅

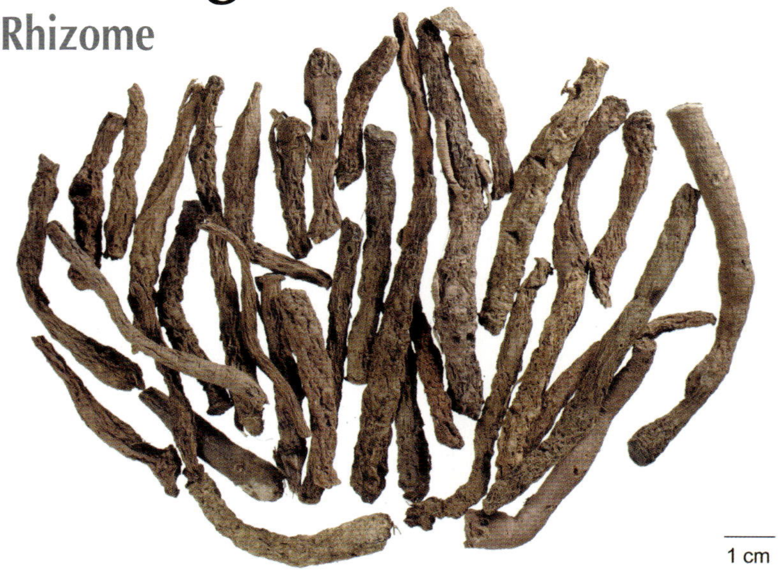

Crude drug

Source The rhizome of *Curculigo orchioides* Gaertn. (Fam. Amaryllidaceae).

Distribution Mainly in Chinese provinces such as Sichuan, Guangxi, Yunnan, Guizhou and Guangdong; also in Hong Kong.

Harvest & Processing Collect rhizomes after above-ground parts wilt in October and before buds burst in the following spring; shake off soil; remove leaf remnants and fibrous roots; dry rhizomes under the sun.

Description Cylindrical, slightly curved; 3-10 cm long, 4-8 mm in diameter. Outer surface dull blackish-brown or reddish-brown; rough; marked with longitudinal grooves, transverse wrinkles and fine poriform (pore-like) root scars. Hard and brittle, breaks easily. When broken, surface relatively smooth, slightly cuticular; dull pale brown or reddish-brown; colour darkens near the centre; centre marked with a dark-coloured ring. Odour: slightly fragrant; taste: slightly bitter, acrid.

Indications 1. Impotence, seminal emission, enuresis, urinary frequency 2. Pain and cold feeling of epigastrium, abdomen, loin and knee 3. Anorexia, diarrhoea 4. Arthralgia and muscular spasm.

Chemical Composition Mainly contains curculigoside A, B.

Rhizoma Curculiginis

Rhizoma Curcumae

Zedoary Rhizome

Ezhu

莪朮

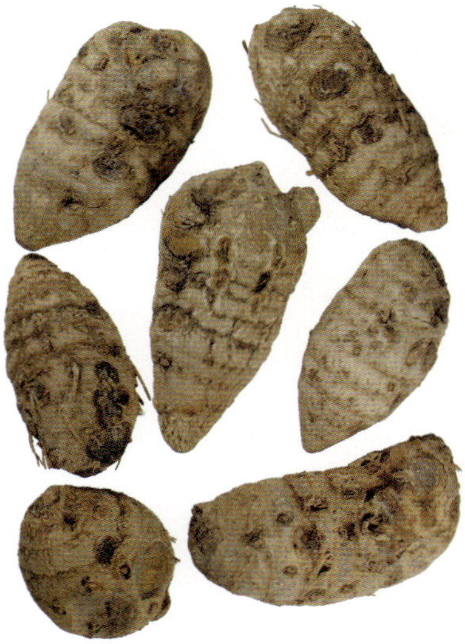

Crude drug

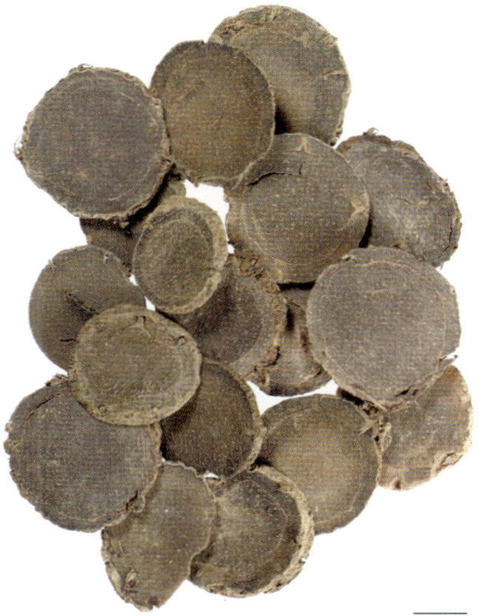

Decoction Pieces

Source The rhizome of *Curcuma aeruginosa* Roxb. (Fam. Zingiberaceae).

Distribution Mainly in Sichuan province in China; also cultivated in small amounts in Chinese provinces such as Guangdong, Guangxi, Yunnan, Zhejiang, Fujian and Hunan.

Harvest & Processing Dig out rhizomes in December when above-ground parts wither; remove soil; wash clean; boil or steam for about 15 minutes; dry under the sun or by heat; remove fibrous roots. Alternatively, soak rhizomes thoroughly in fresh water; scoop up; let drip until dry; cut into thin slices; dry under the sun or by heat.

Description Subspherical, ovoid (egg-shaped), or oblong and spherical, top end usually obtuse; 2-5 cm long, 1.5-2.5 cm in diameter. Outer surface earthy to greyish-yellow in colour; upper part with prominent annular (ring-like) nodes; 1 row of dented bud scars and suborbicular (almost round) scars of lateral rhizomes on either side. Heavy; hard and solid. When broken, surface dark greenish-yellow to brown, often with brownish-yellow powder; cortex and stele separate easily. Odour: slightly fragrant; taste: slightly bitter, acrid.

Indications 1. Amenorrhoea, dysmenorrhoea 2. Precordial pain, abdominal distension, pain and mass, trauma 3. Carcinoma of cervix, ovary, liver, lung and breast, lymphosarcoma, fibroid.

Chemical Composition Mainly contains essential oils with the curzerenone as the main component; also contains curcuminoid.

Note According to *C.P.*, also used for medicinal purposes is the rhizome of *C. kwangsiensis* S. G.. Lee et C. F. Liang and *C. wenyujin* Y. H. Chen et C. Ling.

Rhizoma Curcumae Longae

Turmeric
Jianghuang
薑黃

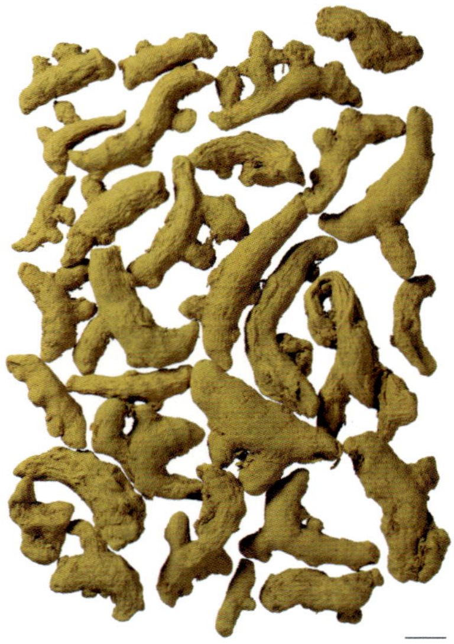

Crude drug

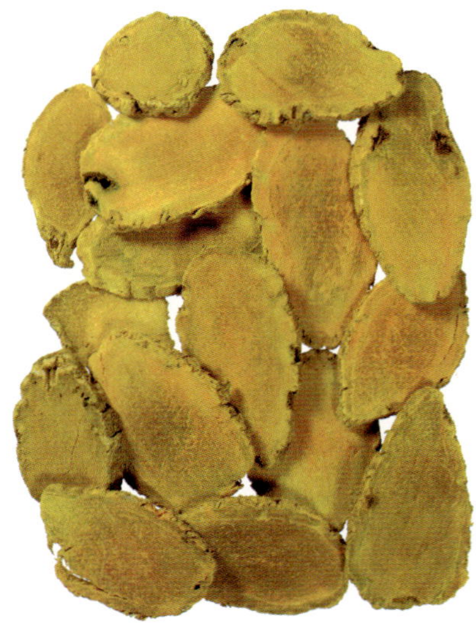

Decoction Pieces

Source The rhizome of *Curcuma longa* L. (Fam. Zingiberaceae).

Distribution Mainly in Chinese provinces such as Sichuan and Fujian; also in Hong Kong.

Harvest & Processing Dig out rhizomes in winter when leaves wilt; wash clean; boil or steam thoroughly; dry under the sun; remove fibrous roots.

Description Irregular and ovoid (egg-shaped), cylindrical or spindle-shaped, often curved, sometimes forked into short branches; 2-5 cm long, 1-3 cm in diameter. Outer surface dark yellow; rough; marked with wrinkles and prominent annular (ring-like) nodes, and with orbicular (round) scars of branches and fibrous roots. Hard and solid, does not break easily. When broken, surface brownish-yellow to golden-yellow, cuticular, with waxy lustre; endodermis ring conspicuous; broken surface scattered with punctiform (dot-like) vascular bundles. Odour: fragrant and distinctive; taste: bitter and acrid.

Indications 1. Chest and abdominal distension 2. Rheumatic arthralgia 3. Menstrual disorders, amenorrhoea 4. Trauma.

Chemical Composition Mainly contains diarylheptanoids such as curcumin.

Rhizoma Cynanchi Stauntonii

Willowleaf Swallowwort Rhizome

Baiqian

白前

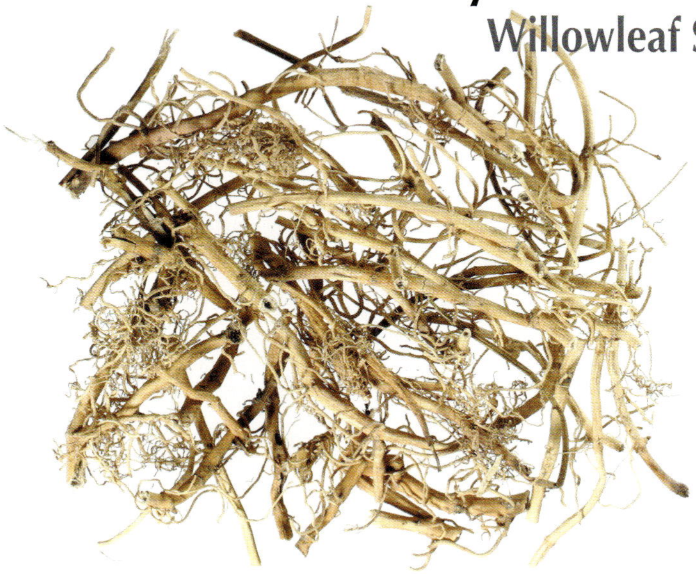

1 cm

Crude drug

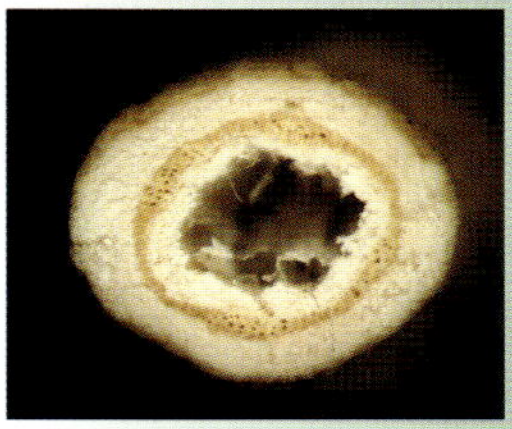

Willowleaf Swallowwort Rhizome Magnified

Source The root and rhizome of *Cynanchum stauntonii* (Decne.) Schltr. ex Lévl. (Fam. Asclepiadaceae).

Distribution Mainly in Chinese provinces such as Zhejiang, Jiangsu and Anhui.

Harvest & Processing Dig up roots and rhizomes in autumn; wash clean and dry under the sun.

Description Rhizome fine, long and cylindrical, rameous (branched), slightly curved; 4-15 cm long, 1.5-4 mm in diameter; outer surface yellowish-white or yellowish-brown; nodes prominent, internodes 1.5-4.5 cm long; top end marked with remnants of stems. Brittle. Transverse section hollow in the middle. Roots fine and curved; multi-branched, hairy and bearded, usually coiled into a mass. Odour: faint; taste: slightly sweet.

Indications Cough and cold, bronchitis, bronchial asthma characterized by copious expectoration.

Chemical Composition Mainly contains glaucoside A, B, C, D.

Note According to *C.P.*, also used for medicinal purposes is the rhizome and root of *C. glaucescens* (Decne.) Hand.-Mazz.

Rhizoma Cyperi

Nutgrass Galingale Rhizome
Xiangfu

香附

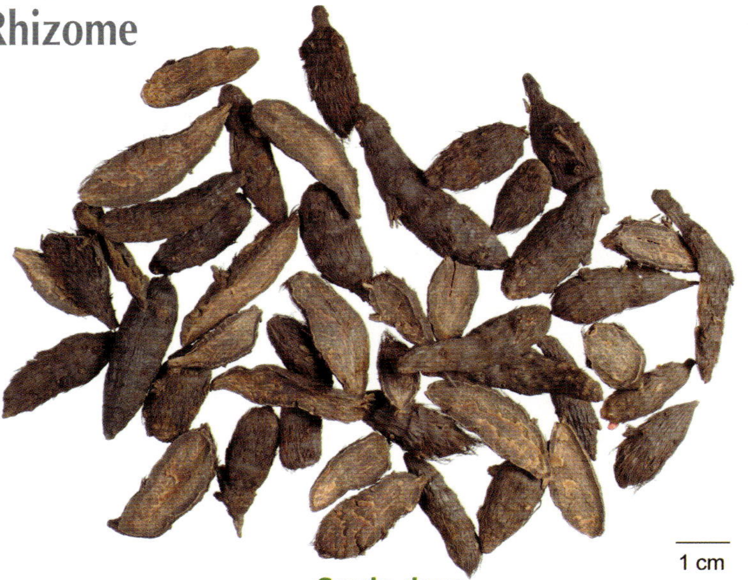

Crude drug

Source The rhizome of *Cyperus rotundus* L. (Fam. Cyperaceae).

Distribution Mainly in Chinese provinces such as Shandong, Zhejiang and Hunan; also in Hong Kong.

Harvest & Processing Dig out rhizomes in autumn; scorch away pubescence; blanch in boiling water or steam thoroughly; dry under the sun. Alternatively, dry under the sun straight after scorching.

Description Mostly spindle-shaped, or slightly curved; 2-3.5 cm long, 0.5-1 cm in diameter. Outer surface reddish-brown or dull blackish-brown; marked with longitudinal wrinkles and several slightly bulgy annular (ring-like) nodes. '*Mao Xiangfu*'(Hairy Nutgrass Galingale Rhizome) often with brown fibres and scars of fibrous root on nodes; '*Guang Xiangfu*'(Glabrous Nutgrass Galingale Rhizome) smoother, with indistinct annular (ring-like) nodes. Hard. For rhizomes boiled or steamed, broken surface yellowish-brown or reddish-brown, cuticular; for those dried under the sun directly after scorching, broken surface white and starchy, with a conspicuous endodermis ring, darker stele and scattered punctiform (dot-like) vascular bundles. Odour: aromatic; taste: slightly bitter.

Indications 1. Distension and pain of the hypochondria and breast, menstrual disorders 2. Headache, epigastric pain, vomiting and acid regurgitation 3. Morning sickness, threatened abortion.

Chemical Composition Mainly contains 0.65%-1.4% essential oils with β-pinene, and camphene as the main components; also contains flavonoid glycosides.

Rhizoma Dioscoreae

Common Yam Rhizome

Shanyao

山藥

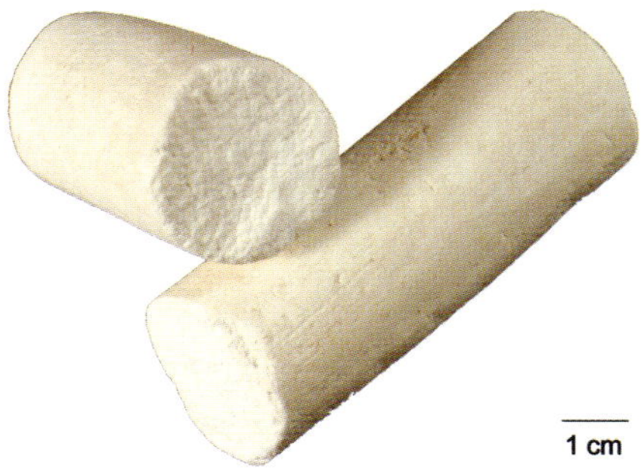

Crude drug

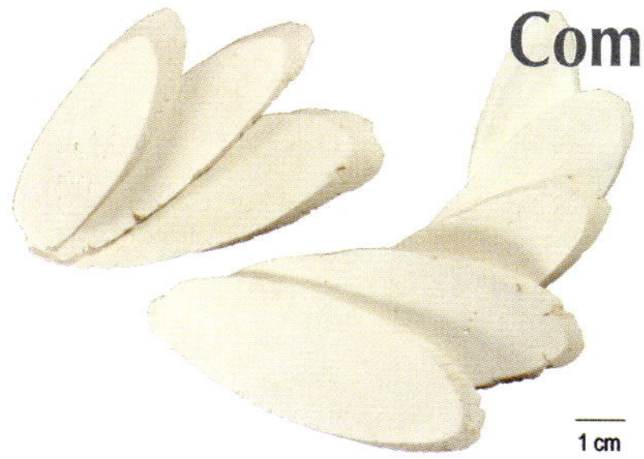

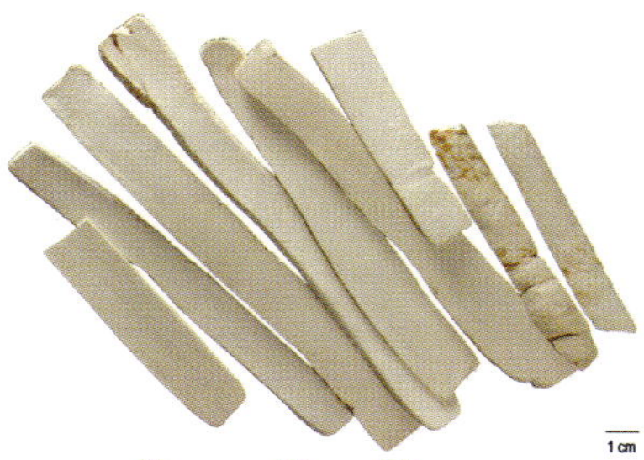

Decoction Pieces

Source The rhizome of *Dioscorea opposita* Thunb. (Fam. Dioscoreaceae).

Distribution Mainly in Chinese provinces such as Henan, Hebei, Shaanxi, Hunan and Jiangxi. Cultivated.

Harvest & Processing Dig out rhizomes in winter; cut off top part of roots; remove cork and fine roots; wash clean; dry under the sun to produce '*Mao shanyao*'(Hairy Common Yam Rhizome). Alternatively, choose the plump and uncurved *Mao shanyao* and put into fresh water; soak thoroughly; knead on wooden boards until cylindrical; cut both ends cleanly; dry under the sun and polish to produce '*Guang shanyao*'(Glabrous Common Yam Rhizome).

Description *Mao shanyao*: Slightly cylindrical, curved and slightly flattened; 15-30 cm long, 1.5-6 cm in diameter; outer surface yellowish-white or pale yellow, marked with longitudinal grooves, longitudinal wrinkles and scars of fine roots, and occasionally with remnants of light brown cork. Heavy; hard and solid, does not break easily; when broken, surface white and starchy. Taste: mild and slightly sour, sticky when chewed.
Guang shanyao: Cylindrical, both ends even; 9-18 cm long, 1.5-3 cm in diameter; outer surface smooth, white or yellowish-white. Commonly seen in the form of angled-cut and length-wise cut slices.

Indications 1. Protracted diarrhoea, chronic enteritis 2. Cough and dyspnoea. 3. Seminal emissions, leukorrhagia.

Chemical Composition Mainly contains dioscin, allantoin.

Rhizoma Dioscoreae Bulbiferae

Airpotato Yam Rhizome
Huangyaozi

黃藥子

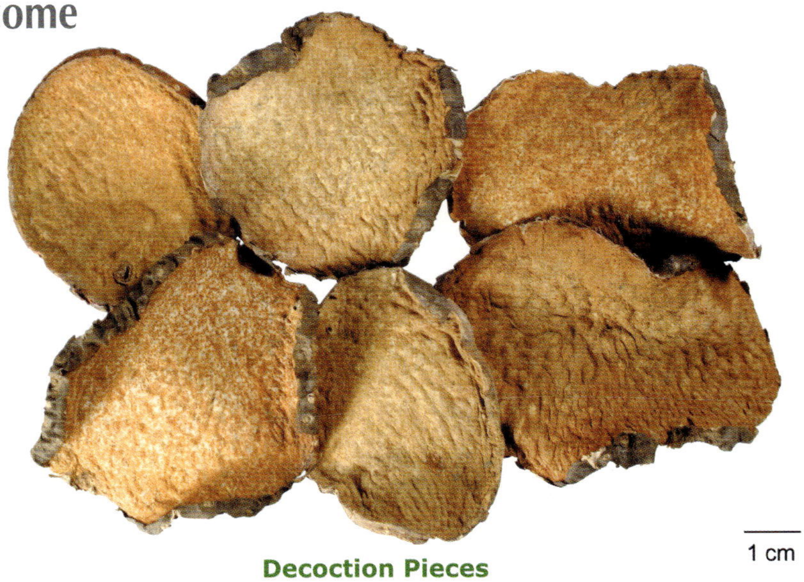

Decoction Pieces

Source The rhizome of *Dioscorea bulbifera* L. (Fam. Dioacoreaceae).

Distribution Mainly in Chinese provinces such as Hubei, Hunan and Jiangsu; also in provinces such as Henan, Shandong, Zhejiang, Anhui and Fujian, and also in Hong Kong.

Harvest & Processing Dig up rhizomes in winter, mostly after 2-3 years of cultivation; pick out those more than 30 cm in thickness, put the rest back into the soil for another year of planting. Wash away soil; clip off rootlets; cross-cut into slices about 1 cm thick; dry slices under the sun or by heat, or use while fresh.

Description Mostly cross-cut thick slices, orbicular (round) or suborbicular (almost round); 2.5-7 cm in diameter, 0.3-1 cm thick. Outer surface brownish-black, shrivelled, marked with numerous punctiform (dot-like) white protuberant scars of fibrous roots, or with curved rootlet remnants; cork easily peels off. Cut surface yellowish-white to yellowish-brown, smooth or uneven. Hard and brittle, breaks easily; when broken, surface granular and scattered with orange-yellow dots. Odour: faint; taste: bitter.

Indications 1. Haemoptysis, epistaxis 2. Pharyngitis 3. Goitre 4. Pyogenic skin infections, scrofula, trauma 5. Orchitis

Chemical Composition Mainly contains diosbulbins A-H.

Rhizoma Dioscoreae Septemlobae

Sevenlobed Yam Rhizome

Mianbixie

綿萆薢

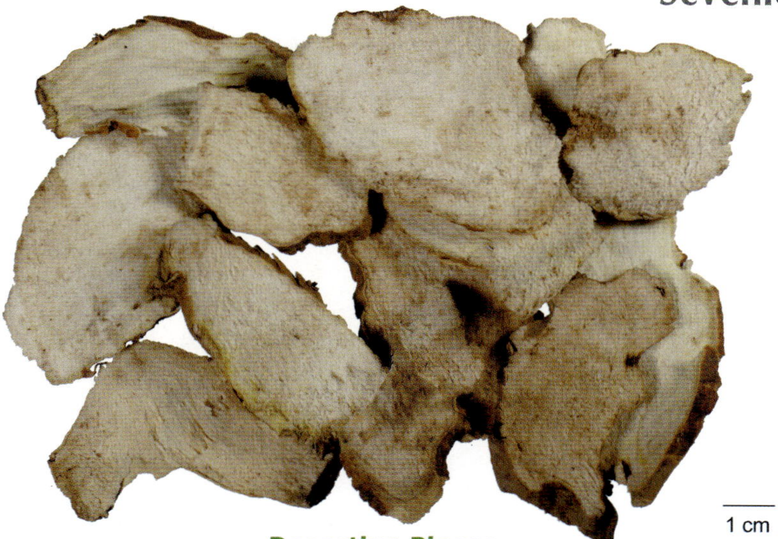

Decoction Pieces

Source The rhizome of *Dioscorea septemloba* Thunb. (Fam. Dioscoreaceae).

Distribution Mainly in Chinese provinces such as Zhejiang, Jiangxi and Fujian.

Harvest & Processing Harvest rhizomes in autumn and winter; remove rootlets; wash rhizomes clean; cut into slices; dry under the sun.

Description Mostly angled-cut or cross-cut orbicular (round) slices, with irregular margin; varying in size, 2-5 mm thick. Bark yellowish-brown or dull yellowish-brown; relatively thick; margin often curled. Cut surface pale yellowish-white, rough, scattered with punctiform (dot-like) yellowish-brown vascular bundles. Texture loose, slightly spongilliform (spongy). Odour: faint; taste: slightly bitter-acrid.

Indications 1. Stranguria complicated by chyluria, turbid urine, leukorrhagia 2. Eczema 3. Rheumatism with swelling and stiffness of joints and numbness of the extremities.

Chemical Composition Contains steroidal spaonins.

Note According to *C.P.*, also used for medicinal purposes is the rhizome of *D. futschauensis* Uline ex R. Kunth.

Rhizoma Drynariae

Fortune's Drynaria Rhizome

Gusuibu

骨碎補

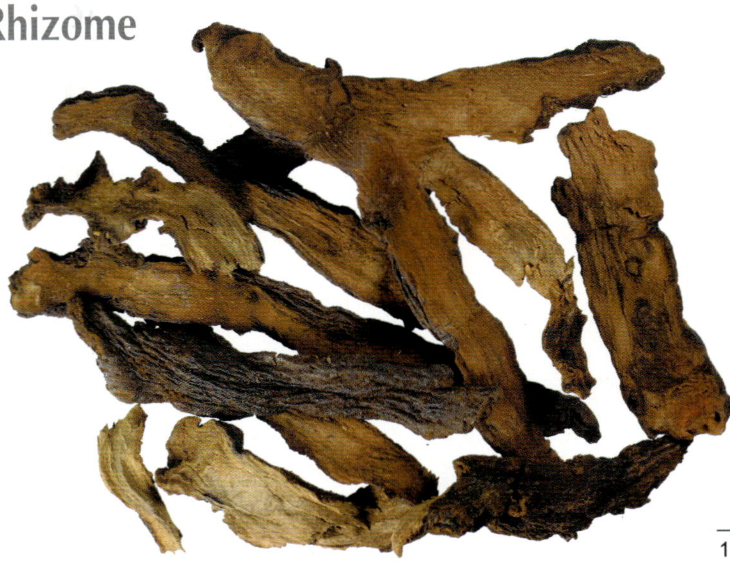

1 cm

Decoction Pieces

Source The rhizome of *Drynaria fortunei* (Kunze) J. Sm. (Fam. Polypodiaceae).

Distribution Mainly in Chinese provinces such as Hubei and Zhejiang, and southwestern China.

Harvest & Processing Dig up rhizomes anytime during the year; remove sand and soil; dry and use, or scorch away pubescence after drying.

Description Flattened, long and thin, mostly curved, rameous (branched); 5-15 cm long, 1-1.5 cm wide, 2-5 mm thick; outer surface densely covered with ramenta dark brown to dull brown and soft as fur. Scorched rhizome reddish-brown or dull brown; upper surface and both sides marked with protuberant or dented orbicular (round) leaf scars, occasionally with remnants of petiole base and of fibrous roots. Light in weight; brittle, breaks easily; broken surface reddish-brown, marked with a ring of punctiform (dot-like) yellow vascular bundles. Odourless; taste: mild, slightly astringent. Commonly used in Hong Kong in the form of lengthwise cut slices.

Indications 1. Rheumatism, weakness of the back and the knee 2. Toothache 3. Dizziness, tinnitus 4. Chronic diarrhoea 5. Tinea (used freshly), baldness (wine preparation)

Chemical Composition Mainly contains naringin, fern-7-ene and filic-3-ene.

Rhizoma Dryopteris Crassirhizomatis

Male Fern Rhizome
Mianmaguanzhong

綿馬貫眾

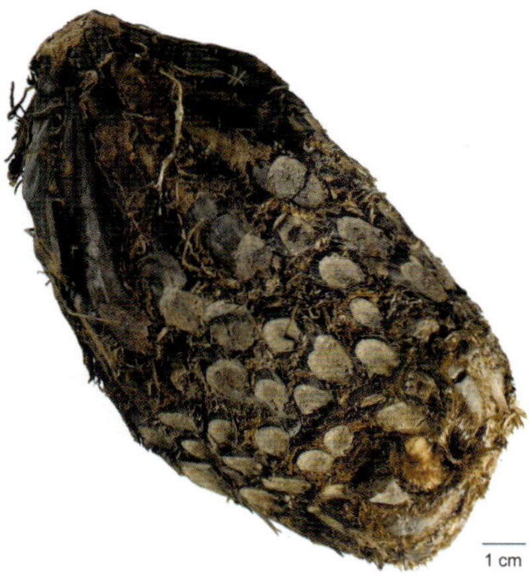

Crude drug (Dryopteris crassirhizoma)

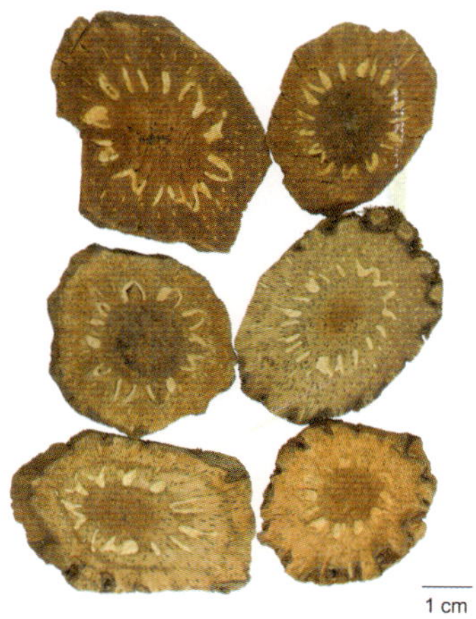

Decoction Pieces (Brainea insignis)

Source The rhizome of *Dryopteris crassirhizoma* Nakai (Fam. Dryopteridaceae).

Distribution Mainly in Chinese provinces such as Inner Mongolia, Hebei and Gansu, and in northeastern China.

Harvest & Processing Harvest whole plants in autumn; remove above-ground parts and fibrous roots; clear away soil and sand; dry rhizomes under the sun.

Description Slightly conical; upper end obtuse, lower end more pointed. Outer surface marked densely with regularly arranged remnants of petiole base, yellowish-brown membranous scales, and curved antrorse (directed forwards or upwards) roots. Petiole base flattened and cylindrical, slightly curved; hard; broken surface brown, with a ring of 5-10 (-13) small meristeles near the margin. Rhizome exposed when base remnants of petiole removed; hard; when broken transversely, surface reveals a ring of 5-13 yellowish-white meristeles. Odour: distinctive; taste: slightly astringent, bitter.

Indications 1. Pestilence and seasonal febrile diseases with eruption such as influenza, epidemic meningitis, mumps, measles, viral pneumonia 2. Bleeding 4. Intestinal parasitosis 5. Sores.

Chemical Composition Mainly contains filixic acid BBB, PBB; also contains diploptene and filicene.

Note In Hong Kong, commonly used for medicinal purposes is the rhizome of *Brainea insignis* (Hook.) J. Smith (Fam. Blechnaceae).

Rhizoma et Radix Baphicacanthis Cusiae

Baphicacanthus Root
Nanbanlangen

南板藍根

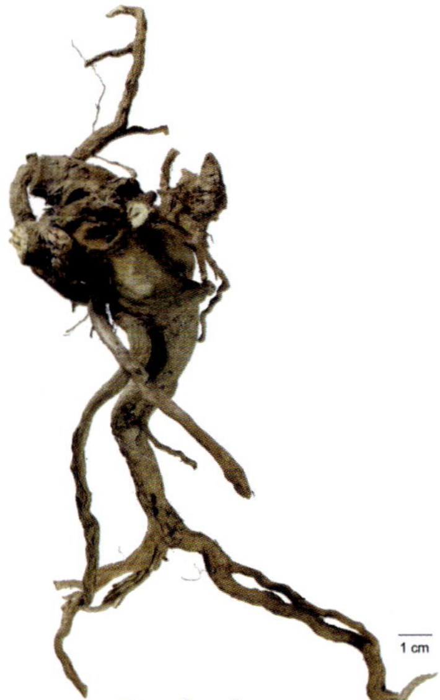

Crude drug

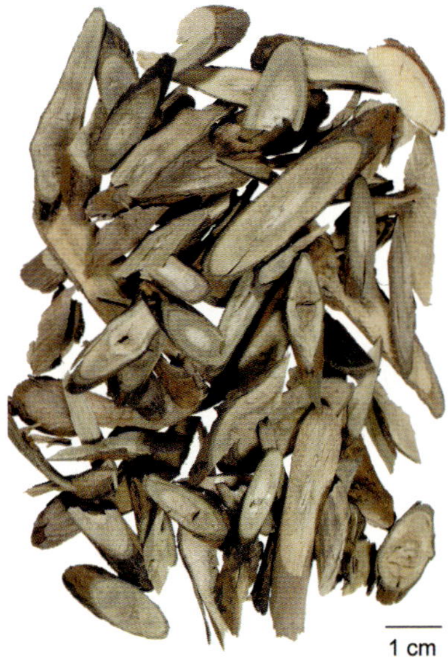

Decoction Pieces

Source The root and rhizome of *Baphicacanthus cusia* (Nees.) Bremek. (Fam. Acanthaceae).

Distribution Mainly in Chinese provinces such as Fujian, Sichuan, Zhejiang, Hunan, Guangdong, Guangxi, Guizhou and Yunnan.

Harvest & Processing Dig up roots and rhizomes in spring and autumn; remove above-ground parts, soil and sand; dry under the sun.

Description Cylindrical, mostly curved, occasionally rameous (branched); 5-10 cm long, 1-5 mm in diameter. Outer surface greyish-brown, with slender, slightly curved roots on bulgy nodes; short stem remnants, with opposite (borne in pairs) branches at the upper part of nodes. Hard and brittle, breaks easily; when broken, surface uneven, with pith at the centre. Rootlets fairly pliable. Odour: faint; taste: mild.

Indications 1. Epidemic eruptive exanthem 2. Erysipelas 3. Influenza 4. Epidemic meningitis.

Chemical Composition Mainly contains indigo and indirubin.

Note Also sold are the above-ground stem of *Baphicacanthus cusia (Nees)* Bremek.

Rhizoma et Radix Notopterygii

Incised Notopterygium Rhizome and Root

Qianghuo

羌活

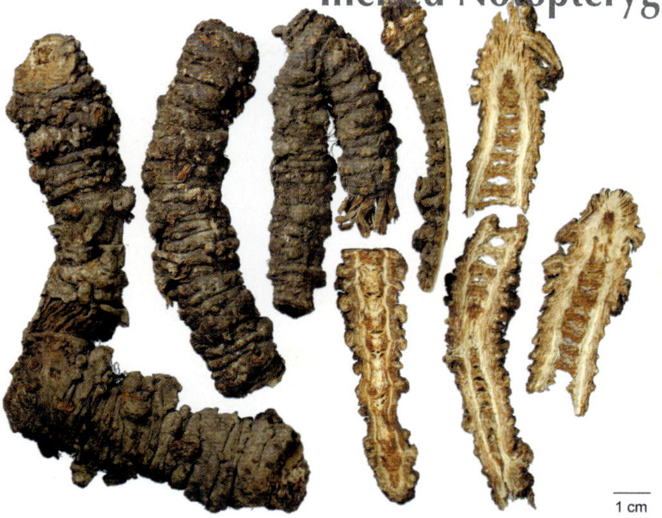

Crude drug　　Decoction Pieces

Source The rhizome and root of *Notopterygium incisum* Ting ex H. T. Chang (Fam. Umbelliferae).

Distribution Mainly in Chinese provinces such as Sichuan, Yunnan, Qinghai and Gansu.

Harvest & Processing Dig out rhizomes and roots in spring and autumn; remove leaves, fibrous roots and soil; dry under the sun. Commonly used in Hong Kong in the form of length-wise cut slices.

Description Rhizome slightly curved, with dense annular (ring-like) nodes resembling those of silkworms, commonly known as "*Canqiang*" (Silkworm Incised Notoptergium); 4-13 cm long, 0.6-2.5 cm in diameter. Outer surface reddish-brown to brownish-black, marked with punctiform (dot-like) root scars and brown broken scales; brownish-yellow where cork has fallen off. Light in weight, brittle, breaks easily. Broken surface uneven, with radial clefts; cortex brownish-yellow, with yellow secretory cavities; xylem yellowish-white; pith yellow to yellowish-brown. Odour: fragrant; taste: slightly bitter, acrid. Rhizome with sparse annular nodes like those of a bamboo is commonly known as "*Zhujie qiang*" (Bamboo Nodes Incised Notoptergium).

Indications 1. Common cold, headache, generalized pain 2. Rheumatism

Chemical Composition Mainly contains coumarins and essential oils.

Note According to *C.P.*, also used for medicinal purposes is the rhizome and root of *N. forbesii* Boiss.

Rhizoma et Radix Notopterygii

Rhizoma Gastrodiae

Tall Gastrodia Tuber
Tianma

天麻

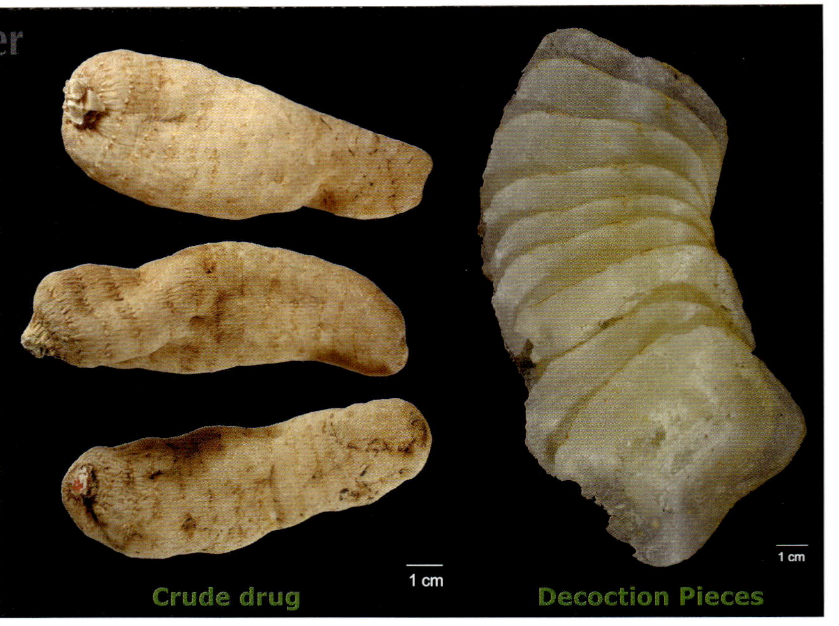

Rhizoma Gastrodiae

Source The tuber of *Gastrodia elata* Bl. (Fam. Orchidaceae).

Distribution Mainly in Chinese provinces such as Sichuan, Yunnan and Guizhou. Cultivated now in many places in China.

Harvest & Processing Dig up root tubers from early November to early April; wash clean immediately; remove cork; steam root tubers thoroughly; dry below 60℃. Commonly used in Hong Kong in the form of length-wise cut slices.

Description Ellipsoid (elliptical in long-section and circular in cross-section), or long and suborbicular (almost round), flattened and shrunken, slightly curved. Top end often with withered reddish-brown to dark brown gemmae or with remnants of caudex; the other end marked with orbicular (round) and umbilicate (with a depression in the middle, like a navel) scars formed after detachment from main tuber. Cork fallen off or partially attached. Outer surface yellowish-white to pale yellowish-brown, with punctiform (dot-like) protuberances forming numerous rings of transverse striae and longitudinal wrinkles; sometimes with reddish-brown mycorrhiza. Hard, does not break easily. When broken, surface relatively smooth; yellowish-white to pale brown. When sliced, surface translucent and cuticular. Odour: faint; taste: sweet.

Indications 1. Vertigo, dizziness, headache 2. Hypertension 3. Facial palpsy, hemiplegia, cerebral vascular accident, numbness of extremities 4. Infantile convulsions, epilepsy.

Chemical Composition Mainly contains gastrodin and gastrodioside.

Rhizoma Homalomenae

Obscured Homalomena Rhizome

Qiannianjian

千年健

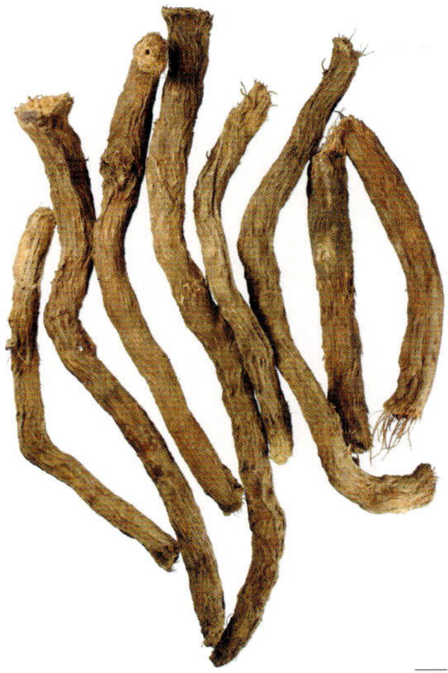

Crude drug

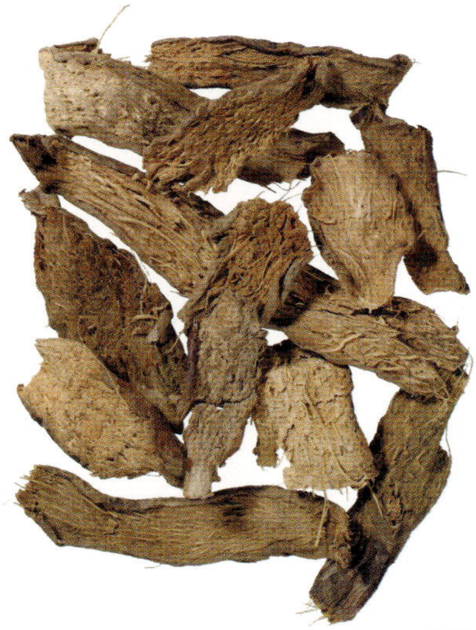

Decoction Pieces

Source — The rhizome of *Homalomena occulta* (Lour.) Schott (Fam. Araceae).

Distribution — Mainly in Chinese provinces such as Guangxi and Yunnan.

Harvest & Processing — Harvest plants in autumn and winter; cut off rhizomes; remove stem tips and fibrous roots; wash away soil; dry rhizomes under the sun.

Description — Cylindrical, or slightly flattened and a little curved; 15-40 cm long, 0.8-1.5 cm in diameter. Outer surface reddish-brown or yellowish-brown, rough, marked with numerous twisted longitudinal grooves and yellowish-white fibre bundles. Brittle, breaks easily; when broken, surface reddish-brown and resinoid (resin-like), with many protruding fibre bundles and lustrous orbicular (round) oil dots. Odour: aromatic; taste: acrid and slightly bitter. Customarily used in Hong Kong in the form of slant-cut slices.

Indications — 1. Rheumatoid arthritis 2. Pain and cold sensation in the loins and knees 3. Muscular contracture and numbness of the lower extremities

Chemical Composition — Mainly contains aromatic compounds such as α - and β -pinene, linalool and limonene.

Rhizoma Imperatae

Lalang Grass Rhizome
Baimaogen

白茅根

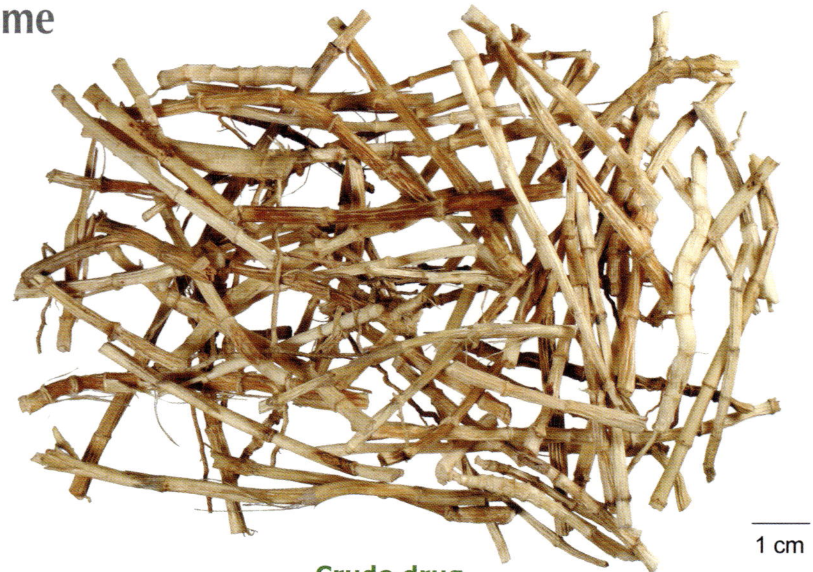

Crude drug

Source The rhizome of *Imperata cylindrical* Beauv. *var. major* (Nees) C. E. Hubb. (Fam. Gramineae).

Distribution In most regions in China, including Hong Kong.

Harvest & Processing Dig out rhizomes in spring and autumn; wash clean; dry under the sun; remove fibrous roots and membranous leaf sheaths.

Description Long and cylindrical; 30-60 cm long, 2-6 mm in diameter. Outer surface yellowish-white or pale yellow, slightly lustrous, marked with longitudinal wrinkles; nodes conspicuous and slightly protuberant; internodes vary in length, usually 1.5-3 cm long. Light in weight; slightly brittle; when broken, cortex white, mostly with cracks arranged in a radial pattern; stele pale yellow, detaches from cortex easily. Odourless; taste: slightly sweet.

Indications 1. Bleeding such as haematuria, haemoptysis, haematemesis, and epistaxis 2. Oedema, dysuria 3. Diabetes, febrile diseases with polydipsia 4. Vomiting, jaundice 5. Cough

Chemical Composition Mainly contains arundoin, cylindrin, fernenol, simiarenol, isoarborinol and anemonin.

Rhizoma Ligustici

Chinese Lovage

Gaoben

藁本

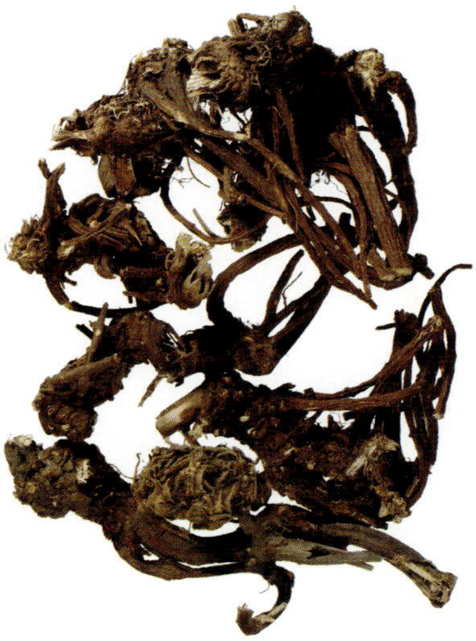

Crude drug 1 cm

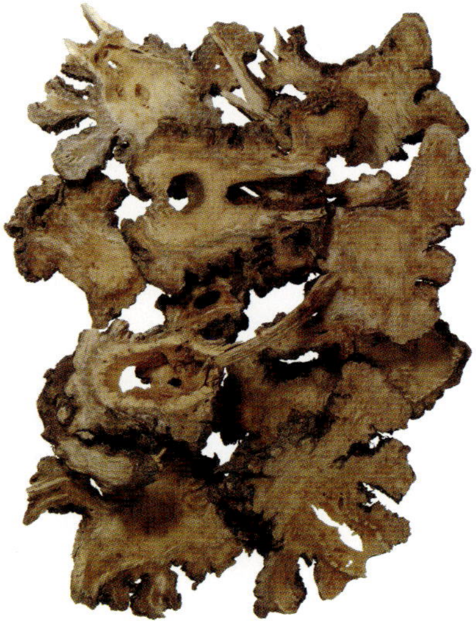

Decoction Pieces 1 cm

Source The rhizome and root of *Ligusticum sinense* Oliv. (Fam. Umbelliferae).

Distribution Mainly in Chinese provinces such as Shaanxi, Gansu, Henan and Sichuan.

Harvest & Processing Dig out rhizomes and roots in autumn when leaves wither, or in the following spring when plants put forth shoots; remove soil and sand; dry under the sun or by heat.

Description Rhizome somewhat nodular and cylindrical, slightly twisted, rameous (branched); 3-10 cm long, 1-2 cm in diameter. Outer surface reddish-brown or dull brown, rough, marked with longitudinal wrinkles; upper surface with several dented, orbicular (round) caudexes; underside with numerous protuberant, punctiform (dot-like) root scars and root remnants. Light in weight; relatively hard, breaks easily; broken surface yellow or yellowish-white, fibrous. Odour: heavily aromatic; taste: acrid, bitter and slightly numbing.

Indications 1. Common cold 2. Headache, especially parietal and occipital headache 3. Toothache 4. Arthralgia.

Chemical Composition Mainly contains essential oils with neocnidilide as the main component.

Note According to *C.P.*, also used for medicinal purposes is the rhizome and root of *L. jeholense* Nakai et Kitag.

Rhizoma Menispermi

Asiatic Moonseed Rhizome

Beidougen

北豆根

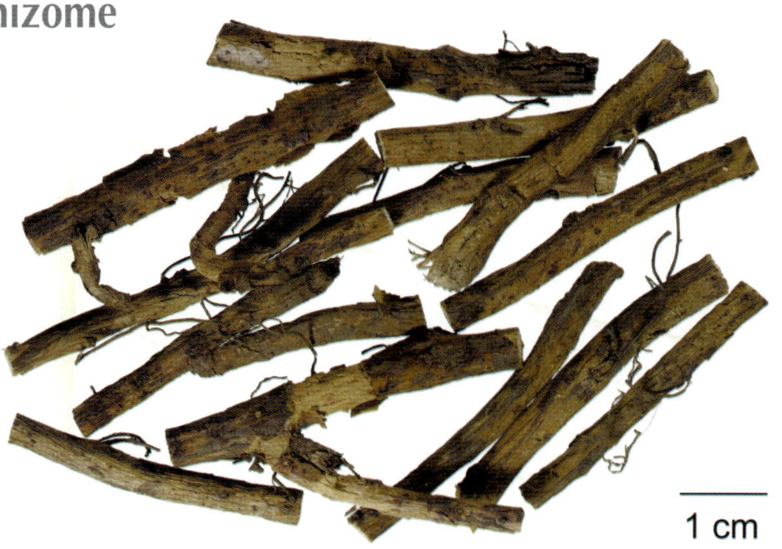

Crude drug

Source The rhizome of *Menispermum dauricum* DC. (Fam. Menispermaceae).

Distribution Mainly in Chinese provinces such as Hebei, Shandong and Shanxi, and in northeastern China.

Harvest & Processing Collect rhizomes in spring and autumn; remove rootlets, soil and sand; dry rhizomes.

Description Slender and cylindrical, curved, rameous (branched); up to 50 cm long; 3-8 mm in diameter. Outer surface yellowish-brown to dark brown; mostly with curved rootlets; surface marked with protuberant root scars and longitudinal wrinkles; bark falls off easily. Pliable; does not break easily. Transverse section uneven and fibrous; xylem pale yellow, arranged in a radial pattern; with pith in the centre. Odour: faint; taste: bitter.

Indications 1.Sore throat 2. Colitis, dysentery 3. Rheumatic arthralgia

Chemical Composition Mainly contains alkaloids such as dauricine and daurinoline.

Note Listed as slightly toxic in *C.P.*

Rhizoma Panacis Japonici

Japanese Ginseng
Zhujieshen

竹節參

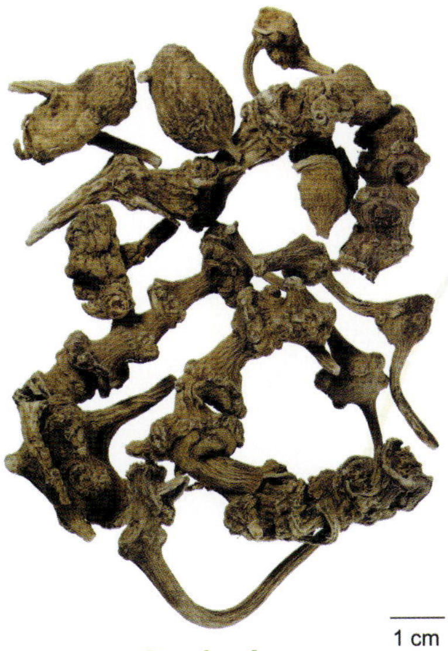

Crude drug

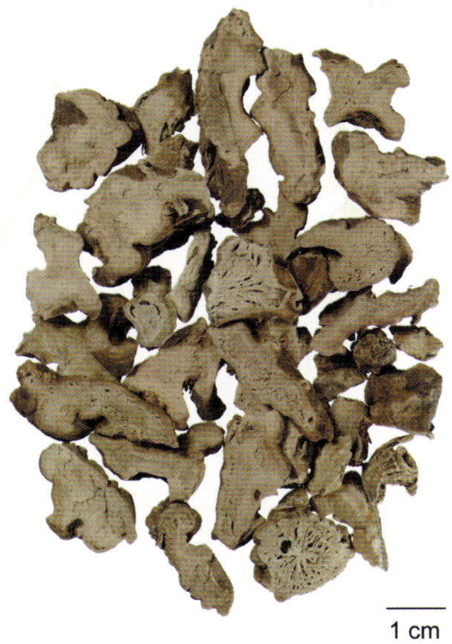

Decoction Pieces

Source The rhizome of *Panax japonicus* C. A. Mey. (Fam. Araliaceae).

Distribution Mainly in Chinese provinces such as Yunnan, Sichuan, Guizhou, Shaanxi and Guangxi.

Harvest & Processing Dig up rhizomes in September and October; remove rootlets; wash away soil; dry rhizomes under the sun or by heat.

Description Shaped like the subterranean stem of bamboo, flattened and cylindrical, slightly curved; 5-22 cm long, 0.8-2.5 cm in diameter. Nodes dense, internodes 0.8-2 cm long, with an orbicular (round) dented stem scar above each node. Outer surface greyish-brown or dull yellowish-brown; rough; marked with dense longitudinal wrinkles and root scars. Hard and brittle, breaks easily. When broken, surface relatively even; yellowish-white to pale yellow; with a ring of numerous punctiform (dot-like) pale yellow scars of vascular bundles. Odour: slightly fragrant; taste: bitter and slightly sweet.

Indications 1. Debility after an attack of disease 2. Cough with copious expectoration, haemoptysis in pulmonary tuberculosis 3. Trauma.

Chemical Composition Mainly contains triterpene saponins such as chikusetsusaponins I, Ia, Ib, III, IV.

Rhizoma Panacis Majoris

Japanese Ginseng Majoris
Zhuzishen

珠子參

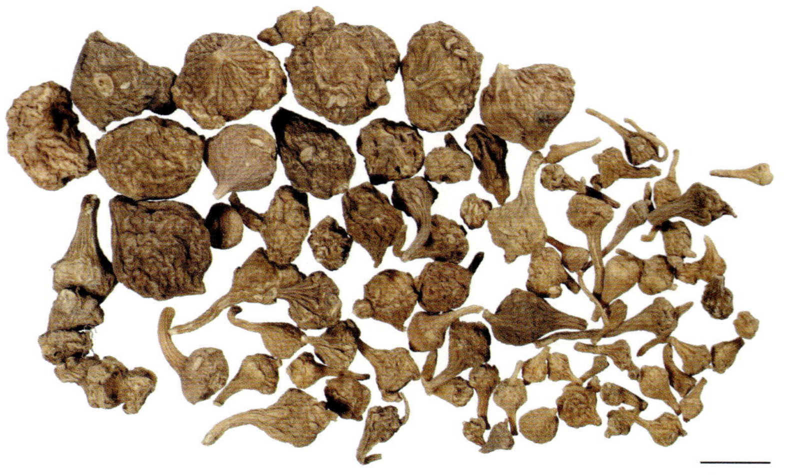

Crude drug

Source The rhizome of *Panax japonicus* C. A. Mey. *var.* major (Burk.) C. Y. Wu et K. M. Feng (Fam. Araliaceae).

Distribution Mainly in Yunnan province in China.

Harvest & Processing Dig up rhizomes in autumn; remove bark and rootlets; dry, or steam thoroughly and then dry under the sun.

Description Flattened and spherical, or conical, or irregular and rhomboid, occasionally torose (cylindrical with alternate swellings and constrictions); 0.5-2.8 cm in diameter. Outer surface brownish-yellow or dull yellowish-brown; marked with conspicuous verruciform (wart-shaped) protuberances and wrinkles, occasionally with orbicular (round) dented stem scars; in some cases surface marked with remnants of fine internodes at one or both lateral sides. Hard; broken surface uneven, pale yellowish-white, starchy. Odour: faint; taste: bitter, slightly sweet, throat-irritating when chewed. Steamed (or boiled) ones with slightly cuticular, yellowish-white or yellowish-brown broken surface; taste: slightly bitter, slightly sweet, not throat-irritating when chewed.

Indications 1. Fever, thirst and cough in wasting diseases 2. Trauma, arthralgia 3. Bleeding such as haemoptysis, haematemesis, traumatic bleeding.

Chemical Composition Mainly contains triterpene saponins such as chikusetsu saponins IVa, V, and ginsenosides Rd, Re, and majonosides R1, R2.

Note According to *C.P.*, also used for medicinal purposes is the rhizome of *P. japonicus* C. A. Mey. *var.* bipinnatifidus (Seem.) C. Y. Wu et K. M. Feng.

Rhizoma Paridis

Paris Rhizome
Chonglou
重樓

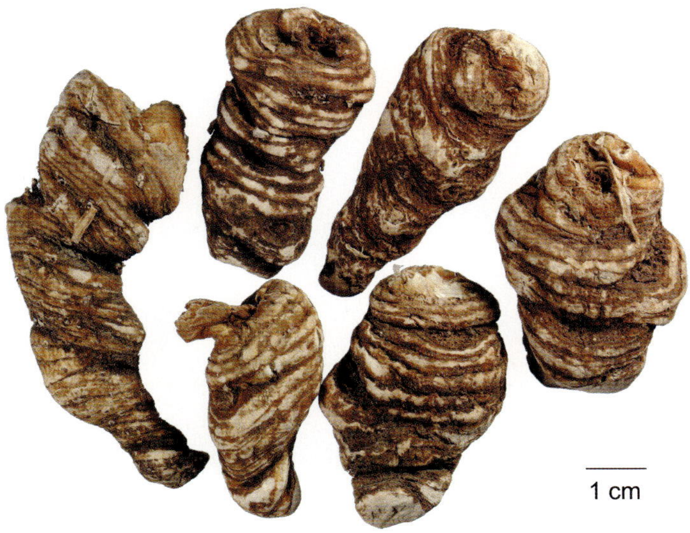

Crude drug

Source
The rhizome of *Paris polyphylla* Smith var. *chinensis* (Franch.) Hara (Fam. Liliaceae).

Distribution
Mainly in Chinese provinces such as Yunnan, Sichuan, Guangxi and Shaanxi.

Harvest & Processing
Dig up rhizomes in autumn; remove fibrous roots; wash clean; dry under the sun.

Description
Nodular, flattened and cylindrical, slightly curved; 5-12 cm long, 1-4.5 cm in diameter. Outer surface yellowish-brown or greyish-brown, white where bark has fallen off; surface densely covered with laminiform (consisting of layers), wide and protuberant annulations; one side of annulations with prominent nodes and elliptical, dented stem scars, the other side with sparsely grown fibrous roots or verruciform (wart-shaped) scars of fibrous roots; apex with scale leaves and caudex remnants. Hard and solid; broken surface smooth, white to light brown, starchy or gummy. Odour: faint; taste: slightly bitter-numbing.

Indications
1. Sore throat, skin infection, snakebite 2. Febrile diseases 3. Convulsion due to high fever, especially infantile convulsion 4. Cough and dyspnoea 5. Ecchymosis and traumatic bleeding.

Chemical Composition
Mainly contains a variety of steroidal saponins.

Note
According to *C.P.*, also used for medicinal purposes is the rhizome of P. polyphylla Smith var. yunnanensis (Franch) Hand.-Mazz.

Rhizoma Phragmitis

Reed Rhizome
Lugen
蘆根

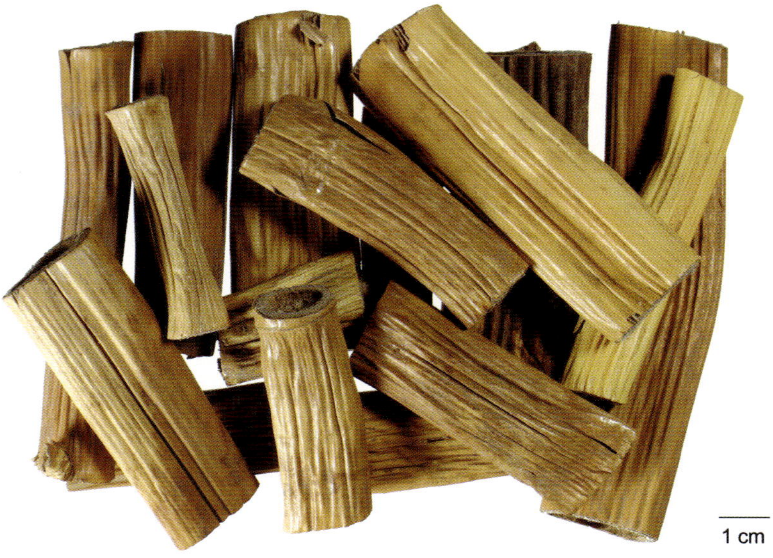

Crude drug

Source The rhizome of *Phragmites communis* Trin. (Fam. Gramineae).

Distribution Mainly in Chinese provinces such as Anhui, Jiangsu, Zhejiang and Hubei.

Harvest & Processing Dig out rhizomes anytime during the year; remove soil; cut away fibrous roots; cut rhizomes into sections; dry under the sun or use while fresh.

Description Fresh rhizome: Long and cylindrical, sometimes slightly flattened; varying in length, 1-2 cm in diameter. Outer surface yellowish-white, lustrous; bark loose, can fall off. Nodes annular (ring-like), marked with root remnants and bud scars. Light in weight; pliable, does not break easily. Broken surface yellowish-white, hollow; wall 1-2 mm thick, with small pores arranged in a ring. Odourless; taste: sweet.
Dried rhizome: Flattened, long and cylindrical. Outer surface lustrous, yellowish-white; nodes relatively hard, reddish-yellow; internodes marked with longitudinal wrinkles. Light in weight; soft and pliable. Odourless; taste: slightly sweet.

Indications 1. Polydipsia 2. Vomiting 3. Fever due to measles.

Chemical Composition Mainly contains p-hydroxybenzaldehyde, ferulic acid and tricin.

Rhizoma Picrorhizae

Figwortflower Picrorhiza Rhizome
Huhuanglian
胡黃連

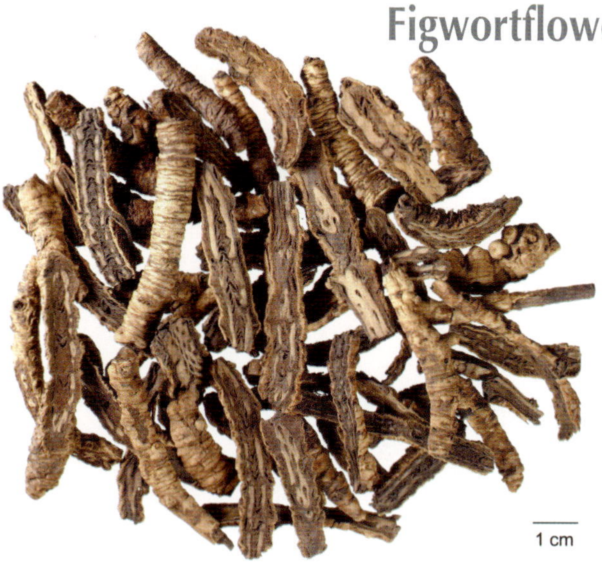

Decoction Pieces

Source The rhizome of *Picrorhiza scrophulariiflora* Pennell (Fam. Scrophulariaceae).

Distribution Mainly in regions such as southern Tibet, northwestern Yunnan provice and western Sichuan provice in China.

Harvest & Processing Dig up rhizomes when above-ground parts wither; remove above-ground parts and soil; wash rhizomes clean; dry under the sun. Commonly used in Hong Kong in the form of length-wise cut slices.

Description Cylindrical and slightly curved, occasionally rameous (branched); 3-12 cm long, 0.3-1.4 cm in diameter. Outer surface greyish-brown to dull brown; rough; marked with relatively dense annular (ring-like) nodes and verruciform (wart-shaped), protuberant scars of buds and roots. Top end often densely covered with squamiform (scale-like) remnants of petiole base. Light in weight; hard and brittle, breaks easily. When broken, surface fairly even; pale brown to dull brown; with a ring of 4-10 punctiform (dot-like) off-white vascular bundles; pith in the centre greyish-black. Odour: faint; taste: extremely bitter.

Indications 1. Late stage of febrile disease with hectic fever, infantile malnutrition with fever 2. Diarrhoea, dysentery, haemorrhoid 3. Carbuncle 4. Conjunctivitis.

Chemical Composition Mainly contains iridoid glycosides such as picroside I, II, III.

Rhizoma Pinelliae

Pinellia Tuber
Banxia

半夏

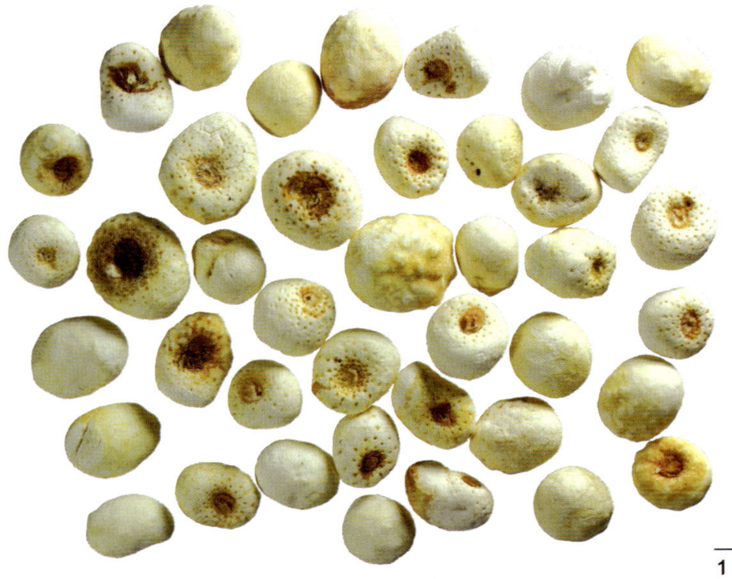

1 cm

Crude drug

Rhizoma Pinelliae

Source The tuber of *Pinellia ternate* (Thunb.) Breit. (Fam. Araceae).

Distribution Mainly in Chinese provinces such as Sichuan, Hubei, Henan, Anhui and Shandong. Also in provinces such as Hunan, Jiangsu, Zhejiang, Jiangxi and Yunnan.

Harvest & Processing Dig out tubers in summer and autumn; remove foreign matter; wash clean; remove cork and fibrous roots; dry under the sun or dry by heat.

Description Subspherical, some slightly slanted; 0.8-1.5 cm in diameter. Outer surface white or light yellow; top end with a dented stem scar in the centre; dense punctiform (dot-like) and dented brown root scars all over; bottom end obtuse, relatively smooth. Hard; when broken, surface white and starchy. Odour: faint; taste: pungent, numbs the tongue and irritates the throat.

Indications 1. Productive cough, chest pain 2. Vomiting 3. Subcutaneous nodule, goiter 4. Skin infection, scrofula, snakebite.

Chemical Composition Contains essential oils with 3-acetoamino-5-methylisooxazole as the main constituent; also contains shogaol and baicalin.

Note According to *C.P.*, also used for medicinal purposes is a processed Rhizoma Pinelliae called '*Fa banxia*'(Prepared Pinellia Tuber). Rhizoma Pinelliae is listed in Hong Kong as Category I (Toxic/ Potent) Chinese Materia Medica, and the processed Rhizoma Pinelliae, Category II.

Rhizoma Polygonati

Solomonseal Rhizome

Huangjing

黄精

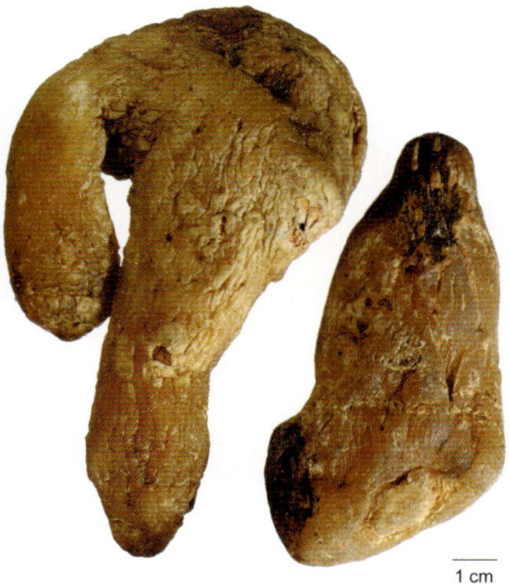

Crude drug

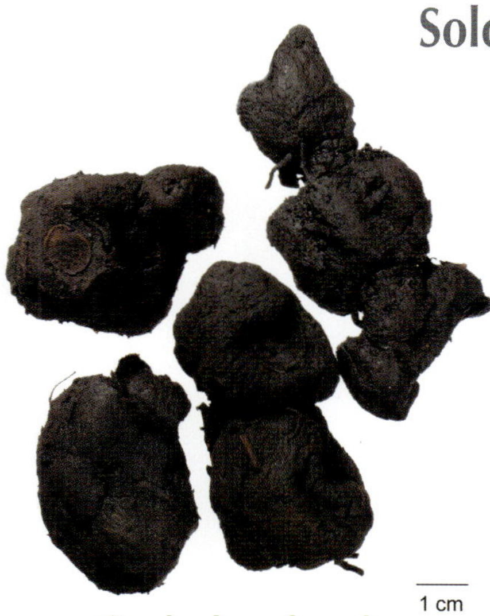

Crude drug (used in Hong Kong)

Source: The rhizome of *Polygonatum sibiricum* Red. (Fam. Liliaceae). Customarily called '*Jitou huangjing*' (Chicken-Head Solomonseal Rhizome).

Distribution: Mainly in Chinese provinces such as Hebei and Shaanxi, and in Inner Mongolia.

Harvest & Processing: Dig up rhizomes in spring and autumn; remove fibrous roots; wash rhizomes clean; blanch in boiling water or steam thoroughly; dry. Commonly used in Hong Kong are the steamed and dried rhizomes.

Description: Nodular and curved; 3-10 cm long, 0.5-1.5 cm in diameter. Nodes 2-4 cm long, slightly conical, often rameous (branched). Outer surface yellowish-white or greyish-yellow, translucent, marked with longitudinal wrinkles; stem scars orbicular (round), 5-8 mm in diameter. Strong and pliable; when broken, surface pale yellowish-brown or pale brown, slightly cuticular. Odour: faint; taste: sweet. Chewy.

Indications: 1. Dry cough, thirst 2. General weakness.

Chemical Composition: Mainly contains steroidal saponins such as sibiricoside A.

Rhizoma Polygonati Odorati

Fragrant Solomonseal Rhizome

Yuzhu

玉竹

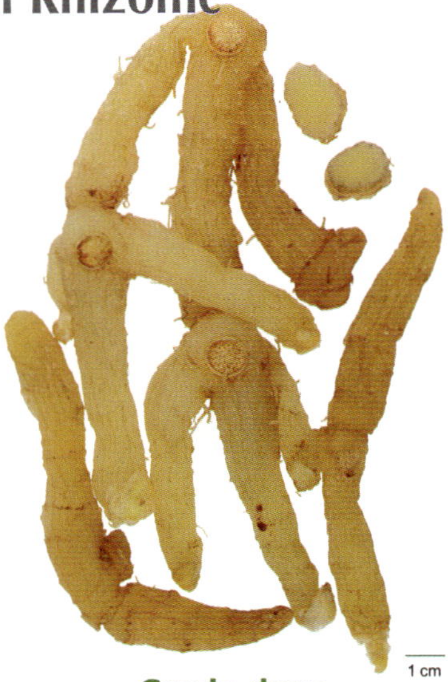

Crude drug

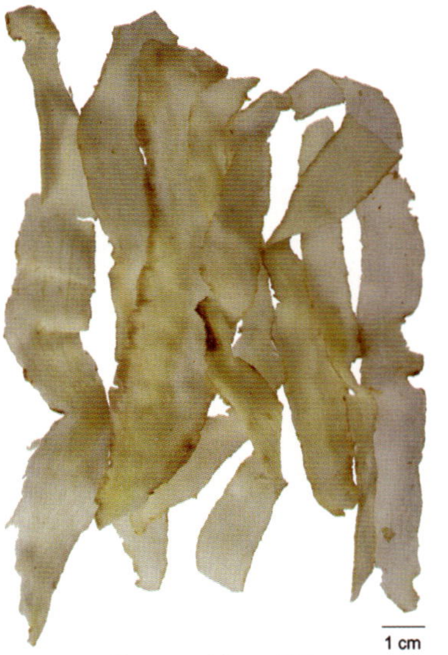

Decoction Pieces

Source The rhizome of *Polygonatum odoratum* (Mill.) Druce (Fam. Liliaceae).

Distribution Mainly in Chinese provinces such as Hunan, Henan, Jiangsu and Zhejiang.

Harvest & Processing Dig up rhizomes in autumn; remove fibrous roots; wash rhizomes clean. Dry until soft; knead repeatedly; dry thoroughly under the sun. Alternatively, steam thoroughly, knead until translucent and dry under the sun.

Description Long and cylindrical, slightly flattened, seldom rameous (branched); 4-18 cm long, 0.3-1.6 cm in diameter. Outer surface yellowish-white or pale yellowish-brown; translucent; with longitudinal wrinkles and slightly protuberant annular (ring-like) nodes, punctiform (dot-like) white scars of fibrous roots, and disciform (disc-like) stem scars. Hard and brittle, pliable when moistened; breaks easily; when broken, surface cuticular or granular. Odour: faint; taste: sweet. Chewy.

Indications 1. Dry cough, fever and cough 2. Dry throat, polydipsia, dehydration due to febrile disease, diabetes 3. Dizziness, muscular spasm 4. Hyperlipidemia, angina pectoris

Chemical Composition Mainly contains odoratan and polyfuroside.

Rhizoma Polygoni Cuspidati

Giant Knotweed Rhizome and Root

Huzhang

虎杖

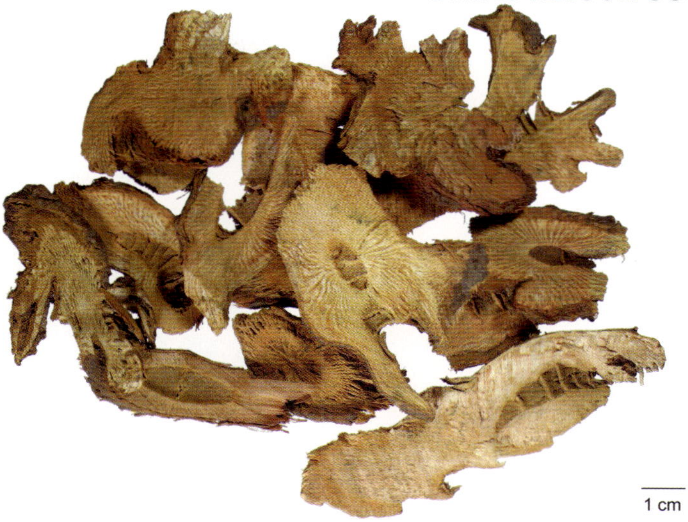

Decoction Pieces

Source The root and rhizome of *Polygonum cuspidatum* Sieb. et Zucc. (Fam. Polygonaceae).

Distribution Mainly in Chinese provinces such as Jiangsu, Zhejiang, Anhui and Guangdong; also in Hong Kong.

Harvest & Processing Collect roots and rhizomes in spring and autumn; remove rootlets; wash clean; cut into short sections or thick slices while fresh; dry under the sun.

Description Mostly cylindrical and in short sections or irregular and in thick slices; 1-7 cm long, 0.5-2.5 cm in diameter. Outer surface reddish-brown; marked with longitudinal wrinkles and scars of rootlets. Cut surface shows relatively thin cortex and wide, brownish-yellow xylem with radial rays; cortex and xylem relatively easy to separate; rhizome pith with septa or cavity. Hard. Odour: faint; taste: slightly bitter, astringent.

Indications 1. Jaundice, hepatitis, cholelithiasis, cholecystitis 2. Dysuria, leucorrhoea 3. Burn, carbuncles, snakebite, trauma 4. Amenorrhoea 5. Cough with yellow sputum

Chemical Composition Mainly contains emodin, chrysophanol and resveratrol.

Rhizoma Smilacis Chinensis

Chinaroot Greenbier Rhizome

Baqia

菝葜

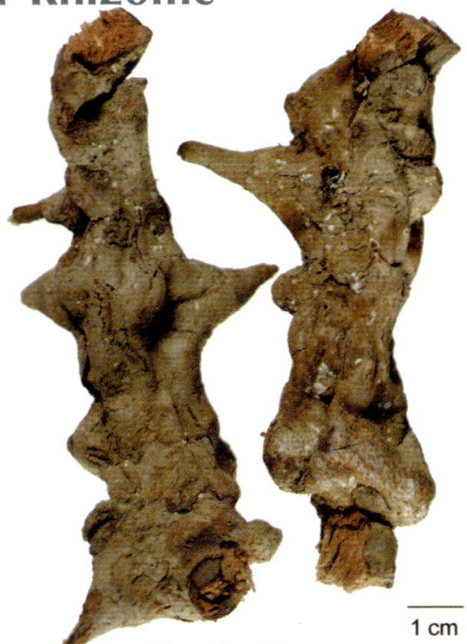

Crude drug

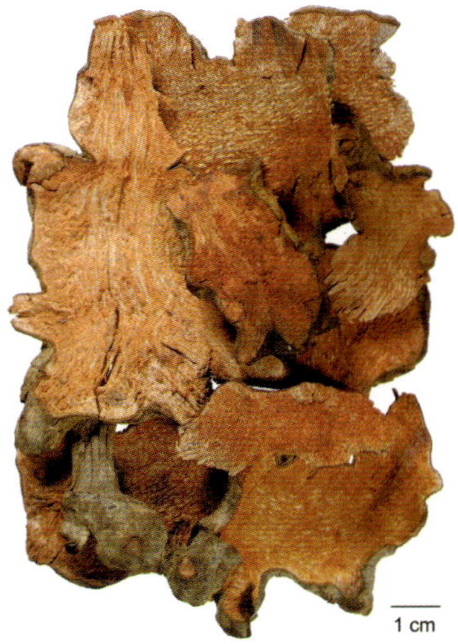

Decoction Pieces

Rhizoma Smilacis Chinensis

Source The rhizome of *Smilax china* L. (Fam. Liliaceae).

Distribution Mainly in Chinese provinces such as Zhejiang, Jiangsu and Guangxi; also in Hong Kong.

Harvest & Processing Dig up rhizomes in February or August; remove soil and fibrous roots; slice and then dry under the sun.

Description Flattened, cylindrical and slightly curved, or irregular; 10-20 cm long, 2-4 cm in diameter. Outer surface yellowish-brown or purplish-brown; internodes marked with conical protuberant stem scars, bud scars and scars of broken rootlets, or with hard but broken spiniform (spine-shaped) rootlets; nodes covered with scale leaves; apex sometimes marked with remnants of above-ground stem. Hard; broken surface brownish-yellow or reddish-brown, coarsely fibrous. Odour: faint; taste: slightly bitter.

Indications 1. Arthralgia, lumbago and pain of the lower extremities, sciatica, rheumatic arthritis 2. Stranguria with turbid urine, leukorrhagia 3. Skin infection, psoriasis, burn 4. Diarrhoea

Chemical Composition Mainly contains flavonoids such as smilaxin and isoengeletin, and steroidal saponins such as dioscin and gracillin.

Rhizoma Smilacis Glabrae

Glabrous Greenbrier Rhizome

Tufuling

土茯苓

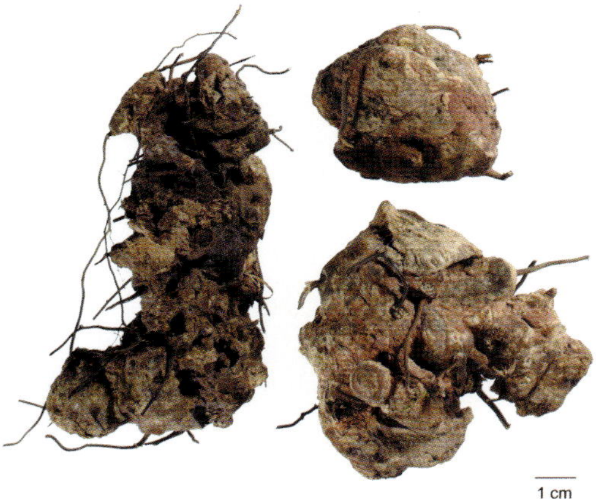

Crude drug

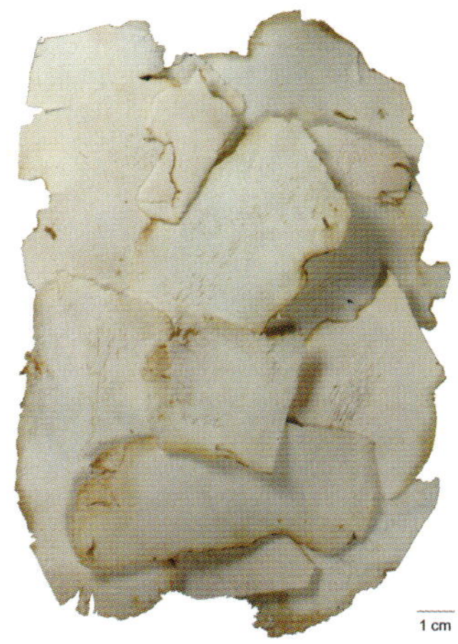

Decoction Pieces

Source The rhizome of *Smilax glabra* Roxb. (Fam. Liliaceae).

Distribution Mainly in Chinese provinces such as Guangdong, Hunan, Hubei, Zhejiang, Sichuan and Anhui; also in Hong Kong.

Harvest & Processing Collect rhizomes anytime during the year; wash clean; slice while fresh and then dry under the sun; or put in boiling water for several minutes; slice and dry under the sun.

Description Irregular pieces; with nodular protuberances and many fine fibrous roots; 5-22 cm long, 2-5 cm in diameter. Outer surface yellowish-brown or dull greyish-brown, rough, uneven; apex protuberant with hard remnants of base of fibrous roots, top end with stem scars. Hard; do not break easily. When sliced, surface off-white to reddish-brown; with faint vascular bundle dots in the centre; small gleaming spots of mucilaginous substance visible under sunlight; starchy; viscid and slippery when moistened with water. Odour: faint; taste: mild and astringent.

Indications 1. Syphilis 2. Arthralgia, muscular spasm 3. Genitourinary infection, oedema, leukorrhagia 4. Carbuncle, scrofula, skin ulcer 5. Leptospirosis

Chemical Composition Mainly contains flavonoids such as astilbin and engeletin.

Rhizoma Sparganii

Common Burreed Tuber

Sanleng

三棱

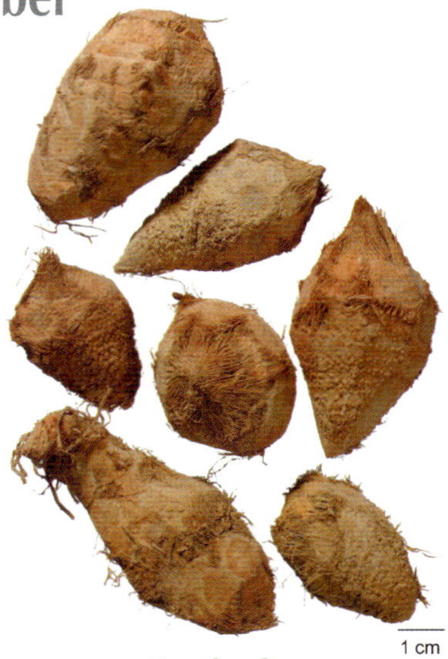

Crude drug

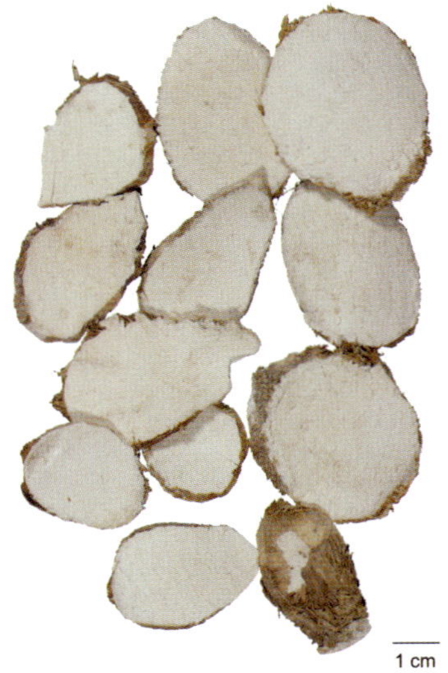

Decoction Pieces

Source The tuber, with bark shaved off, of *Sparganium stoloniferum* Buch.-Ham. (Fam. Sparganiaceae).

Distribution Mainly in Chinese provinces such as Jiangsu, Henan, Shandong, Jiangxi and Anhui.

Harvest & Processing Dig up tubers in winter and spring; remove stem remnants and fibrous roots; wash away soil; shave off cork; dry tubers under the sun. Commercial product is called '*Jing sanleng*' (Jingzhou Common Burreed Tuber).

Description Conical; slightly flat; 2-6 cm long, 2-4 cm wide. Outer surface yellowish-white or greyish-yellow, marked with knife scars; scars of fibrous root punctiform (dot-like), arranged in a slightly transverse and annular (ring-like) manner. Heavy; hard and solid; when broken, surface yellowish-white. Odourless; taste: mild, but hot-numbing when chewed.

Indications 1. Amenorrhoea, dysmenorrhea, postpartum abdominal pain 2. Abdominal mass, fibroid, hepatosplenomegaly 3. Dyspepsia, fullness and pain in the chest and abdomen.

Chemical Composition Mainly contains essential oils with benzeneethanol and 1, 4-benzenediol as the main components.

Rhizoma Typhonii

Giant Typhonium Rhizome

Baifuzi

白附子

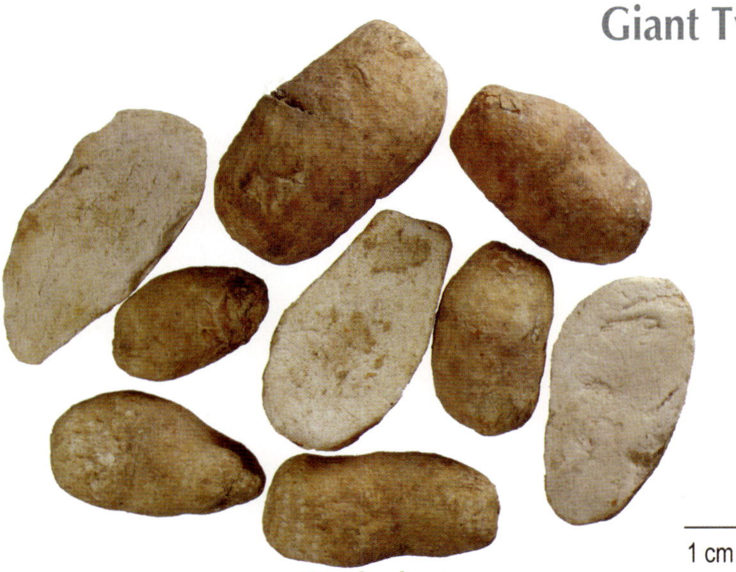

Crude drug

Source	The root tuber of *Typhonium giganteum* Engl. (Fam. Araceae). Customarily called '*Yu Baifu*' (Giant Typhonium Rhizome from *Yu Xian*).
Distribution	Mainly in Chinese provinces such as Henan, Gansu, and Hubei.
Harvest & Processing	Dig out tubers in autumn; remove fibrous roots and cork; dry under the sun.
Description	Ovoid (egg-shaped) or ellipsoid (elliptical in long-section and circular in cross-section); 2-5 cm long, 1-3 cm in diameter. Outer surface white or pale yellow, fairly smooth, marked with annulations and punctiform (dot-like) root scars; top end with scars of stems or buds. Hard; when broken, surface white and starchy. Odourless; taste: mild but hot-numbing and tongue-pricking.
Indications	1. Dizziness 2. Facial palsy, hemiplegia, Cerebral vascular accident 3. Scrofula 4. Snakebite
Chemical Composition	Contains typhonoside, dipalmitin and 2,6-diamino-9- β -D-ribofuranosylpurine.
Note	The unprocessed tuber of *T. giganteum* Engl. and the unprocessed root tuber of *Aconitum coreanum* (Lévl.) Raipaics (Fam. Ranunculaceae) are listed in Hong Kong as Category I (Toxic/Potent) Chinese Materia Medica, and the processed crude drug of the two species mentioned above, Category II.

Rhizoma Zingiberis

Dried Ginger
Ganjiang
乾薑

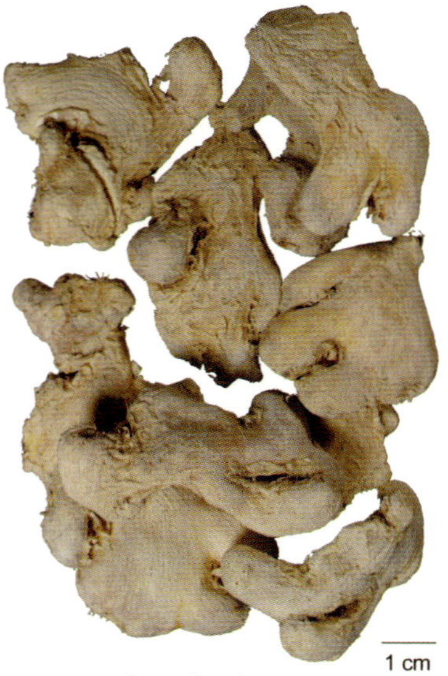

Crude drug

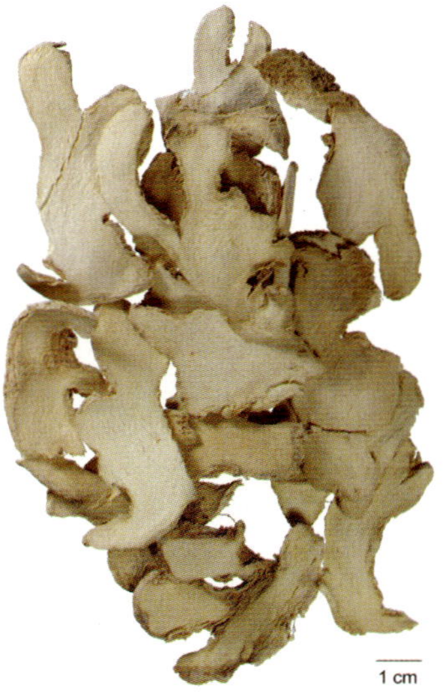

Decoction Pieces

Source The rhizome of *Zingiber officinale* (Wild.) Rosc. (Fam. Zingiberaceae).

Distribution Mainly in Chinese provinces such as Sichuan and Guizhou.

Harvest & Processing Dig out rhizomes in winter when leaves wither; remove leaves, fibrous roots, soil and sand; dry under the sun or at low temperatures. The ones sliced while fresh and dried under the sun or at low temperatures are called '*Ganjiang pian*' (Dried Ginger Slices).

Description Flattened lumps, ramose (with many branches) and digitate (arranged like fingers); 3-7 cm long, 1-2 cm thick. Outer surface greyish-yellow or light greyish-brown; rough; marked with longitudinal wrinkles and conspicuous annulations. Top part of branches with stem scars or buds. Commonly sold in the form of irregular, length-wise cut or angled-cut slices, also rameous (branched) and digitate. Cut surface greyish-yellow or greyish-white; slightly starchy; with relatively more longitudinal fibres, some piliform (hair-like). Hard and solid; broken surface fibrous. Odour: fragrant and distinctive; taste: pungent.

Indications 1. Pain and cold feeling in the lower abdomen, diarrhoea, vomiting 2. Cough with thin sputum 3. Shock

Chemical Composition Mainly contains essential oils with α-zingiberene as the major component.

Sanguis Draxonis

Dragon's Blood
Xuejie
血竭

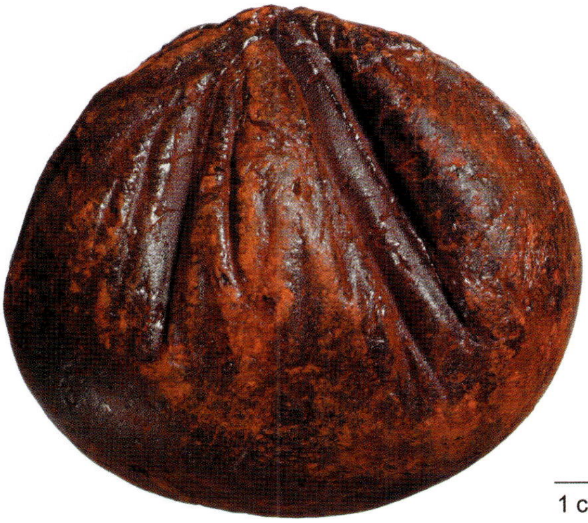

1 cm

Crude drug

Source The processed product of the resin secreted from the fruits of *Daemonorops draco* Bl. (Fam. Palmae).

Distribution Mainly in Kalimantan and Sumatra, Indonesia, and countries such as India and Malaysia.

Harvest & Processing Collect mature fruits, i.e. those with dense small hard scales on the surface and covered almost entirely by red resin secreted from between the scales. Dry the fruits thoroughly under the sun; put in a basket together with shells; shake hard so that the loose and crisp resin flakes of the fruits come off; sieve away foreign matter; wrap the flakes with cloth and put into hot water to soften into a blob; take out and let cool to produce '*Yuanzhuang Xuejie*' (Processed Dragon's Blood). Resin of *Daemonorops draco* mixed with supplementary materials like dammar is called '*Jiagong Xuejie*' (Processed Dragon's Blood with supplements).

Description Processed Dragon's Blood with supplements: Slightly subspherical cube; 6-8 cm in diameter, about 4 cm thick, 250-280 g in weight. Outer surface dull red or dark red, lustrous; base flat and orbicular (round), top end shows longitudinal marks caused by bundling. Hard and brittle; surface of broken-section red; when ground into powder, brick-red. When broken, surface lustrous, or in some cases rough, lustreless, and dark red; when ground into powder, blood-red. Odourless; taste: mild.

Indications 1. Post traumatic swelling, bruises and pain 2. Chronic ulcer, wound pain 3. Amenorrhoea

Chemical Composition Mainly contains dracorubin and dracorhodin.

Semen Abri Precatorii

Coralhead Plant Seed

Xiangsizi

相思子

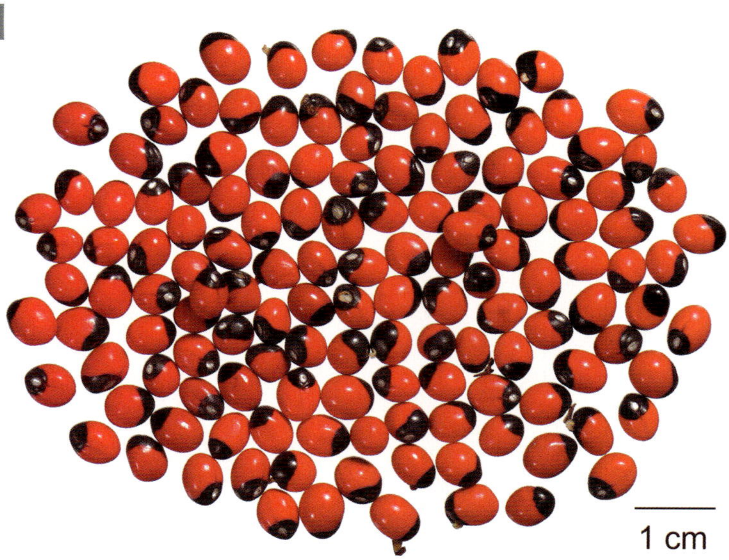

Crude drug

Source The mature seed of *Abrus precatorius* L. (Fam. Leguminosae).

Distribution Mainly in Chinese provinces such as Guangdong, Guangxi, Fujian and Yunnan; also in Hong Kong.

Harvest & Processing Pick mature fruits in batches in summer and autumn; dry under the sun; thresh to get seeds; remove foreign matter.

Description Ellipsoid (elliptical in long-section and circular in cross-section), occasionally subspherical; 5-7 mm long, 3-5 mm in diameter. Outer surface red; hilum linear and slightly protuberant, in an elliptical white pit located at one end of the ventral side. Hard, does not break easily; when cracked open, pale yellow radicle and 2 semi-circular cotyledons revealed. Odour: grassy; taste: slightly bitter-astringent.

Indications Scabies and tinea (external use).

Chemical Composition Contains abricin, stigmasterol and abridin.

Semem Abutili

Chingma Abutilon Seed

Qingmazi

苘麻子

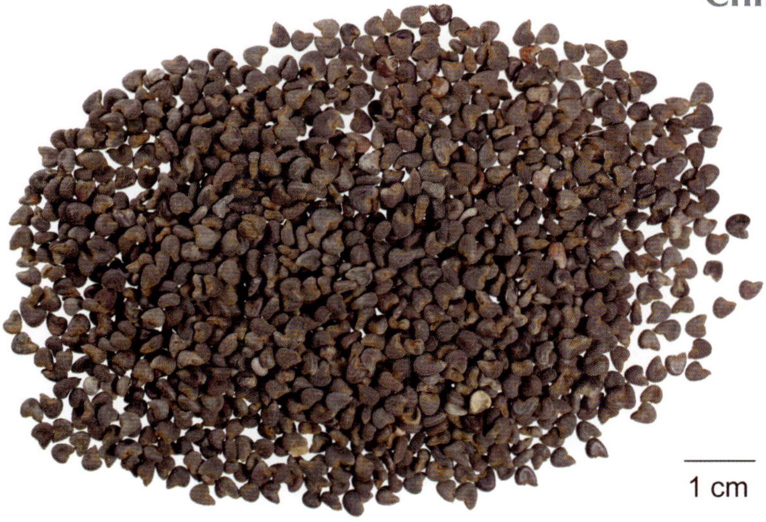

Crude drug

Source The mature seed of *Abutilon theophrasti* Medic. (Fam. Malvaceae).

Distribution Mainly in Chinese provinces such as Sichuan, Henan, Jiangsu and Hubei; also in provinces such as Anhui, Jiangxi, Hunan and Hebei.

Harvest & Processing Collect fruits at maturation in autumn; dry under the sun; thresh to get seeds; sieve away foreign matter; dry the seeds under the sun again.

Description Triangular, flattened and reniform (kidney-shaped); 3.5-6 mm long, about 2.5-4.5 mm wide, 1-2 mm thick. Outer surface greyish-black or dull brown; sparsely covered with white villi; indentation at margin with a sub-elliptical pale brown hilum; under magnification hilum encircled by radial fine striae. Testa hard; cotyledons 2, overlapping and folded, highly oleaginous (oily). Odour: faint; taste: mild.

Indications 1. Dysentery 2. Dysuria, urinary tract infection 3. Carbuncle, gangrene, mastitis 4. Blurred vision

Chemical Composition Mainly contains 15%-17% oils, in which 58% is linoleic acid.

Semen Allii Tuberosi

Tuber Onion Seed
Jiucaizi

韭菜子

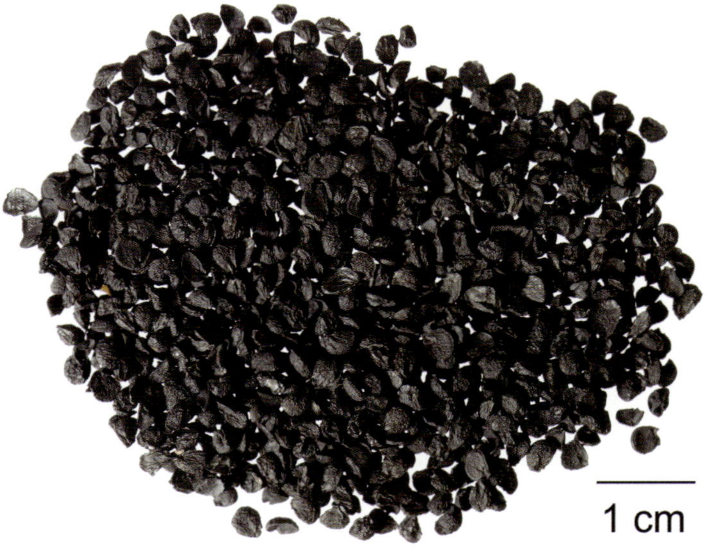

Crude drug

Source The mature seed of *Allium tuberosum* Rottl. (Fam. Liliaceae).

Distribution Mainly in Chinese provinces such as Hebei, Shanxi, Jilin, Jiangsu, Shandong, Anhui and Henan; also in Hong Kong.

Harvest & Processing Cut off fruits in batches when seeds start to mature and harden in autumn; tie up in small bundles; put in well-ventilated places, or on mattresses under the sun; thresh to get seeds; dry under the sun.

Description Seed flattened and ovoid (egg-shaped); slightly dented on one side, bulgy on the other; apex obtuse, base slightly pointed; 3-4 mm long, 2-3 mm wide. Outer surface black; conspicuous reticulate (netted) wrinkles on bulgy side, those on dented side rather indistinct. Base with 2 tiny protuberances, the shorter one with a greyish-brown or greyish-white hilum at apex, the longer one with a micropyle at apex. Longitudinal-section reveals thin testa, greyish-white endosperms, curved white embryo, and 1 cotyledon. Hard. Odour: distinctive; taste: like Chinese chives when chewed.

Indications 1. Impotence, nocturnal emission, loin and knee pain 2. Enuresis, urinary frequency 3. Morbid leukorrhoea

Chemical Composition Mainly contains steroidal saponins such as tuberoside M.

Semen Allii Tuberosi

Semen Alpiniae Katsumadai

Katsumade Galangal Seed

Caodoukou

草豆蔻

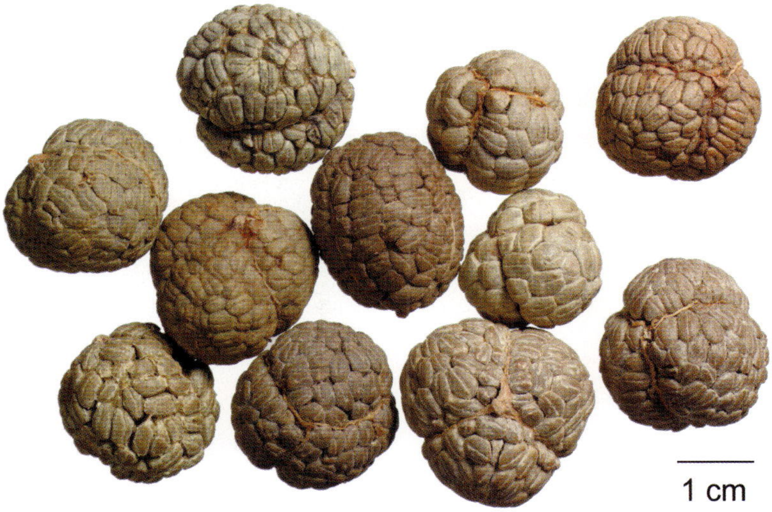

Crude drug

Source The near-mature seed of *Alpinia katsumadai* Hayata (Fam. Zingiberaceae).

Distribution Mainly in Chinese provinces such as Guangdong and Guangxi; also in Hong Kong.

Harvest & Processing Harvest near-mature seeds in summer and autumn; dry under the sun until nearly dry; remove pericarp and take out seed clusters; dry under the sun again. Alternatively, blanch in boiling water; dry under the sun until half-dry; remove pericarp and take out seed clusters; dry under the sun.

Description Seed cluster subspherical; 1.5-2.7 cm in diameter. Outer surface dull greyish-brown, slightly lustrous; with yellowish-white septa in the middle dividing each seed cluster into 3 cloves, each bearing 13-110 seeds stuck fast together. Seeds in the form of ovoid (egg-shaped) polyhedrons; 3-5 mm long, about 3 mm in diameter; covered with pale brown membranous aril; raphe in the form of a longitudinal groove; with a hilum at one end; hard. When seeds are cut longitudinally in half along the raphe, surface slanted and cordate (heart-like) in shape; the part of testa extending along the raphe into the inner part accounts for about 1/2 the length of the whole seed; endosperms greyish-white. Odour: fragrant; taste: acrid and slightly bitter.

Indications Fullness and distending pain in the abdomen, nausea, vomiting, anorexia.

Chemical Composition Mainly contains diarylheptanoids such as katsumadain A, B.

Semen Arecae

Areca Seed
Binglang
檳榔

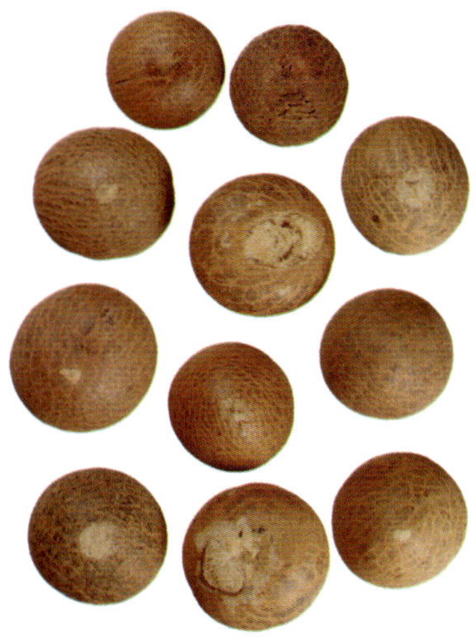

Crude drug

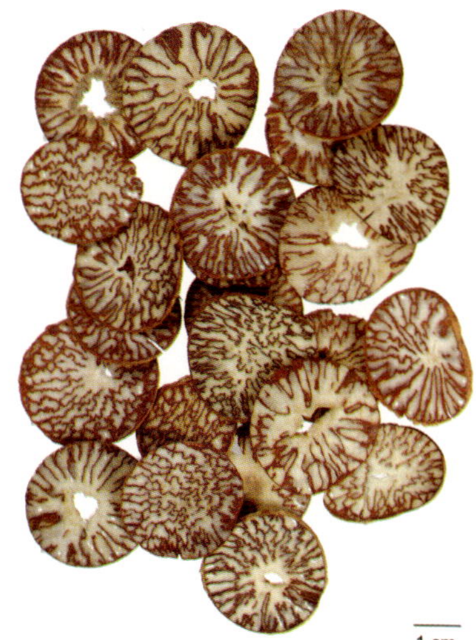

Decoction Pieces

Source The mature seed of *Areca catechu* L. (Fam. Palmae).

Distribution Mainly in Chinese provinces such as Hainan, Yunnan, Guangdong, Fujian, Guangxi and Taiwan.

Harvest & Processing Harvest mature fruits from late spring to early autumn; cook in boiling water; dry over low heat; strip off pericarp; take out seeds; dry again.

Description Flattened and spherical, or conical; 1.5-3.5 cm thick, 1.5-3 cm in diameter at the base. Outer surface pale yellowish-brown or pale reddish-brown; rough; marked with slightly dented reticulate (netted) grooves; often with a small quantity of greyish-white endocarp fragments still attached. Base marked in the centre with an orbicular (round), dented micropyle; beside micropyle lie 1 lunate (crescent-shaped) or triangular scar-like hilum and scars of vascular bundles. Cross-section shows a marble-like pattern of alternating brown and white encircled by a pale yellowish-brown or reddish-brown rim. Hard and brittle, breaks easily. Odour: faint; taste: astringent and slightly bitter.

Indications 1. Tapeworm and roundworm infestation, fasciolopsiasis 2. Abdominal pain 3. Dyspepsia, diarrhoea, tenesmus 4. Oedema 5. Glaucoma (prepared as eyedrops for external use).

Chemical Composition Mainly contains alkaloids such as arecoline; also contains condensed tannins.

Semen Armeniacae Amarum

Bitter Apricot Seed
Kuxingren
苦杏仁

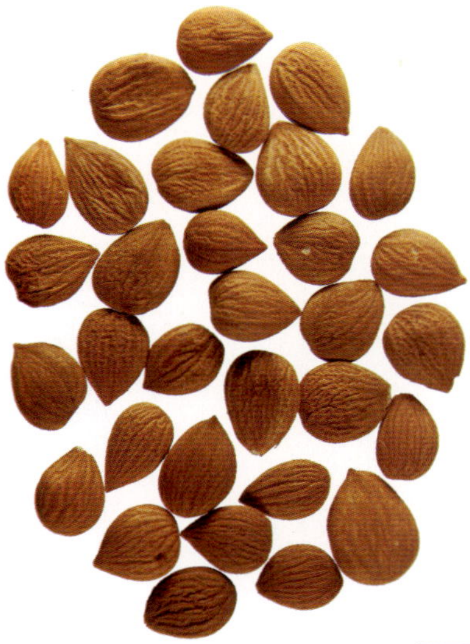
Crude drug 1 cm

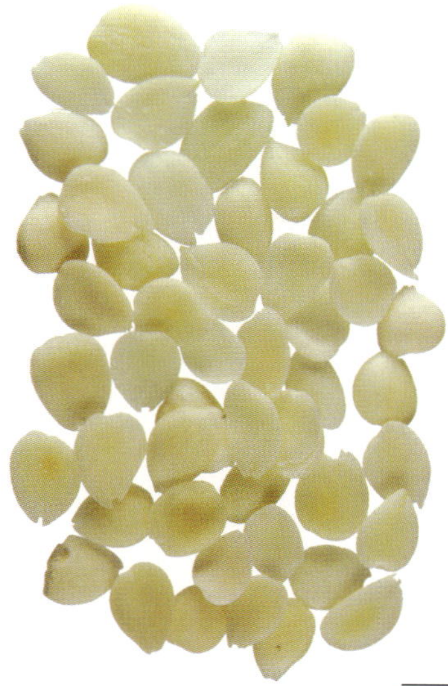
Crude drug 1 cm

Source The mature seed of *Prunus armeniaca* L. var. *ansu* Maxim. (Fam. Rosaceae).

Distribution Mainly in Chinese provinces such as Liaoning, Hebei,and Shandong, and in Inner Mongolia. Mostly naturally grown; also cultivated.

Harvest & Processing Collect fruits after maturation in summer; remove sarcocarp and husks; take out seeds; dry under the sun. Commonly used in Hong Kong are the seeds with the testa removed, called '*Beixing*' (North Bitter Apricot Seed).

Description Flattened and cordate (heart-shaped); 1-1.9 cm long, 0.8-1.5 cm wide, 5-8 mm thick. Apex slightly pointed; base obtuse; two sides asymmetrical. Testa thin, brown to dull brown, with irregular wrinkles; one edge of the apex with a hilum, base with an elliptical chalaza; between hilum and chalaza is a raphe; numerous dark brown venous (vein-like) striae radiating from chalaza. When seeds are soaked in warm boiled water and testa removed, 2 white cotyledons are exposed; cotyledons highly oleaginous (oily), with relatively small radicle and plumule at apex. Odourless; taste: bitter.

Indications 1. Cough 2. Constipation

Chemical Composition Mainly contains amygdalin, chlorogenic acid, 3′-feruloylguinic acid, 3′-p-coumaroylquinic acid etc.

Note According to *C.P.*, also used for medicinal purposes is the mature seed of P. sibirica L., of P. *mandshurica* (Maxim.) Koehne and of P. *armeniaca* L.

Semen Astragali Complanati

Flatstem Milkvetch Seed

Shayuanzi

沙苑子

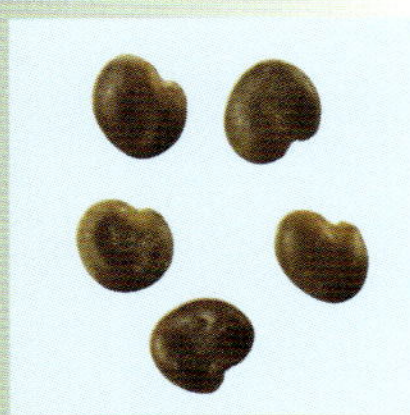

Flatstem Milkvetch Seed Magnified

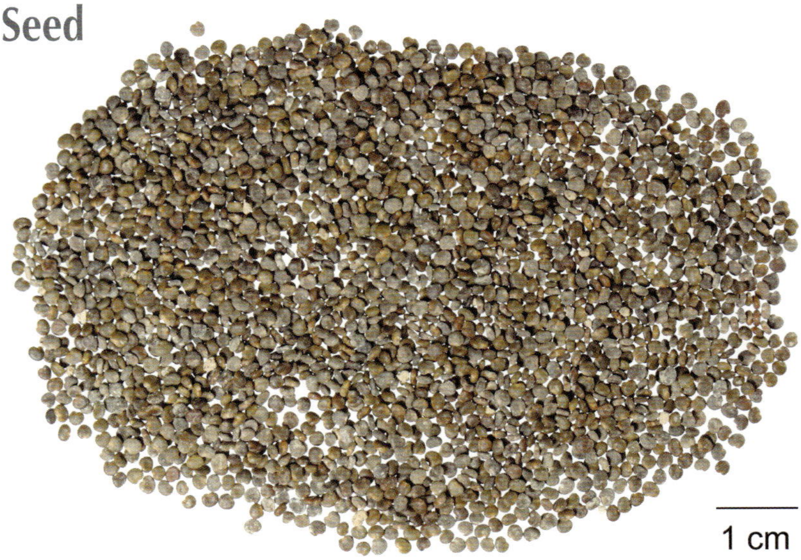

Crude drug

Source The mature seed of *Astragalus complanatus* R. Br. (Fam. Leguminosae).

Distribution Mainly in Chinese provinces such as Shaanxi; also in provinces such as Hebei, Liaoning, Shanxi, and in Inner Mongolia.

Harvest & Processing Cut off above-ground parts in late autumn and early winter when seeds are mature but fruits have not dehisced (split open at maturity); dry under the sun; take seeds; remove foreign matter; dry under the sun again.

Description Somewhat reniform (kidney-shaped) but slightly flattened; 2-2.5 mm long, 1.5-2 mm wide, about 1 mm thick. Outer surface smooth, dull brownish-green or dull greyish-brown; indentation at the edge on one side with a conspicuous hilum. Hard; 2 pale yellow cotyledons exposed when testa removed; radicle curved, about 1 mm long. Odourless; taste: mild, bean-like when chewed.

Indications 1. Back pain 2. Nocturnal emission, premature ejaculation
3. Turbid discharge with urination, dribbling after urination
4. Leukorrhagia 5. Dizziness, blurred vision.

Chemical Composition Mainly contains copmplanatuside.

Semen Benincasae

Chinese Waxgourd Seed
Dongguazi
冬瓜子

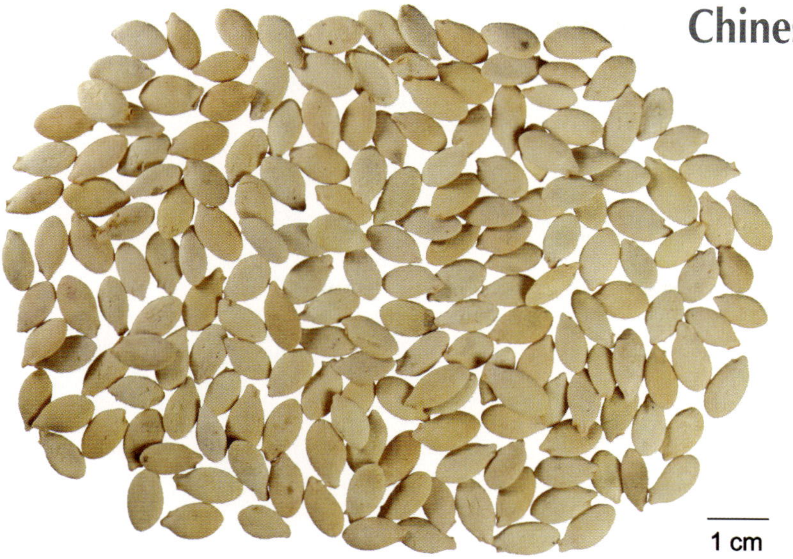

Crude drug

Source The seed of *Benincasa hispida* (Thunb.) Cogn. (Fam. Cucurbitaceae).

Distribution Mainly in Chinese provinces such as Hebei, Henan, Anhui, Jiangsu, Zhejiang and Sichuan.

Harvest & Processing Collect mature seeds when eating Chinese waxgourd; wash clean; dry under the sun.

Description Oblong and elliptical, or ovate (egg-shaped), flat; 1-1.5 cm long, 0.5-1 cm wide, about 2 mm thick. Outer surface yellowish-white; slightly rough; smooth at margin, or with 1 annulation near the margin on each side. One end slightly pointed, with 2 small protuberances, the larger one with a micropyle on raised surface, the smaller one the hilum; the other end obtuse. Testa slightly hard, brittle; on removal of testa, 2 white plump cotyledons visible; radicle short and small. Light in weight; highly oleaginous (oily). Odourless; taste: slightly sweet.

Indications 1. Productive cough with yellowish sputum, lung abscess 2. Appendicitis 3. Morbid leukorrhoea.

Chemical Composition Contains sterol and triterpenes.

Semen Cassiae

Cassia Seed
Juemingzi
決明子

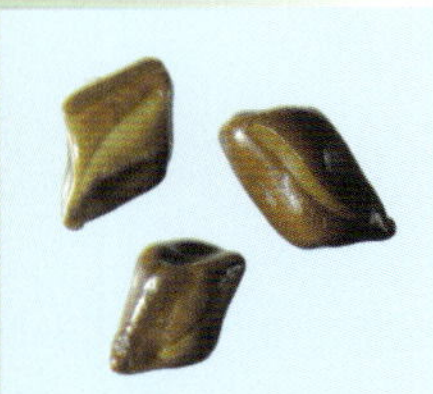

Cassia Seed Magnified

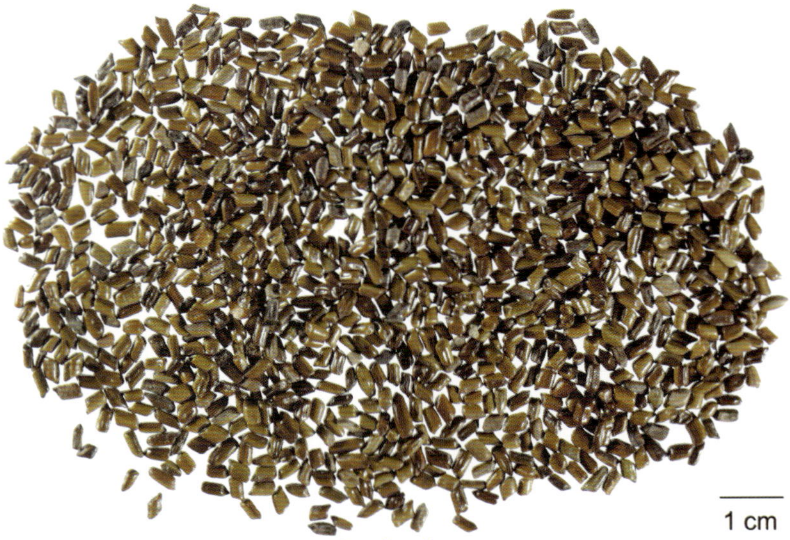

Crude drug

Source The dried mature seed of *Cassia obtusifolia* L. (Fam.).

Distribution Cultivated in most regions of China; also grown in Hong Kong.

Harvest & Processing Collect mature fruits in autumn; dry under the sun; thresh to get seeds; remove foreign matter.

Description Slightly rhomboid, or short and cylindrical; two ends parallel and slanting, hippocrepiform (horseshoe-shaped); 3-7 mm long, 2-4 mm wide. Outer surface greenish-brown or dull brown, smooth and lustrous. One end even, the other end pointed and slanting. Dorsal and ventral sides each marked with a protuberant ridge; on either side of each ridge are 2 symmetrical, slanting dented lines lighter in colour. Hard, does not break easily. Cross-section shows a thin testa, with 2 S-shaped yellow cotyledons overlapping in the middle. Odour: faint; taste: slightly bitter.

Indications 1. Acute conjunctivitis, corneal ulcer, night blindness, glaucoma 2. Dizziness due to hypertension 3.Ascites from cirrhosis 4. Habitual constipation 5. Infant malnutrition.

Chemical Composition Mainly contains anthraquinones such as emodin, obtusen and chryso-obtusin.

Note According to *C.P.*, also used for medicinal purposes is the mature seed of *C. tora* L.

Semen Cassiae Occidentalis

Coffee Senna Seed

Wangjiangnanzi

望江南子

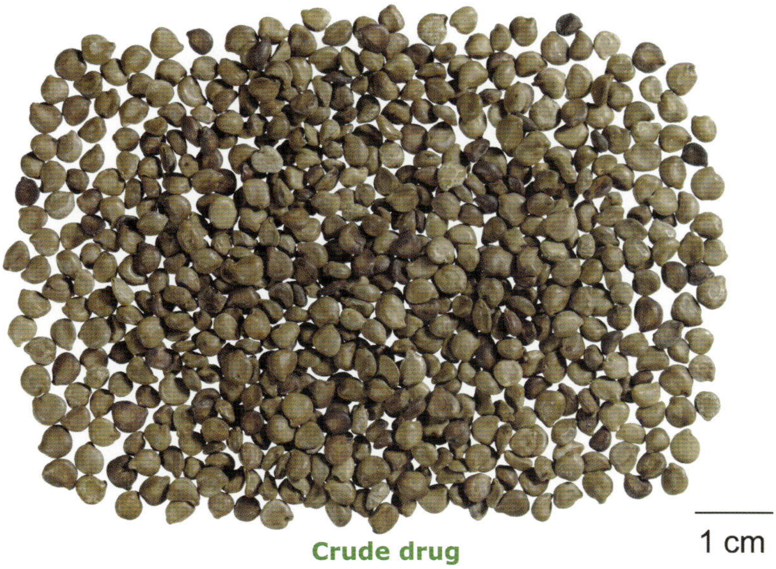

Crude drug

Source The seed of *Cassia occidentalis* L. (Fam. Leguminosae).

Distribution Mainly in Jiangsu province in China; also in provinces such as Zhejiang, Jiangxi, Fujian and Guangxi, and also in Hong Kong.

Harvest & Processing Collect mature fruits in autumn; thresh to get seeds; remove foreign matter and pods; dry seeds under the sun.

Description Flattened and ovoid (egg-shaped), or flattened and peach-shaped; one end acuminate (tapering to a slender point), slanted to one side and with a hilum, the other end slightly dented; 3-5.5 mm long, 3-5 mm wide, 1-2 mm thick. Outer surface dark brown or purplish-brown, slightly lustrous; centre with a pit oblong and orbicular (round), or orbicular; margin with white reticulate (net-like) or radial striae. Taste: slightly bitter.

Indications 1. Red eyes, photophobia with lacrimation, conjunctivitis 2. Dizziness and distension of head, hypertension 3. Dyspepsia, stomachache, dysentery, constipation 4. Carbuncle, mastitis

Chemical Composition Contains 3-methyl-6-methoxy-1, 8-dihydroxyanthraquinone.

Semen Celosiae

Feather Cockscomb Seed
Qingxiangzi
青葙子

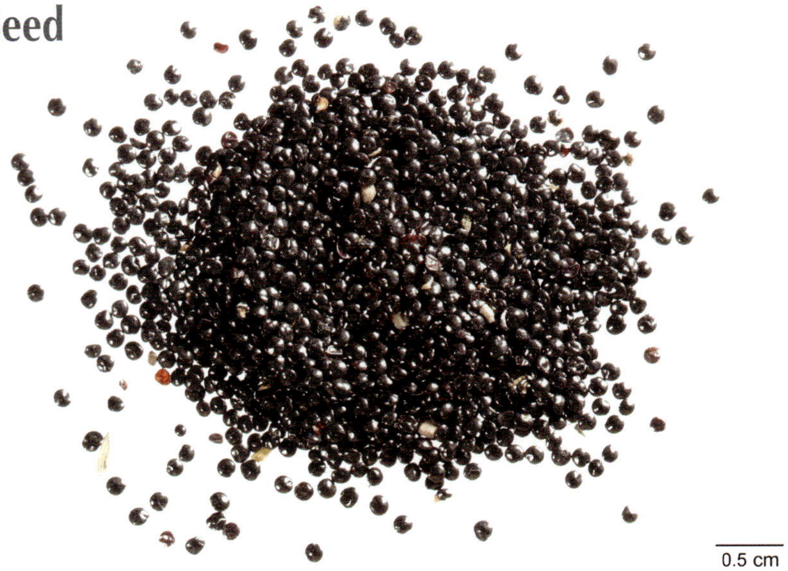

Crude drug

Source The mature seed of *Celosia argentea* L. (Fam. Amaranthaceae).

Distribution In most regions of China, including Hong Kong.

Harvest & Processing Cut off above-ground parts or pick fruit spikes from July to September when seeds ripen; rub out seeds; sieve out foreign matter.

Description Flattened and spherical; 1-1.8 mm in diameter. Outer surface black or reddish-black, shiny; bulgy in the middle; hilum situated at the edge on one side as a slight impression. Seed sticky; testa thin and brittle; endosperms off-white. Odourless; taste: mild.

Indications 1. Acute conjunctivitis, keratitis 2. Chronic uveitis 3. Dizziness due to hypertension.

Chemical Composition Mainly contains celosiaol.

Semen Coicis

Coix Seed

Yiyiren

薏苡仁

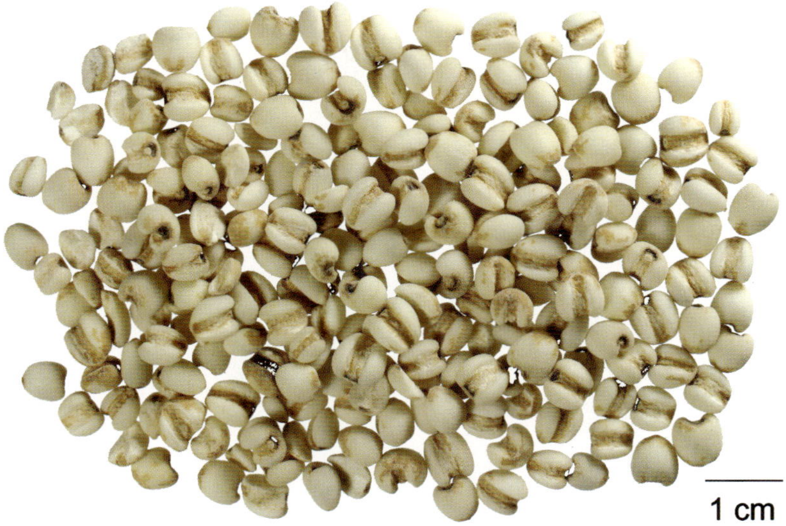

Crude drug

Source The mature kernel of *Coix lacryma-jobi* L. var. *ma-yuen* (Roman.) Stapf (Fam. Gramineae).

Distribution Mainly in Chinese provinces such as Fujian, Hebei, Jiangsu and Liaoning. Cultivated.

Harvest & Processing Harvest plants in autumn when fruits are ripe; dry under the sun; thresh to obtain fruits; dry under the sun again; remove foreign matter; collect kernels.

Description Broad and ovoid (egg-shaped), or oblong and ellipsoid (elliptical in long-section and circular in cross-section); 4-8 mm long, 3-6 mm wide. Outer surface milky-white, smooth, with occasional dull yellowish-brown testa remnants; apex obtuse; base broader and dented, with 1 punctiform (dot-like), pale brown hilum. Dorsal side rounded and protuberant; ventral side with 1 relatively wide and deep longitudinal groove. Hard and solid; broken surface white, starchy. Odour: faint; taste: slightly sweet.

Indications 1. Chronic enteritis, diarrhoea 2. Morbid leukorrhoea 3. Oedema 4. Warts, eczema.

Chemical Composition Mainly contains triglycerides, diglycerides and coixan A, B, C.

Semen Cuscutae

Dodder Seed

Tusizi

菟絲子

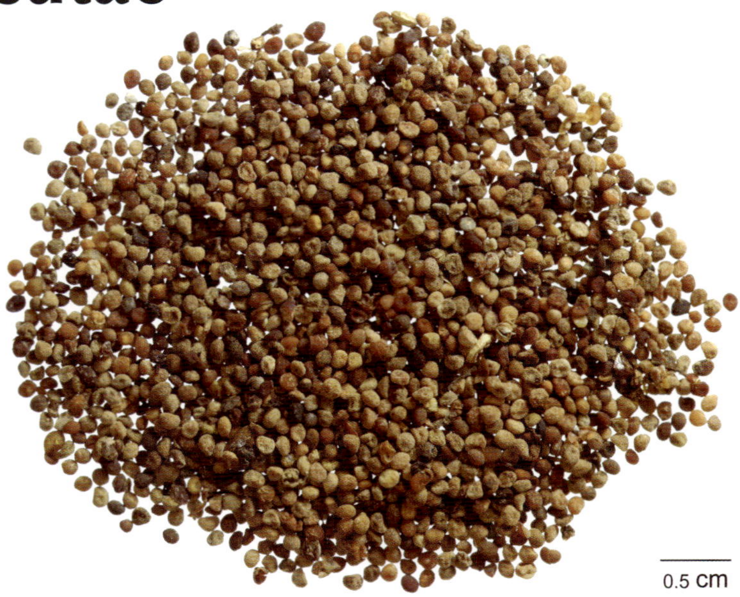

0.5 cm

Crude drug

Source The mature seed of *Cuscuta chinensis* Lam. (Fam. Convolvulaceae).

Distribution Mainly in Chinese provinces such as Jiangsu, Liaoning, Jilin and Hebei.

Harvest & Processing Harvest plants in autumn when fruits ripen; dry under the sun; thresh to get seeds; remove foreign matter.

Description Subspherical; 1-1.5 mm in diameter. Outer surface greyish-brown or yellowish-brown; dense, protuberant small dots visible under magnification; one end with a slightly dented, linear (long and narrow) hilum. Hard, not crushed easily when pressed with fingernails. Surface becomes sticky when soaked in boiling water; testa cracks when water heats up, revealing a white helicoid (coiled like a spiral) embryo. Odour: faint; taste: mild.

Indications 1. Weakness in lower body and legs 2. Impotence, seminal emissions Urinary frequency 3. Vertigo, dizziness 4. Poor vision 5. Threatened abortion

Chemical Composition Contains quercetin and astragalin.

Semen Cuscutae

Semen Sapindi

Chinese Soapberry Seed

Wuhuanzi

無患子

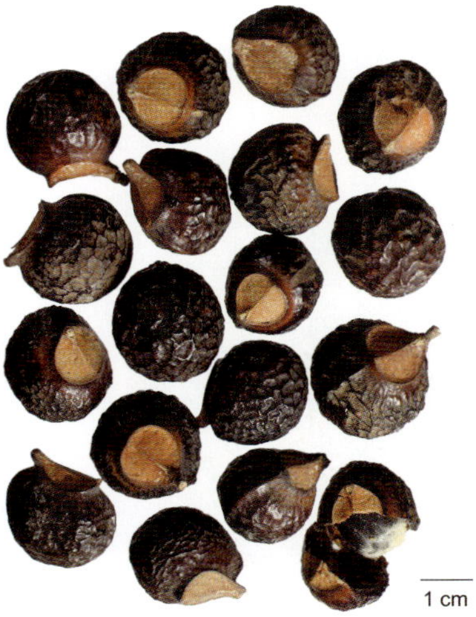

Crude drug (Fruit)

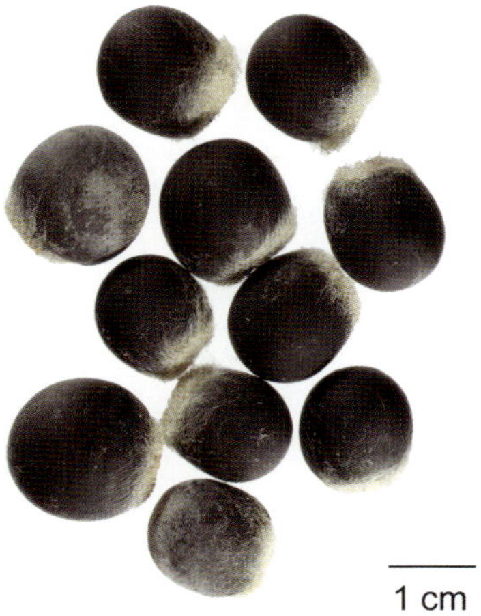

Crude drug (Seed)

Source The fruit or seed of *Sapindus mukorossi* Gaertn. (Fam. Sapindaceae).

Distribution Mainly in Chinese provinces such as Guangdong and Guangxi; also in Hong Kong.

Harvest & Processing Pick mature fruits in autumn; dry under the sun, or remove sarcocarp and dry seeds under the sun.

Description Spherical or ellipsoid (elliptical in long-section and circular in cross-section); about 1.5 cm in diameter. Outer surface black, lustrous; hilum linear, with white villi. Hard. When cut open, 2 cotyledons revealed; cotyledons yellow, plump, superposed (one set on or over another), the one on dorsal side larger, half-surrounding the one on ventral side; embryo short and thick, slightly curved. Odour: faint; taste: bitter.

Indications 1. Pharyngitis, dyspnoeic cough with yellow sputum, hoarseness of voice 2. Dyspepsia, intestinal parasitosis 3. Trichomonas vaginitis 4. Tinea 5. Sores and boils.

Chemical Composition Mainly contains fatty oils.

Note Commonly sold in Hong Kong are the fruits of Chinese Soapberry, but the seeds can also be used for medicinal purposes.

Semen Euphorbiae

Caper Euphorbia Seed
Qianjinzi

千金子

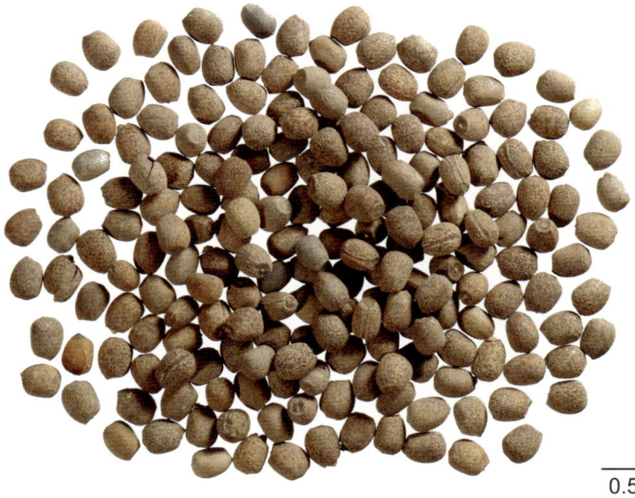

0.5 cm

Crude drug

Source The mature seed of *Euphorbia lathyris* L. (Fam. Euphorbiaceae).

Distribution Mainly in Chinese provinces such as Henan and Zhejiang; also in provinces such as Sichuan, Hebei, Jilin and Liaoning.

Harvest & Processing Collect fruits in summer and autumn when they turn dull dark brown; dry under the sun; take out seeds; remove foreign matter; dry the seeds.

Description Ellipsoid (elliptical in long-section and circular in cross-section) or obovoid (inverse egg-shaped); about 5 mm long, about 4 mm in diameter. Outer surface greyish-brown or dull greyish-brown, marked with irregular reticulate (net-like) wrinkles; indentations in meshes greyish-black, forming minute maculae. One side with a raphe in the form of a longitudinal groove; top end with a protuberant chalaza, bottom end with a linear (long and narrow) hilum; base with a protuberant off-white caruncle or caruncle scar. Testa thin and brittle; kernel white or yellowish-white, highly oleaginous (oily). Odour: faint; taste: acrid.

Indications 1. Oedema and ascites 2. Constipation 3. Amenorrhoea 4. Abdominal mass

Chemical Composition Mainly contains ingenol-20-hexadecanote, lathyrol-3, 15-diacetate-5-benzoate, daphretin and euphorbetin.

Note Semen Euphorbiae is listed in Hong Kong as Category I (Toxic/Potent) Chinese Materia Medica, and the processed Semen Euphorbiae, Category II.

Semen Euryales

Gordon Euryale Seed

Qianshi

芡實

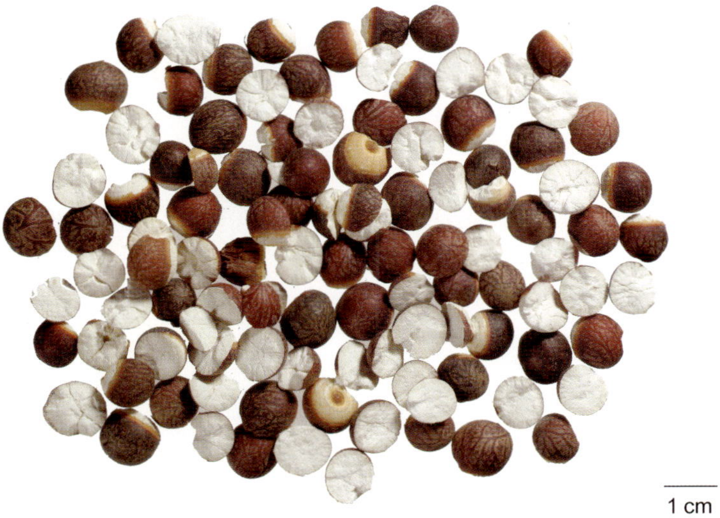

Crude drug

Source The mature kernel of *Euryale ferox* Salisb. (Fam. Nymphaeaceae).

Distribution Mainly in Chinese provinces such as Jiangsu, Shandong, Anhui, Hunan and Hubei.

Harvest & Processing Collect mature fruits in late autumn and early winter; dry under the sun and break the thorny bark; take out seeds and wash clean; dry; grind away husks or remove with a kibbler; sieve away remaining husks and foreign matter.

Description Subspherical; 5-8 mm in diameter; in some cases crumbled into fragments. When intact, outer surface with reddish-brown or dull purple endotesta marked with irregular, venous (vein-like) reticulate (net-like) striae; about 1/3 of one end yellowish-white in colour. Embryo small, located in an orbicular (round) pit at the pale yellow end. Relatively hard; broken surface white and starchy. Odourless; taste: mild.

Indications 1. Nocturnal emission 2. Urinary frequency, enuresis, whitish and turbid urine 3. Leukorrhagia 4. Diarrhoea

Chemical Composition Mainly contains starch, proteins and fatty oils.

Semen Ginkgo

Ginkgo Seed
Baiguo
白果

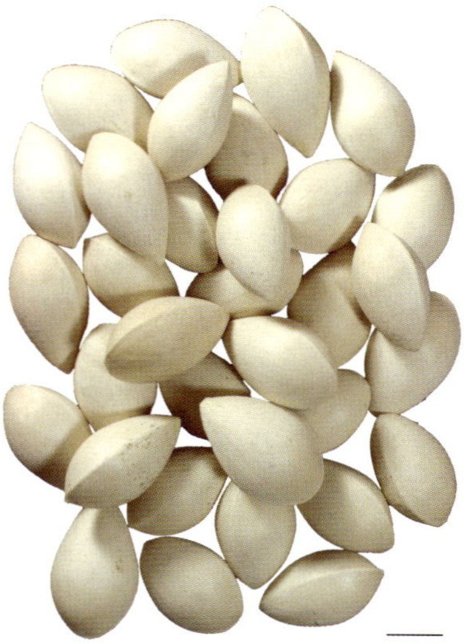

1 cm

Crude drug

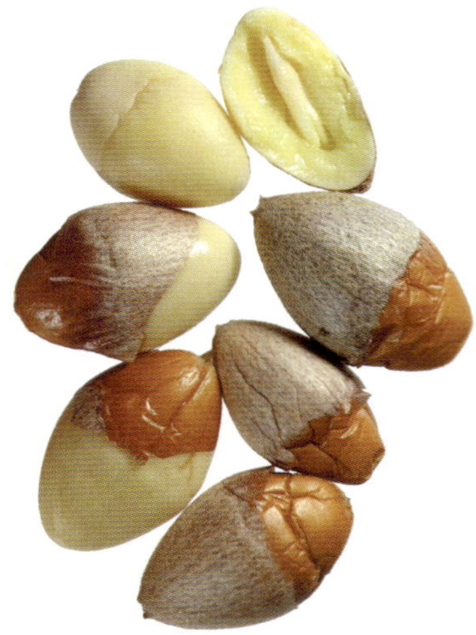

1 cm

Kernel

Source The mature seed of *Ginkgo biloba* L. (Fam. Ginkgoaceae).

Distribution Mainly in Chinese provinces such as Guangxi, Sichuan, Henan, Shandong, Hubei, Liaoning and Jiangsu.

Harvest & Processing Harvest seeds in late autumn after they ripen; remove fleshy exotesta; wash clean; dry under the sun; break shells to get kernels.

Description Seed with exotesta removed: Ovoid (egg-shaped) or ellipsoid (elliptical in long-section and circular in cross-section); 1.5-3 cm long, 1-2.2 cm wide. Outer shell (i.e. mesosperm) bony, smooth; outer surface yellowish-white or pale brownish-yellow; base with an orbicular (round) punctiform (dot-like) protuberance; margin with 1 ridge on each side, occasionally with 3 ridges. Endotesta membranous, dull reddish-brown or pale yellowish-brown; kernel flattened and spherical, pale yellowish-green; endosperms plump, starchy, with clefts in the centre; embryo extremely small. Odourless; taste: slightly sweet, bitter.

Indications 1. Cough and dyspnoea 2. Leukorrhagia, white and turbid urine, urinary frequency, nocturnal emission.

Chemical Composition Contains ginkgotoxin, ginkgolic acid and bilobol.

Semen Hoveniae Dulcis

Japanese Raisin Tree Seed
Zhijuzi
枳椇子

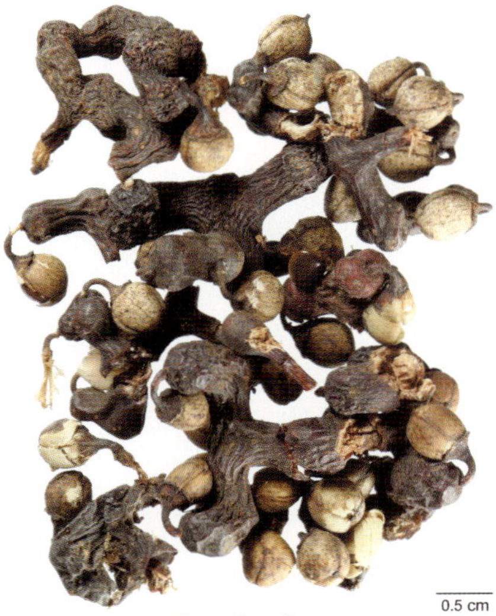

Crude drug
(Fleshy Rachises)

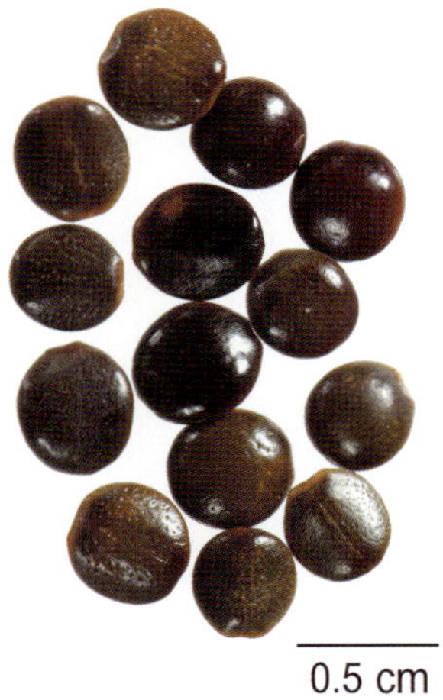

Crude drug
(Seeds)

Source The mature seed of *Hovenia dulcis* Thunb. (Fam. Rhamnaceae). Also used for medicinal purposes is the fleshy rachis.

Distribution Mainly in Chinese provinces such as Shaanxi, Hubei, Jiangsu and Anhui.

Harvest & Processing Harvest fruits together with fleshy rachises in October and November when fruits are ripe; dry under the sun; take out seeds.

Description Seed disc-like; dorsal side slightly protuberant, ventral side relatively flat; 3-5 mm in diameter, 1-1.5 mm thick. Outer surface reddish-brown, brownish-black or greenish-brown, lustrous, scattered pits visible under magnification; indentation at the base with a punctiform (dot-like) hilum pale in colour; apex with a slightly dented chalaza; ventral side with a protuberant, longitudinal raphe. Testa hard; endosperms white; cotyledons pale yellow, plump; endosperms and cotyledons highly oleaginous (oily). Odour: faint; taste: slightly astringent.

Indications 1. Drunkenness 2. Polydipsia 3. Vomiting 4. Dysuria

Chemical Composition Contains alkaloids such as perloyrine and β -carboline.

Note Also used for medicinal purposes is the mature seed of *H. acerba* Lindi and *H. trichocarpa* Chun et Tsiang.

Semen Hyoscyami

Henbane Seed

Tianxianzi

天仙子

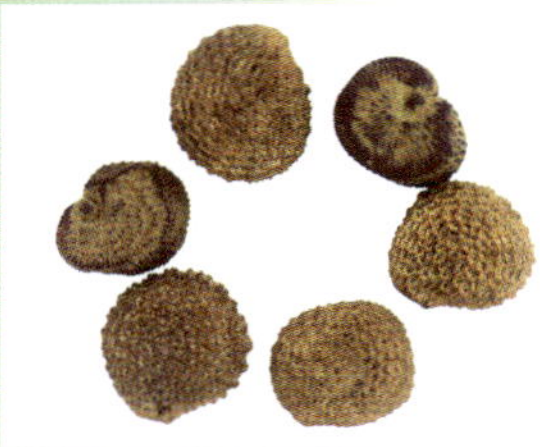

Henbane Seed
Magnified

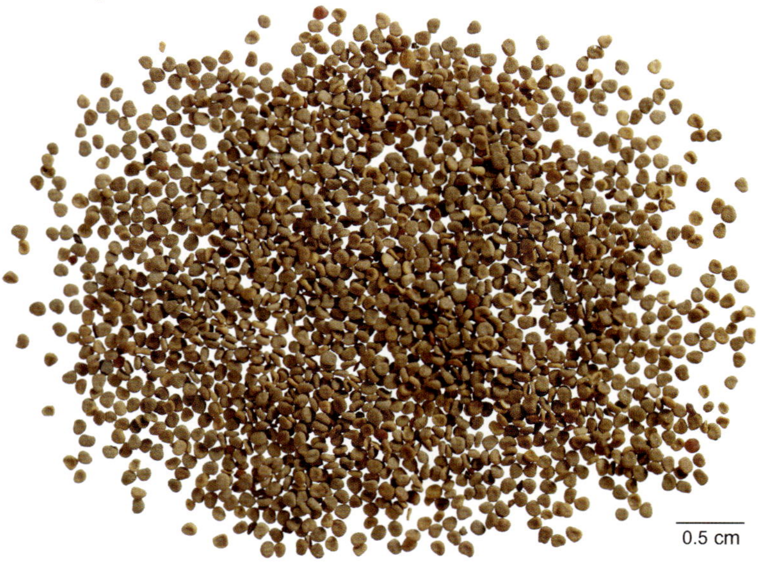

Crude drug

Source The mature seed of *Hyoscyamus niger* L. (Fam. Solanaceae).

Distribution Mainly in Chinese provinces such as Hebei and Henan, and in Inner Mongolia northeastern and northwestern China. Called '*Bei Tianxianzi*' (North Henbane Seed).

Harvest & Processing Pick fruits in summer and autumn when pericarp turns yellow; dry under the sun; thresh to get seeds; sieve away foreign matter; dry seeds under the sun.

Description Somewhat flattened and reniform (kidney-shaped), or flattened and ovoid (egg-shaped); about 1 mm in diameter. Outer surface brownish-yellow or greyish-yellow; dense fine bulgy reticulate (net-like) veins visible under magnification; hilum protuberant. Cross-section greyish-white, oleaginous (oily), with endosperms; embryo curved. Odour: faint; taste: slightly acrid.

Indications 1. Bronchial asthma, chronic bronchitis 2. Epigastric pain, toothache, rheumatic pain, post traumatic pain 3. As anaesthesia.

Chemical Composition Mainly contains hyoscyamine, scopolamine and atropine.

Note Semen Hyoscyami is listed in Hong Kong as Category I (Toxic/Potent) Chinese Materia Medica, and the processed Semen Hyoscyami, Category II.

Semen Impatientis

Garden Balsam Seed

Jixingzi

急性子

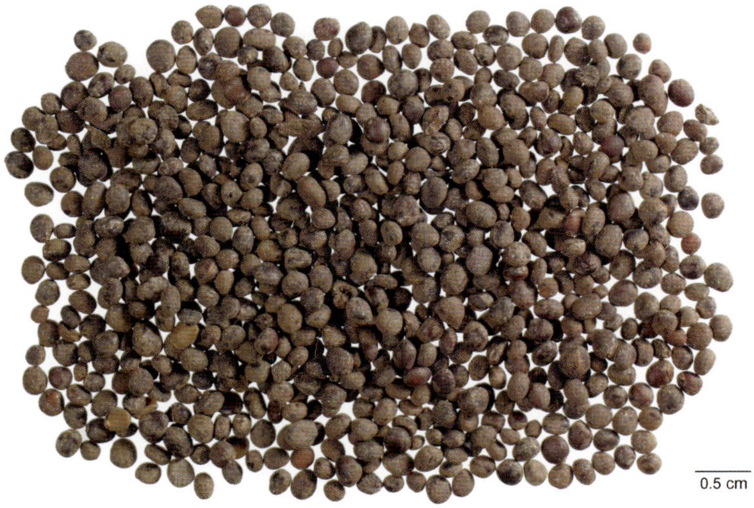

Crude drug

Source The seed of *Impatiens balsamina* L. (Fam. Balsaminaceae).

Distribution Mainly in Chinese provinces such as Jiangsu, Zhejiang, Hebei and Anhui; also in Hong Kong.

Harvest & Processing Pick fruits before maturation throughout August and September; dry under the sun; thresh to get seeds; remove foreign matter.

Description Flattened and spherical, or flattened and ovoid (egg-shaped); 2-3.5 mm long, 2-3 mm wide. Outer surface reddish-brown; rough; densely marked with verruciform (wart-shaped) protuberances and short striae; one end with a protuberant hilum. Hard. When cut open, thin testa revealed; cotyledons 2, greyish-white, plump, translucent, oleaginous (oily). Odour: faint; taste: mild and slightly bitter.

Indications 1. Amenorrhoea, dystocia 2. Dysphagia.

Chemical Composition Mainly contains a peptide Ib-AMP1 which is composed of 20 amino acids.

Note Listed as slightly toxic in *C.P.*

Semen Lablab Album

White Hyacinth Bean
Baibiandou

白扁豆

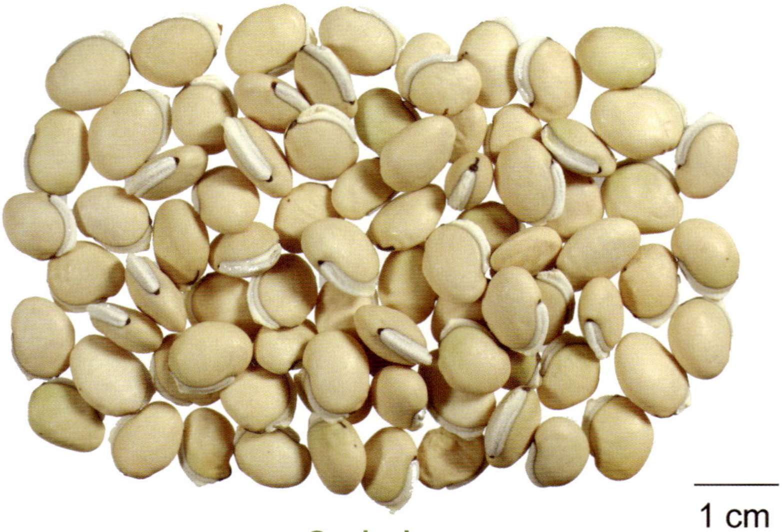

Crude drug

Source The mature seed of *Dolichos lablab* L. (Fam. Leguminosae).

Distribution Mainly in Chinese provinces such as Anhui, Shaanxi, Hunan, Henan, Zhejiang and Shanxi.

Harvest & Processing Pick pods in autumn when seeds are ripe; take out seeds; remove foreign matter; dry under the sun.

Description Flattened and ellipsoid (elliptical in long-section and circular in cross-section), or flattened and ovoid (egg-shaped); 0.8-1.3 cm long, 6-9 mm wide, about 7 mm thick. Outer surface pale yellowish-white or pale yellow, smooth and slightly lustrous, sometimes marked with reddish-brown maculae; margin on one side marked with a protuberant semilunar (half-moon shaped) white caruncle 7-10 mm long; dented hilum exposed when caruncle is peeled off; the end next to the caruncle with a micropyle, the other end with a raphe. Hard; testa thin and brittle; cotyledons 2, plump, yellowish-white. Odour: faint; taste: mild, bean-like when chewed.

Indications 1. Malabsorption and diarrhoea 2. Nausea, vomiting, anorexia 3. Leukorrhagia

Chemical Composition Contains trigonelline, L-2-pipecolic acid and phytoagglutinin.

Semen Lepidii

Pepperweed Seed

Tinglizi

葶藶子

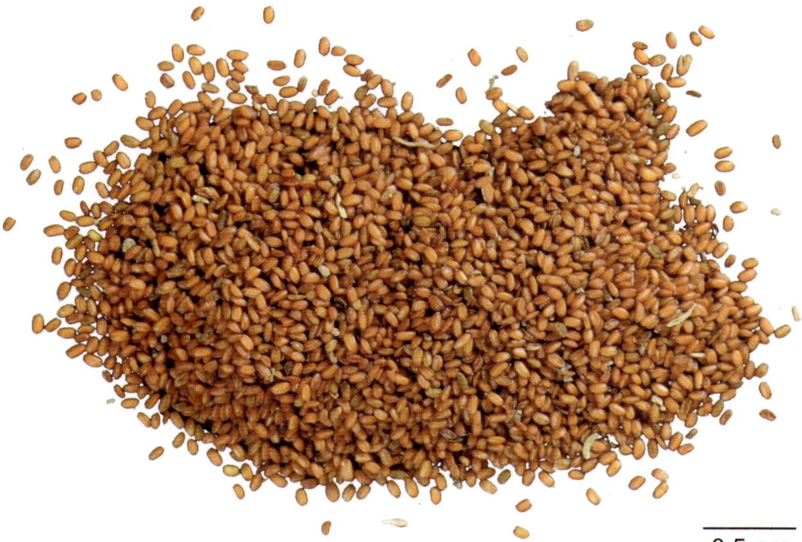

0.5 cm

Crude drug

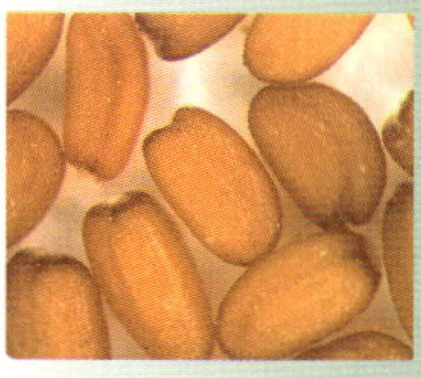

Pepperweed Seed Magnified

Source The mature seed of *Lepidium apetalum* Willd. (Fam. Cruciferae). Customarily called '*Bei tinglizi*' (North Pepperweed Seed).

Distribution Mainly in Chinese provinces such as Hebei and Liaoning, and in Inner Mongolia; also in provinces such as Heilongjiang, Jilin, Shanxi, Shandong, Gansu and Qinghai.

Harvest & Processing Cut off plants promptly in summer and autumn when fruits turn yellowish-green; dry under the sun; thresh to get seeds; remove foreign matter.

Description Flattened and ovoid (egg-shaped); 1-1.5 mm long, 0.5-1 mm wide. Outer surface yellowish-brown or reddish-brown, slightly lustrous, marked with numerous minute granular protuberances and 2 longitudinal shallow grooves, one of the grooves more conspicuous than the other. One end obtuse, the other end acuminate (tapering to a slender point) and slightly dented; indistinct hilum at indentation. Odourless; taste: slightly bitter, acrid. Relatively sticky.

Indications 1. Copious expectoration with cough and dyspnoea 2. Distension in the chest and hypochondrium 3. Oedema 4. Oliguria.

Chemical Composition Contains sinigrin and sinapic acid.

Note According to *C.P.*, also used for medicinal purposes, and commonly known as '*nantinglizi*' (South Pepperweed Seed), is the mature seed of *Descurainia sophia* (L.) Webb ex Prantl, which belongs to the same family as *Lepidium apetalum* Willd.

Semen Lini

Linseed
Yamazi
亞麻子

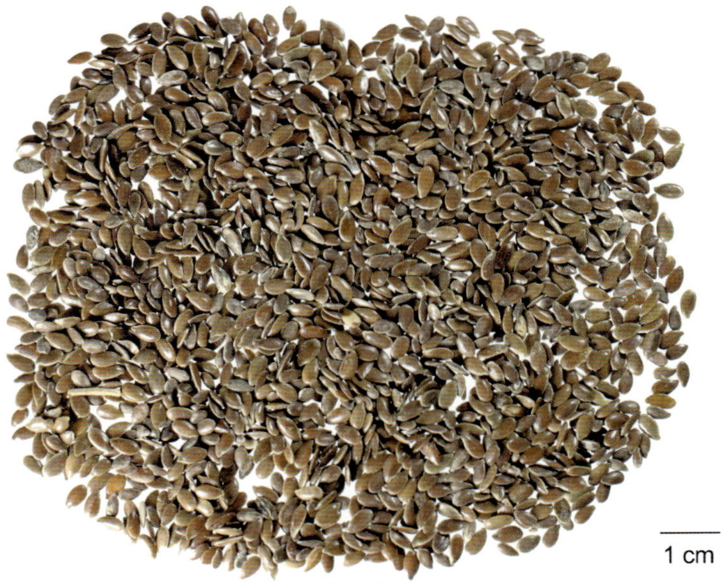

Crude drug

Source The mature seed of *Linum usitatissimum* L. (Fam. Linaceae).

Distribution Mainly in Chinese provinces such as, Heilongjiang, Liaoning and Jilin also in Inner Mongolia.

Harvest & Processing Harvest plants in autumn as fruits ripen; dry under the sun; thresh to get seeds; remove foreign matter; dry seeds under the sun again.

Description Flattened and ovate (egg-shaped); 4-7 mm long, 2-3 mm wide. Outer surface reddish-brown or dull blackish-brown; smooth and lustrous. One end obtuse; the other end, i.e. the apex, with a slightly slanted mucro, and a minute pit visible under magnification. Hilum situated at pit of apex; raphe at margin of one side. Testa thin and brittle; endosperms membranous, brown; cotyledons 2, yellowish-white, highly oleaginous (oily). After being immersed in water, epidermal mucilage of testa swells to form a transparent mucilage membrane enveloping the whole seed. Odourless; taste: bean-like when chewed.

Indications 1. Constipation 2. Dryness and itching of the skin 3. Premature greying of hair, alopecia.

Chemical Composition Contains 30-48% organic acid and trace amounts of linamarin, sterols, triterpenes.

Semen Momordicae

Cochinchina Momordica Seed

Mubiezi

木鱉子

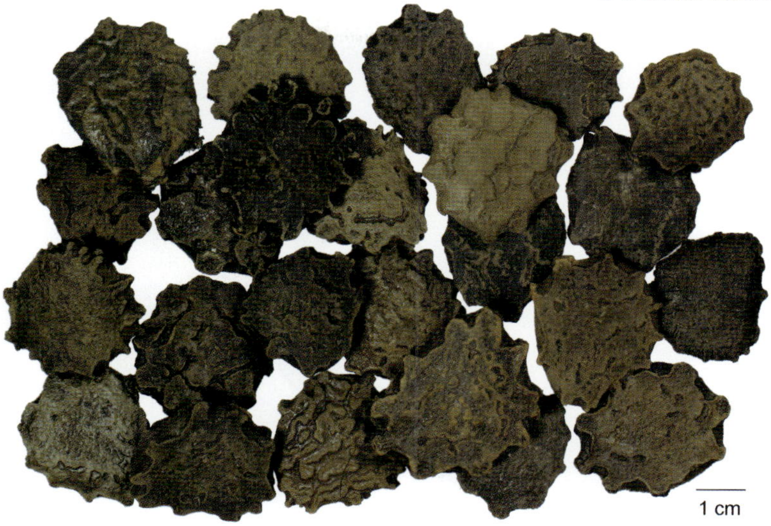

Crude drug

Source The mature seed of *Momordica cochinchinensis* (Lour.) Spreng. (Fam. Cucurbitaceae).

Distribution Mainly in Chinese provinces such as Hubei, Guangxi and Sichuan.

Harvest & Processing Collect fruits in autumn when they are mature; cut open; dry under the sun until half-dry; take out seeds. Alternatively, put fruits in a container, mix with plant ashes and wait until sarcocarp rots away; wash and take out seeds. Dry under the sun or dry by heat. Usually shell is removed to get kernel, which is then pounded into small pieces for use.

Description Flattened, placoid (plate-like), and orbicular (round) or slightly triangular; two sides slightly asymmetrical; slightly bulgy or dented in the centre; 2-4 cm long, 1.5-3.5 cm wide, about 5 mm thick. Outer surface greyish-brown to brownish-black; rough; marked with dented reticulate (net-like) markings or only with fine wrinkles. Margin with over 10 randomly arranged big teeth; the 2 larger teeth marked with a light yellow hilum. Testa hard and brittle; endotesta quite thin, encasing 2 plump, yellowish-white, highly oleaginous (oily) cotyledons. Odour: with a distinctive greasy smell; taste: bitter.

Indications 1. Boils, nodules and swelling of skin 2. Dermatitis

Chemical Composition Mainly contains triterpenes such as momordic acid, gypsogenin.

Note Listed as toxic in *C.P.*

Semen Myristicae

Nutmeg Kernel
Roudoukou

肉豆蔻

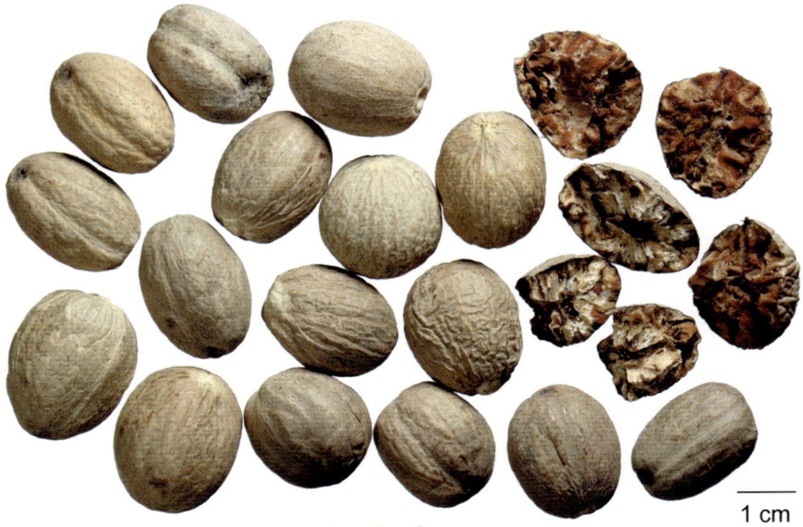

Crude drug

Source The kernel of *Myristica fragrans* Houtt. (Fam. Myristicaceae).

Distribution Mainly in countries like Malaysia, Indonesia and Sri Lanka; also in the West Indies.

Harvest & Processing Pick mature fruits; remove pericarp; peel off aril; dry kernels slowly by roasting at 45°C and turning frequently until they rattle. If roasted at temperatures higher than 45°C, fat will dissolve and evaporate, losing the fragrance and resulting in poorer quality.

Description Ovoid (egg-shaped) or ellipsoid (elliptical in long-section and circular in cross-section); about 3 cm long, about 2 cm in diameter. Outer surface grey or greyish-yellow; marked with reticulate (net-like) grooves; edge on one side marked with a conspicuous longitudinal groove; broad end with a light-coloured orbicular (round) protuberance; narrow end with a dull-coloured indentation. Hard and solid, difficult to break; when broken, surface uneven; longitudinal-section shows a layer of dull brown perisperm on the outside extending inward and intertwining with the off-white endosperm on the inside, forming areca-like markings. Odour: aromatic and strong; taste: pungent and slightly bitter.

Indications 1. Protracted diarrhoea 2. Stomachache 3. Anorexia.

Chemical Composition Monoterpenes, such as α -pinene, (+)-camphene and myristicin exist in its essential oils.

Semen Nelumbinis

Lotus Seed
Lianzi
蓮子

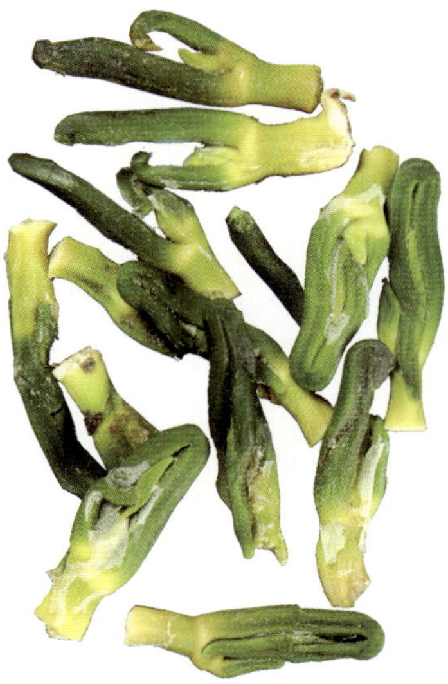

Lotus Plumules 0.5 cm

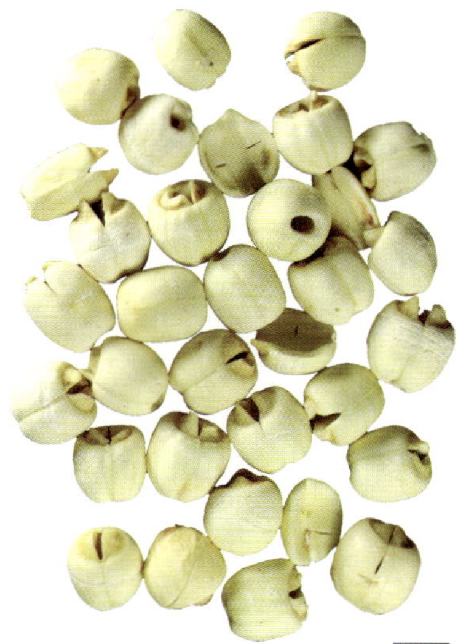

Crude drug 1 cm

Source The mature seed of *Nelumbo nucifera* Gaertn. (Fam. Nymphaeaceae).

Distribution Mainly in Chinese provinces such as Hunan, Hubei, Fujian, Jiangsu and Jiangxi; also in Hong Kong.

Harvest & Processing Cut off lotus seedpods in autumn when fruits ripen; take out fruits; remove fruit shells while fresh; dry seeds under the sun.

Description Slightly ellipsoid (elliptical in long-section and circular in cross-section) or subspherical; 1.2-1.7 cm long; 0.8-1.5 cm in diameter. Outer surface light yellowish-brown to reddish-brown, marked with fine longitudinal striae and relatively thick venous (vein-like) striae; apex with a papilla in the centre; papilla dark brown, often marked with cracks, slightly dented around the edge. Testa thin, stuck fast to cotyledons, does not peel off easily. Hard; 2 plump yellowish-white cotyledons revealed when cut open; centre dented and sulciform (groove-like), with a green lotus plumule. Odourless; taste: sweet and slightly astringent, lotus plumule extremely bitter.

Indications 1. Diarrhoea 2.Nocturnal emission, enuresis, leukorrhagia 3. Palpitation, vexation, insomnia, excessive dreams, tinnitus, soreness and weakness of the back and lower extremities

Chemical Composition The lotus plumule contains alkaloids such as liensinine and pronuciferine and flavonoids such as rutin.

Note Also used as lotus plumule for medicinal purposes are the young leaf and radicle of *Nelumbo nucifera* Gaertn.

Semen Nigellae

Fennelflower Seed
Heizhongcaozi

黑種草子

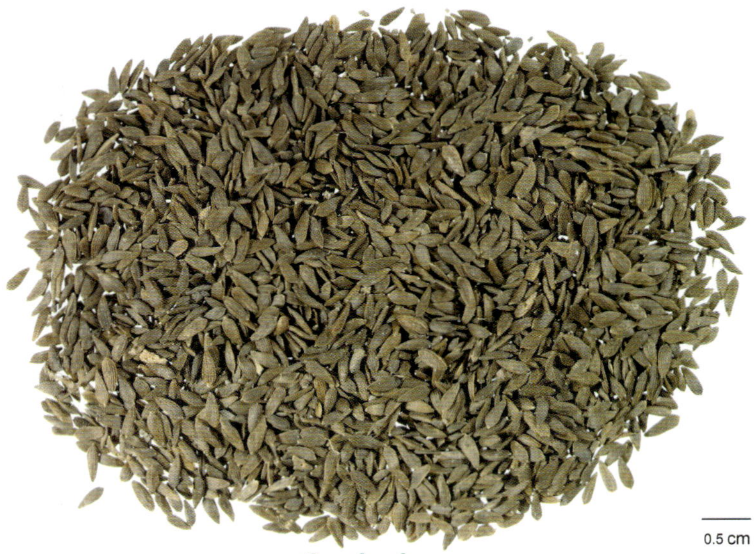

Crude drug

Source The mature seed of *Nigella glandulifera* Freyn et Sint. (Fam. Ranunculaceae).

Distribution Mainly in Xinjiang, China.

Harvest & Processing Harvest mature seeds in autumn; remove sand, soil and pericarp; dry seeds under the sun.

Description Triangular and ovate (egg-shaped); outer surface black; 2.5-3 mm long, 1-2 mm in diameter. Top end narrow and pointed, with a hilar spot; bottom end a little obtuse; outer surface rough, with irregular protuberances. Relatively hard, does not break easily; when broken, surface greyish-white, highly oleaginous (oily). Odour: with a distinctive fragrance; taste: acrid.

Indications 1. Tinnitus and forgetfulness 2. Amenorrhoea, insufficient lactation 3. Urinary infection, urolithiasis.

Chemical Composition Mainly contains flavonoid glycosides such as nigeglanoside.

Semen Oroxyli

Indian Trumptflower Seed
Muhudie
木蝴蝶

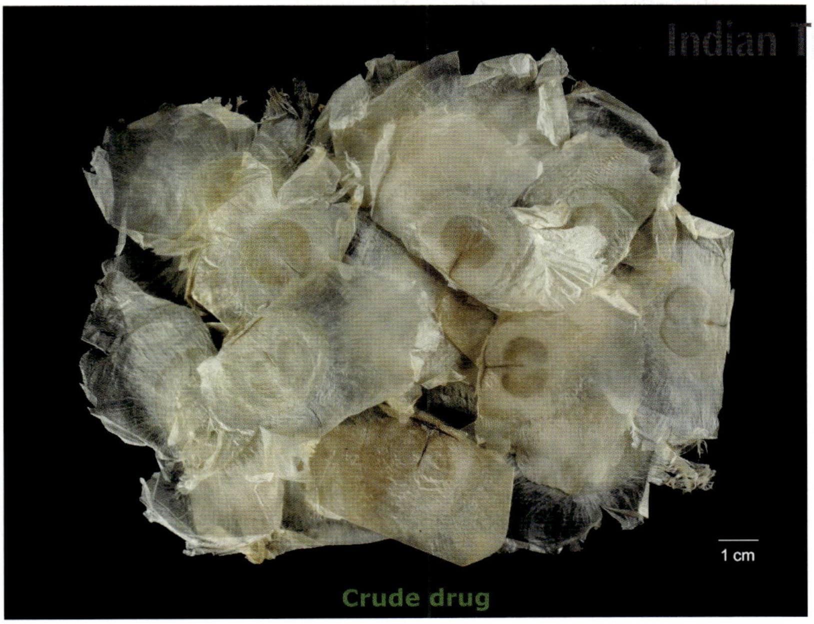

Crude drug

Source The mature seed of *Oroxylum indicum* (L.) Vent. (Fam. Bignoniaceae).

Distribution Mainly in Chinese provinces such as Yunnan, Guangxi and Guizhou; also in provinces such as Fujian, Guangdong and Sichuan, and in Hong Kong.

Harvest & Processing Collect mature fruits in autumn and winter; dry under strong sunlight until fruits crack; take out seeds; dry under the sun.

Description Sub-elliptical and lamellar (like a thin plate); 2-3 cm long, 1.5-2 cm wide. Outer surface light yellowish-white; with silky lustre. Testa extending on three sides, forming wide wings; each wing about 2.5 cm wide, membranous and translucent, marked with radial markings, with margin mostly broken. Upon removal of testa, membranous endosperms can be seen tightly covering the cotyledons. Cotyledons 2, flattened and papilionaceous (butterfly-shaped); yellowish-green or light yellow; long diameter about 1.5 cm, short diameter about 1 cm. Radicle conspicuous. Odour: faint; taste: slightly bitter.

Indications 1. Sore throat 2. Cough.

Chemical Composition Mainly contains oroxin A, B and chrysin.

Semen Persicae

Peach Seed
Taoren

桃仁

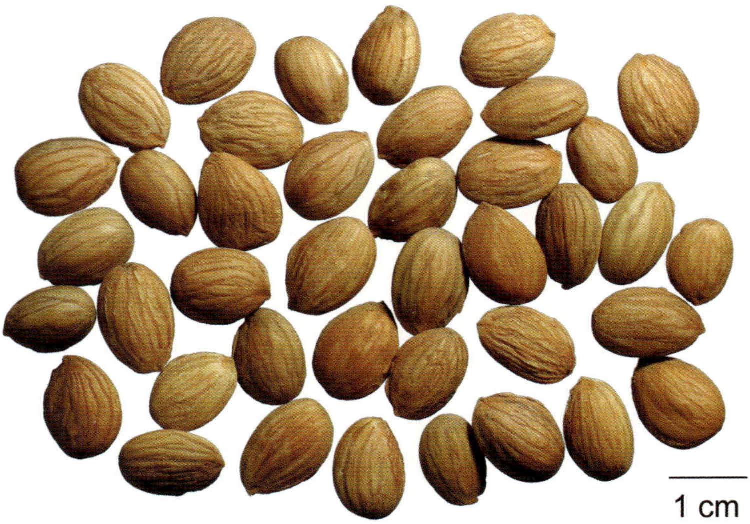

Crude drug

Source The mature seed of *Prunus persica* (L.) Batsch (Fam. Rosaceae).

Distribution Mainly in Chinese provinces such as Sichuan, Shaanxi, Hebei and Shandong; also in Hong Kong.

Harvest & Processing Harvest mature fruits; remove sarcocarp and putamens; take out seeds; dry under the sun.

Description Oblong and ovoid (egg-shaped), flattened; 1.2-1.8 cm long, 0.8-1.2 cm wide, 2-4 mm thick. Top end pointed; middle part bulgy; base obtuse and oblique (with unequal sides); margin thin. Testa yellowish-brown to reddish-brown; marked with longitudinal wrinkles; with numerous venous (vein-like) striae branching out from chalaza at base. One side of pointed end with 1 angular, linear (long and narrow) hilum. Testa thin; peels off easily; containing 2 highly oleaginous (oily) cotyledons. Odour: faint; taste: slightly bitter.

Indications 1. Dysmenorhoea, amenorrhoea 2. Trauma 3. Constipation.

Chemical Composition Mainly contains a variety of glycoside, such as amygdalin.

Note According to *C.P.*, also used for medicinal purposes is the mature seed of *P. davidiana* (Carr.) Franch.

Semen Pharbitidis

Pharbitis Seed
Qianniuzi
牽牛子

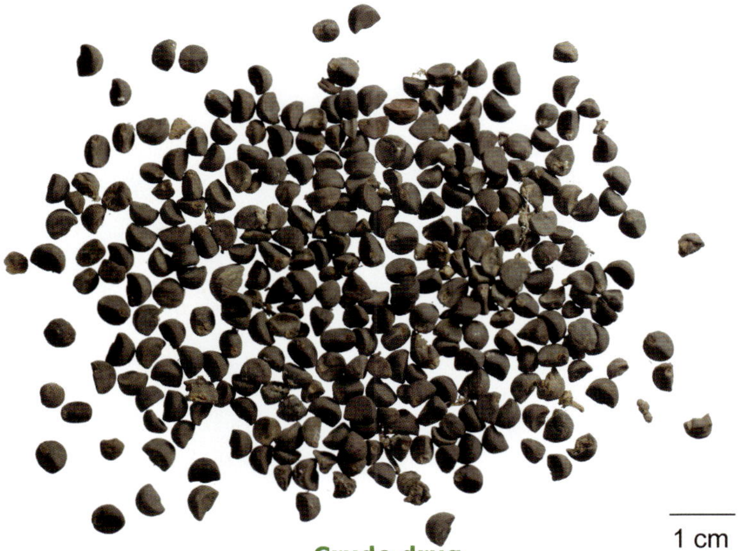

Crude drug

Source The mature seed of *Pharbitis nil* (L.) Choisy (Fam. Convolvulaceae).

Distribution Mainly in Liaoning province in China; naturally grown or cultivated in all provinces in China; also in Hong Kong.

Harvest & Processing Harvest plants in late autumn when fruits have ripened but not yet dehisced (split open at maturity); dry under the sun; thresh to get seeds; remove foreign matter.

Description Seed the shape of a segment of orange; 4-8 mm long, 3-5 mm wide. Outer surface greyish-black or pale yellowish-white; dorsal side with a shallow longitudinal groove, lower end of ridge on ventral side with a slightly dented punctiform (dot-like) hilum. Hard; cross-section shows pale yellow or yellowish-green cotyledons; cotyledons shrivelled, folded and slightly oleaginous (oily). After being soaked in water, testa becomes rimose (with fissures or cracks), viscid and slippery. Odourless; taste: acrid and bitter, tongue-numbing.

Indications 1. Oedema, ascites due to liver cirrhosis 2. Constipation 3. Abdominal pain due to parasitosis

Chemical Composition Mainly contains pharbitin.

Note According to *C.P.*, also used for medicinal purposes and listed as toxic is the mature seed of *P. purpurea* (L.) Voigt.

Semen Phaseoli

Rice Bean
Chixiaodou

赤小豆

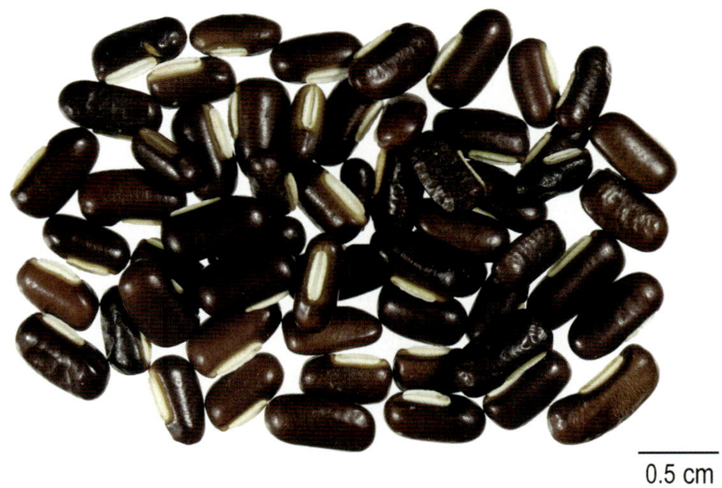

Crude drug

Source The mature seed of *Vigna umbellata* (Thunb.) Ohwi et Ohashi (Fam. Leguminosae).

Distribution Mainly in Chinese provinces such as Jilin, Hebei, Shaanxi, Shandong, Anhui, Jiangsu, Jiangxi, Guangdong and Yunnan.

Harvest & Processing Dig out whole plants in autumn when pods have ripened but not yet dehisced (split open at maturity); dry under the sun and thresh to get seeds; remove foreign matter and dry seeds under the sun again.

Description Cylindrical and slightly flattened; both ends truncate (squared as if cut off) or obtuse; 5-7 mm long, 3-5 mm in diameter. Outer surface purplish-red or dull reddish-brown, smooth, slightly lustrous or lustreless; the edge on one side with a protuberant linear (long and narrow) hilum near one end; hilum white, about 2/3 of seed length, dented in the centre, forming a longitudinal groove; the other edge with an indistinct raphe. Hard; does not break easily. When cut open, thin and brittle testa exposed; cotyledons 2, milky-white, plump; radicle slender and bending towards one end. Odour: faint; taste: slightly sweet; bean-like when chewed.

Indications 1. Dysuria, oedema, ascites 2. Diarrhoea, jaundice 3. Skin infection (orally and external use).S

Chemical Composition Mainly contains triterpene saponins and condensed tannins.

Note According to *C.P.,* also used for medicinal purposes is the mature seed of *V. angularis* (Wild.) Ohwi et Ohashi.

Semen Plantaginis

Plantain Seed
Cheqianzi
車前子

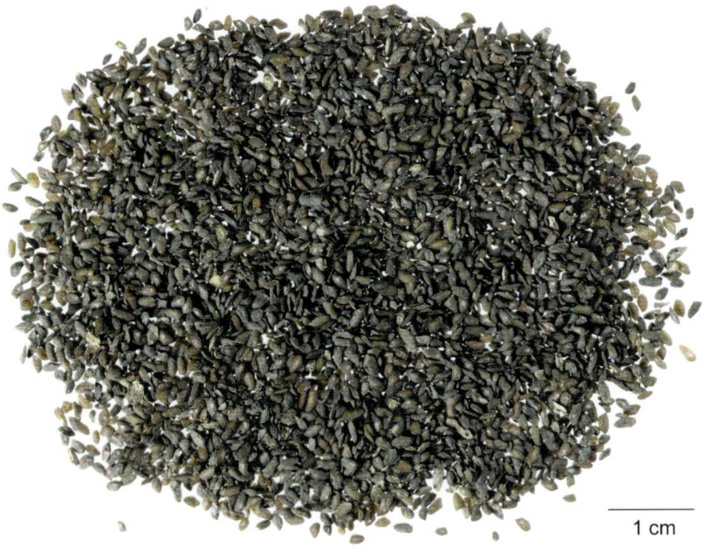

Crude drug

Source The mature seed of *Plantago asiatica* L. (Fam. Plantaginaceae).

Distribution In all parts of China, including Hong Kong.

Harvest & Processing Collect fruit-spikes in summer and autumn when seeds are mature; dry under the sun; rub to get seeds; remove foreign matter.

Description Ellipsoid (elliptical in long-section and circular in cross-section), or somewhat oblong and spherical, or triangular, oblong and spherical; slightly flattened; about 2 mm long, about 1 mm wide. Outer surface yellowish-brown to dull blackish-brown, marked with fine wrinkles; one side with a dented, punctiform (dot-like), greyish-white hilum. Hard. Odour: faint; taste: mild.

Indications 1. Urinary stones and infections, nephritic oedema 2. Diarrhoea 3. Cold, cough, bronchitis 4. Acute conjunctivitis 5. Hypertension

Chemical Composition Mainly contains iridoid glycosides such as aucubin.

Note According to *C.P.*, also used for medicinal purposes is the mature seed of *P. depressa* Willd.

Semen Platycladi

Chinese Arborvitae Kernel

Baiziren

柏子仁

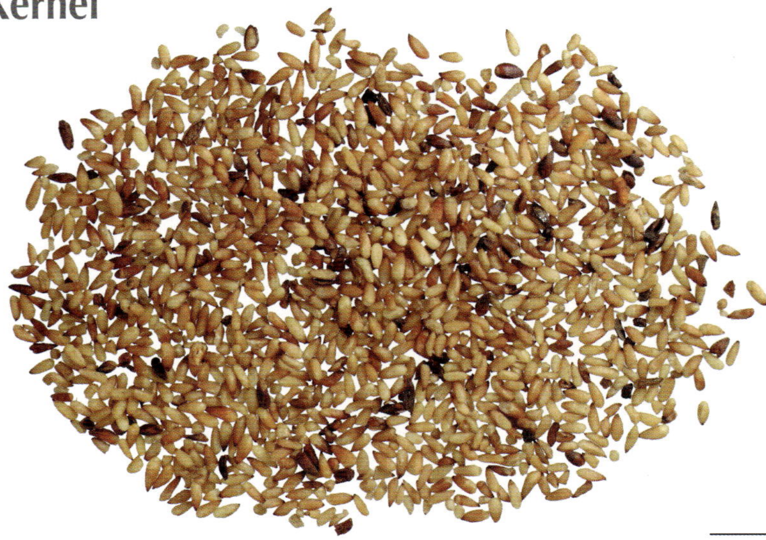

Crude drug 1 cm

Source
The mature kernel of *Platycladus orientalis* (L.) Franco (Fam. Cupressaceae).

Distribution
Mainly in Chinese provinces such as Shandong, Hebei, Henan, Shaanxi, Hubei, Gansu and Yunnan.

Harvest & Processing
Harvest mature cones in autumn and winter; dry under the sun; collect and husk seeds; sieve away testa.

Description
Oblong and ovoid (egg-shaped) to oblong and ellipsoid (elliptical in long-section and circular in cross-section); 3-7 mm long, 1.5-3 mm in diameter. Pale yellow or yellowish-white while fresh; colour darkens and becomes yellowish-brown after long storage. Enveloped in membranous endotesta; apex slightly pointed, orbicular (round) and triangular, marked with dark brown dots; base obtuse, lighter in colour. When broken, surface milky-white to yellowish-white; endosperms relatively well-developed; cotyledons 2 or more, highly oleaginous (oily). Odour: slightly fragrant; taste: mild. Greasy.

Indications
1. Apprenhension, severe palpitation, excessive dreams, forgetfulness and night sweating, anxiety, neurasthenia 2. Constipation.

Chemical Composition
Mainly contains cedrol.

Semen Pruni

Chinese Dwarf Cherry Seed

Yuliren

郁李仁

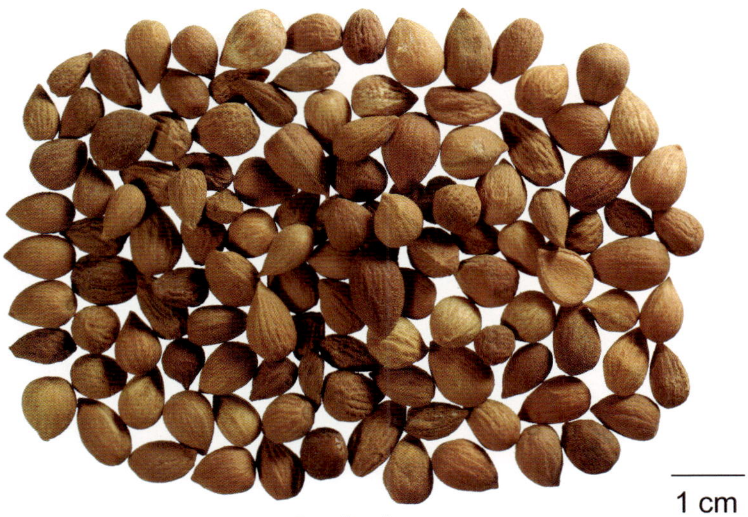

Crude drug

Source The mature seed of *Prunus humilis* Bunge(Fam. Rosaceae).

Distribution Mainly in Chinese provinces such as Liaoning, Heilongjiang, Hebei and Shandong.

Harvest & Processing Harvest mature fruits in summer and autumn; remove sarcocarp and putamens; take out seeds; dry.

Description Ovoid (egg-shaped); 5-8 mm long, 3-5 mm in diameter. Outer surface yellowish-white or light brown; one end pointed, the other obtuse. Pointed end with a linear (long and narrow) hilum on one side; obtuse end with a dark-coloured chalaza in the centre; numerous longitudinal venous (vein-like) striae of vascular bundles branching upwards from chalaza. Testa thin; cotyledons 2, milky-white, highly oleaginous (oily). Odour: faint; taste: slightly bitter.

Indications 1. Constipation, habitual constipation 2. Oedema, dysuria

Chemical Composition Mainly contains amygdalin, prunuside A, B and ursolic acid.

Note According to *C.P.*, also used for medicinal purposes is the mature seed of *P. japonica* Thunb. and *P. pedunculata* Maxim.

Semen Raphani

Radish Seed

Laifuzi

萊菔子

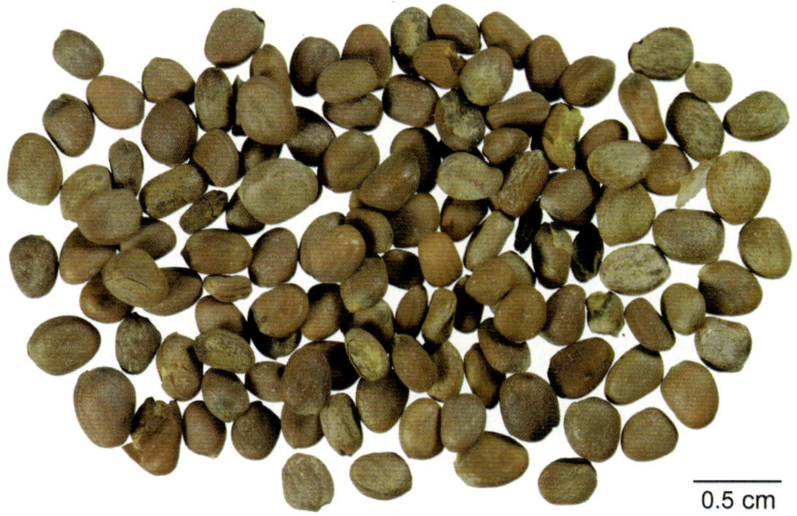

Crude drug

Source The mature seed of *Raphanus sativus* L. (Fam. Cruciferae).

Distribution In all parts of China.

Harvest & Processing Harvest plants in summer when fruits are ripe; thresh to get seeds; remove foreign matter; dry under the sun.

Description Suborbicular (almost round) or ellipsoid (elliptical in long-section and circular in cross-section), slightly flattened; 2-4 mm long, 2-3 mm wide. Testa thin. Outer surface reddish-brown, yellowish-brown or dark greyish-brown, with fine, dense reticulate (net-like) striae visible under magnification; seed marked with several longitudinal grooves along the edge on one side and a black hilum at one end. Cotyledons 2, milky-yellow, plump, longitudinally folded; oleaginous (oily). Odour: faint; taste: slightly acrid.

Indications 1. Severe dyspepsia with feeling of oppression in the chest, abdominal distension, belching, acid regurgitation, diarrhoea 2. Constipation 3. Productive cough and dyspnoea

Chemical Composition Contains sinapine and raphanin.

Semen Ricini

Castor Seed
Bimazi
蓖麻子

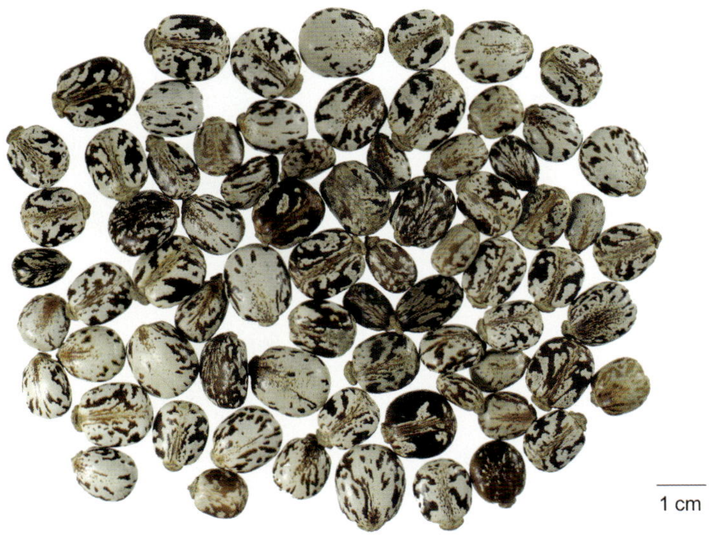

Crude drug

Source The mature seed of *Ricinus communis* L. (Fam. Euphorbiaceae).

Distribution In most regions of China, including Hong Kong.

Harvest & Processing Harvest fruits which have ripened but not yet dehisced (split open at maturity) in autumn; spread out and dry under the sun; take out seeds; remove foreign matter.

Description Ellipsoid (elliptical in long-section and circular in cross-section) or ovoid (egg-shaped), slightly flattened; 0.9-1.8 cm long, 0.5-1 cm wide. Outer surface smooth, marked with alternating greyish-white and dull blackish-brown or alternating yellowish-brown and reddish-brown striae. One side relatively flat, the other relatively bulgy; the flatter side with 1 protuberant raphe; one end with a protuberant greyish-white or light brown caruncle. Testa thin and brittle; endosperms plump, white, highly oleaginous (oily); cotyledons 2, thin. Odourless; taste: slightly bitter-acrid.

Indications 1. Dermatitis (external use) 2. Constipation (castor oil is used as purgative).

Chemical Composition Mainly contains fatty oils.

Semen Sesami Nigrum

Black Sesame
Heizhima

黑芝麻

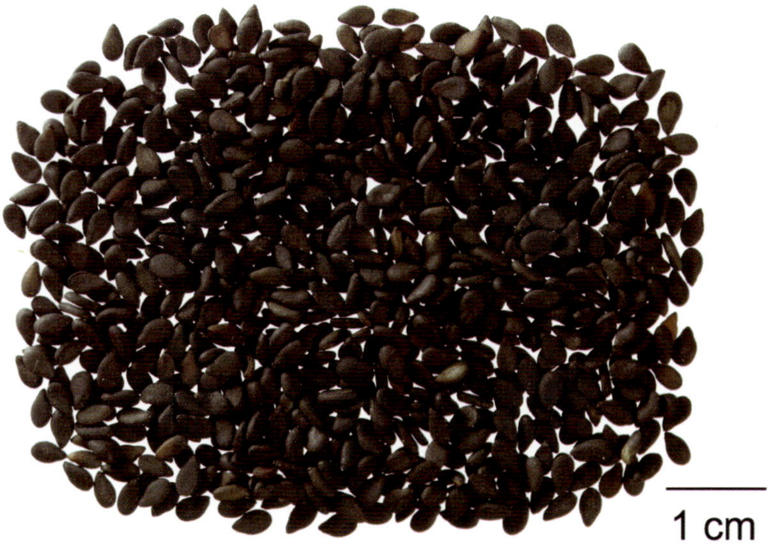

Crude drug

Source The black seed of *Sesamum indicum* L. (Fam. Pedaliaceae).

Distribution Mainly in Chinese provinces such as Shandong, Henan, Hubei, Sichuan, Anhui, Jiangxi and Hebei.

Harvest & Processing Cut off whole plants in August and September when fruits turn yellowish-black; tie up in small bundles with top end pointing upwards; dry under the sun; thresh to get seeds; remove foreign matter; dry under the sun again.

Description Flattened and ovate (egg-shaped); 2-4 mm long, 1-2 mm in diameter, about 1 mm thick. Outer surface black, smooth or marked with reticulate (net-like) wrinkles, verruculose (with small wart-shaped protuberances) under magnification; margin smooth or angular; apex with a punctiform (dot-like) brown hilum. Testa papery; endosperms white, fleshy, enveloping embryo in a thin layer; embryo relatively well-developed, erect; cotyledons 2, white, highly oleaginous (oily). Odour: faint; taste: mild, but fresh and fragrant when chewed.

Indications 1. Dizziness, blurred vision, tinnitus, impaired hearing 2. Premature greying of hair, alopecia after a severe disease 3. Constipation.

Chemical Composition Mainly contains lignans such as sesamin and sesamolin.

Semen Sinapis

Mustard Seed

Jiezi

芥子

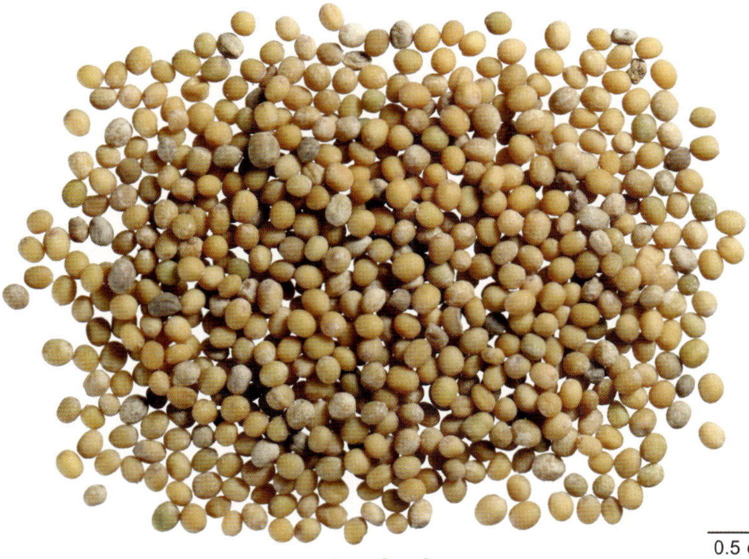

0.5 cm

Crude drug

Source The mature seed of *Sinapis alba* L. (Fam. Cruciferae). Customarily called '*Bai Jiezi*' (White Mustard Seed).

Distribution Mainly in Chinese provinces such as Anhui, Henan, Sichuan and Shaanxi.

Harvest & Processing Harvest plants in late summer and early autumn when fruits ripen; dry under the sun, thresh to get seeds, remove foreign matter.

Description Spherical; 1-2.5 mm in diameter. Outer surface greyish-white to yellowish-white; fine reticulate (net-like) striae visible under magnification; one end with a dull punctiform (dot-like) hilum. When cracked open, folded, highly oleaginous (oily), yellowish-white cotyledons revealed. Odourless; taste: acrid and hot.

Indications 1. Distension in the chest and hypochondrium 2. Dyspnoea 3. Arthralgia, neuralgia

Chemical Composition Mainly contains glucosinolate.

Note According to *C.P.*, also used for medicinal purposes, and customarily known as '*Huang jiezi*' (Yellow Mustard Seed), is the mature seed of *Brassica juncea* (L.) Czern et Coss, which belongs to the same family as *Sinapis alba* L.

Semen Sterculiae Lychnophorae

Boat-fruited Steculia Seed

Pangdahai

胖大海

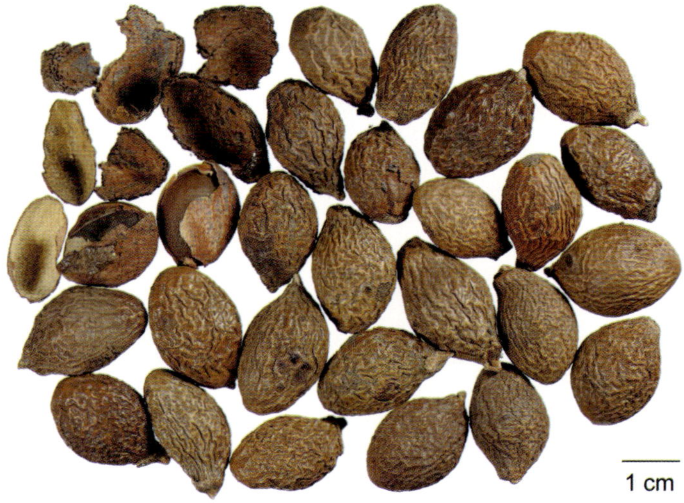

Crude drug

Source The mature seed of *Sterculia lychnophora* Hance (Fam. Sterculiaceae).

Distribution Mainly in countries such as Vietnam, Thailand and Indonesia.

Harvest & Processing Collect mature seeds from April to June when fruits dehisce (split open at maturity); dry under the sun. Since boat-fruited sterculia seeds will germinate when the exotesta swells upon contact with water, they must be harvested promptly once the fruits ripen.

Description Spindle-shaped or ellipsoid (elliptical in long-section and circular in cross-section). Apex obtuse; base slightly pointed, slanted and with an orbicular (round) light-coloured hilum; outer surface brown or dull brown, slightly lustrous, with irregular shrivelled wrinkles. Exotesta extremely thin; brittle; falls off easily. Mesosperm thicker; dull dark brown; loose, breaks easily; swells up to become spongilliform (sponge-like) upon contact with water. When broken, surface shows scattered resinoid (resin-like) dots. Endotesta detachable from mesosperm, slightly coriaceous (leathery), containing 2 plump, broad and ovate (egg-shaped) endosperms; 2 thin cotyledons attached to the inner side of endosperms, each the same size as endosperms. Odour: faint; taste: mild, sticky when chewed.

Indications 1. Hoarseness of voice, dry cough, dry and sore throat 2. Constipation 3. Headache 4. Conjunctivitis.

Chemical Composition Bassorin exist in the external layer of the seeds; galactose exists in the fruits.

Semen Strychni

Nux Vomica
Maqianzi
馬錢子

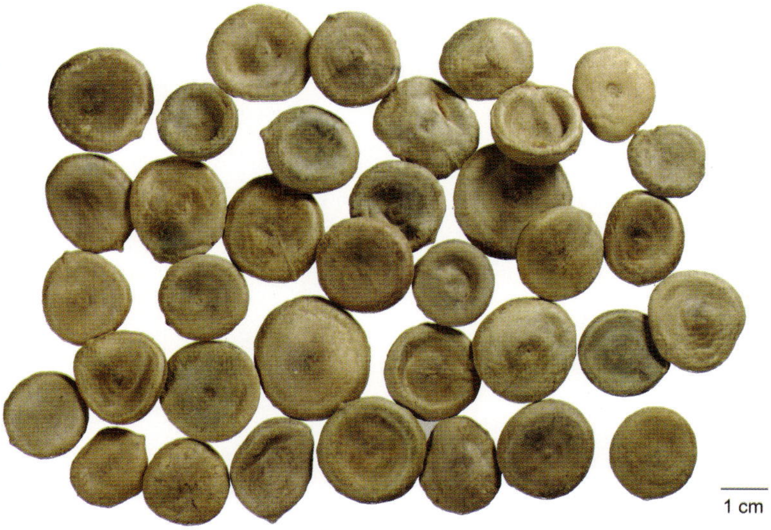

Crude drug

Source The mature seed of *Strychnos nux-vomica* L. (Fam. Loganiaceae).

Distribution Mainly in countries such as India, Vietnam and Thailand; also in Chinese provinces such as Fujian, Gaungdong and Taiwan.

Harvest & Processing Harvest mature fruits in winter; take out seeds; wash away attached sarcocarp; dry the seeds under the sun.

Description Button-shaped or disc-shaped, usually slightly bulgy on one side and slightly dented on the other; 1.5-3 cm in diameter, 3-6 mm thick. Outer surface densely covered with greyish-brown or greyish-green pubescence silky in texture and lustre and radiating from the centre. Margin slightly bulgy and thicker, with a protuberant micropyle; centre of underside with a protuberant, punctiform (dot-like), orbicular (round) hilum. Hard. When cut open along margin, surface shows pale yellowish-white cuticular endosperms; cotyledons cordate (heart-shaped), with 5-7 veins and a short radicle. Odourless; taste: extremely bitter.

Indications 1. Chronic arthritis, rheumatoid arthralgia, numbness and paralysis of limbs, sequela of poliomyelitis, post traumatic pain 2. Boils and sores.

Chemical Composition Mainly contains alkaloids such as strychnine and brucine.

Note According to *C.P.*, also used for medicinal purposes is a processed Semen Strychni called '*Maqianzi fen*' (Nux Vomica Powder). Semen Strychni and *S. wallichiana* Stead. cx DC. are listed in Hong Kong as Category I (Toxic/Potent) Chinese Materia Medica, and the processed Semen Strychni, Category II.

Semen Trichosanthis

Snakegourd Seed
Gualouzi

瓜蔞子

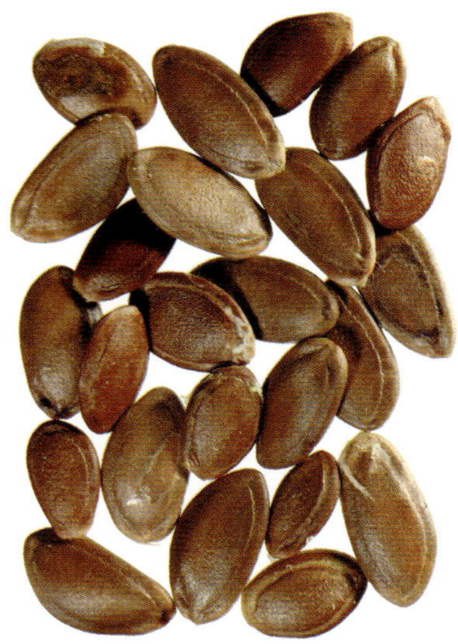

Crude drug 1 cm

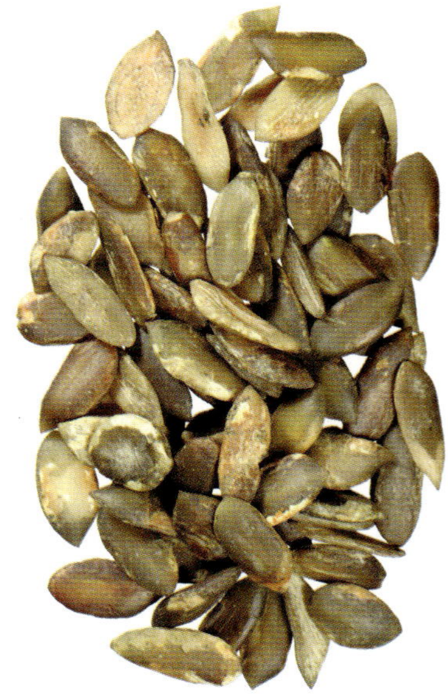

Crude drug 1 cm

Source The mature seed of *Trichosanthes kirilowii* Maxim. (Fam. Cucurbitaceae).

Distribution Mainly in Chinese provinces such as Shandong; also in provinces such as Hebei, Shanxi and Shaanxi.

Harvest & Processing Collect mature fruits in autumn; cut open fruits to get seeds; wash clean; dry under the sun. Alternatively, soak fruits in water for several days; pound open and take out seeds; wash seeds clean; dry under the sun.

Description Ovate (egg-shaped) and elliptical, flat; 1.1-1.6 cm long, 0.8-1.2 cm wide, about 3.5 mm thick. Outer surface yellowish-brown to brown, smooth, marked with a loop of rather indistinct groove near the margin; one end narrower and with a hilum, the other end obtuse. Testa hard; when cracked open, 2 cotyledons exposed; kernel yellowish-white or greenish, highly oleaginous (oily). Odour: faint; taste: mild.

Indications 1. Cough with sticky sputum, feeling of oppression in the chest 2. Constipation 3. Abscess.

Chemical Composition Contains sterols, fatty acids and triterpenes.

Note According to *C.P.*, also used for medicinal purposes and commonly used in Hong Kong is the mature seed of *T. rosthornii* Harms.

Semen Trigonellae

Common Fenugreek Seed

Huluba

胡蘆巴

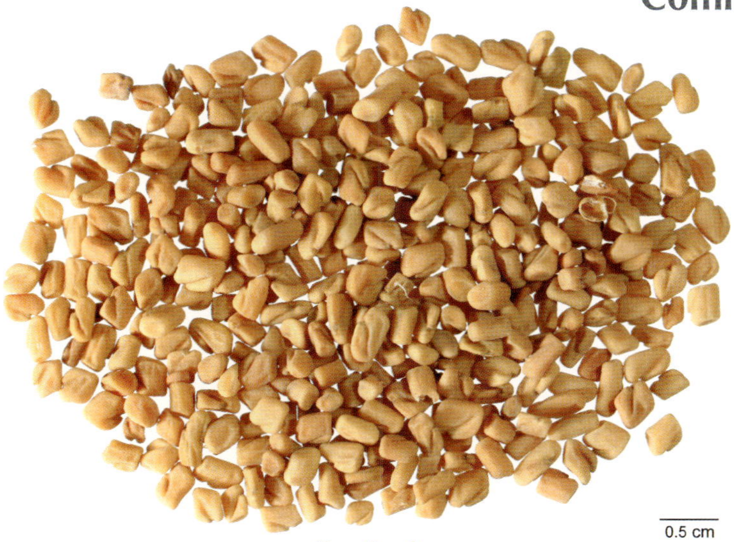

Crude drug

Source The mature seed of *Trigonella foenum-graecum* L. (Fam. Leguminosae).

Distribution Mainly in Chinese provinces such as Anhui, Sichuan and Henan.

Harvest & Processing Harvest whole plants when fruits are ripe; dry under the sun; take out seeds; remove foreign matter; dry seeds under the sun.

Description Slightly rhombic, slightly pointed at one end; 3-4 mm long, 2-3 mm wide, about 2 mm thick. Outer surface pale yellowish-brown to pale brown, smooth, with a deep groove on each side sloping towards and meeting at the punctiform (dot-like) hilum. Hard, does not break easily. When cut longitudinally, thin testa revealed; endosperms translucent, viscid upon contact with water; cotyledons 2, pale yellow; radicle thick, long and curved. Odour: faint; taste: slightly bitter.

Indications 1. Pain and cold feeling in the lower abdomen 2. Hernia 3. Weakness and oedema of the legs.

Chemical Composition Contains trigonelline, vitexin and diosgenin.

Semen Vaccariae

Cowherb Seed
Wangbuliuxing

王不留行

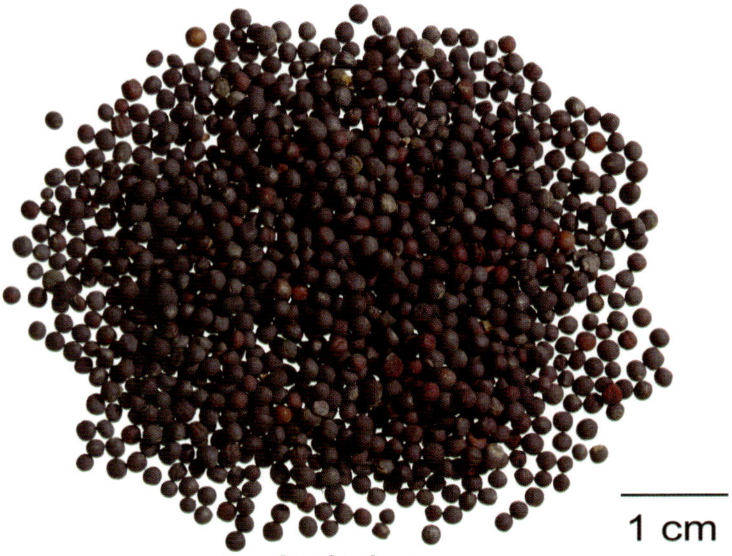

Crude drug

Source The mature seed of *Vaccaria segetalis* (Neck.) Garcke (Fam. Caryophyllaceae).

Distribution Mainly in Chinese provinces such as Jiangsu, Hebei, Henan and Shaanxi.

Harvest & Processing Harvest plants in summer when fruits are mature but pericarp has not yet dehisced (split at maturity); dry fruits under the sun; thresh to get seeds; remove foreign matter; dry under the sun again.

Description Spherical; about 2 mm in diameter. Outer surface black, a few immature ones brownish-red; slightly lustrous. Evenly distributed granular protuberances visible on testa surface under magnification; hilum suborbicular (almost round) and dented, with a shallow taenioid (ribbon-like) groove on one side. Hard; milky-white endosperms exposed when cracked open; embryo curved like a ring; cotyledons 2. Odourless; taste: mild.

Indications 1. Acute mastitis, insufficient lactation, galactostasis 2. Dysmenorrhoea, amenorrhoea, dystocia 3. Carbuncle 4. Stranguria with haematuria.

Chemical Composition Mainly contains vacsegoside A, B, C, D and flavonoid glycosides.

Semen Ziziphi Spinosae

Spina Date Seed

Suanzaoren

酸棗仁

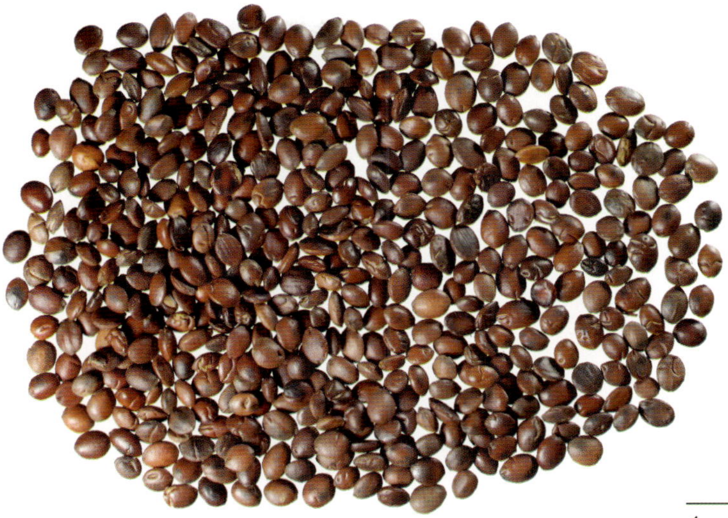

Crude drug

Source The mature seed of *Ziziphus jujuba* Mill. var. *spinosa* (Bunge) Hu ex H. F. Chou (Fam. Rhamnaceae).

Distribution Mainly in Chinese provinces such as Hebei, Shaanxi, Liaoning and Henan.

Harvest & Processing Harvest mature fruits in late autumn and early winter; remove sarcocarp and putamens; collect seeds; dry under the sun.

Description Flattened and spherical, or flattened and ellipsoid (elliptical in long-section and circular in cross-section); 5-9 mm long, 5-7 mm wide, about 3 mm thick. Outer surface purplish-red or dull purplish-brown; smooth and lustrous; sometimes marked with cracks. Under magnification, one side relatively smooth and with a protuberant longitudinal wrinkle in the centre, the other side slightly bulgy. One end dented, with a linear (long and narrow) hilum; the other end with a small protuberant chalaza. Testa relatively brittle; endosperms white; cotyledons 2, light yellow, highly oleaginous (oily). Odour: faint; taste: mild.

Indications 1. Neurasthenia, insomnia, forgetfulness 2. Palpitations 3. For general debility with spontaneous sweating and night sweating.

Chemical Composition Mainly contains alkaloids and triterpene saponins.

Spica Prunellae

Common Selfheal Fruit-Spike
Xiakucao

夏枯草

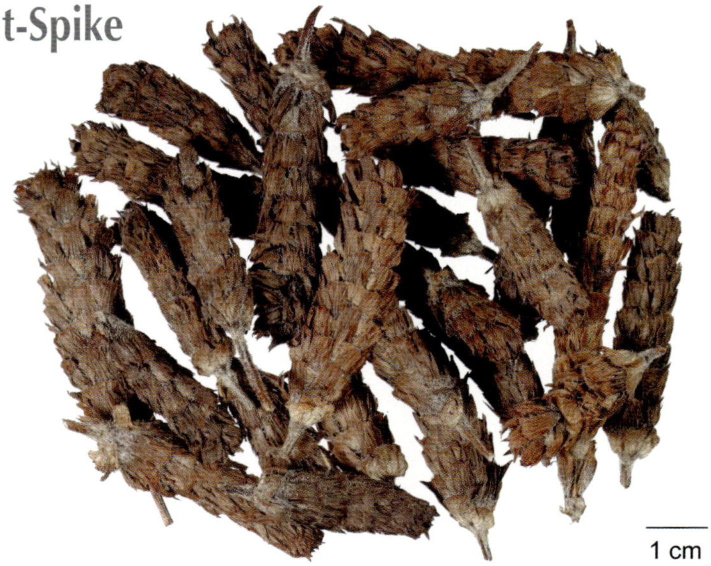

Crude drug

Source

The fruit spike of *Prunella vulgaris* L. (Fam. Labiatae).

Distribution

Mainly in Chinese provinces such as Jiangsu, Anhui and Henan.

Harvest & Processing

Harvest fruit spikes in summer when they turn brownish-red; remove foreign matter; dry under the sun.

Description

Baculiform (rod-shaped), slightly flattened; 1.5-8 cm long, 0.8-1.5 cm in diameter; pale brown to brownish-red. A whole spike contains several to more than 10 whorls of persistent calyx and bracts; each whorl with 2 opposite (borne in pairs at each node) bracts; each bract flabellate (fan-shaped), apex the shape of a pointed tail, veins prominent, outer surface covered with white hairs. 3 flowers in each bract; corolla mostly fallen off; persistent calyx bilabiate (two-lipped), with 4 small nutlets inside; nutlets ovoid (egg-shaped), brown, with a white protuberance at apex. Light in weight. Odour: faint; taste: mild.

Indications

1. Dizziness due to hypertension, headache, tinnitus 2. Red eyes, photophobia with lacrimation, conjunctivitis 3. Dry cough 4. Dermititis and boils.

Chemical Composition

Mainly contains ursolic acid, oleanolic acid and their saponins.

Spina Gleditsiae

Chinese Honeylocust Spine

Zaojiaoci

皂角刺

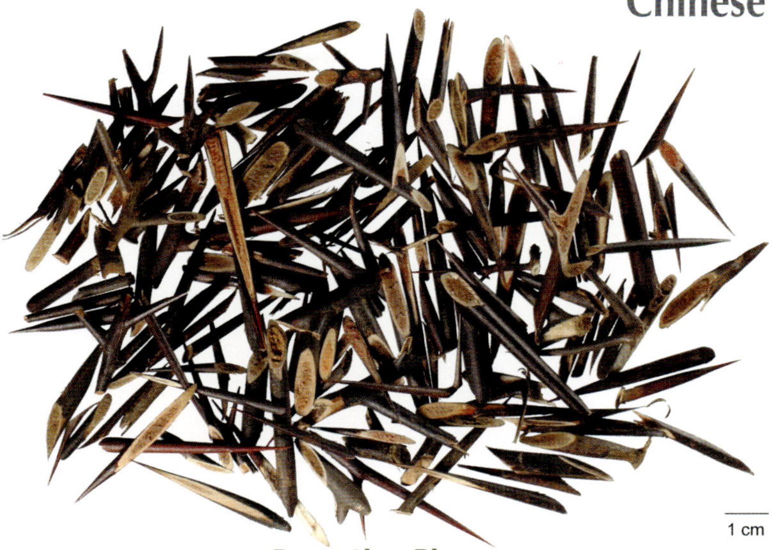

Decoction Pieces

Source The spine of *Gleditsia sinensis* Lam. (Fam. Leguminosae).

Distribution Mainly in Chinese provinces such as Henan, Jiangsu, Hubei and Guangxi.

Harvest & Processing Collect spines anytime during the year, preferably from September to March. Cut off spines; dry under the sun; alternatively slice length-wise or at an angle while fresh and dry the slices under the sun.

Description A full spine contains a main spine and 1-2 branch spines; purplish-brown all over; smooth or with fine wrinkles, occasionally with greyish-white lichen maculae. Main spine flattened and cylindrical; 5-18 cm long, base about 8-12 mm thick; tip acute. Branch spines arranged in a spiral, stretching out from main spine at angles of 60°-80°; about 1-7 cm long in general; often with even smaller spines; inner side of base often raised like mounds. Light in weight; hard, does not break easily.

Indications 1. Carbuncle 2. Tinea 3. Leprosy

Chemical Composition Mainly contains a variety of triterpene saponins.

Spora Lygodii

Japanese Climbing Fern Spore

Haijinsha

海金沙

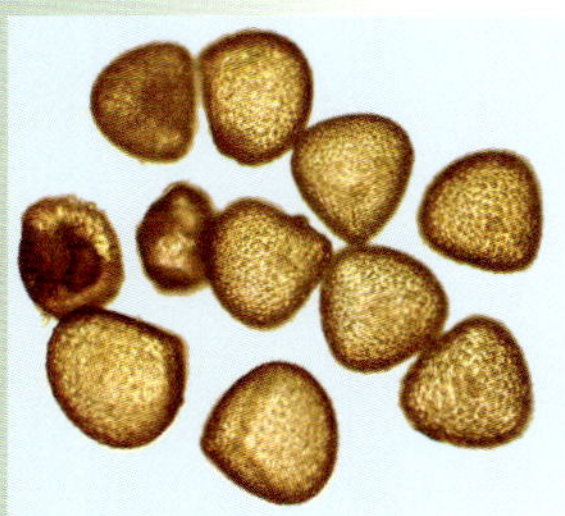

Japanese Climbing Fern Spore Magnified

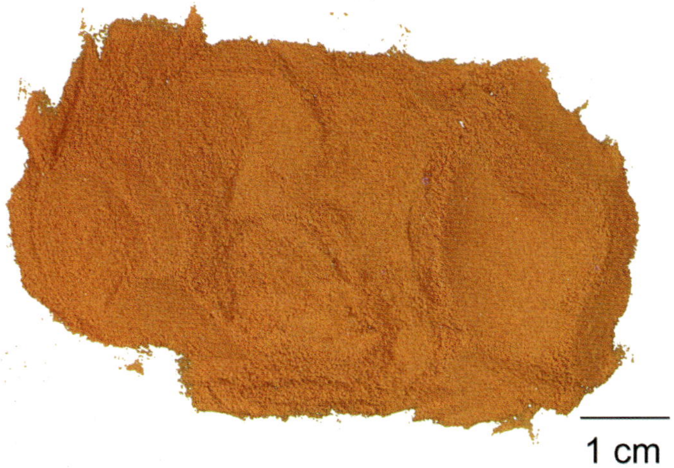

Crude drug

Source The mature spore of *Lygodium japonicum* (Thunb.) Sw. (Fam. Lygodiaceae).

Distribution Mainly in Chinese provinces such as Guangdong, Zhejiang, Jiangsu, Hubei and Hunan; also in Hong Kong.

Harvest & Processing Collect sporophylls in autumn before spores fall off; dry under the sun; rub or thresh to get spores; remove sporophylls.

Description Powdery, brownish-yellow or light brownish-yellow. Light in weight; smooth in texture when twiddled with fingers; slip through fingers easily when placed in hands. Odour: faint; taste: mild. Spores float when scattered over water, sink gradually when heated. Burn ealily when cast into fire, produce sparks and crackle, leaving no dregs.

Indications 1. Urinary tract infection and stones, nephritic oedema 2. Cold, fever 3. Mastitis.

Chemical Composition Mainly contains fatty oils and methylester of gibberellin A_{73}.

Stamen Nelumbinis

Lotus Stamen

Lianxu

蓮鬚

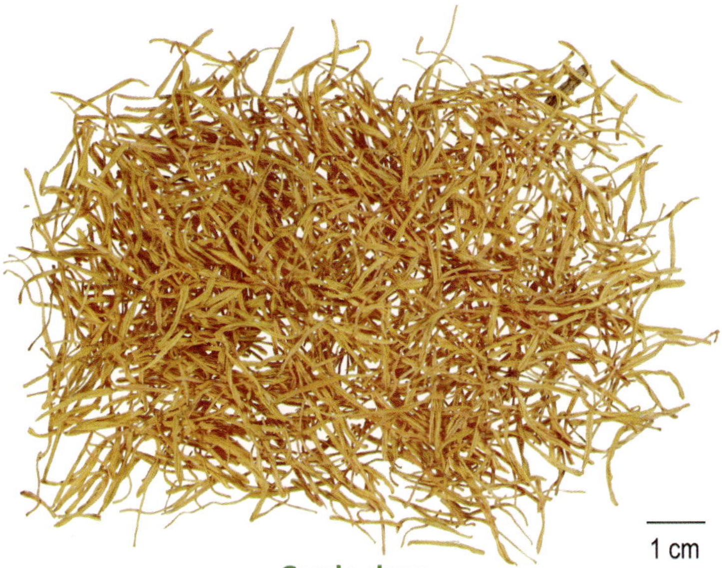

Crude drug

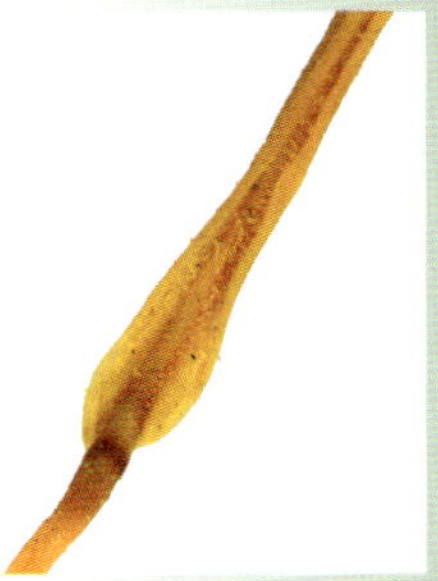

Lotus Stamen Magnified

Source The stamen of *Nelumbo nucifera* Gaertn. (Fam. Nymphaeaceae).

Distribution In most regions of China, including Hong Kong.

Harvest & Processing Pick stamens in summer when flowers are in full bloom; dry in shaded areas.

Description Linear (long and narrow), often twisted in a spiroid (spiral-like) form. Anther 1.2-1.5 cm long; pale yellowish-brown; longitudinally parted into 2 locules containing numerous yellow pollens. Filament filiform (thread-like), slightly flattened, slightly curved; 1-1.5 cm long; brownish-yellow or reddish-brown. Light in weight. Odour: faint; taste: slightly astringent.

Indications 1. Nocturnal emission, spermatorrhoea 2. Leukorrhagia 3. Urinary frequency.

Chemical Composition Mainly contains luteolin and quercetin.

Stigma Croci

Saffron
Xihonghua
西紅花

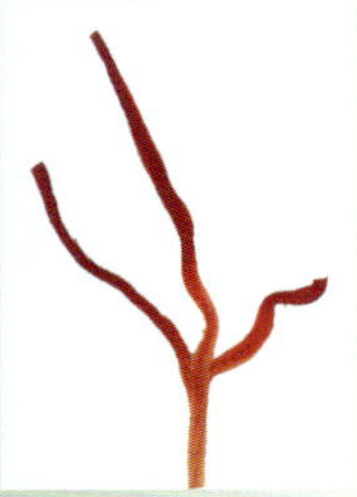

Saffron Magnified

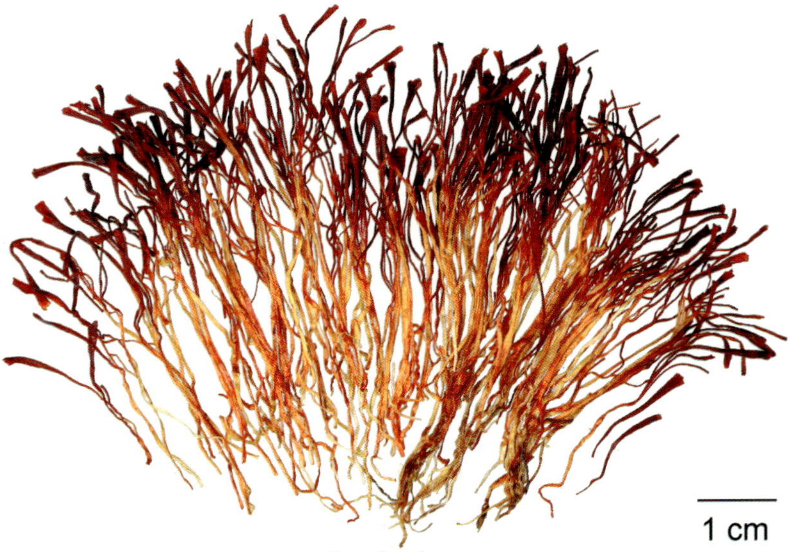

1 cm

Crude drug

Source The stigma of *Crocus sativus* L. (Fam. Iridaceae).

Distribution Mainly in Spain, Greece, France and the central and western Asia region of Russia. Cultivated in small amounts in China.

Harvest & Processing Collect flowers on sunny mornings in flowering season; pick stigmas; spread out in round, shallow bamboo baskets; cover with a thin sheet of water-absorbent paper; dry under the sun or by heat at 40-50℃, or by airing in well-ventilated places.

Description Dried stigma curled and filiform (thread-like) or linear (long and narrow); trifurcate (forked into three divisions); 2-3 cm long; dull red. Each division with a relatively broad and slightly flat upper part; top end margin irregular and dentate (tooth-edged), inner side with a short cleft; bottom end occasionally with a small section of yellow style remnant. Light in weight; texture loose and soft; no oily lustre; brittle and breaks easily when dried. Odour: distinctive, slightly pungent; taste: slightly bitter.

Indications 1. Amenorrhoea with abdominal mass, lochiostasis 2. Post traumatic swelling, bruises and pain 3. Depression, mania. 4. Eruptions in infectious diseases

Chemical Composition Mainly contains crocin, crocetin and β -carotene.

Styrax

Storax
Suhexiang
蘇合香

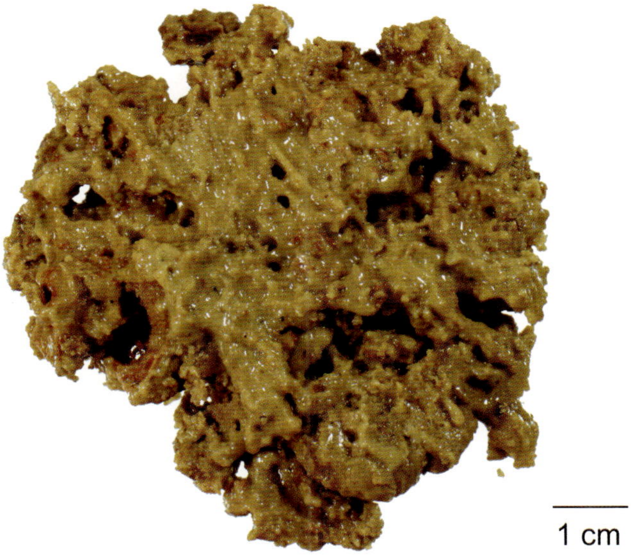

Crude drug

Source The balsam secreted from the trunk of *Liquidambar orientalis* Mill. (Fam. Hamamelidaceae).

Distribution Mainly in southern Turkey and countries like Syria, Egypt and Somalia. Introduced into China and cultivated in Guangxi and Yunnan provinces.

Harvest & Processing In early summer, choose trees 3-4 years old and cut open bark until xylem is revealed so that balsam is secreted and seeps into the bark. In autumn, cut off bark and the outer layer of sapwood; boil in water; filter by compressing in a cloth bag to produce Common Storax; dissolve it in 95% ethanol, filter and evaporate the ethanol from filtrate to produce Refined Storax.

Description A semi-fluid viscous liquid; brownish-yellow to dull drown; translucent. Fine texture; extremely viscous; gelatinous and dribs continuously when scooped up. Heavier than water. Odour: aromatic; taste: bitter, hot. Sticky when chewed.

Indications 1. Impairment of consciousness 2. Angina pectoris 3. Distension, pain and cold feeling of the chest and abdomen.

Chemical Composition Mainly contains essential oils.

Agkistrodon

Long-Nosed Pit Viper

Qishe

蘄蛇

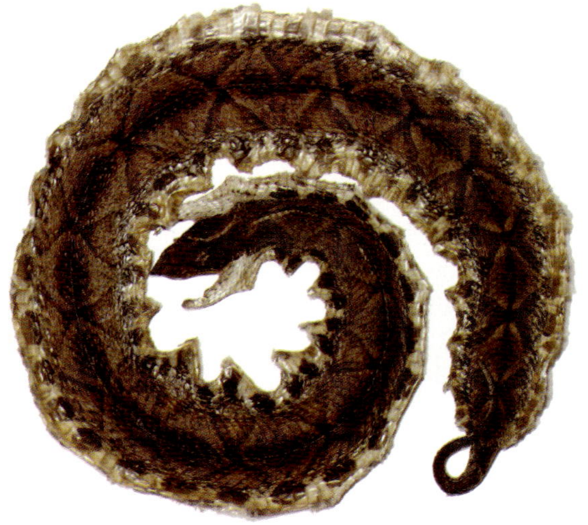

Crude drug

Source The dried body, with the viscera removed, of *Agkistrodon acutus* (Guenther) (Fam. Viperidae).

Distribution Mainly in Chinese provinces such as Zhejiang, Jiangxi, Fujian, Hunan and Guangdong.

Harvest & Processing Catch snakes, mostly in summer and autumn; cut open the abdomen; remove the viscera; wash clean; keep the cut open by backing the snake body with bamboo strips; curl into a coil and dry; remove the bamboo strips when dried.

Description Curled into a coil; body up to 2 m long. Head in the centre, slightly curled up, triangular and flattened; snout tip pointing upwards. Upper jaw with fistular (hollow and cylindrical), sharp fangs. Either side of dorsum marked with 17-25 V-shaped markings in dull blackish-brown and light brown, with the two upper ends of the Vs joining from both sides at the dorsal line, forming quadrate (square-shaped) markings. Abdomen cut kept open or not open, greyish-white; scales relatively large, marked with black suborbicular (almost round) maculae. Tail tapering abruptly, with 1 triangular, dark grey corneous (of horn-like texture) scale at end. Odour: fishy; taste: slightly salty.

Indications 1. Chronic rheumatic or rheumatoid arthritis with numbness and contracture of limbs, hemiplegia in stroke 2. Convulsion, tetanus 3. Leprosy 4. Scabies, ringworm infection.

Chemical Composition Contains three toxic proteins: AaT-I, AaT-II and AaT-III.

Note Listed as toxic in *C.P.*

Aspongopus

Stink-bug
Jiuxiangchong

九香蟲

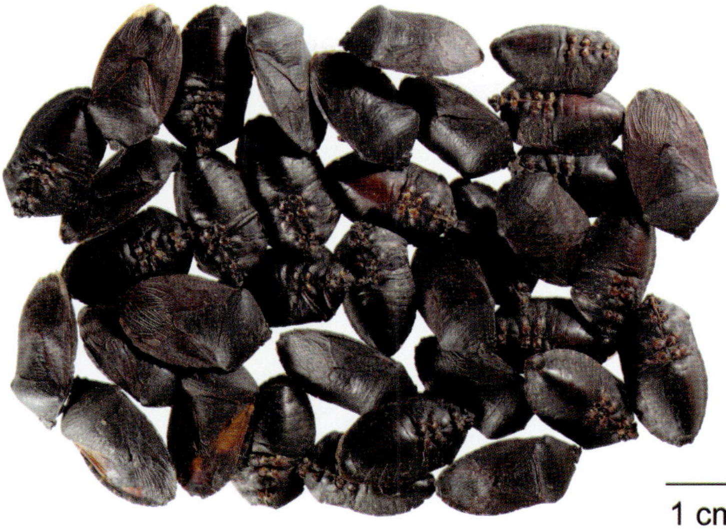

Crude drug

Source The body of *Aspongopus chinensis* Dallas (Fam. Pentatomidae).

Distribution Mainly in Chinese provinces such as Sichuan and Guizhou.

Harvest & Processing Catch whole insects in spring and autumn; scald to death in boiling water; dry under the sun.

Description Slightly hexagonal, flattened and elliptical; 1.6-2 cm long, about 1 cm wide. Outer surface reddish-brown or brownish-black; slightly lustrous. Head small; head and thorax together form a roughly triangular shape; compound eyes protuberant, egg-shaped; simple eyes 1 pair; antennae 1 pair, each in five segments, mostly broken off. Abdomen brownish-red to brownish-black, with tiny protuberant dots near the edges of each segment. Brittle; when broken, light brown contents revealed in abdomen. Odour: distinctive; taste: slightly salty.

Indications 1. Epigastric pain with distension 2. Impotence, loin and knee pain.

Chemical Composition Mainly contains fats, proteins and chitin.

Asteriscus Pseudosciaenae

Yellow Croaker Ear-Stone
Yunaoshi

魚腦石

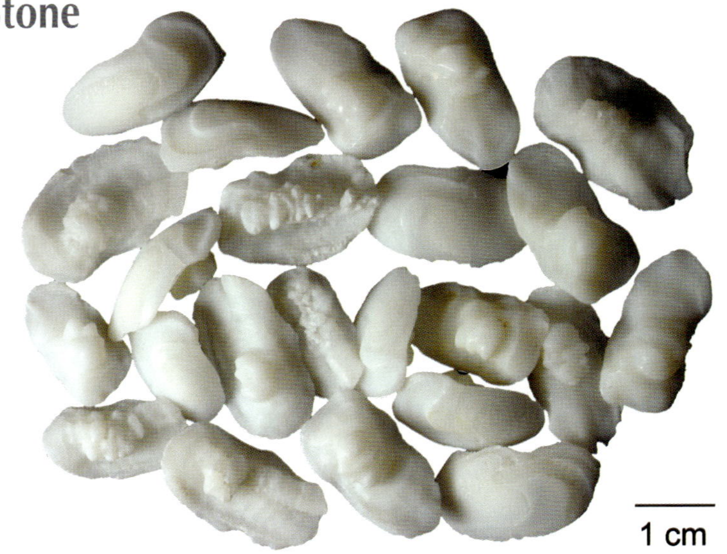

Crude drug

Source The otolith in the internal ear of *Pseudosciaena crocea* (Rich.) (Fam. Sciaenidae) and other species of the same family.

Distribution Mainly in coastal regions in China such as those near the East China Sea and the Yellow Sea.

Harvest & Processing During the yellow croaker season in May and June, catch the fishes; cut open the head and take out the otolith. Alternatively, while consuming fresh yellow croakers collect the otoliths; wash clean and dry under the sun.

Description Slightly flattened, oblong and egg-shaped, with 3 ridges; 1.5-2.3 cm long, 0.8-1.8 cm wide. Pale white or yellowish-white all over; one end broad and rounded; the other end narrow and pointed, slightly curled towards the exterior margin, with 1 slanted groove near the pointed end. Dorsal side slightly bulgy, marked with granular protuberances and fine layered striae (i.e. growth lines); ventral side relatively even, with a conspicuous orbicular (round) scar and grooves. Hard, does not break easily. Odour: faint; taste: slightly astringent.

Indications 1. Renal stone, dysuria 2. Otitis media, rhinitis, rhinorrhoea.

Chemical Composition Mainly contains proteins, fat and thiamine.

Bombyx Batryticatus

Stiff Silkworm

Jiangcan

僵蠶

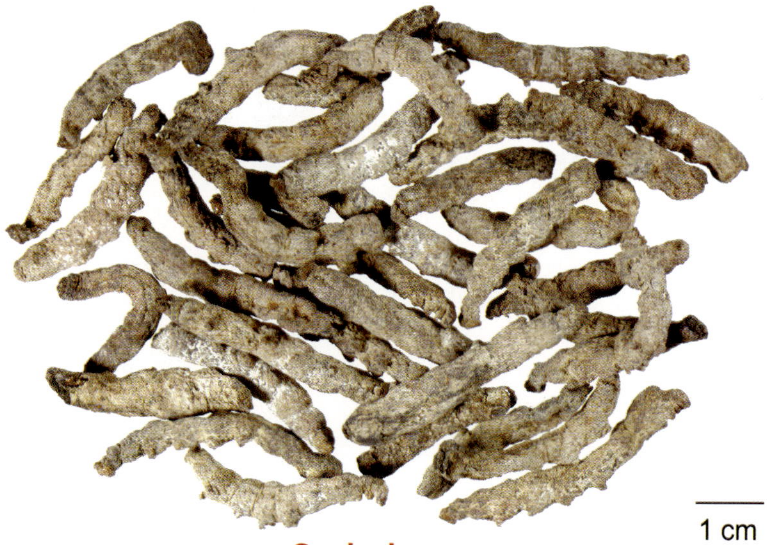

1 cm

Crude drug

Source The body of 4th-5th stage larvae of *Bombyx mori* L. (Fam. Bombycidae) which have died of infection (or artificial infection) by *Beauveria bassiana* (Bals.) Vuillant.

Distribution Mainly in Chinese provinces such as Jiangsu, Zhejiang, Sichuan and Guangdong.

Harvest & Processing Mostly processed in spring and autumn. Collect silkworm larvae which have died of infection by *Beauveria bassiana* (Bals.) Vuillant; dry under the sun or over a gentle fire.

Description Subcylindrical, mostly curved and shrivelled; 2-5 cm long, 5-7 mm in diameter. Outer surface greyish-yellow, covered with white powdery aerial mycelia and conidia. Head relatively round, yellowish-brown; 8 pairs of protuberant legs on ventral side; somites conspicuous; tail slightly bifurcate (forked into two divisions). Hard and brittle, breaks easily. Broken surface smooth; outer layer white, middle part with 4 rings of lustrous brown or lustrous black silk glands. Odour: slightly fishy; taste: slightly salty.

Indications 1. Convulsion, epilepsy, tetanus, infantile convulsion, cerebral vascular accident with hemiplegia 2. Headache, ocular pain, sore throat, prurigo 3. Subcutaneous nodules and scrofula.

Chemical Composition Mainly contains 3-hydroxy kynurenine and 6-N-hydroxy ethyl adenine.

Bombyx Batryticatus

Calculus Bovis

Cow-Bezoar
Niuhuang

牛黄

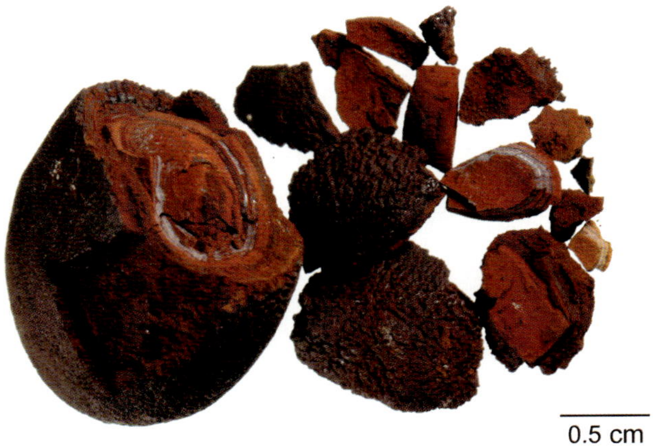

Crude drug

Source The gallstone of *Bos taurus domesticus* Gmelin (Fam. Bovidae).

Distribution Mainly in Chinese provinces such as Hebei, Jiangsu, Zhejiang, Guangxi and Guangdong; also in northwestern China, Inner Mongolia, and cities such as Beijing and Tianjin. Large volumes are also imported from Brazil.

Harvest & Processing Check cows' gall bladder, bile duct and hepatic duct during slaughter. If gallstones are found, take out immediately; remove the attached membrane; wrap up with cotton or stem pith strips of Medulla Tetrapanacis; put in shaded areas until half-dried; fasten thread around the gallstones to prevent breaking; dry in shaded areas. Customarily called "*Tianran niuhuang*"(Natural Cow-Bezoar).

Description Mostly ovoid (egg-shaped), subspherical, cubical or triangular; varying in size. Outer surface yellowish-red to brownish-yellow, in some cases with a layer of lustrous black membrane; usually fine, smooth and slightly lustrous; verrucose (with wart-shaped protuberances). Light in weight; crisp and brittle, peels off in layers easily; when broken, surface golden-yellow, marked with fine and dense concentric layered annulations, and sometimes with a white core. Odour: fresh and fragrant; taste: bitter at first, then slightly sweet; mint-like. Breaks easily when chewed, not sticky. A small amount mixed with water can dye fingernails yellow.

Indications 1. High fever with convulsion or impairment of consciousness, delirium, heavy expectoration 2. Infantile convulsion, epilepsy and stroke 3. Sore throat 4. Carbuncles, boils, breast cancer

Chemical Composition Natural Cow-Besoar Mainly contains bilirubin and cholic acid.

Carapax et Plastrum Testudinis

Tortoise Carapace and Plastron

Guijia

龜甲

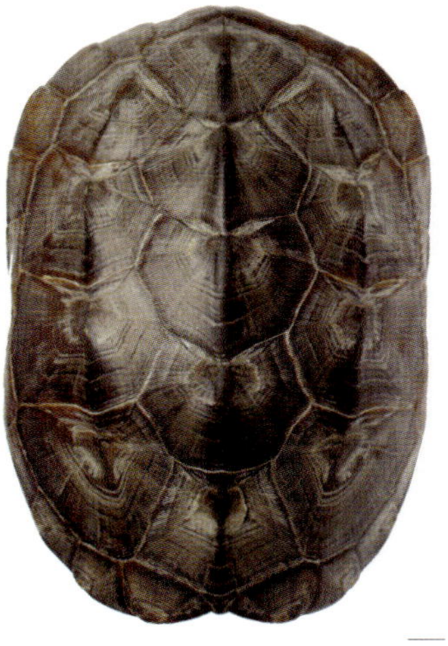

Crude drug (Guijia)

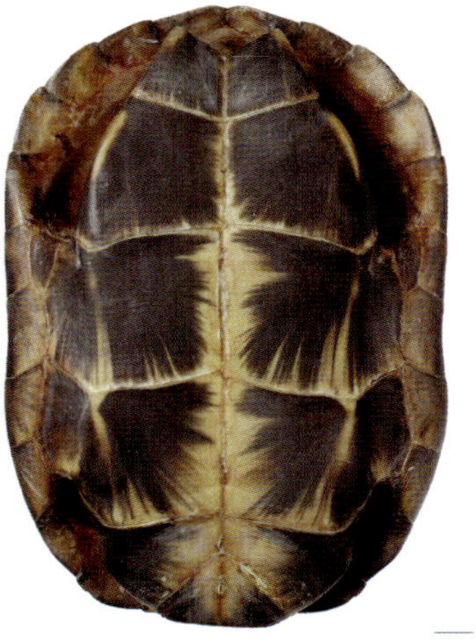

Crude drug (Guiban)

Source The carapace and plastron of *Chinemys reevesii* (Gray) (Fam. Testudinidae).

Distribution Mainly in Chinese provinces such as Zhejiang, Anhui, Hubei and Hunan. Harvested from both wild and domestic tortoises.

Harvest & Processing Catch tortoises anytime during the year, but mostly in autumn and winter; and kill; strip off carapaces and plastrons; remove flesh remnants; dry under the sun. There are two kinds of processed products: '*Xueban*' (Blood Plate), and '*Tangban*' (Scalded Plate).

Description Carapace and plastron linked by a bridge; carapace slightly longer than plastron and often detached from it. Plastron placoid (plate-like), rectangular and elliptical. Outer surface pale yellowish-brown to brownish-black; scutes 12, each often marked with dull purplish-brown radial markings; median sutures on ventral, pectoral and femoral scutes are long, those on gular and anal scutes shorter, the ones on humeral scutes the shortest. Inner surface yellowish-white to greyish-white. Hard. Odour: slightly fishy; taste: slightly salty.

Indications 1. Hectic fever and night sweating 2. Nocturnal emission 3.Dizziness, tinnitus, convulsion 4. Weakness of the waist and lower limbs, maldevelopment in infants 5. Menstrual disorders

Chemical Composition Mainly contains collagen and amino acids.

Note Plastrons are usually used in Hong Kong and are customarily called '*Guiban*' (Tortoise Plate).

Carapax Trionycis

Turtle Carapace
Biejia
鱉甲

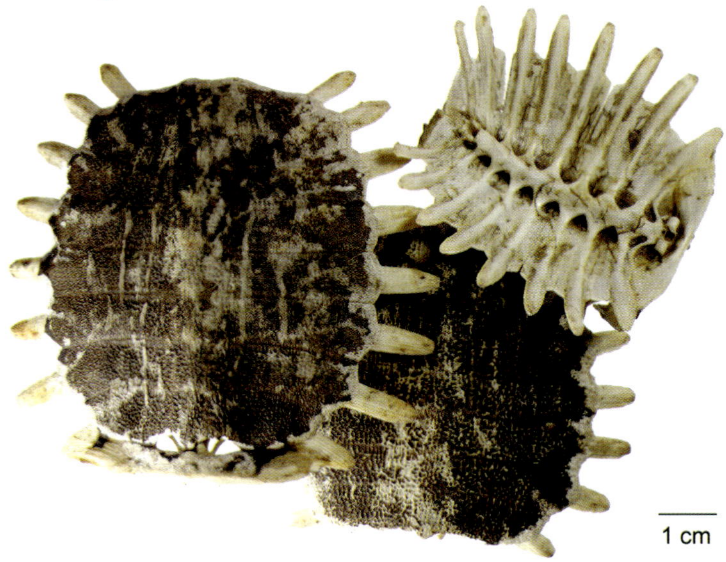

Crude drug

Carapax Trionycis

Source The carapace of *Trionyx sinensis* (Wiegmann) (Fam. Trionychidae).

Distribution Mainly in Chinese provinces such as Hubei, Anhui, Jiangsu and Henan. Now mostly harvested from cultivated turtles.

Harvest & Processing Catch turtles anytime during the year, but mostly in autumn and winter; kill and scald in boiling water until the scleroderm on the carapaces can be peeled off; take out and strip off carapaces; remove flesh remnants; dry under the sun.

Description Elliptical or ovate (egg-shaped in outline), dorsal side bulgy; 10-15 cm long, 9-14 cm wide. Outer surface dull blackish-brown or dark green, slightly lustrous, marked with reticulate (net-like) wrinkles and greyish-yellow or greyish-white maculae; centre with a longitudinal ridge; 8 pairs of transverse dented lines running symmetrically on both sides of the ridge; when outer skin is removed, serrate (saw-like) joint sutures along the dented lines revealed. Inner surface off-white, with vertebrae protruding from the middle; cervical vertebra curving inwards; each side with 8 ribs extending beyond the edges. Hard. Odour: slightly fishy; taste: mild.

Indications 1. Hectic fever, night sweating 2. Late stage of febrile diseases 3. Convulsion 4. Abdominal mass, hepatosplenomegaly.

Chemical Composition Mainly contains collagen and a variety of amino acids.

Cera Chinensis

Insect Wax
Chongbaila
蟲白蠟

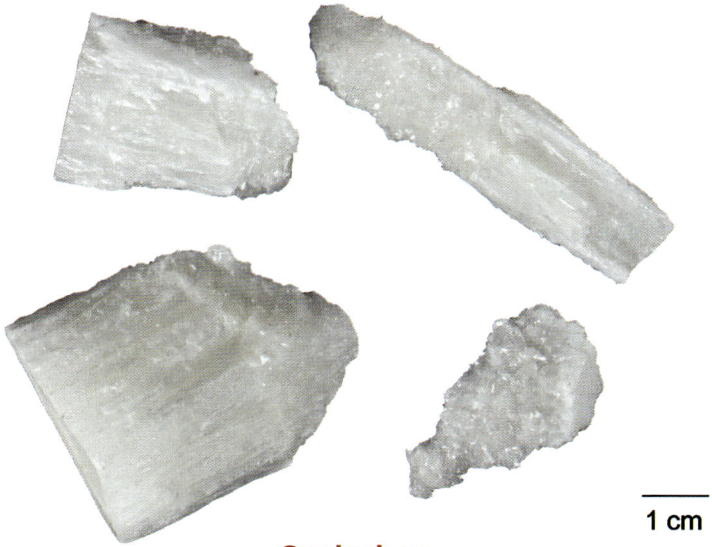

Crude drug

Source The wax secreted by male *Ericerus pela* (Chavannes) Guerin (Fam. Coccidae) inhabiting gregariously in the stems and branches of *Fraxinus chinensis* Roxb. and *Ligustrum lucidum* Ait. (both belouging to Fam. Oleaceae) and other species of the genus *Ligustrum*.

Distribution Mainly in Chinese provinces such as Sichuan, Hunan, Guizhou and Yunnan.

Harvest & Processing Collect insect wax around late August and early September. If possible, process the wax on the day of collection; boil in water and compress into pieces.

Description Irregular pieces, white or off-white. Outer surface smooth or slightly wrinkled, with waxy lustre. Light in weight; hard and slightly brittle, crumble when rubbed or twiddled. Broken surface in linear (long and narrow) or granular pattern. Odour: faint; taste: mild.

Indications Excipient and lubricant for making pills and tablets.

Chemical Composition Mainly contains ceryl montanate, ceryl ceratate and melissyl alcohol.

Colla Corii Asini

Donkey-Hide Glue

Ejiao

阿膠

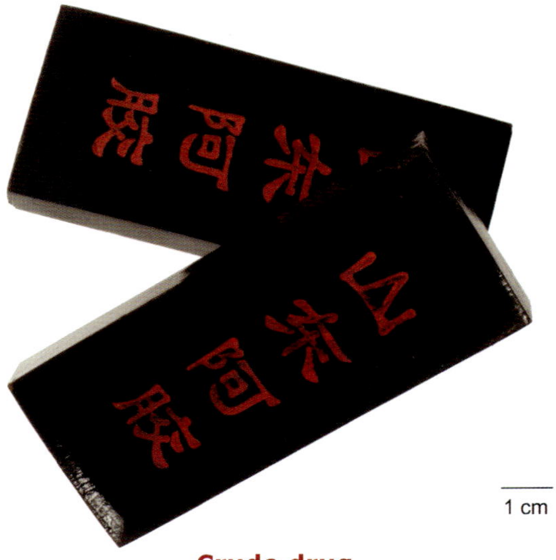

Crude drug

Source The solid glue obtained through decoction and concentration from the skin, with hair removed, of *Equus asinus* (Fam. Equidae).

Distribution Mainly in Chinese provinces such as Shandong, Henan, Jiangsu, Zhejiang and Hebei.

Harvest & Processing Harvest donkey-hide anytime during the year; put in water to soften, and then rinse; remove hair; cut into small pieces; soften in water and rinse clean again; decoct the pieces in separate portions in water; filter; add all the filtrates together and reduce over a gentle fire until concentrated into a thick paste; cool; cut into pieces; dry in shaded areas.

Description Solid glue in rectangular pieces, or flattened and quadrate (square-shaped); dull blackish-brown; lustrous. Hard and brittle; broken surface shiny. Fragments amber in colour and translucent when held against the light. Odour: faint; taste: slightly sweet.

Indications 1. Anaemia, leukopenia, thrombocytopenia purpura 2.Bleeding
3. Amenorrhoea, menstrual disorders, threatened abortion
4. Vexation, insomnia, 5. Muscular spasm 6. Cough and thirst.

Chemical Composition Mainly contains gelatin proteins.

Concha Arcae

Ark shell
Walengzi
瓦楞子

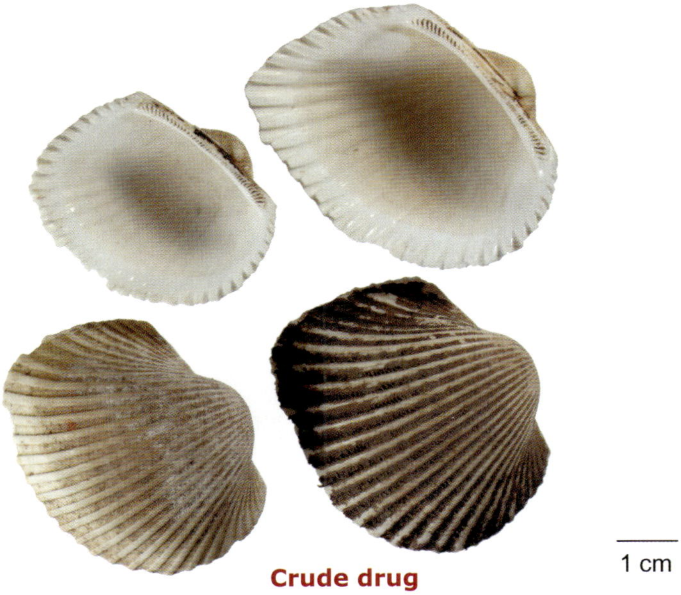

Crude drug

Source The shell of *Arca inflate* Reeve (Fam. Arcidae).

Distribution Mainly along the coast of Chinese provinces such as Jiangsu, Shandong and Hebei.

Harvest & Processing Collect shells from sand at the bottom of shallow waters or from nets anytime during the year; wash clean; boil until cooked; remove flesh; dry shells under the sun.

Description Oblique and ovate (egg-shaped in outline); left valve and right valve identical in shape, with the left one slightly larger in size; about 8 cm long, about 6 cm wide. Dorsal side slightly bulgy, marked with 42-48 straight, corrugated ridges (i.e. radial ribs) radiating from umbo; ribs prominent, dull greyish-brown, with white streaks between ridges, without conspicuous nodes, covered with fine brown hairs. Interior of shell milky-white and smooth; brim with notches corresponding to the ribs, forming about 70 protuberant teeth (i.e. hinge teeth). Hard, can be pounded to pieces; when broken, surface white. Odourless; taste: mild.

Indications 1. Thick sputum with difficult expectoration 2. Goiter, scrofula, abdominal masses 3. Stomachache with acid regurgitation.

Chemical Composition Mainly contains calcium carbonate ($CaCO_3$).

Note According to *C.P.*, also used for medicinal purposes is the shell of *A. granosa* Linnaeus and *A. subcrenata* Lischke.

Concha Mauritiae Arabicae

Arabic Cowry Shell
Zibeichi

紫貝齒

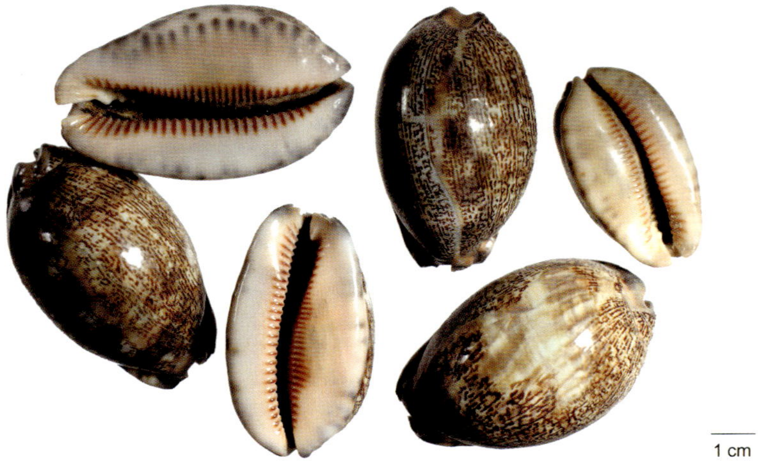

Crude drug

Source The shell of *Mauritia arabica* (L.) (Fam. Cypraeidae).

Distribution Mainly in Chinese provinces such as Fujian, Taiwan, Guangdong, Hainan and Guangxi.

Harvest & Processing Catch cowries between May and July every year; remove flesh; wash shells clean; dry under the sun.

Description Oblong and egg-shaped shell; hard. Dorsum bulgy and orbicular (round), with the two lateral sides tapering towards base; margin relatively thick. Outer surface shiny and fine; dull brown or light brown; marked with criss-crossing, irregular, interrupted reddish-brown striae and numerous stellate (star-like) markings; almost completely covered by enamel. Dorsum with faint dull brown or greyish-blue transverse striae. Both lateral margins dull greyish-brown, marked with dull purplish-brown maculae extended into the base. Aperture narrow and long, slightly curved, wider at anterior end; 2 lips, each with about 32 teeth dull purplish-brown in colour. Inner surface of shell pale purple.

Indications 1. Nebula 2. Infantile eyes affected by eruptive exanthem, infantile irritability and insomnia.

Chemical Composition Contains around 90% calcium phosphate [$Ca_3(PO_4)_2$].

Concha Meretricis seu Cyclinae

Clam Shell

Geqiao

蛤殼

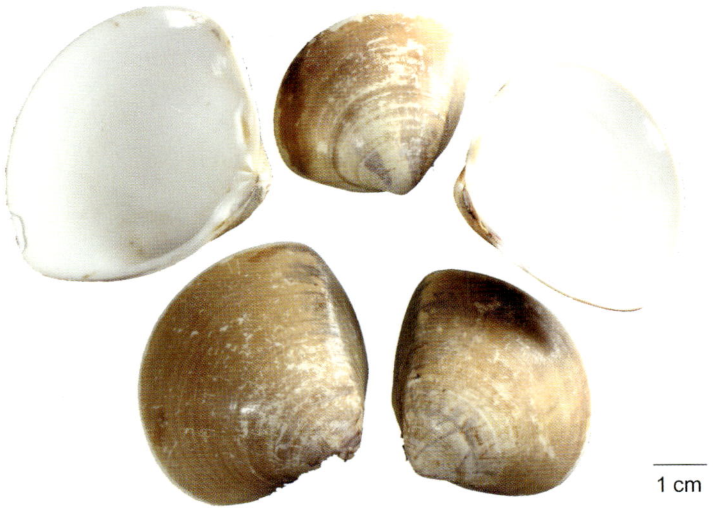

Crude drug

Source The shell of *Meretrix meretrix* Linnaeus (Fam. Veneridae).

Distribution In all coastal regions of China.

Harvest & Processing Harvest clams in spring and autumn; remove flesh; wash clean; dry under the sun.

Description Flabellate (fan-shaped) or suborbicular (almost round); dorsal brim somewhat triangular, ventral brim arch-like; 3-10 cm long, 2-8 cm wide. Umbo prominent, on the dorsal side, slightly nearer the anterior. Outer surface of shell smooth, dull yellowish-brown, marked with conspicuous concentric growth striae; dorsal side usually marked with dull brown striae in the form of serrations or waves; anterior and posterior margins slightly purple in some cases; hinge relatively broad. Right valve with 3 cardinal teeth and 2 anterior lateral teeth; left valve with 3 cardinal teeth and 1 anterior lateral tooth. Hard; broken surface shows layered striae. Odourless; taste: mild.

Indications 1. Cough, chest pain and blood stained sputum 2. Goiter, scrofula 3. Epigastric pain with acid regurgitation 4. Eczema, burn and scalds (external use).

Chemical Composition Mainly contains $CaCO_3$ chitin etc.

Note According to *C.P.*, also used for medicinal purposes is the shell of *Cyclina sinensis* (Gmelin), which belongs to the same family as *Meretrix meretrix* Linnaeus.

Concha Meretricis seu Cyclinae

Concha Ostreae

Oyster Shell
Muli
牡蠣

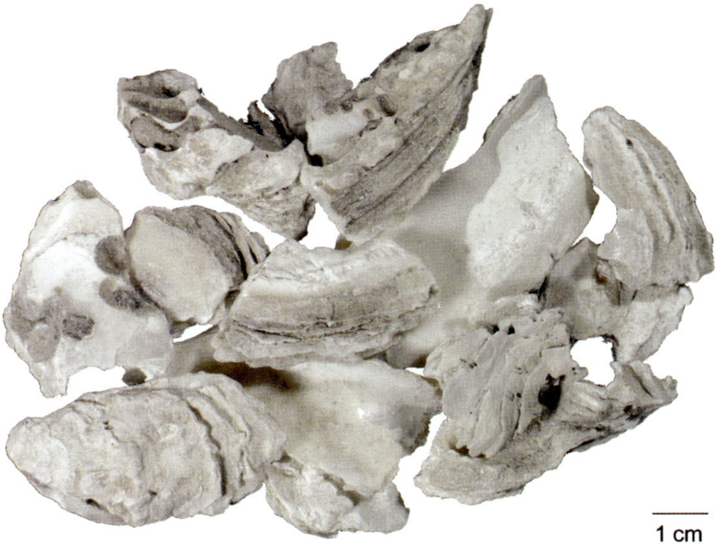

Crude drug

Concha Ostreae

Source The shell of *Ostrea gigas* Thunberg. (Fam. Ostreidae).

Distribution Mainly from the northern part of Shandong province in China to the northeastern coast of China. Mostly harvested from wild oysters, also from cultivated ones.

Harvest & Processing Collect oysters anytime during the year; remove flesh for food; wash shells clean; dry under the sun.

Description Elongated and thin, dorsal and ventral brims almost parallel; 10-50 cm long, 4-15 cm thick. Right valve relatively flat, like a lid; scales thick and hard, laminiform (consisting of layers) or forming layered striae; outer surface even or with several depressions, pale purple, greyish-white or dull yellowish-brown in colour; inner surface porcelain-white, with no denticles at either side of umbo. Left valve. Left valve with a deep hollow; scales thicker than those of right valve. The area of the umbo where the two valves are joined together is small. with a deep hollow; scales thicker than those of right valve. Hard; broken surface laminiform, pure white. Odourless; taste: slightly salty.

Indications 1. Dizziness, tinnitus, irritability and insomnia, convulsion, febrile diseases 2. Subcutaneous nodule, scrofula 3. Emission, enuresis, 4. Menstural disorders 5. Sweating 6. Peptic ulcer

Chemical Composition Contains over 90% calcium carbonate ($CaCO_3$).

Note According to *C.P.*, also used for medicinal purposes is the shell of *O. talienwhanensis* Crosse and *O. rivularis* Gould.

Corium Erinacei

Hedgehog Hide
Ciweipi
刺猬皮

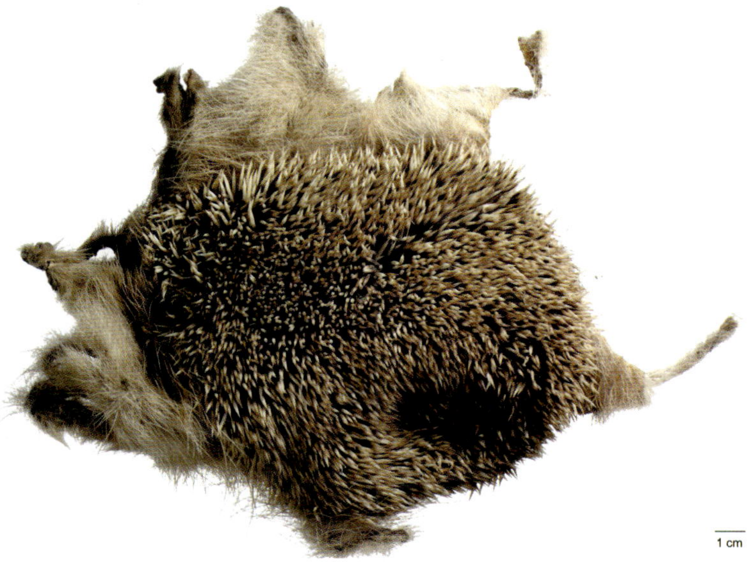

Crude drug

Source — The skin of *Erinaceus europaeus* L. (Fam. Erinaceidae).

Distribution — Mainly in Chinese provinces such as Hebei, Shandong, Jiangsu, Henan, Shaanxi, Gansu, Zhejiang and Anhui, and in Inner Mongolia.

Harvest & Processing — Catch and kill hedgehogs, mostly in spring; strip off skin; remove fat and flesh remnants; stretch skin out with bamboo strips; hang to dry in cool, well-ventilated places.

Description — Polygonal, brush-like or slab-like; some with rolled-up tubular or discoid (disc-like) edges. Outer surface densely covered with criss-crossing spines, each 1.5-2 cm long and hard as a needle; spines greyish-white, yellow or dull greyish-brown. Abdominal skin covered with dull greyish-brown soft fur; inner side greyish-white or reddish-brown. Odour: with a distinctive fishy stench.

Indications — 1. Regurgitation 2. Pain in abdomen and hernia 3. Haemorrhoidal bleeding 4. Nocturnal emission.

Chemical Composition — The spines mainly contain keratin; the dermis Mainly contains collagen and elastin.

Cornu Bubali

Buffalo Horn

Shuiniujiao

水牛角

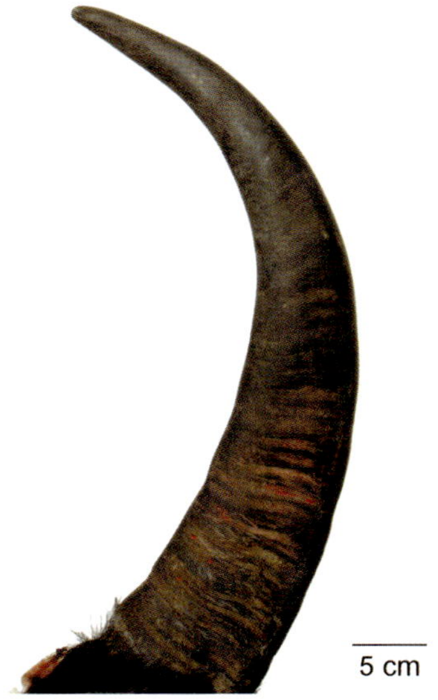

Crude drug

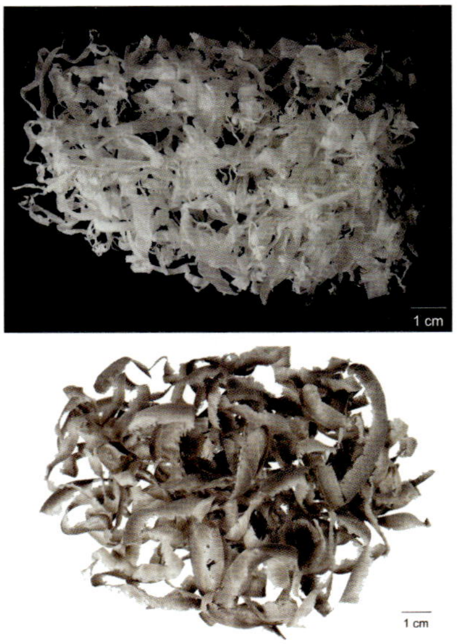

Decoction Pieces

Source ▶ The horn of *Bubalus bubalis* L. (Fam. Bovidae).

Distribution ▶ In all regions of China south of the Yangtze River.

Harvest & Processing ▶ Collect horns anytime during the year; boil in water; remove horn cores; dry horns.

Description ▶ Somewhat flattened and curved, subulate (awl-shaped); varying in length. Outer surface brownish-black or greyish-black, with several transverse grooves on one side and a cluster of transverse dented striae on the other. Upper part acuminate (tapering to a slender point), marked with longitudinal striae; base somewhat triangular, hollowed. Corneous (of horn-like texture); hard. Odour: slightly fishy; taste: mild. Commercially sold buffalo horns in two forms—shavings and slices.

Indications ▶ 1. Hyperpyrexia, delirium and eruptive exanthem in epidemic diseases 2. Haematemesis, epistaxis 3. Convulsion, mania.

Chemical Composition ▶ Mainly contains sterols and amino acids.

Cornu Cervi

Deerhorn

Lujiao

鹿角

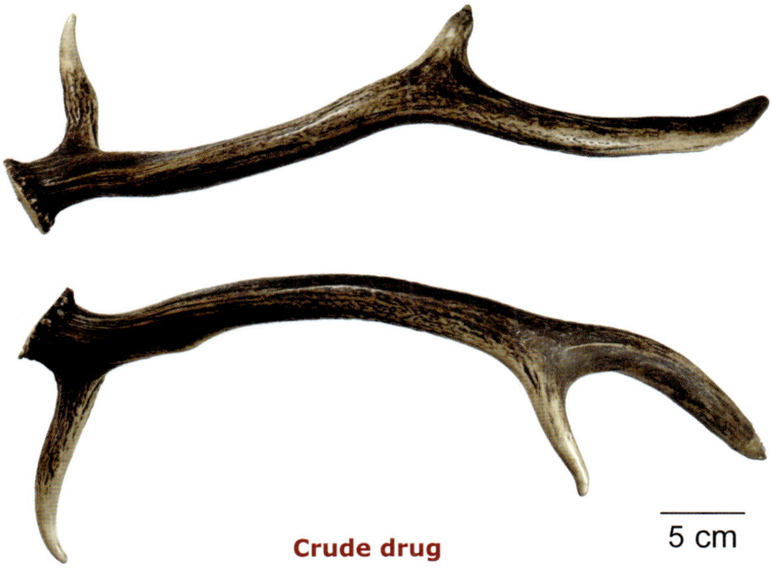

Crude drug

Source The ossified antler, or the antler base shed in the year after the sawing of the pilose antler of *Cervus Nippon* Temminck (Fam. Cervidae).

Distribution Mainly in Chinese provinces such as Heilongjiang, Jilin, Liaoning, Sichuan and Qinghai, and in Inner Mongolia and Xinjiang.

Harvest & Processing Chop off antlers together with cranium or saw at the base, usually in winter or early spring; wash clean; dry by wind to produce '*Kanjiao*' (Chopped-off Antler). Alternatively, in late spring collect antlers shed naturally — called '*Tuijiao*' (Shed Antler).

Description Usually divided into 3-4 branches; 30-60 cm in full length, 2.5-5 cm in diameter. Lateral branches mostly extending sideways, with the first one nearer to the base the second one relatively far away from the first one. Tip of main branch divided into two branchlets. Outer surface yellowish-brown or greyish-brown; tips greyish-white. The part near tips with conspicuous intermittent protuberances forming a longitudinal ridge; ridge top greyish-white or greyish-yellow, lustrous. Odourless; taste: slightly salty.

Indications 1. Impotence, nocturnal emission, back pain with cold sensation 2. Chronic ulcer and sores 3. Early stage mastitis

Chemical Composition Mainly contains collagen, calcium phosphate [$Ca_3(PO_4)_2$], calcium carbonate ($CaCO_3$) and a variety of amino acids.

Note According to *C.P.*, also used for medicinal purposes, and commonly known as '*Malujiao*' (Red Deer Horn), is the ossified antler, or the antler base shed in the year after the sawing of the pilose antler of *C. elaphus* Linnaeus.

Cornu Cervi Pantotrichum

Pilose Antler
Lurong
鹿茸

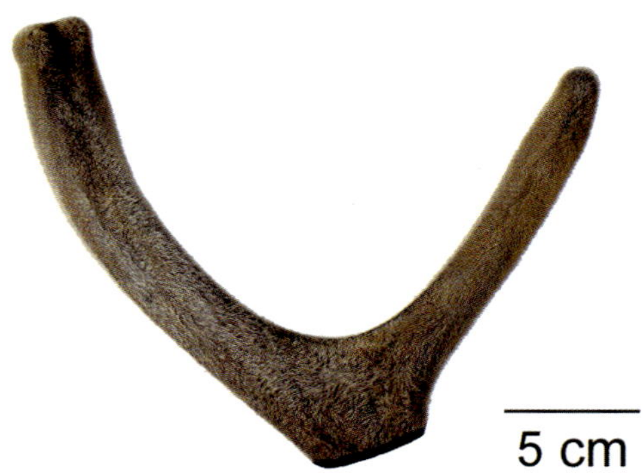

Crude drug

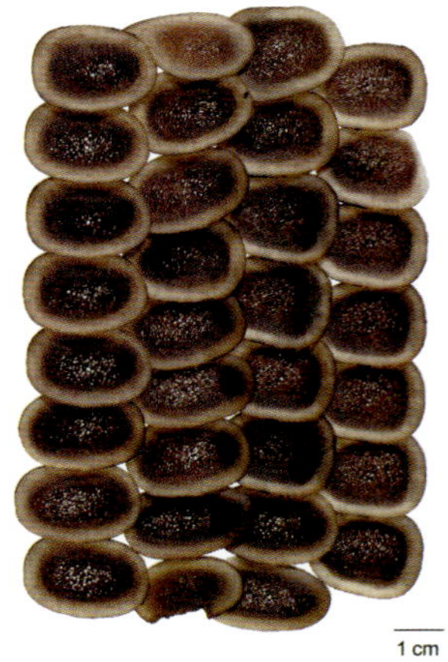

Decoction Pieces

Source The young, non-ossified pilose antler of male *Cervus nippon* Temminck (Fam. Cervidae).

Distribution Mainly in Chinese provinces such as Jilin, Liaoning and Heilongjiang. Deer are now mostly raised in farms.

Harvest & Processing Harvesting usually begins with three-year-old deer. Two rounds of harvesting a year, the first mostly in early April, i.e. 45-50 days after the antler base is shed; the second about 50-60 days later. Saw off sika antlers, then start processing: nail the antler, cauterize the cut surface, drain blood from antler, wash clean, boil and dry.

Description Sawn-off antler: Cylindrical and ramous (branched); antler with 1 branch commonly known as '*ergang*' (double sticks). Side branch obtuse at tip, slightly thinner than main branch. Outer skin reddish-brown or brown, covered with reddish-yellow or brownish-yellow fine pubescence; pubescence denser in upper part, comparatively sparse in lower part; skin between main branch and side branch marked with a greyish-black vein. Cut surface yellowish-white, with dense honeycomb-like holes in the middle; rim not bony. Light in weight. Odour: slightly blood-like; taste: slightly salty.

Indications 1. Cold extremities, fatigue, backache, impotence, emission, enuresis, sterility 2. Menstrual disorders, leukorrhagia 3. Dyspnoea 4. Maldevelopment in infants 5. Unhealed skin lesions.

Chemical Composition Mainly contains amino acids, sterol and polyamine.

Note According to *C.P.*, also used for medicinal purposes, and commonly known as *'Malurong'* (Red Deer Pilose Antler), is the young, non-ossified pilose antler of male *C. elaphus* Linnaeus.

Crinis Carbonisatus

Carbonized Hair
Xueyutan
血餘炭

Crude drug

Source The human hair.

Distribution In all parts of China.

Harvest & Processing Gather together human hair; remove foreign matter; wash away grime with alkaline solution, then rinse with fresh water; scoop up and dry under the sun. Put hair into a calcination pot, then place a same-sized pot upside-down on top, completely covering the original one; seal up the crevice between the two pots with mud to form an airtight container; lay a sheet of white paper on the bottom of the inverted pot; calcine until the paper turns scorched yellow; let cool and then take out hair.

Description Pieces irregular in shape; varying in size. Jet black, shiny; outer surface poriferous (with numerous holes), spongiform (spongy). Light in weight; brittle, breaks easily; when broken, surface alveolate (honeycombed). Odour: like scorched hair when burnt in fire; taste: bitter.

Indications 1. Bleeding such as epistaxis, haemoptysis, haematuria, gastrointestinal bleeding, dysfunctional uterine bleeding 2. Dysuria, stranguria.

Chemical Composition Mainly contains eukeratin.

Endoconcha Sepiae

Cuttlebone
Haipiaoxiao

海螵蛸

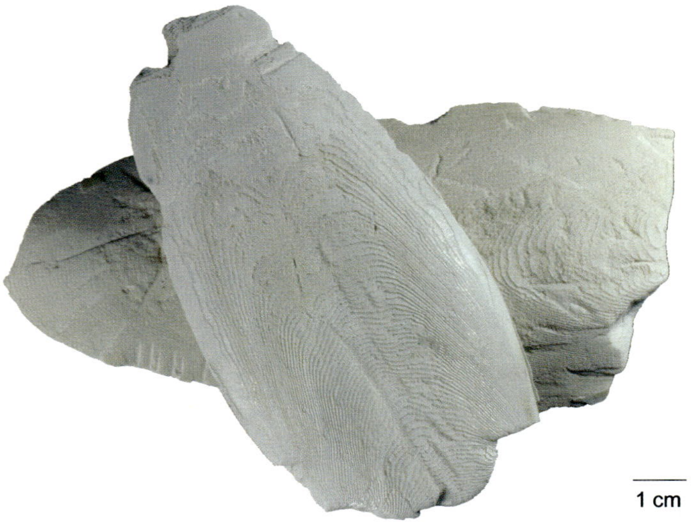

Crude drug

Source The internal shell of *Sepiella maindroni* de Rochebrune (Fam. Sepiidae).

Distribution Mainly in Chinese provinces such as Zhejiang, Jiangsu and Guangdong.

Harvest & Processing Tear off osseous (bone-like) internal shells from cuttlefish, or collect cuttlefish internal shells floating near the coast between April and August; rinse clean; dry under the sun.

Description Oblong and elliptical, flat, thin around the edge and thick in the middle; 9-14 cm long, 2.5-3.5 cm wide, 1.2-1.5 cm thick. Dorsal side with a pale white, ridge-like protuberance, both sides of protuberance tinged with light red and marked with faint minute tubercles arranged in near-parallel semi-annular striae; ventral side white, with fine, dense, undulate (wavy), and transverse layered striae from caudal end to middle portion; corneous (of horn-like texture) edge translucent; tail broader and flat, with no spicule. Light in weight; texture loose, breaks easily; broken surface starchy, with sparse layered striae. Odour: slightly fishy; taste: slightly salty.

Indications 1. Bleeding 2. Nocturnal emission, leukorrhagia 3. Peptic ulcer, stomachache with acid regurgitation 4. Goiter 5. Pyogenic skin infection, unhealed skin lesion, eczema.

Chemical Composition Contains over 85% calcium carbonate ($CaCO_3$), and a variety of amino acids.

Note According to *C.P.*, also used for medicinal purposes is the internal shell of *Sepia esculenta* Hoyle, which belongs to the same family as *Sepiella maindroni* de Rochebrune.

Endothelium Corneum Gigeriae Galli

Chicken Gizzard-Skin

Jineijin

雞內金

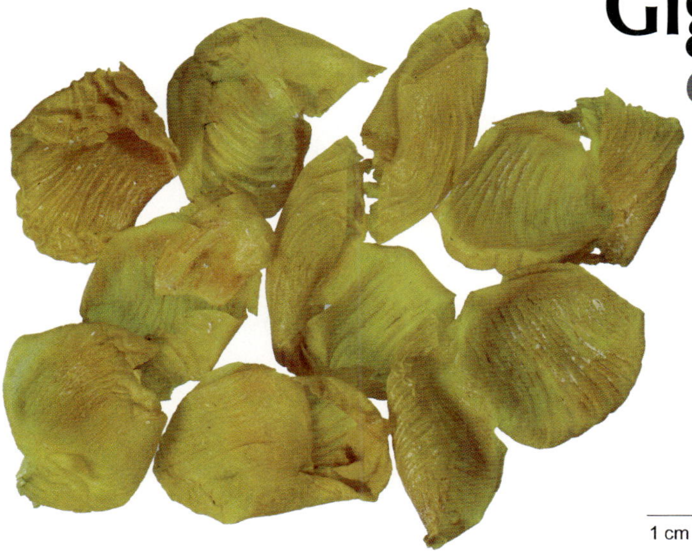

Crude drug

Source The endothelium of the gizzard of *Gallus gallus domesticus* Brisson (Fam. Phasianidae).

Distribution In all parts of China.

Harvest & Processing Collect chicken gizzards; immediately peel off the endothelium; wash clean; dry.

Description Shrivelled sacciform (sac-form) pieces irregular in shape; when intact, up to 6-7 cm long, about 3 cm wide, 0.5-2 mm thick. Outer surface yellow, yellowish-green or dull yellowish-brown; thin and translucent; marked with numerous ridge-like wrinkles, undulate (wavy) when viewed laterally. Brittle, breaks easily; when broken, surface cuticular and lustrous. Odour: slightly fishy; taste: slightly bitter.

Indications 1. Dyspepsia, infantile malnutrition, anaemia 2. Enuresis, nocturnal emission 3. Urinary and biliary stones 4. Hepatospleenomegaly

Chemical Composition Mainly contains ventriculin, karatin and a variety of amino acids.

Eupolyphaga seu Steleophaga

Ground Beetle
Tubiechong
土鱉蟲

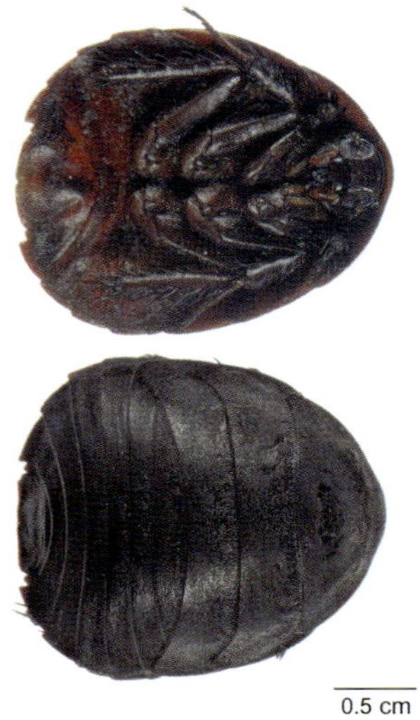

Crude drug

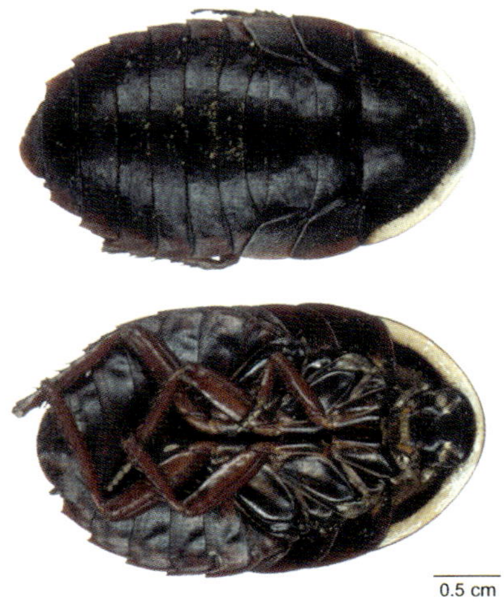

***Opisthoplatia orientalis* Burmeister**

Source The body of female *Eupolyphaga sinensis* Walker (Fam. Corydiidae).

Distribution Mainly in Chinese provinces such as Jiangsu, Anhui, Henan, Hubei and Sichuan. Harvested from wild or domestic ground beetles.

Harvest & Processing Catch ground beetles anytime in spring, summer and autumn; scald to death in boiling water; dry under the sun or by heat.

Description Flattened and egg-shaped; 1.3-3 cm long, 1.2-2.4 cm wide. Anterior end relatively narrow, posterior end broader. Dorsum light purplish-brown, lustrous, apterous (wingless); tergum of prothorax relatively well-developed, covering the head; ventral shields 9, imbricate (overlapping like tiles on a roof). Ventral side reddish-brown; head relatively small, with a pair of filiform (thread-like) antennae; antennae often fallen off; thorax with 3 pairs of legs covered with fine hairs and prickles. Abdomen with transverse annular somites. Texture loose and brittle, breaks easily; when broken, greyish-black soil found in abdomen. Odour: with a fishy stench; taste: slightly salty.

Indications 1. Bone fracture 2. Amenorrhoea 3. Abdominal mass.

Chemical Composition Mainly contains essential oils, fatty acids and amino acids.

Note According to *C.P.*, also used for medicinal purposes is the body of female *Steleophaga Plancyi* (Boleny), which belongs to the same family as *E. sinensis* Walker. Eupolyphaga seu Steleophaga is listed as slightly toxic. Commonly used in Hong Kong is the body of female *Opisthoplatia orientalis* Burmeister (Fam. Epilampidae).

Faeces Trogopterori

Trogopterus Dung

Wulingzhi

五靈脂

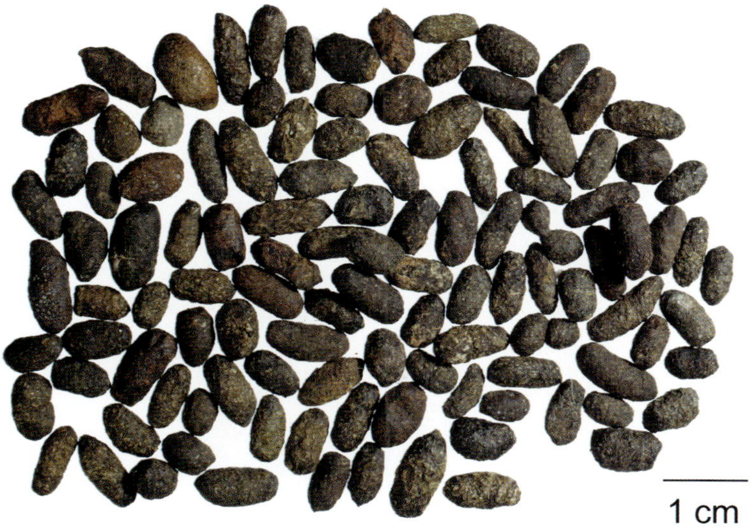

1 cm

Crude drug

Source The faeces of *Trogopterus xanthippes* Milne-Edwards (Fam. Petauristidae)

Distribution Mainly in Chinese provinces such as Hebei and Shanxi; also in provinces such as Hubei and Sichuan. Some harvested from cultivated trogopterus.

Harvest & Processing Collect faeces in caves or crevices of rocks anytime during the year, more frequently in spring and autumn; remove foreign matter; dry under the sun.

Description Oblong and elliptical, both ends obtuse; 0.5-1.5 cm long, 3-6 mm in diameter. Outer surface relatively smooth or slightly rough; dull blackish-brown or greyish-brown. Light in weight; texture loose; when broken, surface yellowish-green or blackish-brown, fibrous; when twiddled, breaks easily and becomes pulverulent (powdery). Odour: the fragrance of cypress leaves; taste: slightly bitter.

Indications 1. Dysmenorrhoea, menorrhagia, dysfunctional uterine bleeding 2. Trauma, angina pectoris, peptic ulcer 3. Snake, scorpion and centipede bites (both orally and external use)

Chemical Composition Mainly contains goreishic acid, catechol, benzoic acid, allantoin and uracil.

Gecko

Tokay Gecko
Gejie

蛤蚧

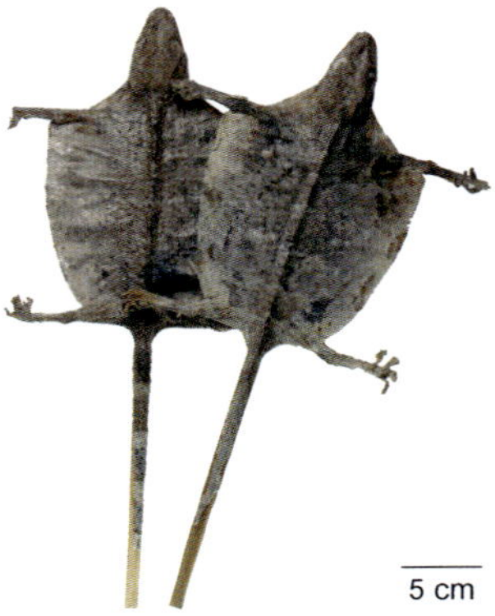

Crude drug
(Tokay gecko)

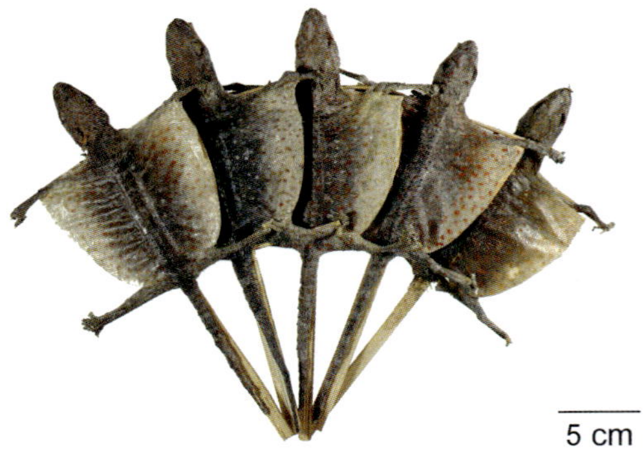

Crude drug
(Imported Tokay gecko)

Source The body of *Gekko gecko* L. (Fam. Gekkonidae).

Distribution Mostly in Chinese provinces such as Guangxi and Jiangsu, and harvested from cultivated tokay geckos. Also imported from Vietnam, Thailand, Cambodia and Indonesia. Commonly used in Hong Kong are imported tokay geckos.

Harvest & Processing Catch geckos, usually from May to September; cut open the abdomen to remove viscera; wipe off blood (do not wash); stretch out with bamboo strips and sticks to keep the body flattened and the legs straightened; dry at low temperatures.

Description Flattened. Head, neck and trunk together 9-18 cm long, with head and neck taking up about one-third the length; tail 6-12 cm long. Head rather flat, somewhat triangular in shape; two eyes mostly sunken into holes; tiny corneous (of horn-like texture) teeth in mouth grown closely along the jaw; one supranasal scale on each side of nose. Abdomen and dorsum elliptical, abdomen thin. Dorsum greyish-black or silver-grey, scattered with maculae; maculae on imported tokay geckos usually brick-red. Each of the four limbs with five toes, with only rudimentary web between toes; all toes with suckers on the underside. Tail long, thin and firm. Whole body densely covered with small suborbicular (almost round), slightly lustrous scales. Strong and pliable. Odour: fishy; taste: slightly salty.

Indications
1. Dyspnoea, asthma, cough and haemoptysis in wasting diseases
2. Impotence, nocturnal emission.

Chemical Composition Mainly contains choline and amino acids.

Hippocampus

Sea Horse
Haima

海馬

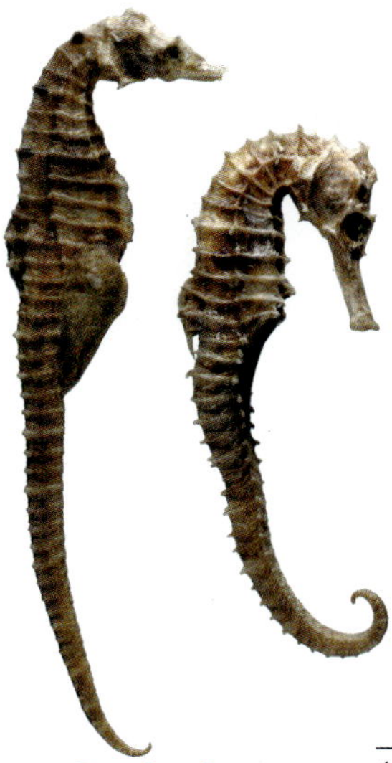

1 cm

Crude drug
(Unskinned)

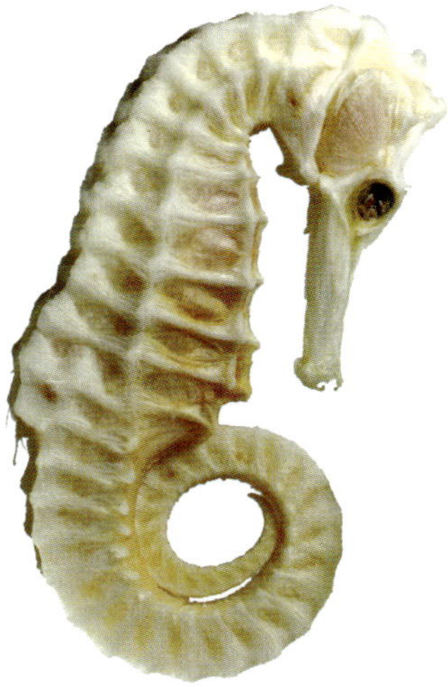

1 cm

Crude drug
(Skinned)

Source The body of *Hippocampus kuda* Bleeker (Fam. Syngnathidae).

Distribution Mainly in Chinese provinces such as Guangdong, Fujian and Taiwan; also in the Malaysian peninsula, the Philippines, Indonesia, and the coastal regions of Australia and Africa. Also cultivated.

Harvest & Processing Collect sea horses from the sea in summer and autumn; wash clean; dry under the sun; or remove skin and viscera; then dry under the sun.

Description Long, flat and curved; about 11-25 cm long. Outer surface yellowish-white. Head somewhat like that of a horse, with a coronary (crown-shaped) protuberance; eyes sunken. Trunk heptangular (seven-angled); tail quadrangular (four-angled), tapered and coiled. Body segmented by corrugations, with thick and short spines. Known for its features of 'horse head, snake tail and corrugated body'. Light in weight; bony; hard. Odour: slightly fishy; taste: slightly salty.

Indications 1. Soreness and weakness of the loin and knees 2. Impotence, sterility, enuresis 3. Dyspnoea 4. Abdominal mass, scrofula, goiter 5. Trauma

Chemical Composition Mainly contains arginine and other amino acids.

Note According to *C.P.*, also used for medicinal purposes is the body of *H. kelloggi* Jordan et Snyder, of *H. histrix* Kaup, of *H. trimaculatus* Leach, and of *H. japonicus* Kaup.

Hirudo

Leech

Shuizhi

水蛭

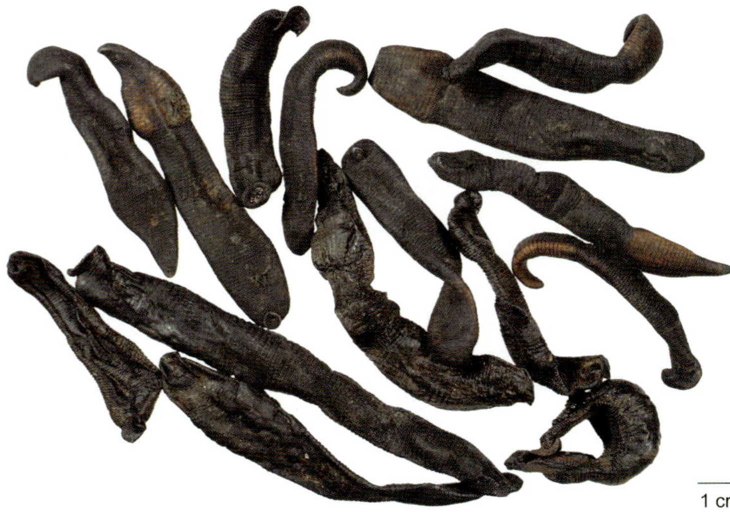

Crude drug

Source The body of *Whitmania pigra* Whitman (Fam. Hirudinidae).

Distribution In all parts of China.

Harvest & Processing Catch leeches in summer and autumn; wash clean; scald to death in boiling water, or suffocate to death with lime powder or ashes of grass and wood; dry under the sun or at low temperatures.

Description Flattened and spindle-shaped; 4-10 cm long, 0.5-2 cm wide. Whole body formed by many somites; anterior sucker inconspicuous, posterior sucker larger. Dorsum slightly bulgy, dull blackish-brown or blackish-brown; when soaked in water, 5 longitudinal rows formed by many black maculae become visible; ventral and lateral sides brownish-yellow. Ventral side smooth; anterior end slightly pointed, posterior end obtuse. Brittle, breaks easily; when broken, surface gelatinous. Odour: slightly fishy.

Indications 1. Amenorrhoea, abdominal mass, trauma 2. Angina pectoris, pulmonary heart diseases 3. Acute conjunctivitis and nebula (eyedrop preparation).

Chemical Composition Mainly contains proteins, heparins and antithrombin.

Note According to *C.P.*, also used for medicinal purposes is the body of *Hirudo nipponica* Whitman and *W. acranulata* Whitman, both of which belong to the same family as *W. pigra* Whitman. *Hirudo* is listed as slightly toxic.

Huechys

Red Lady-Bug

Hongniangchong

紅娘蟲

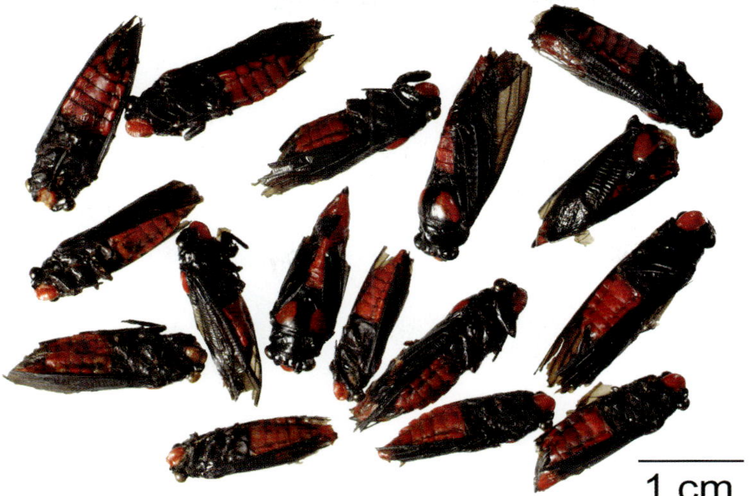

Crude drug

Source The whole body of *Huechys sanguinea* De Geer (Fam. Cicadidae).

Distribution Mainly in Chinese provinces such as Guangdong, Guangxi, Sichuan, Fujian, Taiwan, Zhejiang and Jiangsu.

Harvest & Processing Catch bugs in summer and autumn; dry under the sun or by heat.

Description Oblong and orbicular (round), tapering towards tail, cicada-like in shape but smaller; 1.5-2.5 cm long, 5-7 mm wide. Head black; mouth red; compound eyes large and protuberant. Neck brownish-black. Two shoulders red. Dorsum with 2 pairs of blackish-brown membranous wings; under-wings thinner and transparent; both types of wings with conspicuous fine striae. Thorax brownish-black; legs in 3 pairs, mostly fallen off. Abdomen red, in 8 somites; tail pointed. Texture loose; light in weight; cross-section pale yellow in colour when cut open. Odour: with a slightly stink; taste: slightly acrid. Extremely toxic.

Indications 1. Amenorrhoea 2. Rabies 3. Scrofula, carbuncle 4. Scabies.

Chemical Composition Mainly contains fatty acids and hydrocarbons.

Note Listed in Hong Kong as Category I (Toxic/Potent) Chinese Materia Medica.

Lytta

Mung Bean Bristle Beetle
Qingniangchong

青娘蟲

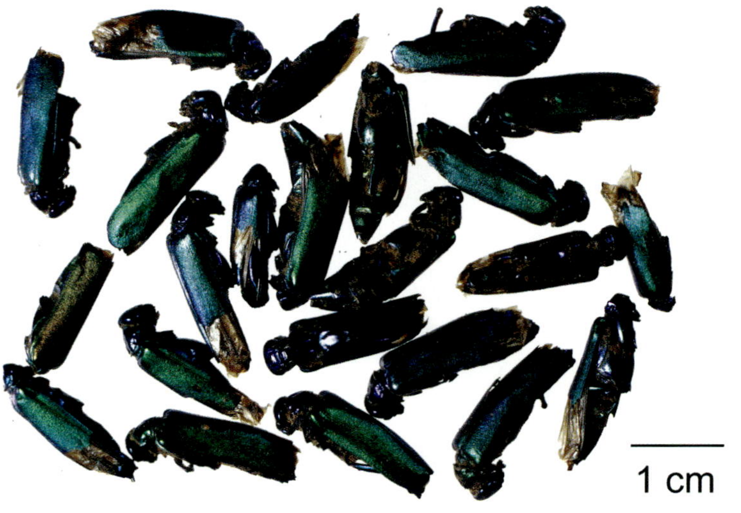

Crude drug

Lytta

Source The whole body of *Lytta caragana* Pallas (Fam. Meloidae).

Distribution Mainly in Chinese provinces such as Jiangsu; also in provinces such as Zhejiang.

Harvest & Processing Catch beetles in April and May; kill by scalding in boiling water; dry under the sun or by heat.

Description Body oblong and orbicular (round); 1-2 cm long, 4-5 mm wide. Head slightly triangular, blue, lustrous; eyes small, slightly protuberant. 1 pair of elytra at dorsum, bright green, bluish-purple or reddish-purple, shiny and beautiful; 1 pair of membranous wings beneath elytra, pale brown, marked with 4 conspicuous venous (vein-like) striae. Thorax protuberant; abdomen in 5 somites; legs mostly broken, emerald-green; antennae mostly fallen off. Odour: slightly unpleasant; taste: hot; powder will cause blisters upon contact with skin.

Indications 1. Abdominal mass 2. Scabies, carbuncles 3. Lymphadenities, tuberculous of lymph nodes.

Chemical Composition Mainly contains cantharidin.

Note Listed in Hong Kong as Category I (Toxic/Potent) Chinese Materia Medica.

Mylabris

Blister Beetle

Banmao

斑蝥

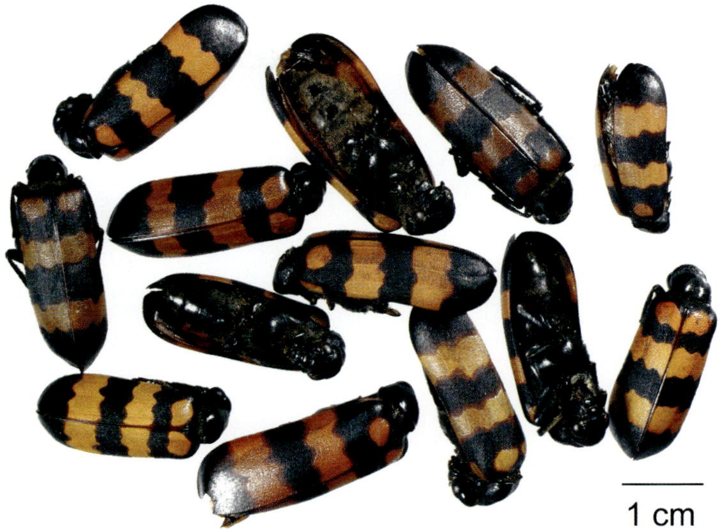

Crude drug

Source The body of *Mylabris phalerata* Pallas (Fam. Meloidae).

Distribution Mainly in Chinese provinces such as Henan, Anhui, Jiangsu, Hunan, Guizhou and Guangxi.

Harvest & Processing Put on protection gear and catch blister beetles in summer or autumn, mostly early in the morning. Kill by scalding in boiling water; dry under the sun or by heat, or stir-fry with grains of rice.

Description Oblong and orbicular (round); 1.5-2.5 cm long, 0.5-1 cm wide. Head and mouthpart pointing downward; head with 1 relatively large pair of compound eyes and 1 pair of antennae, the latter usually dropped off. 1 pair of black, coriaceous (leathery) elytra on dorsum, marked with 3 yellow or brownish-yellow transverse stripes; 2 pieces of transparent, reddish-brown, membranous under-wings under elytra. Thorax and abdomen jet black; thorax with 3 pairs of legs. Odour: with a distinctive stink.

Indications 1. Scrofula, rabies, carbuncle, scabies, leukoplakia vulvae 2. Facial palsy (external use), rheumatism 3. Cancer of liver, oesophagus, stomach 4. Chronic hepatitis 5. Tuberculosis

Chemical Composition Contains 1-1.2% cantharidin.

Note According to *C.P.*, also used for medicinal purposes is the body of *M. cichorii* Linnaeus. The body of *M. phalerata* Pallas and that of *M. cichorii* Linnaeus are listed in Hong Kong as Category I (Toxic/ Potent) Chinese Materia Medica.

Nidus Vespae

Honeycomb
Fengfang

蜂房

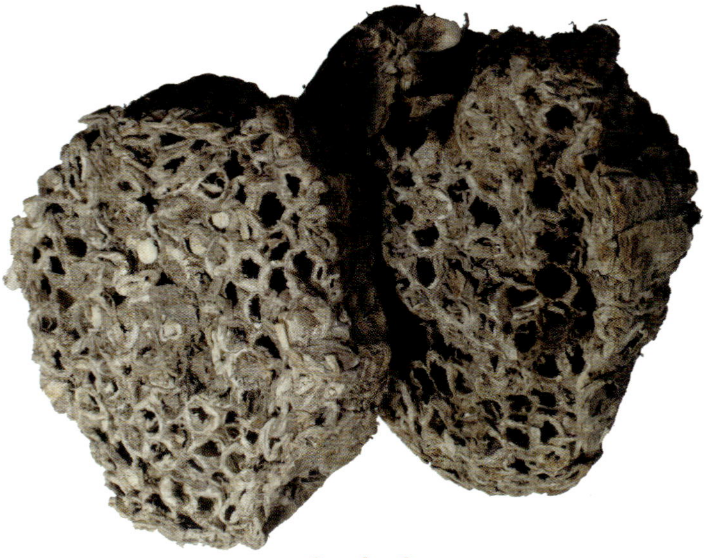

Crude drug

Nidus Vespae

Source The nest of *Polistes olivaceous* (DeGeer) (Fam. Vespidae).

Distribution Mainly in southern China.

Harvest & Processing Collect honeycombs in autumn and winter; dry under the sun; alternatively steam briefly, remove dead bees and pupae and then dry honeycombs under the sun.

Description Disc-like or irregular flattened pieces, some resembling lotus seedpods; varying in size. Outer surface greyish-white or dull greyish-brown. Ventral side with numerous hexagonal cell openings with diameters ranging from 3-4 mm to 6-8 mm. Dorsal side with 1 or several short black stalks. Light in weight; pliable, slightly elastic. Odour: faint; taste: acrid and mild.

Indications 1. Toothache due to caries 2. Sores, ulcers, mastitis, scrofula 3. Ringworm infection, tinea unguium

Chemical Composition Mainly contains honeycomb oils, beeswax and resin.

Note According to *C.P.*, also used as Nidus Vespae is the honeycomb of *P. japonicus* Saussure and *P. varia Fabricius*.

Oötheca Mantidis

Mantis Egg-case
Sangpiaoxiao

桑螵蛸

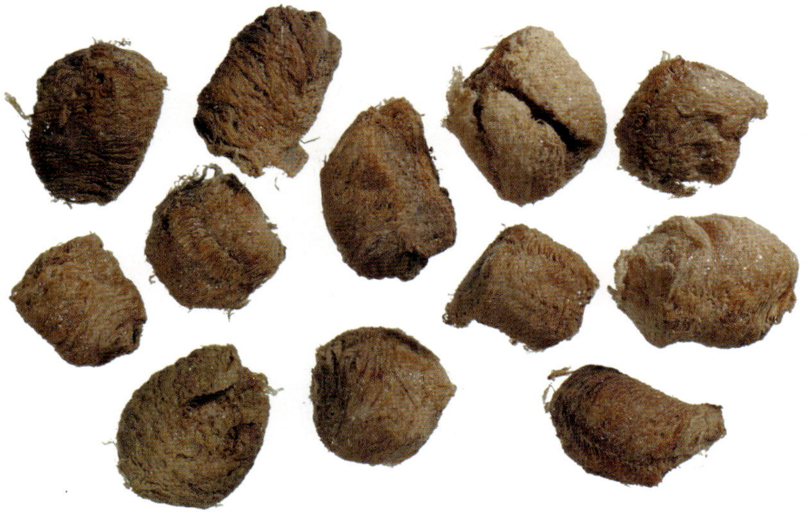

Crude drug

Source The oötheca of *Tenodera sinensis* Saussure (Fam. Mantidae), commonly known as '*Tuan piaoxiao*' (Round Mantis Egg-case).

Distribution An most regions in China.

Harvest & Processing Collect oöthecae from late autumn to the following spring; steam until eggs are killed and then dry. (The eggs must be steamed thoroughly as they can survive heat up to 100℃.)

Description Short and semi-cylindrical, or semi-spherical, laminated with numerous thin membranous layers; 2.5-4.6 cm long, 2-3 cm wide, 1.5-3.1 cm thick. Outer surface light yellowish-brown; dorsal side with an inconspicuous taenioid (ribbon-like) protuberance; underside even or grooved. Light in weight; texture loose but pliable. When broken transversely, surface shows spongiform (spongy) outer layer; inner layer divided into numerous ooecia arranged in a radial pattern, each ooecium with 1 minute, lustrous, elliptical, dark brown egg. Odour: slightly fishy; taste: mild or slightly salty.

Indications 1. Urinary frequency, enuresis 2. Nocturnal emission, impotence, premature ejaculation 3. Leukorrhagia

Chemical Composition Mainly contains glycoproteins and lipoproteins.

Note According to *C.P.*, also used for medicinal purposes is the otheca of *Statilia maculata* Thunberg (customarily called '*Changpiaoxiao*' [Long Mantis Egg-case]) and that of *Hierodula patellifera* (Serville) (customarily called '*Heipiaoxiao*' [Black Mantis Egg-case]), both of which belong to the same family as *Tenodera sinensis* Saussure.

Oviductus Ranae

Forest Frog's Oviduct
Hamayou

哈蟆油

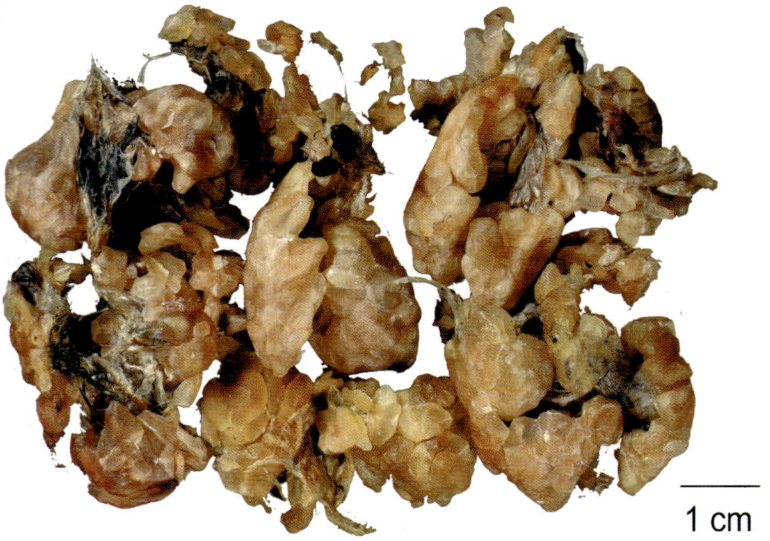

Crude drug

Source The oviduct of female *Rana temporaria Chensinensis* David (Fam. Ranidae).

Distribution Mainly in Chinese provinces such as Jilin, Liaoning and Heilongjiang, and in Inner Mongolia.

Harvest & Processing Choose female frogs; string up through the mouth and dry by wind in open areas; dip dried frogs into hot water to moisten and then scoop up immediately; leave overnight in a bag; cut open the abdomen the next day to take out the oviduct and remove the eggs and other viscera; dry oviduct in cool and well-ventilated places.

Description Lumps irregular in shape, with overlapping folds; 1.5-2 cm long, 1.5-5 mm thick. Outer surface yellowish-white, with lipoidal (fat-like) sheen; occasionally with greyish-white membranous dry skin. Greasy to the touch. Swell up when soaked in warm water. Odour: fishy; taste: slightly sweet, slimy when chewed.

Indications 1. Weakness, palpitation, insomnia and night sweating in debility or in convalescence 2. Haemoptysis in wasting diseases and pulmonary tuberculosis.

Chemical Composition Mainly contains amino acids, cholesterol, and vitamin A and E.

Periostracum Cicadae

Cicada slough
Chantui

蟬蛻

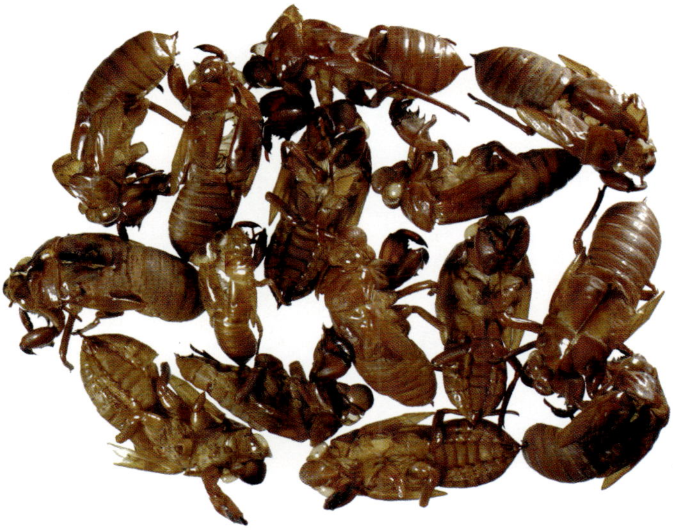

1 cm

Crude drug (Cicada flammta)

Source The slough left during eclosion by larvae of *Cryptotympana pustulata* Fabricius (Fam Cicadidae).

Distribution Mainly in Chinese provinces such as Zhejiang, Shandong, Jiangsu and Hebei.

Harvest & Processing Collect sloughs on the ground or from trees in cicada habitats in summer and autumn; remove soil and other foreign matter; dry under the sun and pack in bamboo baskets; avoid crushing and moistening.

Description Slightly elliptical and curled. Outer surface yellowish-brown, translucent, lustrous. Head with 1 pair of filiform antennae and protruding compound eyes; antennae usually dropped off. Frons protruding; labrum wide and short, labium extended and fistular. Dorsal side of thorax with a cruciform, inward-curling crack in the middle, and 2 pairs of winglets on the lateral sides. Ventral side with 3 pairs of legs; legs covered with fine yellowish-brown pubescence. Abdomen obtuse, divided into 9 somites marked with alternating black and reddish-brown striae. Light in weight; hollow; crumbles easily. Odourless; taste: mild.

Indications 1. Seasonal febrile diseases, sore throat and hoarseness, 2. Eruptive exanthem, pruritus 3. Tetanus, convulsion due to high fever, infantile convulsion 4. Conjunctivitis, nebula, cataract

Chemical Composition Mainly contains chitin, proteins, amino acids and organic acids.

Note In Hong Kong, commonly used for medicinal purposes, and called '*Jin Chanyi*' (Golden Coats of Cicada), is the slough left by eclosion by larvae of *Cicada flammata Dist.*, which belongs to the same family as *Cryptotympana pustulata* Fabricius.

Pheretima

Earthworm

Dilong

地龍

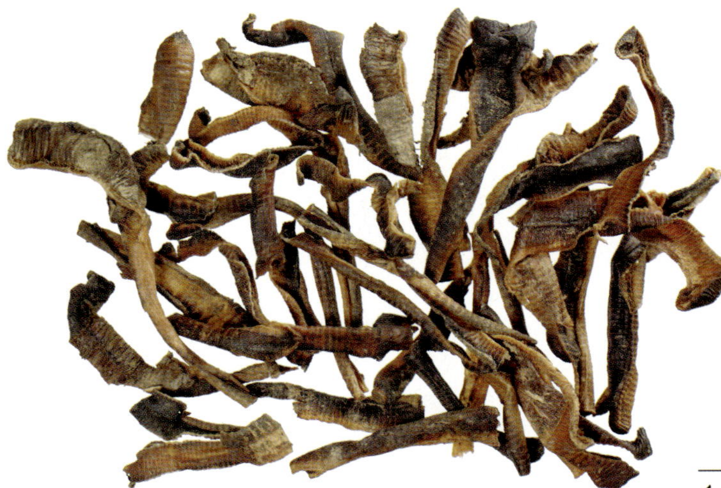

1 cm

Crude drug

Pheretima

Source The body of *Pheretima aspergillum* (E. Perrier) (Fam. Megascolecidae). Known as '*Guang dilong*' (Guangdong Earthworm).

Distribution Mainly in Chinese provinces such as Guangdong, Guangxi and Fujian.

Harvest & Processing Gather earthworms from spring to autumn; promptly cut open abdomen and remove organs, soil and sand; wash clean; dry under the sun or at low temperatures.

Description Long thin strip, slightly curled at margin. With somites down the whole length; dorsal side reddish-brown to purplish-grey, ventral side light yellowish-brown; the 14th to the 16th somites are slightly more shiny and contain the clitellum. Anterior end slightly pointed, caudal end obtuse, setae rings stiff and coarse. Male gonopore located on ventral side at the 18th segment as a small protruding aperture in the setae ring; rim surrounded by several shallow skin folds; setae ring at the inner side of gonopor bulges thicker; in front of gonopore are rows of papillules, 10-20 on either side. Light in weight; slightly coriaceous (leathery), does not break easily. Odour: fishy; taste: slightly salty.

Indications 1. Convulsion, dizziness, headache, epilepsy and insanity 2. Asthma 3. Rheumatism, hemiplegia after stroke 4. Dysuria, retention of urine 5. Hypertension.

Chemical Composition Contains hemolysing lumbritin and amino acids.

Note According to *C.P.*, also used for medicinal purposes, and customarily called '*Hudilong*' (Shanghai Earthworm), is the body of *P. vulgaris* Chen, of *P. guillelmi* Michaelsen and of *P. pectinifera* Michaelsen.

Scolopendra

Centipede
Wugong
蜈蚣

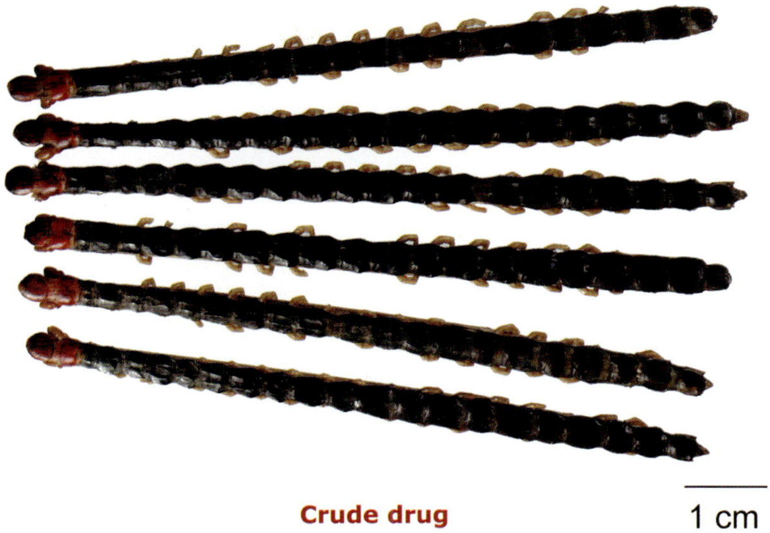

Crude drug

Source The body of *Scolopendra subspinipes mutilans* L. Koch (Fam. Scolopendridae).

Distribution Mainly in Chinese provinces such as Zhejiang, Hubei, Jiangsu and Anhui.

Harvest & Processing Capture centipedes in spring and summer; stretch and straighten by inserting a thin bamboo stick through the head to the tail; dry.

Description Flat slat-shaped strip. The whole body contains head and trunk divided into 22 somites. Head dull red or dull reddish-brown, slightly lustrous, covered by a cephalic plate. First tergum of trunk same colour as cephalic plate, the other 20 terga brownish-green or dark green with lustre, the 4th to the 20th terga often marked with two longitudinal grooves; ventral side pale yellow or brownish-yellow, shrivelled; ambulatory legs yellow or dull reddish-brown, occasionally yellowish-white, hook-shaped, last pair caudate (with a tail-like appendage or end) and breaks off easily. Brittle; broken surface shows clefts. Odour: slightly fishy, with a distinctive nose-irritating stink; taste: acrid and slightly salty.

Indications 1. Tetanus, convulsion, Infantile convulsion, hemiplegia 2. Headache 3. Rheumatism 4. Skin infection, scrofula, subcutaneous nodules, abcesses, snake and insect bites.

Chemical Composition Mainly contains calcium phosphate [$Ca_3(PO_4)_2$] and chitin.

Note Listed as toxic in *C.P.*

Scopio

Scorpion
Quanxie
全蠍

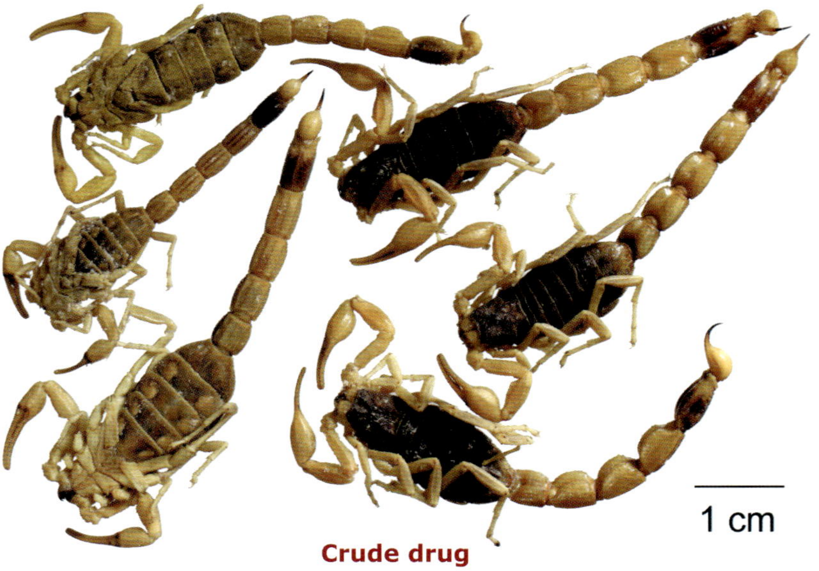

Crude drug

Source The body of *Buthus martensii* Karsch (Fam. Buthidae).

Distribution Mainly in Chinese provinces such as Henan and Shandong.

Harvest & Processing Catch scorpions from late spring to early autumn; put in clear water to wash away soil and sand; scoop out and soak in clear or slightly salty water for 30 minutes to two hours; boil for 20-30 minutes until scorpions become hard and stiff; take out; dry in cool, ventilated places.

Description Cephalothorax and preabdomen flattened, oblong and elliptical; postabdomen caudate, shrivelled and curved; when intact, whole body about 6 cm long. Cephalothorax greenish-brown, anterior part with 1 pair of short, small chelicerae and 1 pair of longer, larger cheliform (pincer-like) pedipalps resembling crab pincers. Dorsal side covered with a scalariform (ladder-like) carapace; ventral side with 4 pairs of legs, each in 7 segments and with 2 claw hooks at the tip. Preabdomen consisting of 7 somites, with the 7th somite darker in colour; carapace with 5 ridges; dorsal side dull greenish-brown. Postabdomen brownish-yellow, consisting of 6 somites; surface of each somite marked with longitudinal grooves; the last somite bearing a sharp unciform (hook-shaped) poisonous sting. Breaks easily. Odour: slightly fishy; taste: salty.

Indications 1. Tetanus, acute and chronic infantile convulsion, cerebral vascular accident, hemiplegia, facial palsy 2. Headche, rheumatism 3. Skin infection, scrofula, subcutaneous nodules.

Chemical Composition Mainly contains katsutoxin, buthotoxin and taurine.

Note Listed as toxic in *C.P.*

Syngnathus

Pipe-Fish
Hailong

海龍

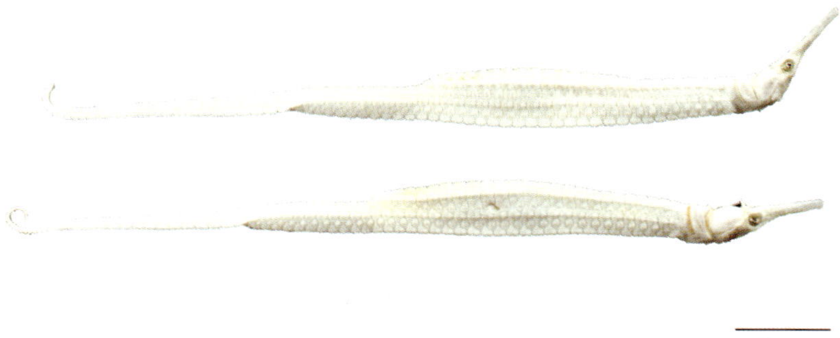

5 cm

Crude drug

Source The body of *Solenognathus hardwickii* (Gray) (Fam. Syngnathidae)

Distribution Mainly in the coastal areas of Guangdong and Fujian provinces in China.

Harvest & Processing Harvest pipe-fish from the sea in summer and autumn; remove skin and viscera; wash clean pipe-fish bodies; dry under the sun.

Description Long and narrow, flat on both sides; 30-50 cm long. Outer surface yellowish-white or dull greyish-brown. Head with a long fistular (hollow and cylindrical) snout, a small mouth, no teeth, and orbicular (round), sunken eyes; head set at an obtuse angle from body axis. Trunk 3 cm wide, pentagonal; upper part of tail hexangular (six-angled), tapering to a quadrangular (four-angled), coiled caudal end. Each side of dorsal ridge with 1 row of greyish-black maculae. Whole body ringed by scleromata with markings, and covered with fine transverse striae; each scleroma with protuberant granular spines. Pectoral fins broad and short; dorsal fins longer but in some cases indistinct; no caudal fin. Bony and hard. Odour: slightly fishy; taste: slightly salty.

Indications 1. Impotence, nocturnal emission 2. Abdominal mass 3. Trauma 4. Scrofula 5. Carbuncles and sores (external use).

Chemical Composition Mainly contains cholesterol and a variety of fatty acids.

Note According to *C.P.*, also used for medicinal purposes is the body of *Syngnathoides biaculeatus* (Bloch), of *Syngnathus acus* Linnaeus, and of other species which all belong to the same family as *Solenognathus hardwickii* (Gray).

Zaocys

Black-tail Snake
Wushaoshe

烏梢蛇

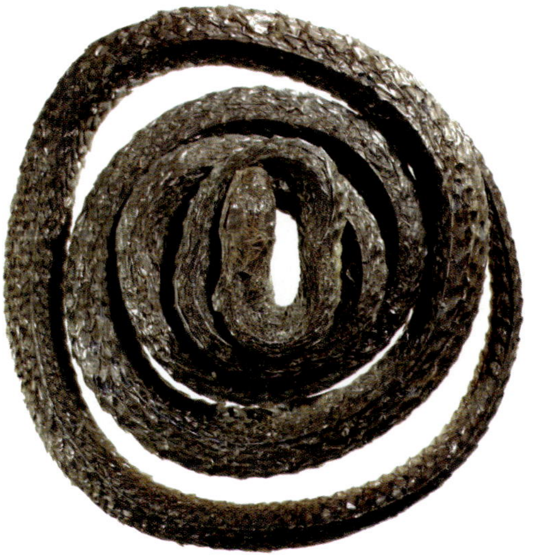

Crude drug

Source The dried, whole body, with the viscera removed, of *Zaocys dhumnades* (Cantor) (Fam. Colubridae)

Distribution Mainly in Chinese provinces such as Zhejiang, Jiangsu, Anhui and Jiangxi.

Harvest & Processing Catch snakes, mostly in summer and autumn; cut open the abdomen or strip off the skin except for the head and tail; remove viscera; curl into a coil and dry.

Description A coil in shape. Outer surface dull blackish-brown or greenish-dark, covered densely with rhombic scales. Dorsal scale in rows of even number; 2-4 rows of scales at the centre of the dorsum ridged, forming two black striae through the whole length of the body. Head in centre of coil, flat and orbicular (round); eyes big and sunken. Upper labial scales 8, with the 4th and 5th reaching the eye socket; 1 loreal scale; 1 preocular scale, relatively small; 2 postocular scales. Spinal column raised, forming a high ridge. Edges of the cut abdomen curling inwards; spinal musculature thick, yellowish-white or pale brown; ribs orderly. Tail long and tapering, with two rows of subcaudal scales. Odour: fishy; taste: mild.

Indications 1. Rheumatism, hemiplegia after cerebral vascular accident 2. Infantile convulsion, tetanus 3. Pruritus caused by scabies, tinea, infection, urticaria 4. Severe skin infection, scrofula.

Chemical Composition Mainly contains amino acids.

Actinolitum

Actinolite
Yangqishi
陽起石

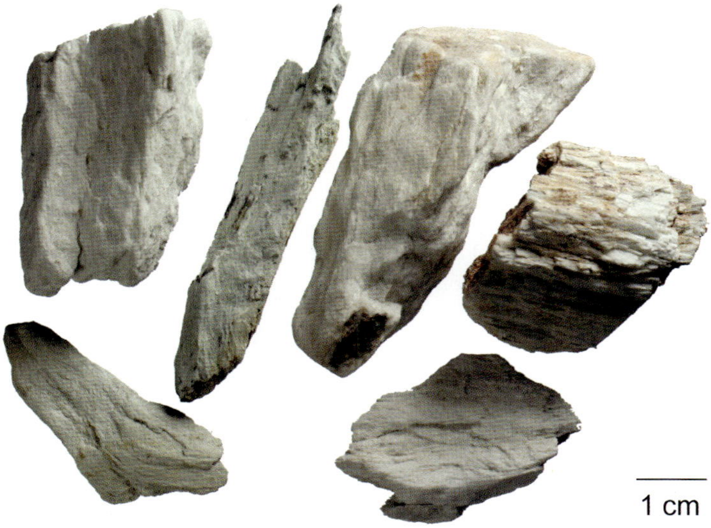

Crude drug

Source A group of silicate minerals called actinolite, which belongs to the amphibole group.

Distribution Mainly in Chinese provinces such as Hubei, Hunan, Henan and Shanxi.

Harvest & Processing Dig out actinolite; remove foreign matter.

Description Aggregates in irregular lumps, or slab-like, or columnar (column-shaped). Outer surface uneven; light greyish-green, green to dull green; with silky or glassy lustre. Heavy; relatively hard and brittle, crushed easily; broken surface fibrous. In some cases relatively loose in texture, twiddled into fibrous powder easily. Odourless; taste: mild.

Indications 1. Impotence 2. Weakness of the loins and knees.

Chemical Composition Mainly contains $Ca_2Mg_5(Si_4O_{11})_2.(OH)_2$.

Arsenicum

Arsenic Trioxide

Pishuang

砒霜

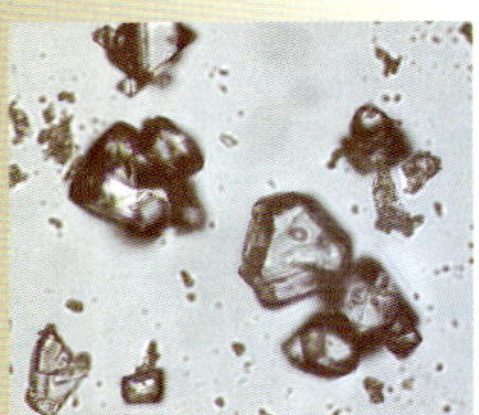

Arsenovs Oxide
Magnified

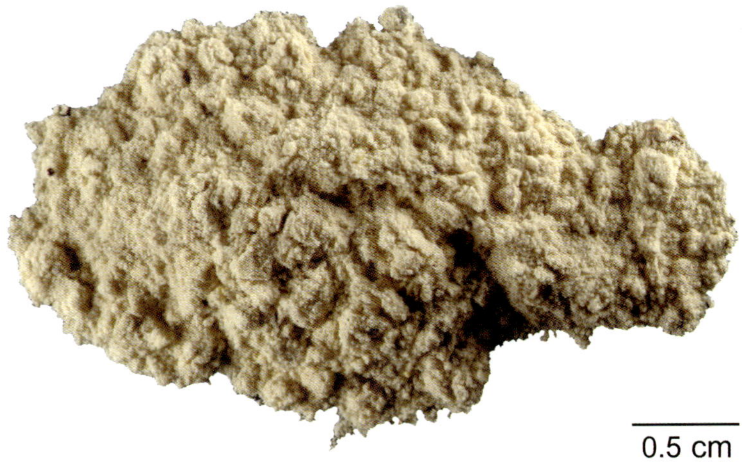

Crude drug

Source Arsenic trioxide obtained through sublimation of *arsenolite*.

Distribution Mainly in Chinese provinces such as Hunan, Jiangxi and Guizhou.

Harvest & Processing Crush arsenolite into pieces; put in a tin, cover the opening with the bottom of an iron bowl; seal the joint with saline soil; fill the iron bowl with water; heat up the tin with a gentle fire for 2-3 hours to produce sublimates on the bowl bottom; let cool; collect the sublimates and remove the remnants in the tin; put sublimates back into the tin and repeat the heating process 2-3 times to produce extremely pure arsenic trioxide.

Description Placoid (plate-like) or pulverulent (powdery). White or pale yellowish-white. Heavy. Odourless and tasteless. Extremely toxic; must not be tasted in the mouth.

Indications 1. Dyspnoeic cough with whitish sputum, asthma 2. Malaria 3.Scrofula, tuberculosis 4. External use for haemorrhoid, fistula, chronic uclers, chronic tinea infection.

Chemical Composition Mainly contains arsenic (III) oxide (As_2O_3).

Note Listed in Hong Kong as Category I (Toxic/Potent) Chinese Materia Medica.

Arsenicum Sublimatum

Arsenolite
Pishi
砒石

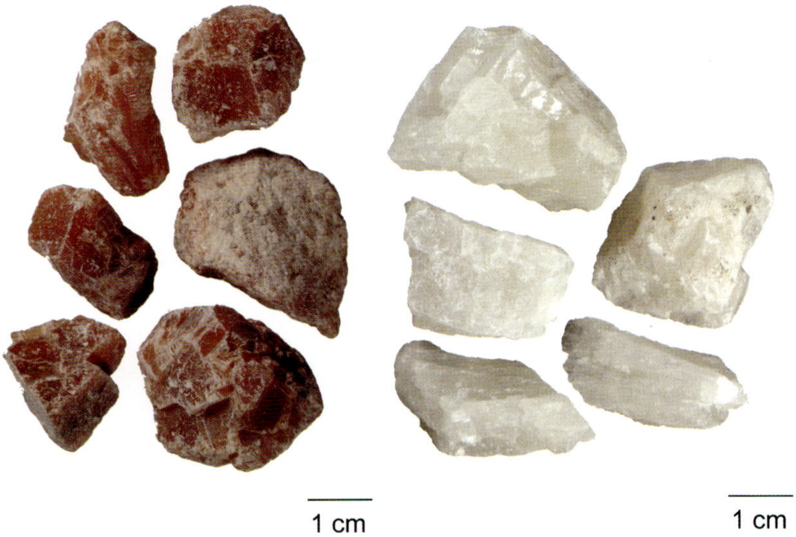

Red Pishi   White Pishi

Source
An oxide mineral called arsenolite; existing naturally, or formed from arsenopyrite, realgar or orpiment, all of which are sulphide minerals.

Distribution
Mainly in Chinese provinces such as Jiangxi, Hunan, Guangdong and Guizhou.

Harvest & Processing
In most cases, process arsenopyrite, realgar or orpiment to produce As_2O_3 and SO_2. In rare cases, collect natural arsenolite ore and remove foreign matter.

Description
Pishi is classified into red *Pishi* and white *Pishi*; red *Pishi* is the main type used for medicinal purposes. Red *Pishi*: Irregular lumps; pale red, pale yellow or a mixture of red and yellow; slightly transparent or opaque; with glassy or silky lustre, or lustreless. Brittle; crushed easily; broken surface uneven or laminiform (consisting of layers). Odourless; when being burned, produce a garlic-like stink. Extremely toxic; must not be tasted in the mouth. White *Pishi*: Colourless or white; in some cases transparent. Purer and more toxic than red *Pishi*.

Indications
1. Dyspnoeic cough with whitish sputum, asthma 2. Malaria 3.Scrofula, tuberculosis 4. External use for haemorrhoid, fistula, chronic uclers, chronic tinea infection.

Chemical Composition
Mainly contains arsenic (III) oxide (As_2O_3).

Note
Listed in Hong Kong as Category I (Toxic/Potent) Chinese Materia Medica.

Calamina

Calamine
Luganshi
爐甘石

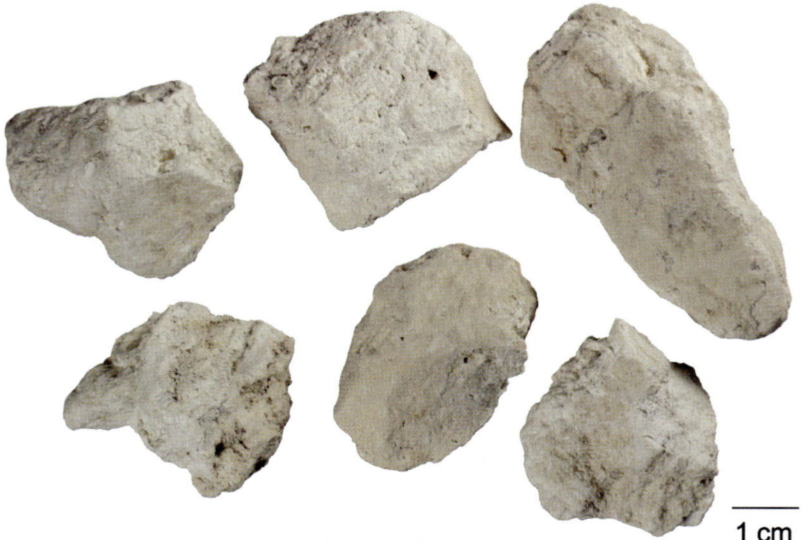

Crude drug

Source A group of carbonate minerals called smithsonite.

Distribution Mainly in Chinese provinces such as Hunan, Guangxi and Sichuan.

Harvest & Processing Mine calamine anytime during the year; remove foreign minerals and soil.

Description Irregular pieces; outer surface greyish-white, pale red or dull yellowish-brown, rough and uneven, poriferous (with numerous pores) and alveolate (honeycombed); pulverulent (powdery). Light in weight; loose in texture, break easily; broken surface greyish-white or pale brown, granular, marked with pores; hygroscopic (water-absorbent). Odourless; taste: slightly astringent.

Indications 1. Conjunctivitis, blepharitis, photophobia, lacrimation, nebula, pterygium 2. Eczema, purulent skin lesion, skin ulcer (external use).

Chemical Composition Mainly contains zinc carbonate ($ZnCO_3$).

Calomelas

Calomel
Qingfen
輕粉

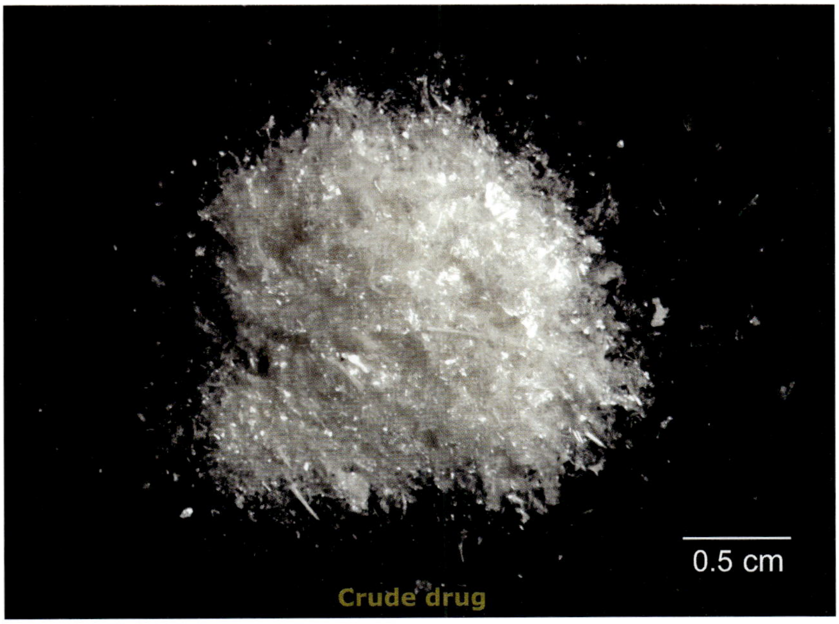

Crude drug

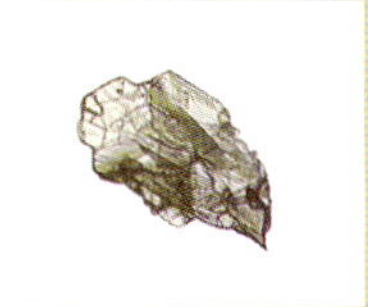

Calomel Magnified

Source The crystal of mercurous chloride obtained through sublimation.

Distribution Mainly in Chinese provinces such as Tianjin, Hubei and Hunan.

Harvest & Processing Mix bluestone, table salt and mercury, put in an airtight container and heat up to sublimate. Alternatively, mix mercuric sulphate and mercury to form mercurous sulphate, add in table salt and sublimate; or, mix table salt solution with mercurous nitrate and nitric acid to produce mercurous chloride precipitates.

Description Lustrous, white squamiform (scale-like) or snow flake-like crystal, or crystalline powder. Light in weight. Odourless and tasteless. Colour gradually turns dull upon exposure to light.

Indications 1. Oedema, ascites, oliguria and constipation 2. Ringworm infection 3. Scabies, ulcus cruris, syphilis, ulcers, eczema (external use).

Chemical Composition Mainly contains mercurous chloride (Hg_2Cl_2).

Note Listed in Hong Kong as Category I (Toxic/Potent) Chinese Materia Medica.

Fossilia Ossis Mastodi

Fossil Bone

Longgu

龍骨

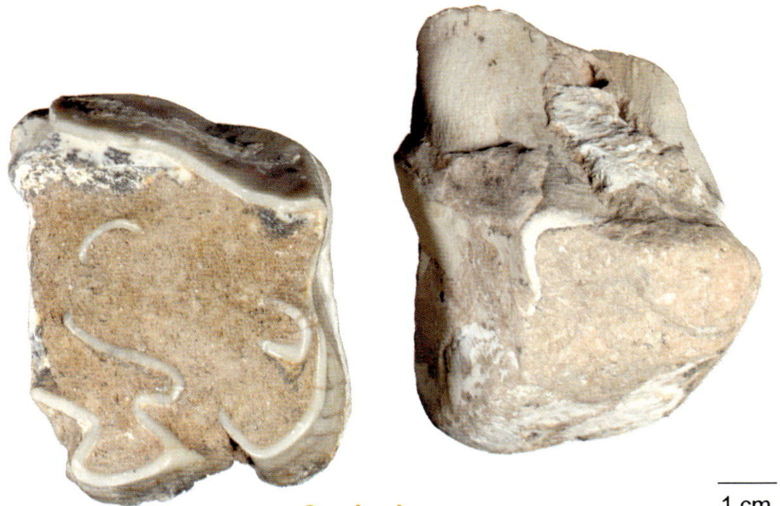

Crude drug

1 cm

Source The bone fossil of ancient mammals such as *Hipparion*, rhinoceros, deer, bovid and elephant.

Distribution Mainly in Chinese provinces such as Shanxi and Shaanxi, and in Inner Mongolia.

Harvest & Processing Dig out bone fossils; remove soil and foreign matter. Since the bone fossils of "*Wuhua long*"(Five-Flower Dragon) are crisp and brittle and break extremely easily upon exposure to air, they are often wrapped with water-absorbent paper.

Description Osseous (bone-like), or irregular fragments; varying in size. Outer surface white or greyish-white, mostly relatively smooth; in some cases marked with longitudinal clefts or brown striae and maculae. Hard, do not break easily; when broken, surface uneven, occasionally hollow in the centre; highly hygroscopic (water-absorbent); sticky when licked. Odourless and tasteless. *Wuhua long* bone fossils: irregular pieces; pale greyish-white or pale yellowish-brown all over, with bluish-grey and reddish-brown markings varying in shade and fineness.

Indications 1. Dizziness, headache, hypertension, irritability, palpitation, insomnia, epilesy, insanity 2. Nocturnal emission, enuresis 3. Menstrual disorders 4. Sweating 5. Exudative prurigo, chronic ulcer.

Chemical Composition Mainly contains calcium carbonate ($CaCO_3$) and calcium phosphate [$Ca_3(PO_4)_2$].

Gypsum Fibrosum

Gypsum
Shigao
石膏

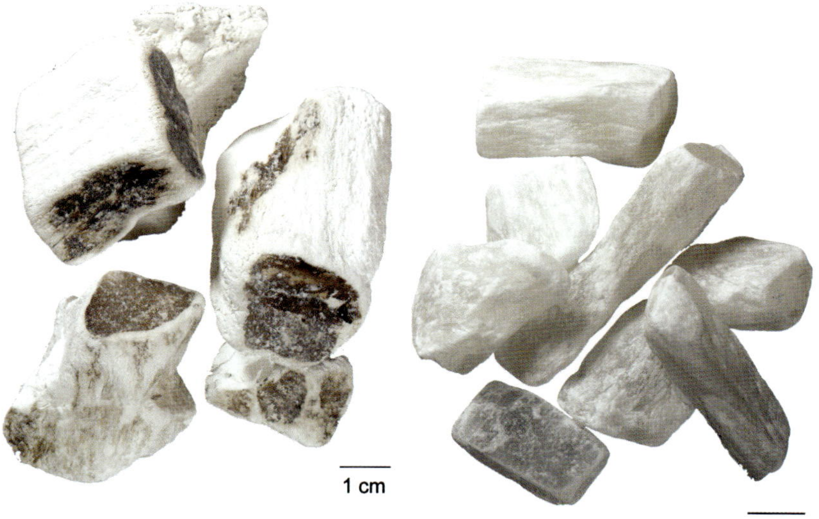

Different forms of Gypsum

Source A group of sulphate minerals called plaster stone.

Distribution Mainly in Chinese provinces such as Hubei.

Harvest & Processing Mine plaster stone anytime during the year, mostly in winter; remove soil and foreign minerals.

Description Slab-like or irregular aggregates of fibrous crystals; varying in size. Off-white all over; often with sandwich layers containing greenish-grey or greyish-yellow placoid (plate-like) foreign matter. Heavy; soft, break easily along the length; length-wise broken surface marked with fibrous markings and silky lustre. Odourless; taste: mild.

Indications 1. Hyperpyrexia, polydipsia, eruptive exanthem, headache 2. Gingivitis 3. Diabetes 4. Osteoarthritis deformans 5. Unhealed skin lesions, eczema, burns (external use).

Chemical Composition Mainly contains hydrated calcium sulphate ($CaSO_4.2H_2O$).

Note According to *C.P.*, also used for medicinal purposes is a processed *Gypsum Fibrosum* called "*Duan shigao*"(Calcined Gypsum).

Haematitum

Hematite
Zheshi

赭石

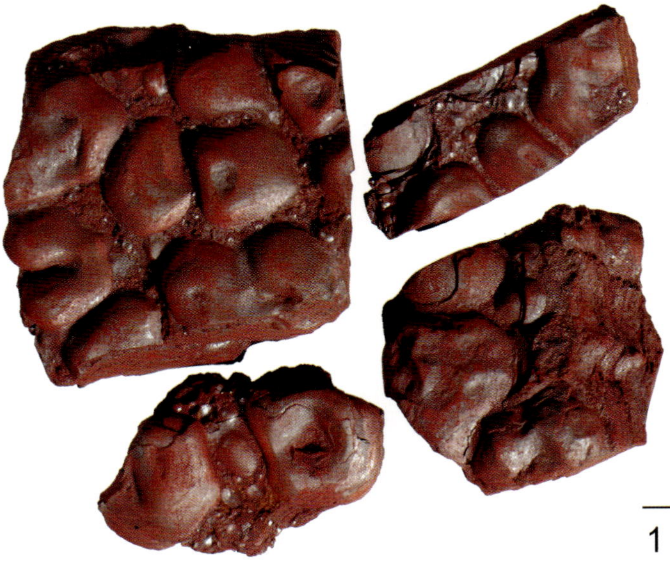

1 cm

Crude drug

Source A group of oxide minerals called hematite.

Distribution Mainly in Chinese provinces such as Shanxi, Hebei and Guangdong.

Harvest & Processing Mine hematite anytime during the year; remove soil and foreign minerals; pick the ones with nail-head shaped protuberances—commonly called "*Dingtou daizheshi*"(Nail-Head Hematite).

Description Mostly irregular and flat; varying in size. Brownish-red or iron-black all over; outer surface with a small amount of brownish-red powder, and in some cases with metallic lustre. One side with orbicular (round), nipple-like 'nail heads' the other side with indentations corresponding in size and position to the protuberances. Hard; not easily cracked; broken surface laminiform (consisting of layers), each layer with undulate (wavy) curves in accordance with the 'nail heads'. Reddish-brown powder sticks to the hand upon contact; hematite turns cherry-red when rubbed against rock. Odour: faint; taste: mild.

Indications 1. Vertigo, tinnitus 2. Vomiting, belching, hiccup 3. Dyspnoea 4. Bleeding such as haemoptysis, epistaxis, dysfunctional uterine bleeding.

Chemical Composition Mainly contains iron (III) oxide (Fe_2O_3).

Halloysitum Rubrum

Red Halloysite
Chishizhi

赤石脂

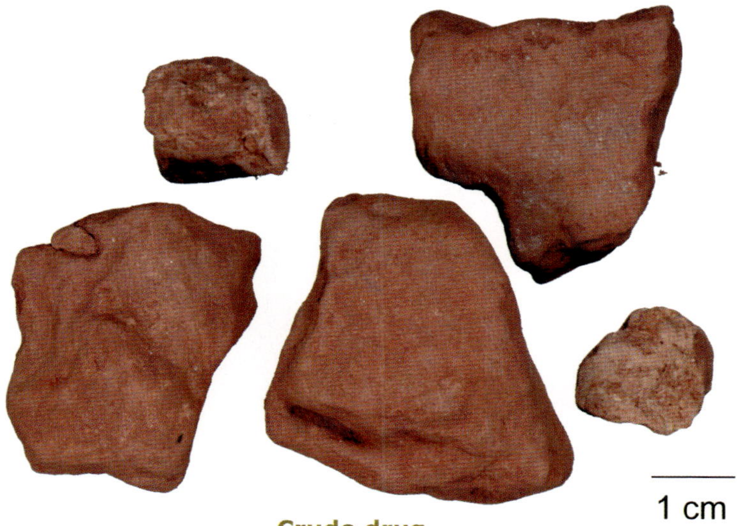

Crude drug

Source A group of silicate minerals called halloysite.

Distribution Mainly in Chinese provinces such as Fujian, Henan and Jiangsu.

Harvest & Processing Dig out red halloysite; remove foreign matter and soil; choose red lumps smooth as grease for medicinal purposes.

Description Lumps irregular in shape. Pink, red to purplish-red, or with alternating red and white striae. Relatively soft, smooth as grease, break easily. Broken surface sometimes with waxy lustre. Highly hygroscopic (water-absorbent). Odour: clay-like; taste: mild; not gritty when chewed.

Indications 1. Chronic diarrhoea, chronic dysentery 2. Bleeding such as haematochezia, dysfunctional uterine bleeding 3. Leukorrhagia 4. Chronic ulcer, eczema with exudation (external use).

Chemical Composition Mainly contains hydrated aluminum silicate $[Al_4(Si_4O_{10})(OH)_8\text{-}H_2O]$; also contains iron oxide (Fe_2O_3).

Hydrargyri Oxydum Rubrum

Red Mercuric Oxide

Hongfen

紅粉

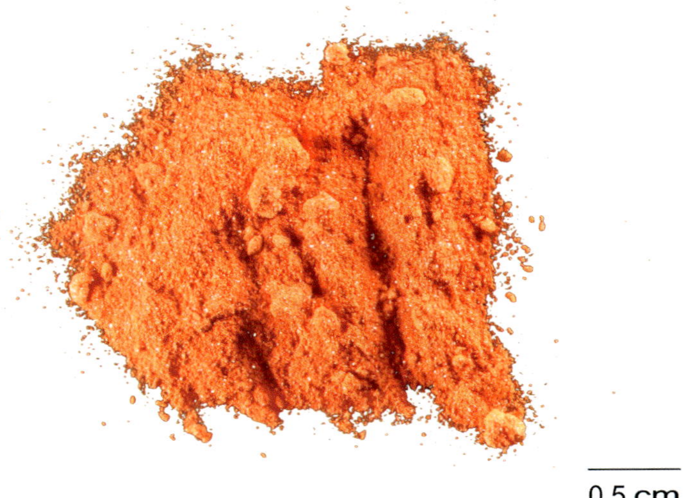

Crude drug

Source Red mercuric oxide processed from mercury, saltpetre and alum, or from mercury and nitric acid.

Distribution Mainly in Chinese provinces such as Hebei, Tianjin, Hubei, Hunan and Jiangsu.

Harvest & Processing Conventional method: put saltpetre and alum in a pot; grind into fine powder and mix well; melt; let cool to solidify; spray mercury onto the surface; cover the pot, often with a porcelain bowl turned face down; refine to get the sublimate called "*Hongsheng*"(Red Sublimate). Nowadays, the synthesis method is also used.

Description Placoid (plate-like) or pulverulent (powdery) crystal; orange or orange-red. Placoid crystals smooth and slightly lustrous on one side; the other side rougher, as if covered with a layer of powder, lustreless. Heavy; hard and brittle. Placoid crystals break easily; broken surface rough, often scattered with sparse pores. Odourless. Colour gradually darkens upon exposure to light.

Indications 1. Chancre 2. Sores, carbuncles (with darkcoloured putrid tissues, constant discharge of pus and difficult to heal up) with possible complications such as fistula and sinuses formation

Chemical Composition Mainly contains mercury oxide (HgO).

Note Listed in Hong Kong as Category I (Toxic/Potent) Chinese Materia Medica.

Hydrargyrum

Quicksilver Hydrargyrum

Shuiyin

水銀

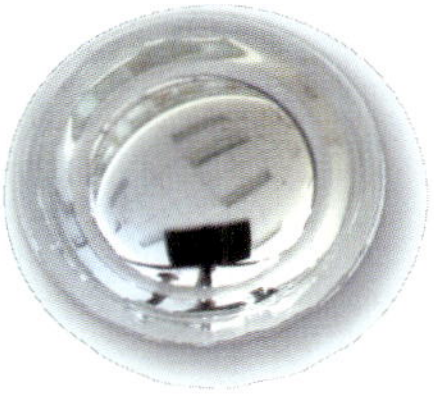

Crude drug

Source A liquid mineral mainly processed from cinnabar ore.

Distribution Mainly in Chinese provinces such as Guizhou, Hunan, Hubei, Sichuan, Guangxi and Yunnan.

Harvest & Processing Collect cinnabar ore, process and refine it into a liquid mineral called mercury.

Description Takes the form of heavy liquid at ordinary temperatures. Silver-white; opaque; with metallic lustre; flows or splits into small balls easily Volatile under heat; becomes gas at 357℃, hardens into tin-like solid at -39℃. Insoluble in water, ethanol and hydrochloric acid; dissolves in nitric acid and hot sulphuric acid, forming mercuric salts. Odourless.

Indications 1. Scabies, tinea 2. Syphilis chancre 3. Skin lesion of leprosy 4. Carbuncles and sores, chronic ulcer. 5. Haemorrhoid and fistula.

Chemical Composition Contains mercury (Hg), and trace amounts of silver (Ag).

Note Listed in Hong Kong as Category I (Toxic/Potent) Chinese Materia Medica.

Lapis Chloriti

Chlorite Schist

Qingmengshi

青礞石

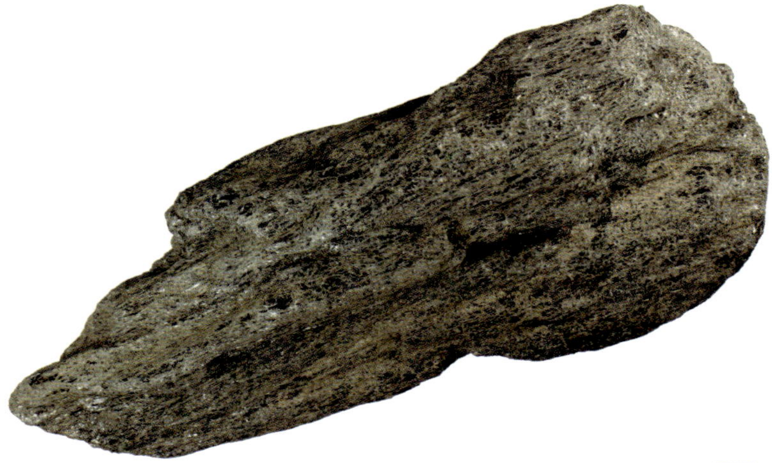

1 cm

Crude drug

Source A black mica schist of the metamorphic group.

Distribution Mainly in Chinese provinces such as Henan, Hebei and Hunan.

Harvest & Processing Quarry schist anytime during the year; remove foreign rocks, soil and sand.

Description Aggregates in irregular, slat-like lumps or long and slanted lumps; without prominent ridges or angles. Dull brownish-black or greenish-black, with glassy lustre. Soft, break easily; broken surface marked with relatively conspicuous layers. Powder with starry lustre. Odour: faint; taste: mild.

Indications 1. Cough, dyspnoea 2. Epilepsy, mania, convulsion, restlessness with feeling of oppression in the chest.

Chemical Composition Black mica schist Mainly contains silicates of potassium, magnesium and aluminum.

Note According to *C.P.*, also used for medicinal purposes is a carbonate schist of chlorite mica.

Lapis Micae Aureus

Mica-Schist
Jingmengshi

金礞石

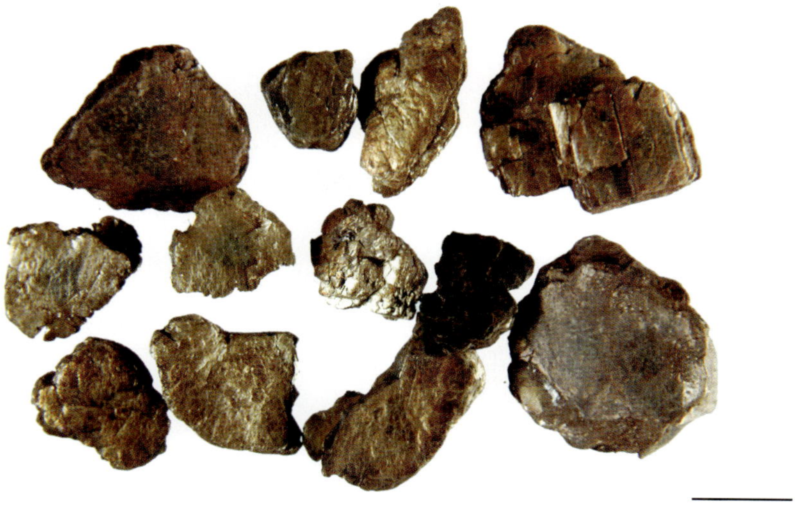

Crude drug

Source A rock schist of the metamorphic group.

Distribution Mainly in Chinese provinces such as Henan, Shanxi and Hebei.

Harvest & Processing Quarry schist anytime during the year; remove foreign minerals; clean off soil.

Description Aggregates mostly in the form of irregular fragments or slats; fragments 1-8 mm in diameter; slats 2-10 cm long, 0.6-1.5 cm thick. Neither ridged nor angular; when broken, surface laminiform (consisting of layers). Pale brown or brownish-yellow, with golden-yellow lustre. Relatively soft; can be used for writing on hard paper, leaving pale brown markings. Odour: earthy; taste: mild.

Indications 1. Cough, dyspnoea 2. Epilepsy, mania, convulsion, restlessness with feeling of oppression in the chest.

Chemical Composition Mainly contains silicates of potassium, magnesium and aluminum.

Note According to *C.P.*, also used as *Lapis Micae Aureus* for medicinal purposes is Black Schist.

Limonitum

Limonite
Yuyuliang
禹餘糧

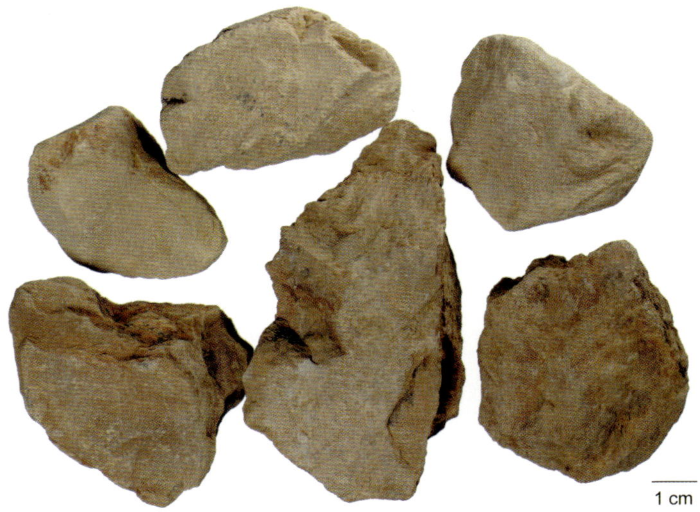

Crude drug

Source A mineral of hydroxides called limonite, containing mainly goethite and hydrous goethite.

Distribution Mainly in Chinese provinces such as Henan, Jiangsu, Zhejiang, Guangdong and Sichuan.

Harvest & Processing Mine ore anytime during the year; remove foreign minerals and soil.

Description Aggregates roughly in the form of rhomboid lumps; 5-10 cm long, 1-3 cm thick. Outer surface reddish-brown, greyish-brown or light brown; usually rugged or with yellow powder. Broken surface usually layered with alternating dark brown and pale brown or light yellow striae; hardness varies between layers, the softer parts can be scratched with fingernails. Heavy and hard. Odourless; tasteless, not gritty when chewed.

Indications 1. Chronic diarrhoea, chronic dysentery 2. Dysfunctional uterine bleeding 3. Morbid leukorrhoea.

Chemical Composition Mainly contains $Fe_2O_3 \cdot xH_2O$, $Fe_2O_3 \cdot OH$ and $Fe_2O_3 \cdot xH_2O \cdot OH$.

Hygrargyrum Chloratum Compositum

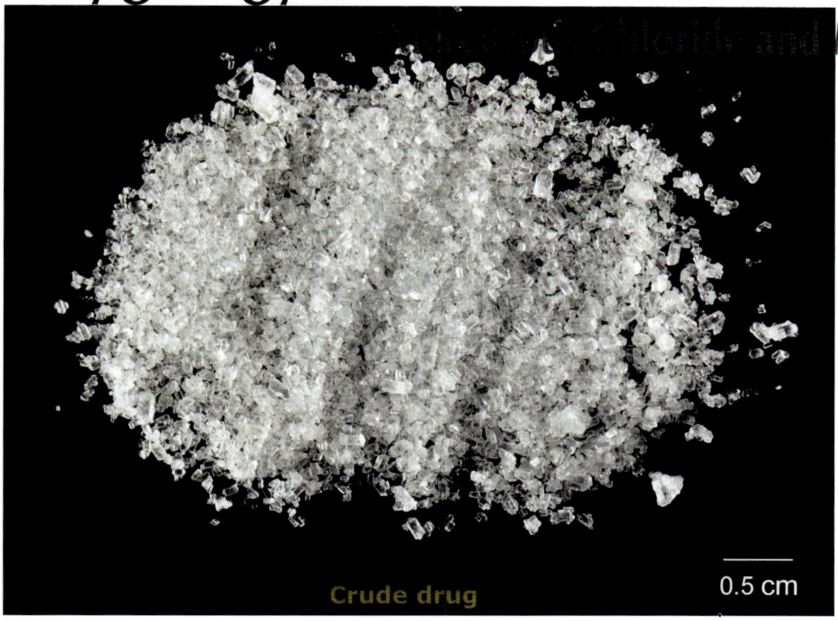

Mercurous Chloride and Mercuric Chloride

Baijiangdan

白降丹

Source The mixed crystal of mercuric chloride and mercurous chloride.

Distribution Mainly in Chinese provinces such as Hunan, Hubei and Jiangxi.

Harvest & Processing Grind saltpetre, melanterite and table salt each 45 g into fine powder, add 30 g of mercury and mix well; mix with the fine powder of 6 g of cinnabar, 6 g of realgar and 15 g of borax; put in an earthen jar and melt over a gentle fire; then dry over gentle heat, do not stop until the jar can be turned upside down and the powder still stays inside - a process called "*jietai*"(base forming). Mix with calcined gypsum powder into a paste and seal the jar tightly; burn with high heat and then gentle heat, stop heating and let cool—a process called "*jiangdan*"(pill finishing). Open the jar and scrape off the white crystals.

Description Placoid (plate-like) aggregates, thick in the middle and thinning towards the brim; 0.2-1.2 cm thick. White or extremely pale yellowish-white. One side smooth, the other rougher; crystals shaped like a bundle of needles visible when viewed from the side, varying in length, unevenly arranged. Opaque; with pearly lustre. Heavy; soft, break easily; broken powder acerose (needle-shaped) or columnar (column-shaped). Odourless; taste: acrid. Extremely toxic.

Indications 1. Carbuncles, furuncles and sores 2. Scrofula 3. Chronic ulcer 4. Eczema, scabies and tinea

Chemical Composition Mainly contains mercury (II) chloride ($HgCl_2$) and mercury (I) chloride (Hg_2Cl_2).

Note Listed in Hong Kong as Category I (Toxic/Potent) Chinese Materia Medica.

Natrii Sulfas

Sodium Sulfate

Mangxiao

芒硝

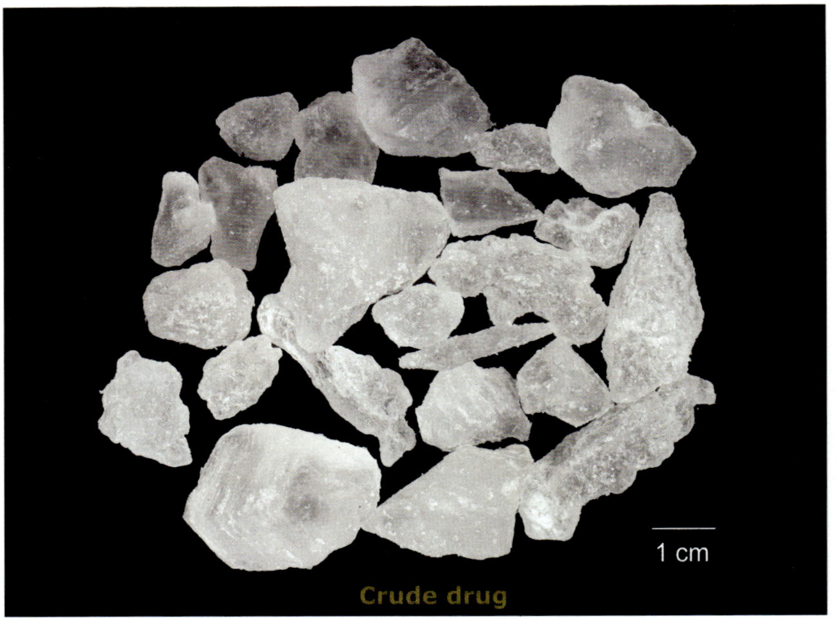

Crude drug

Source The crystal of a group of sulphate minerals called Glauber's salts.

Distribution In most regions of China. Mostly in alkaline-earth coastal regions, areas near mineral springs and salterns, and the interior of damp caves.

Harvest & Processing Dissolve natural sodium sulphate (customarily called '*Tuxiao*', which means crude sodium sulphate) in water; leave to precipitate; filter. Condense the filtrate by boiling; let cool to crystallize; separate out crystals (usually known as '*Poxiao*' or '*Pixiao*', or mirabilite); let the crystals re-crystallize to get *Mangxiao*.

Description Crystals prismatic, oblong and cubical, or irregular in shape, with uneven ends; varying in size. Colourless and transparent; upon exposure to air, surface gradually becomes covered with white powder of anhydrous sodium sulphate as a result of weathering; with glassy lustre. Brittle, break easily; surface marked with white striae. Broken surface rugged. Odourless; taste: bitter and salty.

Indications 1. Constipation with abdominal pain 2. Appendicitis 3.Mastitis 4. Painful swollen haemorrhoid (external use).

Chemical Composition Mainly contains sodium sulphate (Na_2SO_4).

Note Dried, weathered *Mangxiao* is called *Xuanmingfen*, *Natrii Sulfas Exsiccatus*.

Ophicalcitum

Ophicalcite
Huaruishi

花蕊石

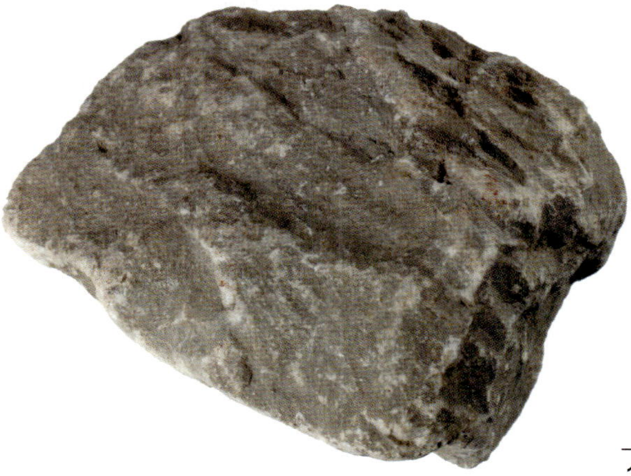

1 cm

Crude drug

Source A serpentine marble of the metamorphic group.

Distribution Mainly in Chinese provinces such as Sichuan, Henan, Jiangsu, Zhejiang, Shanxi, Shaanxi and Hebei.

Harvest & Processing Quarry marble; remove foreign minerals; choose for medicinal purposes small pieces with pale yellow or yellowish-green dot-like or stripe-like serpentine markings.

Description Irregular lumps of aggregates, ridged and angular but not sharp. White or pale greyish-white; marked with what is customarily called '*caiyun*'('halos of colours'); i.e. pale yellowish-green dot-like or stripe-like serpentine markings with wax-like lustre; marble acquires a starry lustre under illumination. Heavy and hard. Broken surface rugged; can be scratched with a carving knife. Odourless; tasteless.

Indications 1. Haemoptysis, haematemesis 2. Traumatic bleeding and pain.

Chemical Composition Mainly contains mineral salts of calcium (Ca), magnesium (Mg), trace amounts of iron salts and aluminum salts.

Orpimentum

Orpiment
Cihuang
雌黃

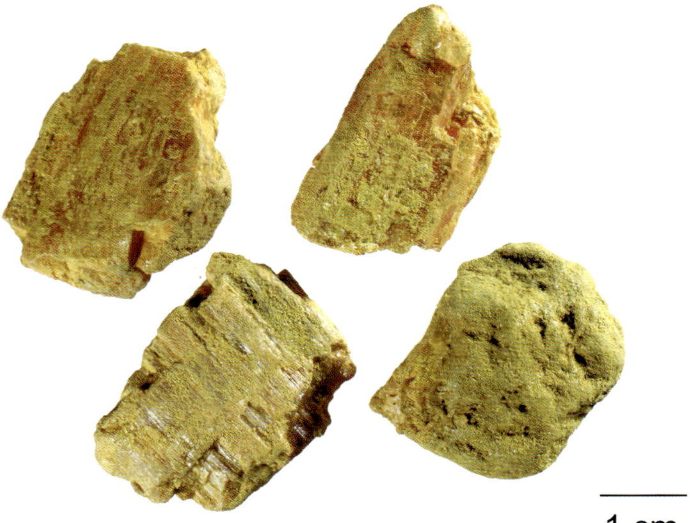

Crude drug

Source A group of sulphide minerals called orpiment.

Distribution Mainly in Chinese provinces such as Hunan and Guizhou; also in provinces such as Yunnan, Sichuan and Hubei.

Harvest & Processing Mine orpiment; remove soil, sand and other minerals.

Description Aggregates in irregular lumps. Yellow, sometimes orange-yellow when mixed with realgar. Outer surface often covered with a layer of yellow powder; marked with lemon-yellow striae; slightly lustrous; transparent; can be scratched with fingernails. Relatively heavy; brittle, break easily; when broken, surface marked with resin-like lustre. Fairly smooth to the touch; stains the fingers. Those with foreign matter greyish-green, opaque, lustreless. Odour: with a garlic-like stench.

Indications 1. Dyspnoeic cough with whitish sputum, asthma 2. Convulsion, epilepsy 3. Intestinal parasitosis 4. Scabies, tinea, sores, carbuncles, snake and insect bites (external use).

Chemical Composition Mainly contains arsenic (III) oxide (As_2O_3).

Note Listed in Hong Kong as Category I (Toxic/Potent) Chinese Materia Medica.

Pumex

Pumice
Fushi

浮石

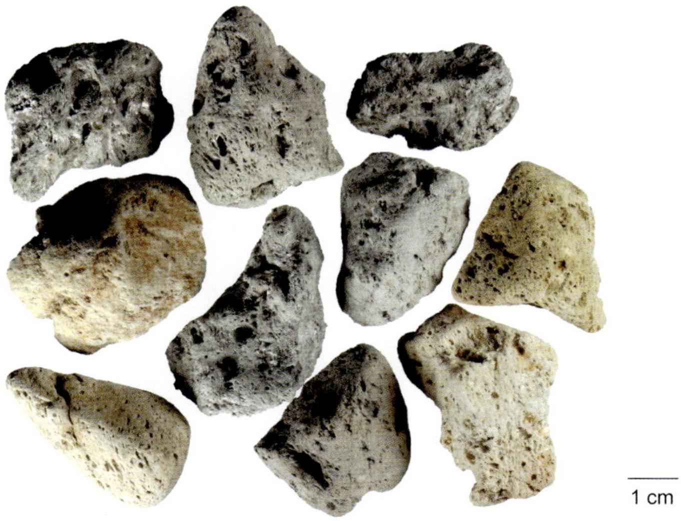

Crude drug

Source The lava from volcanoes.

Distribution Mainly in Guangdong and Guangxi provinces in China; also in Hainan, Liaoning and Shandong provinces.

Harvest & Processing Dredge up pumice stones from the sea in summer and autumn; wash away saline, soil and sand with water; dry stones under the sun.

Description Irregular pieces; varying in size; 2-7 cm in diameter or bigger. Outer surface rough; greyish-white, greyish-yellow or pale brown. With innumerable canals of different sizes, forming a poriferous (with numerous holes), spongilliform (spongy) structure. Hard and brittle; broken surface porous, some with silky lustre. Light in weight; float in water. Odour: faint; taste: mild.

Indications 1. Cough with thick and yellowish sputum, chronic cough 2. Subcutaneous nodules, scrofula 3. Stranguria caused by renal stone.

Chemical Composition Mainly contains silicon oxide (SiO_2), and trace elements.

Realgar

Realgar
Xionghuang
雄黃

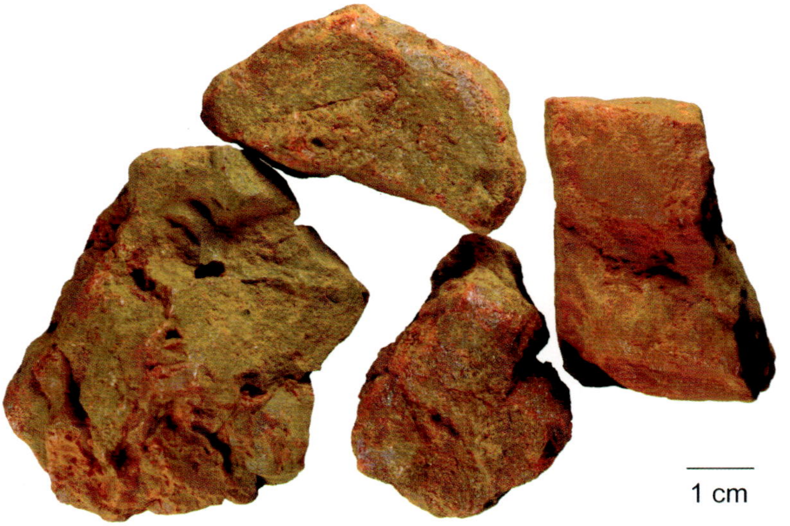

Crude drug

Source: A group of sulphide minerals called realgar, consisting mainly of arsenic sulphide.

Distribution: Mainly in Hunan province in China; also in Chinese provinces such as Guizhou, Hubei, Gansu, Yunnan and Sichuan.

Harvest & Processing: Mine anytime during the year; remove foreign minerals and soil.

Description: Aggregates mostly in irregular lumps. Dark red or orange-red in colour; outer surface often with orange-yellow powder, fingers stained upon touching the powder; surface marked with orange streaks. Slightly transparent or translucent; broken surface lustrous. Relatively crisp and brittle, easily cracked; broken surface red to dark red, marked with resinoid (resin-like) lustre. Odour: with a faint but distinctive stench. Refined ore powder: pulverulent (powdery), or aggregates of powder; aggregates loose in texture, brittle, turn immediately into powder when twiddled with fingers; orange-yellow; lustreless.

Indications:
1. Ascariasis, schistosomiasis, malaria, epidemic diseases
2. Snakebite, insect bite, herpes zoster, scabies, tinea, furuncle, carbuncles with fistule and sinuses formation (external use).

Chemical Composition: Mainly contains arsenic (II) oxide (As_2O_2).

Note: Listed in Hong Kong as Category I (Toxic/Potent) Chinese Materia Medica.

Chinese Index

五畫

六畫

七畫

八畫

九畫

十畫

十一畫

十二畫

十三畫

十四畫

十五畫

十六畫

十七畫

十八畫

十九畫

二十畫或以上

English Index

PinYin Index

Latin Index

Epilogue

Chinese medicine is gaining popularity, status and support, both in Hong Kong and other parts of the world. This must be happy news to all who care about the growth and development of this unique form of Chinese cultural practice. But if Chinese medicine is to be internationally accepted, more work must be done. Every effort must be made to ensure that the strictest safety standards are met. The health hazards posed by counterfeit products must be removed. There must be an end to the incorrect administration of Chinese crude drugs and decoction pieces (known collectively as Chinese materia medica) caused by the lack of standardized nomenclature and other factors. At the same time, every effort must be made to ensure that translations of Chinese medical texts - an important vehicle for the dissemination of Chinese medicine to the western world - meet the expectations and demands of the international community for quality and standard. As they stand now, translations of Chinese medical texts are sometimes marred by errors, or they are rendered in a way which readers with little or no knowledge of Chinese culture, let alone of Chinese medicine, would find foreign, awkward, peculiar, alien, abstruse, uncompromisingly technical, or downright unapproachable. More must be done to improve the situation.

This translation, *An Illustrated Chinese Materia Medica in Hong Kong,* together with its source text, is an effort to improve the situation - both to sort out confused nomenclature and to contribute to quality in translation. The source text, which covers 506 items of commonly used Chinese materia medica in Hong Kong, contributes to the correct identification of these items by listing all the names by which they are known - Chinese common names, *pinyin* of Chinese common names, Latin names, English names, and alternative names (i.e. names by which some crude drugs are customarily known, in Hong Kong and/or certain parts of China, and which account partly for the confused nomenclature [see 'Introduction', Section 5 'Custom-drugs and confused nomenclature' for details]). In addition, the source text provides descriptions of each of the species under the following headings, 'Source', 'Distribution', 'Harvest & Processing', 'Description', 'Nature and Action', 'Chemical Composition' and, if necessary, 'Notes' carrying information pertinent to the requirements of identification, including information on the degree of toxicity, if any, of these crude drugs, and the customary substitutes of these crude drugs. The source text aims to establish an industry platform on standardization and to serve the purpose of setting the benchmark for the Chinese materia medica commonly used in Hong Kong. At the same time, the source text aims to assist in the further education of the practitioners and to nurture more interested participants in Chinese medicine. The translated version shares the same aims. In addition, the translation hopes to contribute to the popularization of Chinese medicine in the English-speaking communities in different parts of the world.

Despite the similarity in aims, *An Illustrated Chinese Materia Medica in Hong Kong* envisages a readership different from that of its source text. While the main body of readers for the source text will be the practitioners of Chinese medicine and professionals in the field, or those who would join the field, this English version is likely to appeal only to people from this group who are interested in the problems or methods of translating Chinese medical texts into English, the rest of the group probably would have no need for it, their working language being Chinese. In view of this, this English version aims to target at two additional groups of readers. The first comprises doctors and medical personnel who are trained in Western medicine and have English as their working language, but who wish to receive training in Chinese medicine or are engaged in the work of standardization of Chinese medicine in an environment with a bilingual language policy. Together with those practitioners of Chinese medicine interested in the translating of Chinese medical texts into English, this group forms what could be called the specialist readers. The second group comprises laymen who know English, and who are interested in getting acquainted, through English, with Chinese medicine, or in joining the profession. Rather than specialists, they could be profiled as the fairly sophisticated and intellectually curious common reader.

Are the demands and expectations of these two groups of readers compatible? What does one have to do to satisfy both groups of readers?

One must consider carefully the strategies of translation.

For *An Illustrated Chinese Materia Medica in Hong Kong,* a translation strategy has been devised to produce a text that addresses the needs of the specialists and the (intellectually curious) common reader alike. This 'twin-appeal strategy' shapes the overall style of translation and informs the making of decisions at every stage of translation. In tackling the problems involved in the treatment of terminology and of style - the two areas where the demands of the specialists and of the common reader are likely to come into conflict - the 'twin-appeal strategy' works in a bifurcated manner while in dealing with the question of accuracy, the 'twin-appeal strategy' can follow a single track mode of operation.

Terminology

In translating a text the main purpose of which is to establish an industry platform on standardization, the use of terminology is an important consideration. However, a text that is full of technical terms and Latinized names would drive away the common reader. It is necessary, therefore, to make some fairly unconventional editorial decisions.

Where it involves identification, in particular, of the different parts of a species of Chinese materia medica, the NOUNS used to designate the parts will be the technical terms. To help the common reader, a number of pen-and-ink drawings will be included to help them know what these *parts* refer to. As for the ADJECTIVES used to describe the parts, the technical terms will be used, but any technical term that is not included in a commonly used dictionary such as *Collins Cobuild English Language Dictionary* will be followed by a simple English explanation in parenthesis. For a phrase such as '先端漸尖，基部近楔形，敘偏斜，上表面墨綠色，下表面灰綠色', the translation will not be 'Apex acuminate, base somewhat cuneate, often oblique; upper surface dark green, underside greyish-green'. Based on the editorial decision just presented, the sentence is rendered as, 'Apex acuminate (tapering to a slender point), base somewhat cuneate (wedge-shaped), often oblique (with unequal sides); upper surface dark green, underside greyish-green.' (See entry on Caulis et Folium Piperis Hancei [Hance Pepper Stem and Leaf, *Shanju*, 山蒟]). After the first instance, the technical terms will be used all through the rest of the text for the same item. And, if two technical terms, both belonging to the category of 'adjectives', are available, the term likely to be known by more readers will be used, provided that both are equally precise in meaning and both are listed in the authoritative reference work, *Plant Identification Terminology: An Illustrated Glossary* (Beijing: Science Press 2001). For example, 'spindle-shaped' will be used rather than 'fusiform', and 'covered with stellate hairs' will be used rather than 'stelipilous'.

Wouldn't the inclusion of explanations make the writing burdensome? For the common reader envisaged by this translation, i.e. readers who are fairly sophisticated and intellectually curious, the answer should be 'no'. In fact, they should welcome the opportunity to learn more about the specificities of the plants, animals and minerals used in Chinese medicine. As for the specialists, the psychology of reading tells us that since the technical terms come first, and the explanations are bracketed, the readers can always skip the parenthetical parts and their reading will not be unnecessarily slowed down.

For the same reason, when a crude drug is referred to in this translation (e.g. in the 'Introduction', the 'Preface', and the text proper), the Latin name will be given first, followed by the English names, the Chinese common name in *pinyin*, and then the Chinese common name. After the first instance, only the Latin name and English name are provided, unless the context requires other arrangements.

Writing style

The twin-appeal strategy informs also the writing style adopted for the translation. A condensed style is used, as befits the genre to which *An Illustrated Chinese Materia Medica in Hong Kong* belongs. This means that phrases and incomplete sentences are often relied upon for the presentation of information. Care, however, is taken to ensure that the condensed style does not make the information load heavier for the common reader than is necessary. Consequently, a fairly well established method of translation for this type of text will not be adopted, i.e. the literal, word-for-word method of rendering. Under this policy, a description such as the following, '撒於火上易燃燒發生爆鳴聲且有閃光，無殘留灰渣' will not be rendered as 'When sprayed into the fire they burn easily, have "pop" sound and flash light, but no dregs remain'. Instead, effort is made to achieve syntactical smoothness and a smooth flow of words: 'Burn easily when cast into fire, produce sparks and crackle, leaving no dregs' (See entry on Spora Lygodii [Japanese Climbing Fern Spore, *Haijinsha*, 海金沙].

In addition, to ensure that the information load does not become heavier than is necessary, clarity of picture will, if necessary, take precedence over the condensed style. In the section 'Harvest & Processing', that which is being harvested is clearly stated even though in the Chinese text, the object will be omitted if it is the same as that described in the section 'Source'. The reader of the English text will be greeted, for example, with the picture 'Collect mature fruits in winter' rather than the more condensed but lifeless phrase 'Collect in winter'. Of course, the specialists do not need such a reminder, but the common reader will be able to see the picture with greater immediacy than if the object was omitted and the reader had to go back to the section 'Source' and check what is being harvested and processed.

The question of information overload is a real consideration. For this reason, the content of the present translation deviates a little from that of the source text: the section on '性味功效' ('Nature and Action') is replaced by a section on 'Indications', which lists the diseases or symptoms for which the crude drugs and decoction pieces described in this book could provide suitable treatment or remedy. Such a move is necessary because the section on 'Nature and

Action' in the Chinese text describes the Chinese materia medica in terms of the philosophical concepts of the five phases and the theoretical parlance of Chinese medicine and it would be impossible to translate that section without providing an introduction to the fundamental concepts of Chinese medicine, or a glossary of key philosophical and theoretical terms in Chinese medicine. But such padding would make *An Illustrated Chinese Materia Medica in Hong Kong* more loaded with terminology and information than it already is. In order not to overburden the readers, both the editor of the source text and of this translation believe it would be more appropriate, at this particular point in the history of the reception of Chinese medicine in the West, to replace that section with one on 'Indications' and thus present information about Chinese materia medica in a language that is more familiar and recognizable - at least to the specialists.

Accuracy

As for accuracy, both groups of readers would definitely expect a high standard of accuracy from the translation. With this happy congruence of expectations, the twin-appeal strategy can work in unison rather than in a bifurcated manner. The following is a description of such a strategy in action:

(1) When a technical term in the Chinese text can be translated by a term in English that is more specific in designation and meaning, that English term will be used to achieve precision of reference. Take for example the term '鬚根', which is frequently used in the Chinese text in descriptions of roots and rhizomes. Instead of rendering it as 'roots', the term '鬚根' is translated as 'fibrous roots' for monocotyledons (i.e. plants having a single seed-leaf) and as 'rootlets' for dicotyledons.

(2) Terms which have not been used in a precise or accurate manner will be jettisoned, even though they are frequently found in existing translations or bilingual texts. Three terms, in particular, require discussion at some length - '中藥' (*zhongyao*), '中成藥' (*zhongchengyao*), and the term 'drug'. It is true that in this book, the first two terms figure almost solely in the 'Introduction' and not the text proper, nonetheless, they deserve careful attention because they represent two central concepts in Chinese medicine and the existing translations of these terms are either lacking in precision or in uniformity. '中藥' (*zhongyao*) is translated in this book as 'Chinese medicines', which is also the translation adopted by the Chinese Medicine Council of Hong Kong (香港中醫藥管理委員會), even though the more popular and more frequently used translation is 'Chinese herbal medicine'. This decision is best explained by an explication of what is embraced in the category, '中藥' (*zhongyao*). 'Zhongyao' refers to the medicines prescribed in accordance with the principles and theories of orthodox Chinese medicine. It includes three main components: crude drugs (*yuanyaocai*, 原藥材), decoction pieces (*yinpin*, 飲片), and proprietary Chinese medicines (*zhongchengyao*, 中成藥). The crude drugs often come from the kingdom of plants although they also include animals and minerals. The prevailing translation 'Chinese herbal medicine' is based on the principle of using the part to represent the whole. In the days when Chinese medicine was still unknown to the Western world, or known primarily as a kind of curiosity or a somewhat exotic practice, the translation of '*zhongyao*' (中藥) as 'Chinese herbal medicine' has the advantage of highlighting the distinctive feature of Chinese medicine - the predominant use of plants and herbs for medicinal purposes. Now that there is a concerted effort to establish Chinese medicine in the international arena as a separate and independent school of medicine, now that Chinese medicine is getting more widely accepted in the West, it is perhaps time to replace 'Chinese herbal medicine'[1] with a more comprehensive, more exact, and more precise translation - 'Chinese medicines'. The plural form is used to stress that the ingredients are not confined to plants and herbs.

As for '*zhongchengyao*' (中成藥), it is translated as 'Chinese patent medicine' in *Chinese-English Classified Dictionary of Traditional Chinese Medicine and Pharmacology* (1996), and as 'traditional Chinese patent medicine' in *A Comprehensive Chinese-English Dictionary of Traditional Chinese Medicine* (1997).[2] In Webster's Third International Dictionary, 'patent medicine' is explained as meaning 'a packaged nonprescription drug or medicine of secret composition protected by a trademark and with the name of the medicine, directions for use, and name and business of the address of the manufacturer on the label or package'. While the explanation does come close to the meaning of

---

1 'Chinese herbal medicine' in its plural form - 'Chinese herbal medicines' - would serve as a good translation of 中草藥 (*zhongcaoyao*). See footnote 4 of 'Introduction' for a short discussion of this question.

2 The use of the term 'patent Chinese medicines' could perhaps be traced to the 1992 English edition of the authoritative work on Chinese materia medica, the *Pharmacopoeia of the People's Republic of China*. The *Pharmacopoeia* uses the term 'traditional Chinese patent medicines' to translate '成方' and indicates that '中藥成方' is interchangeable with '中成藥'. But this is a complex question that needs further research.

'zhongchengyao' (中成藥), the word 'patent' remains problematic because of the legal implications carried by the word, i.e., the implications contained in the patent laws, both of Britain and of the United States. It is well known that the practice of obtaining patent is not yet very well developed in the Chinese medicine profession. Certainly, not every item included in the *Pharmacopoeia of the People' s Republic of China* has been officially patented. In fact, one of the matters for concern among members of the profession is how the precious discoveries about the medicinal values and potentials of plants, herbs, animals, minerals, etc., made by the Chinese people through the millennia, could be protected. The matter is becoming more urgent as there is now a danger that members of the profession might lose the legal right to the use of some Chinese crude drugs due to their slowness in obtaining patent. Given all these considerations, the translation of '*zhongchengyao*' (中成藥) as 'Chinese patent medicine' or 'traditional Chinese patent medicine' would no longer be appropriate. The term used by the Chinese Medicine Council of Hong Kong, mainly for legislation purpose, is 'proprietary Chinese medicine'. One of the meanings of 'proprietary' listed in *Webster' s Third International Dictionary* is 'a nonprescription drug or medicine designed for self-medication and required to be accompanied by a list of active ingredients and directions for safe use'. Since this is also an accurate description of the characteristic features of '*zhongchengyao*' (中成藥), the term 'proprietary Chinese medicines' is adopted in this book. When the urgent task of obtaining patent for Chinese medicines has been completed, the translation of '*zhongchengyao*' (中成藥) could perhaps revert to 'patent medicines' or 'patent Chinese medicines'. At present, however, the situation makes 'proprietary Chinese medicines' a more appropriate and more precise rendering.

Regarding the term 'drug', it is used, in some existing translations of texts on Chinese materia medica, in the section on harvest and processing to refer to the crude drug that is being collected or harvested. But since the term 'drug' has very specific meanings in Western medicine, and since doctors and students of Western medicine are some of the specialists targeted at by *An Illustrated Chinese Materia Medica in Hong Kong*, the word should be avoided. In its place, the name of the actual thing that is being collected should be given - a point already made above, in the section on 'Writing Style'. In any case, an expression such as 'Collect drug in summer' does not make sense to the specialists since it should be the raw material, for example, the roots, stems, rhizomes, etc., that are being collected. Likewise, the specialists would frown at a phrase such as the following: 'commonly used in Hong Kong are the angled-cut slices of the drug'. The present translation seeks to present this type of information in a more accurate manner, 'Commonly used in Hong Kong in the form of angled-cut slices' (See, for example, the entry on Caulis Sargentodoxae [Sargentgloryvine Stem, *Daxueteng*, 大血藤]).

(3)Ambiguities will be removed to ensure greater clarity of meaning. Generally speaking, there are two kinds of ambiguities to be guarded against:

(a) Ambiguities permitted to exist in Chinese texts because the meanings are already clear to the practitioners of Chinese medicine will be eliminated to achieve precision of meaning. Take for example, the description '多分枝'. Does it mean 'mostly with branches', or 'with many branches', or both? The practitioners of Chinese medicine know the answer, but in translating these two phrases into English, the ambiguities must be resolved and the correct meaning (i. e. 'with many branches') given.

(b)Ambiguities existing inherently in Chinese will be cleared up. An illustrative example is the adjective '破碎' (meaning 'broken-fragmented', with no distinction between the active and passive states). The term is used in the source text to describe the shape of leaves - '葉多皺縮, 有的破碎'. At the same time, it can also be used together with the adjective '易' (easy) to form '易破碎' (easy + broken-fragmented) to describe leaves, testa, flower buds, fruits, and minerals. In the former case, it is translated as 'Leaves mostly shriveled, with some in fragments' (See entry on Caulis et Folium Piperis Hancei [Hance Pepper Stem and Leaf]), and not 'broken', 'crushed' or 'crumpled', even though all three are acceptable translations of '破碎' (broken-fragmented). In the latter case, i.e. '易破碎' (easy + broken-fragmented), since no distinction is drawn in the Chinese expression between the active and passive states, the expression can be rendered as 'easily broken' or 'breaks easily'. However, there is a distinction in meaning between the two renderings. 'Breaks easily' implies that no external force or agent is required to break the thing being referred to while 'easily broken' implies that the thing being referred to is fragile and can be easily broken. In translation, the inherent ambiguities in the Chinese expression are removed and the expression 'breaks easily' is used, except for the description of the slough of cicadas, which is translated as 'crumbles easily' (See entry on Periostracum Cicadae [Cicada Slough, *Chantui*, 蟬蛻]).

Indeed, it is for the purpose of resolving, clarifying and removing the ambiguities in meaning detected in the process of translating that the present version would, when necessary, differ in content from the Chinese version.

(4) Comical expressions found in other translations or bilingual texts will be replaced. Translators who are translating out of their mother tongue do well to be especially alert to this point. Again, just one example will suffice. The expression '不易折斷' is frequently used in Chinese texts on Chinese materia medica to describe roots, rhizomes, etc. In translation, the expression is often rendered as 'uneasily broken'. The specialists would certainly know the correct

meaning (i.e. 'does not break easily'). The common reader, however, might think that the personification technique (i.e. the attribution of human attributes to non-human objects) is used and that the leaves, etc., are feeling uneasy as they are being broken, or that the agent of force feels uneasy over his/her violence. A peculiar rendering. Of course, one might say that inaccuracies of this type are minor. But when different kinds of minor inaccuracies accumulate, the readers may begin to cast doubt on the quality, and hence the reliability, of the translation. This translation attempts to guard against the emergence of such a scenario.

Conclusion

The twin-appeal strategy of translation, described above, is aimed at producing a translation with a readership that goes beyond the circle of specialists. At every stage in the process of translation, the twin-appeal strategy involves decisions and measures that often depart from the conventional ways of thinking about translating. Conventionally, the Chinese version of *An Illustrated Chinese Materia Medica in Hong Kong* would be categorized by its text type and characterized as information-centred and technical in nature. Translating this type of text would be considered to fall into the category of technological translating and all translation decisions will be informed by the principles of technological translating.

Such a mode of thinking has helped generations of translators handle the job of translating and it is still helpful today, for the translating of many different types of texts, including texts on Chinese materia medica. The question is - how widely do we want Chinese medicines to travel? In what manner do we want Chinese medicines to travel? What status do we want it to achieve? Do we want to see Chinese medicines travelling apologetically in the West as one speaking in an esoteric tongue and incapable of communicating with the ordinary people? Or as one inadequate, for whose inadequacies allowances have to be made to be accepted? If the translations that transport the relatively simple information on Chinese materia medica should be wanting, either because they are too technical or because they are burdened with inadequacies and peculiarities, what hopes are there for the more complex philosophical system of Chinese medicine to be safely and happily carried across to another land? Or, for that matter, how would Chinese medicine find a coherent and precise language of its own in a foreign land without being at best subsumed as an appendage to Western medicine? In this light, the task of translating Chinese medical texts has to be undertaken with great care. And the translations thus produced would prioritize fine distinction of meaning, accuracy of information, and, above all, they would aspire to reach a readership that includes not only the converted and the professionals but also the common reader. Of course, not just any common reader - not yet - but those who are ready to venture into a domain of knowledge new to them, and who are intellectually curious and fairly sophisticated.

This is not an attempt to dismiss existing methods of translating. Rather it is an attempt to call for a new way of thinking about what translating entails. The call is for a way of thinking that takes fully into account how well the subject matter (e.g. Chinese medicines) has been received by the target culture at the time when the job of translation is being undertaken. The call is for a careful planning of the strategy of translating. It requires just a mental switch - from the notion of 'principles of translating' to that of 'strategies of translating'. But the effect is significant. 'Principles' provide guidelines for a translator, they serve to tell the translator what methods to use for particular types of texts, or particular types of translation; they have general applicability. 'Strategy', on the other hand, is always purpose-built; it has flexibility as a built-in mechanism, is constantly evolving, and requires constant reassessment of its effectiveness. When the intellectual climate has changed (when, for example, Western understanding of Chinese medicine has deepened) even the same text could be - and probably would be - translated differently, with a different translation strategy.

It is the aspiration of everyone involved in the preparation of *An Illustrated Chinese Materia Medica in Hong Kong* that this translation would contribute, in however modest a manner, to the promotion of Western understanding of Chinese medicines, specifically of Chinese materia medica in Hong Kong.

Martha P. Y. Cheung
Editor-in-Chief of the English translation

Acknowledgements

An interdisciplinary project such as *An Illustrated Chinese Materia Medica in Hong Kong* cannot be completed without the contributions of professionals in both the field of Chinese medicine and of Translation. To colleagues and fellow translators of this project, a very warm thank-you. Without their total dedication and sense of commitment, without their professionalism and infinite patience, this project would still be limping rather painfully along.

A warm thank-you also goes to colleagues in the field of medicine and of Chinese medicine, especially Dr Zhao Zhongzhen, General Editor and the project designer and consultant of this translation. The names of the Chinese materia medica described in this book are provided by him, with the help of Ms Hu Yani and Mr Peng Yong. Dr Zhao has, in addition, provided advice on every single aspect of this book and strengthened the translation and editorial team with manpower - for the sections on 'Indications' and 'Chemical Composition'. The wisdom of such a division of labour is gratefully acknowledged. In particular, Dr. Zhao's expert views and opinions on the accuracy aspect of the content of the 'Introduction' and of the English translation, especially of the sections on 'Harvest & Processing' and 'Description', are deeply appreciated. Also appreciated is the input on these parts offered by Dr Sauris Panda, Ms Wu Wenying and Ms Hu Yani. Dr Jiang Zhihong has kindly taken up the responsibility of translating the section on 'Chemical Composition'. Ms Echo P.W. Lau, a registered nurse and a registered Chinese medicine practitioner in Hong Kong, has undertaken to work on the section on 'Indications' while Mr Tam Hung Pun - a pharmacist for the Hong Kong Hospital Authority, Dr Lee Wai Tsun (MBBS) and Dr Malcolm Taw have been very generous with their time in going over this section and offering their comments. The pen-and-ink drawings by Ms Cheng Xuanxuan are also acknowledged with thanks. And, last but not the least, a very special word of thanks to Ms Rosalind Chan, whose appreciation of the difficulties involved in the job of translating has helped bring this project to fruition.

The professionals are important. Equally important are institutional and corporate support. Eu Yan Sang's sponsorship of this project will be gratefully remembered. The School of Chinese Medicine and the Centre for Translation of the Hong Kong Baptist University have, in more ways than one, provided the translation and editorial team with precious resources.

Martha P. Y. Cheung
Editor-in-Chief of the English translation